Casebook in Clinical Pharmacokinetics and Drug Dosing

NOTICE

Medicine is an ever-changing science. As new research and clinical experience broaden our knowledge, changes in treatment and drug therapy are required. The authors and the publisher of this work have checked with sources believed to be reliable in their efforts to provide information that is complete and generally in accord with the standards accepted at the time of publication. However, in view of the possibility of human error or changes in medical sciences, neither the authors nor the publisher nor any other party who has been involved in the preparation or publication of this work warrants that the information contained herein is in every respect accurate or complete, and they disclaim all responsibility for any errors or omissions or for the results obtained from use of the information contained in this work. Readers are encouraged to confirm the information contained herein with other sources. For example and in particular, readers are advised to check the product information sheet included in the package of each drug they plan to administer to be certain that the information contained in this work is accurate and that changes have not been made in the recommended dose or in the contraindications for administration. This recommendation is of particular importance in connection with new or infrequently used drugs.

Casebook in Clinical Pharmacokinetics and Drug Dosing

Henry Cohen, MS, PharmD, FCCM, BCPP, CGP

Professor of Pharmacy Practice
Arnold & Marie Schwartz College of Pharmacy and Health Sciences
Long Island University
Brooklyn, New York
and
Chief Pharmacotherapy Officer
Director of Pharmacy Residency Programs (PGY-1 & PGY-2)
Kingsbrook Jewish Medical Center
Department of Pharmacy Services
Brooklyn, New York

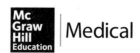

New York   Chicago   San Francisco   Athens   London   Madrid
Mexico City   Milan   New Delhi   Singapore   Sydney   Toronto

Casebook in Clinical Pharmacokinetics and Drug Dosing

1 2 3 4 5 6 7 8 9 0 QVS/QVS 19 18 17 16 15 14

ISBN 978-0-07-162835-8
MHID 0-07-162835-5

This book was set in Minion Pro by Thomson Digital.
The editors were Michael Weitz, Karen Edmonson, and Cindy Yoo.
The production supervisor was Richard Ruzycka.
Project management was provided by Shaminder Pal Singh, Thomson Digital.
The cover designer was Mary McKeon.
Credit: Kenneth Eward/Science Source
Caption: Erlotinib
Quad Graphics/Versailles was printer and binder.

This book is printed on acid-free paper.

Cataloging-in-Publication data for this title is on file with the Library of Congress.

McGraw-Hill Education books are available at special quantity discounts to use as premiums and sales promotions, or for use in corporate training programs. To contact a representative, please visit the Contact Us pages at www.mhprofessional.com.

CONTENTS

CONTRIBUTORS

Ahmed M. Abdelhady, MS

Doctor of Philosophy Candidate
Purdue University College of Pharmacy
West Lafayette, Indiana

Darowan Akajabor, PharmD, BCPS

Clinical Assistant Professor
D'Youville College School of Pharmacy
Buffalo, New York
Syracuse, New York

Antonia Alafris, BS, PharmD, CGP

Associate Director of Pharmacy, Clinical Services
SBH Health System
Bronx, New York

Maurice Alexander, PharmD, BCOP, CPP

Clinical Pharmacist Practitioner
University of North Carolina Medical Center
Chapel Hill, North Carolina

Teresa A. Allison, PharmD, BCPS

Clinical Pharmacist, Neurosciences,
Program Director, PGY2 Critical Care Pharmacy Residency
Memorial Hermann Texas Medical Center
Houston, Texas

Michael Biglow, BS, PharmD, BCPS, BCPP

Doctor of Pharmacy
Assistant Director of Pharmacotherapy
Kingsbrook Jewish Medical Center
Brooklyn, New York

Gretchen M. Brophy, PharmD, BCPS, FCCP, FCCM, FNCS

Professor of Pharmacotherapy & Outcomes Science and Neurosurgery
Virginia Commonwealth University
Medical College of Virginia Campus
Richmond, Virginia

Alice C. Ceacareanu, PharmD, PhD

Assistant Professor of Pharmacy Practice in Oncology
School of Pharmacy and Pharmaceutical Sciences
State University of New York at Buffalo
NYS Center of Excellence in Bioinformatics and Life Sciences
Buffalo, New York

Valery L. Chu, BS, PharmD, BCACP, CACP, AE-C

Pharmacy Clinical Coordinator
Ambulatory Care
SBH Health System
Bronx, New York

Henry Cohen, MS, PharmD, FCCM, BCPP, CGP

Professor of Pharmacy Practice
Arnold & Marie Schwartz College of Pharmacy and Health Sciences
Long Island University,
Chief Pharmacotherapy Officer
Director of Pharmacy Residency Programs (PGY-1 & PGY-2)
Kingsbrook Jewish Medical Center
Department of Pharmacy Services
Brooklyn, New York

Victor Cohen, BS, PharmD, BCPS, CGP

Associate Professor of Pharmacy Practice
Arnold & Marie Schwartz College of Pharmacy and Health Sciences
Long Island University
Clinical Pharmacy Manager/Specialist in Emergency Medicine
Residency Program Director, Pharmacy PGY-1 and
Emergency Medicine PGY-2
Brooklyn, New York

William Darko, BPharm, MPSG, PharmD

Director, PGY 1 Pharmacy Residency Program
Assistant Professor of Medicine
Upstate University Hospital
Syracuse, New York

Amy L. Dzierba, PharmD, FCCM, BCPS

Clinical Pharmacist–Critical Care
New York–Presbyterian Hospital
Columbia University Medical Center
New York, New York

Elizabeth Farrington, PharmD, FCCP, FCCM, FPPAG, BCPS

Pediatrics Clinical Pharmacist
New Hanover Regional Medical Center
Wilmington, North Carolina

Megan Flinchum, PharmD, BCPS

Pharmacist
University of Cincinnati
Linder Center of HOPE
Mason, Ohio

Jeffrey Fudin, BS, PharmD, FCCP

Adjunct Associate Professor of Pharmacy Practice & Pain Management
Albany College of Pharmacy & Health Sciences
Albany, New York
Clinical Pharmacy Specialist in Pain Management
Samuel Stratton VA Medical Center
Albany, New York

Edgar R. Gonzalez, PharmD, FASHP, FASCP

Senior Clinical Consultant
Capital Pharmacy Consultants
Mechanicsville, Virginia

Rebecca B. Gonzalez, PharmD

Chief Executive Officer
Consultant, Infectious Diseases
Certified, Antimicrobial Stewardship Pharmacist
Capital Pharmacy Consultants
Mechanicsville, Virginia

Brian Gulbis, PharmD, BCPS

Cardiovascular Clinical Pharmacist
Program Director, PGY1 Pharmacy Residency
Memorial Hermann Texas Medical Center
Houston, Texas

Tudy Hodgman, PharmD, FCCM, BCPS

Clinical Coordinator/Critical Care Specialist
Northwest Community Hospital
Arlington Heights, Illinois
Associate Professor, Pharmacy Practice
Midwestern University, Chicago College of Pharmacy
Critical Care Residency Director
Downers Grove, Illinois

Samantha P. Jellinek-Cohen, PharmD, BCPS, CGP

Assistant Clinical Professor
St. Johns University
College of Pharmacy and Health Sciences
Queens, New York
Emergency Medicine Clinical Pharmacy Specialist
Mount Sinai Beth Israel
New York, New York

Lesly Jurado, PharmD, BCPS

Critical Care/Nutrition Support Pharmacist
New Hanover Regional Medical Center
Wilmington, North Carolina

Rebecca A. Keel-Jayakumar, PharmD

Assistant Professor of Pharmacy Practice
College of Pharmacy, Roseman University
Henderson, Nevada

Kelly A. Killius, PharmD, BCPS

Clinical Pharmacy Specialist
Emergency Medicine
Boston Medical Center
Boston, Massachusetts

Keri S. Kim, PharmD, MS CTS, BCPS

Clinical Pharmacist
Clinical Assistant Professor
Department of Pharmacy Practice
University of Illinois at Chicago College of Pharmacy
Chicago, Illinois

Sara S. Kim, PharmD, BCOP

Clinical Oncology Pharmacist
Director, PGY-2 Oncology Pharmacy Residency Program
The Mount Sinai Hospital
New York, New York

Vijay Lapsia, MD

Assistant Professor of Medicine and Nephrology
Icahn School of Medicine at Mount Sinai
New York, New York

Arthur G. Lipman, BS, PharmD, FASHP

Professor Emeritus of Pharmacotherapy
Adjunct Professor of Anesthesiology
University of Utah
Editor, Journal of Pain and Palliative Care Pharmacotherapy

Xi Liu-DeRyke, PharmD

Orlando Regional Medical Center
Department of Pharmacy
Orlando, Florida

Erica Maceira, PharmD, BCPS, CACP

Clinical Pharmacy Specialist
Albany Medical Center
Adjunct Experiential Faculty
Albany College of Pharmacy and Health Sciences
Albany, New York

Arkadiy Makaron, PharmD, BCPS

Clinical Staff Pharmacist
Upstate University Hospital
Syracuse, New York

Helene C. Maltz, BS, PharmD, BCPS

Clinical Pharmacy Manager–Transitional Care
New York–Presbyterian Hospital
New York, New York

Erin E. Mancl, PharmD, BCPS

Clinical Pharmacist, Medical ICU
Loyola University Health System
Maywood, Illinois

Kelly E. Martin, PharmD, BCPS

Infectious Diseases Clinical Pharmacy Specialist
Carolinas Medical Center
Charlotte, North Carolina

Karen J. McAllen, PharmD

Clinical Pharmacy Specialist
Surgical and Neurosciences Critical Care
Spectrum Health Hospitals
Grand Rapids, Michigan

Catherine A. Millares-Sipin, PharmD, CGP, BCPS, BCACP

Associate Professor of Pharmacy Practice
Touro College of Pharmacy
New York, New York

Christopher Miller, PharmD, BCPS, AAHIVP

Associate Director of Pharmacy for Clinical Services and Research
Clinical Associate Professor of Medicine
Upstate University Hospital
Syracuse, New York

Maricelle O. Monteagudo-Chu, PharmD, BCPS

Infectious Diseases Clinical Pharmacist
Brookhaven Memorial Hospital Medical Center
Patchogue, New York

Jeffrey J. Mucksavage, PharmD, BCPS

Clinical Pharmacist
Clinical Assistant Professor
Department of Pharmacy Practice
University of Illinois at Chicago College of Pharmacy
Chicago, Illinois

Benyam Muluneh, PharmD, BCOP, CPP

Clinical Pharmacist Practitioner
University of North Carolina Medical Center
Chapel Hill, North Carolina

Timothy Nguyen, PharmD, FASCP, BCPS, CCP

Associate Professor of Pharmacy
Adjunct Clinical Pharmacology Professor
Arnold & Marie Schwartz College of Pharmacy and
Health Sciences
Long Island University
Brooklyn, New York

David P. Nicolau, PharmD, FCCP, FIDSA

Director
Center for Anti-Infective Research & Development
Hartford Hospital
Hartford, Connecticut

John Noviasky, PharmD, BCPS

Clinical Pharmacy Coordinator
Upstate University Hospital, Community Campus
Syracuse, New York

Brian R. Overholser, PharmD, FCCP

Associate Professor
Purdue University College of Pharmacy
West Lafayette, Indiana
Adjunct Associate Professor
Indiana University School of Medicine
Indianapolis, Indiana

Dennis Parker Jr., PharmD, BCPS

Associate Professor Pharmacy Practice
Eugene Applebaum College of Pharmacy and
Health Sciences
Clinical Specialist Neurocritical Care
Detroit Receiving Hospital
Detroit, Michigan

Ruth J. Perkins, BS, MA, PharmD, BCPS

Clinical Pharmacy Specialist
Saratoga Hospital
Saratogsa Springs, New York
Adjunct Faculty
Albany College of Health Sciences
Albany, New York

Danielle Perrodin, PharmD

Pharmacy Clinical Coordinator
Christus St. Frances Cabrini Hospital
Alexandria, Louisiana

Deirdre P. Pierce PharmD, BCPS, CGP

Assistant Professor of Pharmacy Practice
St. John Fisher College
School of Pharmacy
Rochester, New York

Angela M. Plewa, PharmD, BCPS

Clinical Pharmacist Critical Care
John H. Stroger, Jr. Hospital of Cook County
Chicago, Illinois

Liz G. Ramos, BS, PharmD, BCPS

Clinical Manager
Critical Care/Infectious Diseases
New York-Presbyterian Hospital
Weill Cornell Medical Center
New York

Denise H. Rhoney, PharmD, FCCP, FCCM, FNCS

Ron and Nancy McFarlane Distinguished Professor and Chair
Division of Practice Advancement and Clinical Education
UNC Eshelman School of Pharmacy
Chapel Hill, North Carolina

Denise E. Riccobono, PharmD

Clinical Coordinator, Infectious Diseases
Cohen's Children's Medical Center
New Hyde Park, New York

Manny Saltiel, PharmD, FASHP, FCCP

Clinical Regional Director
Comprehensive Pharmacy Services
Adjunct Clinical Professor
University of Southern California
Los Angeles, California

Robert Seabury, PharmD

Clinical Staff Pharmacist
Upstate University Hospital
Syracuse, New York

Dustin Spencer, PharmD, BCPS

Clinical Pharmacy Specialist–Critical Care
Indiana University Health Methodist Hospital
Indianapolis, Indiana

Serina Tart, PharmD

Antimicrobial Stewardship Clinical Pharmacist
Cape Fear Valley Health
Fayetteville, North Carolina
Adjunct Assistant Professor
UNC Eshelman School of Pharmacy,
Chapel Hill, North Carolina
Clinical Associate Professor of Pharmacy Practice
Wingate University School of Pharmacy
Wingate, North Carolina

Eljim P. Tesoro, PharmD, BCPS

Clinical Pharmacist, Neurosciences
Clinical Assistant Professor
College of Pharmacy
University of Illinois Hospital & Health Sciences System
Chicago, Illinois

CONTRIBUTORS

Tracey H. Truesdale, PharmD, BCPS

Clinical Pharmacy Manager
Haywood Regional Medical Center
Clyde, North Carolina

Christy Vaughan, PharmD, BCPS

Clinical Manager of Inpatient Pharmacy
John Peter Smith Hospital
Fort Worth, Texas

Nicole D. Verkleeren, PharmD, BCPS

Clinical Pharmacist-Critical Care
Forbes Regional Hospital
Monroeville, Pennsylvania

Lisa M. Voigt, PharmD, BCPS

Clinical Pharmacy Coordinator
Critical Care/Infectious Disease
Buffalo General Medical Center
Buffalo, New York

Stacy A. Voils, PharmD, MS, BCPS

Clinical Assistant Professor
Department of Pharmacotherapy and Translational Research
University of Florida, College of Pharmacy
Gainesville, Florida

Karen Whalen, BS, Pharm, BCPS

Drug Information Pharmacist
St Josephs Hospital Health Center
Syracuse, New York

Zachary A.P. Wintrob, MSc

Adjunct Instructor
State University of New York at Buffalo
Department of Pharmacy Practice
New York State Center of Excellence in
Bioinformatics and Life Sciences
Buffalo, New York

Dora E. Wiskirchen, PharmD, BCPS

Assistant Professor
Department of Pharmacy Practice & Administration
School of Pharmacy, Saint Joseph College
Hartford, Connecticut

Kimberly T. Zammit, PharmD, BCPS, FASHP

Clinical Pharmacy Coordinator
Critical Care/Cardiology
Kaleida Health/Buffalo General Hospital
Buffalo, New York

PREFACE

Understanding and applying clinical pharmacokinetics and dosing medications safely and appropriately are an essential role of the pharmacist in medication therapy management. Ostensibly, pharmacokinetics and clinical pharmacokinetics are a core part of doctorate of pharmacy program curriculums, and these skills are further honed during pharmacy practice experiences in clerkships and in postgraduate pharmacy residency training programs. Although in the last decade pharmacy has undergone significant specialization, pharmacists are expected to be the drug expert and maintain knowledge of a vast array of agents beyond their area of specialty. Physicians and other prescribers expect the pharmacist to be the expert in pharmacokinetics, drug interactions, and drug dosing. The goal of *Casebook in Clinical Pharmacokinetics and Drug Dosing* is to provide students and clinicians with real-world dosing case scenarios and a step-by-step approach to determining dosing regimens.

Traditionally, clinical pharmacokinetics courses and clinical pharmacokinetic textbooks focus on drugs with readily available therapeutic serum levels such as aminoglycosides, vancomycin, carbamazepine, phenytoin, phenobarbital, valproic acid, lithium, digoxin, amiodarone, immunosuppressants, and antiarrhythmics such as quinidine and procainamide. Many of these agents remain effective and are highly utilized in today's practice; hence, mastering how to dose these agents is an expectation of today's pharmacist. *Casebook in Clinical Pharmacokinetics and Drug Dosing* will provide extensive reviews and cases for these traditional agents with readily available serum levels that are used to determine drug-dosing regimens.

Many drugs in use today do not have readily available therapeutic serum levels, but have narrow therapeutic indexes, sophisticated pharmacokinetics and pharmacodynamics, extensive drug interactions, and complicated dosing schemes, and are classified as high-alert agents. The risk of medication errors and patient harm with these agents is high, but minimal guidance is provided for safely utilizing and dosing these drugs in actual patient case scenarios. Such

agents include the newer second-generation antiepileptics, long-acting antipsychotics, colistin and polymyxin B, dronedarone, direct thrombin inhibitors, neuromuscular blocking agents, oncologic agents, antifungal agents, epoetin alfa, warfarin, heparin and low-molecular-weight heparins, extended-infusion beta-lactams, and opioids for pain management. *Casebook in Clinical Pharmacokinetics and Drug Dosing* provides equal emphasis and focus with these type of agents and traditionally dosed pharmacokinetic agents and offers extensive reviews, cases, and answers to challenging dosing questions.

This casebook is designed to teach and guide the pharmacy student, pharmacist, and clinical pharmacist in dosing drugs and goes beyond agents with readily available and applied therapeutic blood levels. Each drug chapter is written by clinical pharmacists who have expertise and experience in drug dosing. Each chapter provides an overview of the drug's pharmacology including mechanisms of action, indications, toxicities, and pharmacokinetics. A comprehensive review and discussion of the drug's bioavailability, volume of distribution, clearance, half-life, therapeutic drug level monitoring (when applicable), drug interactions, dosing, and availability are provided. Each chapter contains a plethora of patient cases with clear step-by-step answers and explanations. Calculations, equations, and dosing recommendations are provided for each case. Loading doses and maintenance doses using population and actual pharmacokinetics are depicted and reviewed. Challenging cases including drug interactions, alterations in volume of distribution, reduced renal or hepatic function, and overweight and underweight patients are covered extensively.

This casebook is intended for teaching, learning, and clinical practice. The casebook can be used in the classroom by faculty to teach drug dosing, by pharmacy students to practice and learn drug dosing, and by the clinical pharmacist practitioner for daily patient care needs. This casebook will be an invaluable resource providing the clinician with assistance in both routine and challenging drug-dosing cases.

CHAPTER

1

Amiodarone and Dronedarone

AHMED M. ABDELHADY, MS
DUSTIN SPENCER, PharmD, BCPS
BRIAN R. OVERHOLSER, PharmD, FCCP

OVERVIEW

AMIODARONE

Amiodarone is designated as a class III antiarrhythmic drug based on the Vaughan Williams classification. Consistent with other class III antiarrhythmic drugs, amiodarone blocks potassium channels to delay phase 3 repolarization.[1] However, amiodarone possesses electrophysiological (EP) effects similar to all four classes of antiarrhythmic drugs by (1) blocking sodium channels (class I effect)[2], (2) potent nonselective, noncompetitive β-adrenergic receptor blockade (class II effect)[3], and (3) antagonizing calcium channel activity (class IV effect). As a result, amiodarone prolongs action potential duration (APD), resulting in prolongation of the effective refractory period.[1]

Amiodarone is indicated for the treatment of life-threatening, recurrent, refractory ventricular arrhythmias,[4] including recurrent ventricular fibrillation (VF)[5] and recurrent hemodynamically unstable ventricular tachycardia (VT).[6] In addition to these indications, amiodarone is commonly used for treatment of atrial fibrillation (AF) particularly in patients with heart failure.[7-24] According to the 2011 consensus guidelines of the American Heart Association (AHA) and the American College of Cardiology (ACC) for the management of atrial fibrillation,[25] amiodarone can also be used for cardioversion of recent-onset AF.[26] Amiodarone is not only beneficial in terminating AF, but it can be effective at maintaining normal sinus rhythm (NSR) and preventing AF recurrence.[27-37] The Canadian trial of AF (CTAF) reported that amiodarone reduced the incidence of recurrent AF compared to other antiarrhythmic drugs (35% vs. 63%, respectively).[29] Additional studies have demonstrated that amiodarone is effective at preventing AF following cardiovascular and cardiothoracic surgeries.[29,31]

Dosing

Amiodarone dosing varies depending on the clinical indication. Table 1-1 summarizes the dosing recommendations for amiodarone according to AHA recommendations, 2006 guidelines for management of patients with ventricular arrhythmias and the prevention of sudden cardiac death, and its focused update in 2011 on the management of atrial fibrillation. Amiodarone is commercially available as 100 and 200 mg oral tablets or as 50 mg/mL for IV administration.

Adverse Effects and Monitoring

Amiodarone administration has been associated with various cardiac and noncardiac side effects, some life-threatening. (See Table 1-2.) Cardiac adverse effects include bradycardia (2–4%), atrioventricular (AV) block (2–5%), QTc interval prolongation with a mild risk (<1%) of torsades de pointes (TdP) compared to other QTc interval prolonging drugs. Noncardiac adverse effects caused by amiodarone include impaired thyroid function (hypo- 6% or hyper- <1%), which is largely attributed to an iodine moiety on amiodarone resembling the hormone thyroxin.[38] In addition, chronic administration of high doses (>500 mg/day) can result in serious pulmonary fibrosis, which requires treatment discontinuation (2–17%).[39,40] Other adverse effects include skin discoloration, photosensitivity (10%), hepatotoxicity (0.6 %), peripheral neuropathy (0.3%), and corneal deposits (<10%), which may occur with prolonged use. Due to the involvement of multiple organ systems and the potential for serious adverse effects, prolonged use of amiodarone requires close monitoring for these toxicities. Routine monitoring of liver and thyroid function as well as a chest X-ray and electrocardiogram (ECG) is recommended every 6 months.

Pharmacokinetics

Following oral administration, amiodarone absorption is incomplete with highly variable bioavailability reported between 20 to 80 percent.[41,42] This unpredictable and incomplete absorption may be partially attributed to the fact that amiodarone is a substrate for the cytochrome P450 (CYP) 3A metabolizing enzyme and the efflux transport protein, P-glycoprotein (P-gp). Following oral administration, it can take between three to seven hours to achieve maximum plasma concentrations.[43,44] Both the rate and extent of

TABLE 1-1	Amiodarone Dosing		
Clinical Condition		**Initial Dose**	**Follow-Up Dose**
Stable ventricular tachycardia		150 mg IV over 10 min	1 mg/min IV for 6 hours, then 0.5 mg/min IV
Unstable ventricular tachycardia/fibrillation		300 mg IV/IO (Repeat dose with 150 mg IV/IO can be given if persistent)	1 mg/min IV for 6 hours, then 0.5 mg/min IV
Atrial fibrillation			
Conversion to NSR[a]		5 mg/kg IV over 30–60 min	1 mg/min IV for 6 hours, then 0.5 mg/min IV
Maintenance of NSR		400 mg PO BID or TID until 10 g total	200–400 mg PO daily

[a]NSR normal sinus rhythm

TABLE 1-2 Adverse Effects Associated with Dronedarone and Amiodarone

Amiodarone	Dronedarone
Pulmonary fibrosis	**Gastrointestinal toxicity**
Thyroid disorders (hypo- or hyperthyroidism)	Nausea
Peripheral neuropathy	Vomiting
Corneal deposits	Gastroenteritis
Liver enzymes elevation	Liver enzymes elevation
Skin discoloration	Serum creatinine elevation
Cardiac adverse events	
Bradycardia	
QT prolongation	
Low risk (<1%) of TdP	
Gastrointestinal toxicity	
Nausea	
Vomiting	

absorption of amiodarone increase when administered concurrently with food.

Amiodarone is a highly lipophilic compound that results in significant accumulation and an atypical pharmacokinetic profile. (See Table 1-3.) Amiodarone is slowly and extensively distributed to peripheral tissue, especially adipose and cell membranes. This distribution and extensive plasma protein binding (>95%) account for its large volume of distribution (Vd_{ss}) of 50–150 L/kg. Amiodarone is primarily de-ethylated by CYP3A4[45] and CYP2C8[46] into the pharmacologically active metabolite: desethylamiodarone (DEA). Administration of DEA alone suppressed ventricular arrhythmias in dogs, whereas coadministration of DEA and amiodarone suppressed ventricular arrhythmias at lower doses than giving amiodarone alone.[47] Amiodarone and DEA, when given separately, reduced the incidence of ischemia-induced ventricular arrhythmias in rats.[48] Therefore, both amiodarone and DEA are effective, but more DEA may reach cardiac tissue. Similar plasma concentrations of amiodarone and DEA resulted in higher myocardial concentrations of DEA.[47] Renal elimination of both amiodarone and its metabolite is negligible (<1%).

Chronic administration of amiodarone is associated with a long elimination half-life ($t_{1/2} \sim 120$ days). The half-life and volume of distribution appear to be proportional to the duration of therapy, where longer periods of treatment resulted in larger reported values of both pharmacokinetic parameters.

Therapeutic and Toxic Concentrations

A therapeutic plasma concentration range for amiodarone is not clearly defined. However, data suggest that it may be beneficial to maintain concentrations of 1.0–2.5 mg/L, with some studies reporting increased risk of toxicity at plasma concentrations >2.5 mg/L.[1,49,50] Higher plasma concentrations (>2.5 mg/L) are associated with a higher incidence of pulmonary, neurologic, and

gastrointestinal toxicity with no additional antiarrhythmic effect observed. In general, little clinical usefulness comes with monitoring amiodarone plasma concentrations. However, in some cases it may be valuable to measure periodic trough concentrations to determine patient-specific effective concentrations when considering chronic use of the drug. In a multicenter clinical trial in patients with ventricular and supraventricular arrhythmias, amiodarone and DEA concentrations linearly correlated with the administered dose of amiodarone (200, 400, or 600 mg/day).[51] Similarly, the concentration of DEA correlated with observed amiodarone concentrations, whereas drug-to-metabolite ratio remained constant at all studied doses. The patients who experienced adverse events had amiodarone concentrations of 2.9 ± 1.5 mg/L, while drug-to-metabolite ratio was similar (1.8 ± 0.8) whether adverse events occurred or not.[51]

Drug Interactions

Both amiodarone and DEA can inhibit several drug metabolizing enzymes, which is the primary source for drug interactions. Amiodarone itself is a weak inhibitor of CYP2C9, CYP2D6, and CYP3A4. However, DEA is a more potent inhibitor of these enzymes and additionally inhibits the function of CYP1A1, CYP2A6, and CYP2B6.[52] Amiodarone is also a substrate and an inhibitor of P-gp. This primary mechanism of interaction with digoxin results in elevated digoxin plasma concentrations when coadministered with amiodarone.

DRONEDARONE

Dronedarone is a benzofuran derivative that is structurally analogous to amiodarone without an iodine moiety. The structural dissimilarities improve the drug safety profile of dronedarone over amiodarone. The lack of an iodine moiety aims at reducing the incidence and severity of the thyroid toxicity associated with amiodarone.[53] Also, the addition of a methyl-sulfonyl group decreases the lipophilicity of dronedarone, resulting in less tissue distribution and therefore less accumulation compared to amiodarone. Overall, dronedarone has a shorter half-life and more favorable pharmacokinetic profile compared to amiodarone.[53,54]

Similar to amiodarone, dronedarone has electrophysiological effects of all four Vaughan-Williams classes of antiarrhythmic drugs.[55,56] Despite these electrophysiologic similarities, dronedarone is less effective at suppressing AF recurrence (63.5%) compared to amiodarone (42.0%).[57] However, in a large, multicenter, randomized clinical trial, dronedarone was associated with a reduced risk of hospitalizations versus placebo in patients with paroxysmal or persistent AF associated with cardiovascular risk factors.[58] This trial resulted in the U.S. Food and Drug Administration (FDA) approval of dronedarone for the treatment of patients with AF. However, dronedarone has been shown to have detrimental effects in heart failure patients, and postmarketing surveillance has indicated it can prompt life-threatening hepatotoxicity. Therefore, the role of dronedarone in clinical practice remains controversial, and many consider it a second-line agent to amiodarone.[59] Dronedarone has also been investigated for ventricular rate control in permanent AF. In the Efficacy and Safety of Dronedarone for the Control of Ventricular Rate during AF (ERATO) study,[60] a dose of 400 mg twice daily was successful in controlling the ventricular rate compared to placebo; however, dronedarone is not yet approved for rate control.

Dosing

In a dose-ranging study of dronedarone for the prevention of AF (DAFNE), doses of 400, 600, and 800 mg twice daily were assessed.[53]

TABLE 1-3 Key Pharmacokinetic Parameters of Amiodarone and Dronedarone

	Amiodarone	Dronedarone
Bioavailability	20–80%	5–15%
Volume of distribution	50–150 (L/kg)	1,400 L
Protein binding	95%	98%
Clearance	0.2–0.4 (L/kg/h)	130–150 (L/h)
Elimination half-life	Up to 120 days	24 hour
Plasma concentration (mg/L)	1.0–2.5	5–12 (parent drug)

In this trial, 400 mg twice daily increased the time to AF recurrence following cardioversion. This effect on the time to relapse was not statistically significantly for 600 mg and 800 mg twice daily compared to placebo. Moreover, these higher doses (600 and 800 mg twice daily) were not statistically significantly more efficacious in cardioversion to normal sinus rhythm. Additionally, the incidence of drug discontinuation due to adverse events was higher at 600 mg twice daily (7.6%) and 800 mg twice daily (22.6%) versus 400 mg twice daily (3.9%). Therefore, the recommended and approved dose is 400 mg twice daily with meals. Dronedarone exposure is 20–30 percent higher in special populations including females, patients older than 65 years, or patients with moderate hepatic impairment; however, no dosage adjustment in these populations has been reported.

Adverse Events

Drug discontinuation due to adverse events was 3.9 percent with the approved 400 mg twice daily dose.[53] The most frequently reported adverse event is gastrointestinal toxicity (4–20%) in the form of diarrhea, nausea, vomiting, and gastroenteritis.[53]

In clinical trials dronedarone was associated with fewer cases of thyroid toxicity and overall better tolerance compared to amiodarone.[61] (Refer to Table 1-2.) A short-term, randomized, double-blind, parallel-group study to evaluate the efficacy and safety of dronedarone versus amiodarone in patients with persistent atrial fibrillation (DIONYSOS study) directly compared both drugs over a maximum duration of treatment of 13.8 months.[57] Drug discontinuation due to intolerance was 10 percent in dronedarone group versus 13.3 percent in patients receiving amiodarone. Fewer incidences of thyroid, neurologic, ocular, and dermatologic adverse events were reported in patients who were administered dronedarone compared to those who received amiodarone. However, the proportion of patients who experienced gastrointestinal toxicity (12.9% vs. 5.1%) and liver enzymes elevation (12.0% vs. 10.6%) was higher in patients who received dronedarone compared to those who received amiodarone.

Despite an enhanced adverse effect profile compared to amiodarone, dronedarone is largely considered a second-line therapy to amiodarone for a couple of reasons related to adverse effects. First, dronedarone was associated with increased mortality when administered to patients with New York Heart Association (NYHA) class III or IV heart failure. Therefore, current guidelines do not recommend using dronedarone in patients with NYHA class III or IV heart failure or those with a recent exacerbation.[62] Amiodarone remains the agent of choice in heart failure patients. Secondly, severe hepatotoxicity requiring liver transplantation has been reported in two cases.[63] Both patients were female, approximately 70 years of age, and were receiving dronedarone for atrial fibrillation. All other potential causes of hepatic failure were reportedly excluded. Accordingly, the FDA has required the inclusion of this potential risk for hepatotoxicity in the product labeling of dronedarone.

Pharmacokinetics

Dronedarone has less accumulation and exhibits a more traditional pharmacokinetic profile compared to amiodarone. (Refer to Table 1-3.) Dronedarone undergoes extensive first-pass metabolism, which may be attributed to CYP3A metabolism. Consequently, the drug has a low absolute bioavailability (<5%) that increases to approximately 15 percent when administered with food. It takes 3–6 hours to reach peak plasma concentrations following oral administration. Dronedarone is highly bound to plasma proteins (>98%), mainly albumin, with a steady-state volume of distribution of approximately 1,400 L.[64]

Dronedarone is extensively metabolized by CYP3A into an active N-debutyl metabolite, which is three- to tenfold less potent than the parent drug. Following metabolism, the drug is mainly excreted in feces (84%) and a small portion (6%) is excreted in urine. The elimination half-life of dronedarone is approximately 24 hours with steady-state plasma concentrations (85–170 ng/mL) achieved in four to eight days.

Drug Interactions

Dronedarone has a potential for multidrug interactions when coadministered with CYP3A substrates, inducers, or inhibitors. Coadministration with a strong CYP3A inhibitor such as ketoconazole results in greater than a 15-fold increase in dronedarone exposure. Moderate CYP3A inhibitors such as verapamil increase exposure by 40–70 percent. Coadministration with CYP3A inducers such as rifampin reduces exposure by 80 percent.

Dronedarone is also an inhibitor of P-gp, CYP2D6, and CYP3A and can affect the metabolism of other drugs. For example, dronedarone administration causes an approximately fourfold increase in simvastatin exposure and a 1.5-fold increase in verapamil concentration, both substrates of CYP3A. A daily dronedarone dose of 800 mg increases metoprolol (CYP2D6 substrate) C_{max} and exposure by 1.8- and 1.6-fold, respectively.[65] Dronedarone increases exposure of digoxin through P-gp inhibition in a similar manner as with amiodarone.[60] Other drug interactions arise from the electrophysiologic effects of dronedarone. Class I and III antiarrhythmic drugs can potentiate the risk of torsades de pointes (TdP) due to QTc interval prolongation. Similarly, the incidence of bradycardia increases when coadministered with beta blockers.[65]

CASE STUDIES

CASE 1: TRANSITIONING FROM INTRAVENOUS TO ORAL AMIODARONE

MH is a 73-year-old woman (weight = 50 kg) with a past medical history significant for coronary artery disease, hyperlipidemia, hypertension, diabetes mellitus, and chronic kidney disease stage III. She was admitted to the cardiovascular intensive care unit following a three-vessel coronary artery bypass grafting. Her postoperative course was complicated by development of atrial fibrillation on postoperative day 2. She was started on a loading regimen of intravenous amiodarone as a 150 mg intravenous (IV) bolus followed by 1 mg/min for 6 hours. She was switched to and has been on an amiodarone infusion of 0.5 mg/min for approximately 36 hours. The medical team wishes to switch her to an oral regimen to facilitate transfer to a medical floor and eventual discharge.

QUESTION 1

Estimate MH's amiodarone plasma concentration at the end of the six-hour infusion of 1 mg/min of amiodarone.

Answer:

The plasma concentration (C_p) of amiodarone at six hours will reflect both the administered IV bolus (150 mg) and the infused (1 mg/min) amiodarone. To help visually depict the scenario, Figure 1-1 represents a theoretical plasma concentration-time curve for a drug with similar properties to amiodarone that was administered in the same manner as in this clinical case. Point A in Figure 1-1 represents the theoretical concentration of this drug following a bolus dose, and Point B represents a theoretical concentration following a 6-hour infusion. In order to estimate amiodarone concentration after

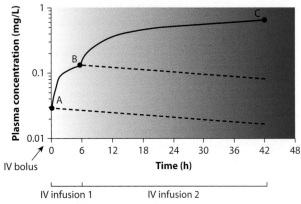

FIGURE 1-1. Amiodarone plasma concentration following IV-injection and infusion at 2 different rates (1.0 mg/min for 6 hours and 0.5 mg/min for 36 hours). A is the amiodarone plasma concentration just after the IV-injection, B is the concentration at 6 hours before starting the second infusion, and C is the concentration at the end of the second infusion. The solid line represents the actual change in plasma concentration, and the dashed line represents the first-order elimination of amiodarone if a second infusion was not started.

six hours, the remaining amount of the IV bolus after 6 hours can be added to the amount accumulated from the 6-hour infusion. To estimate the amount remaining of the IV bolus, the following fundamental first-order elimination kinetics equation can be used:

$$\text{Equation 1: } C_p = (C_p)_0 \times e^{-K_e t}$$

where C_p is the plasma concentration at any time (t), $(C_p)_0$ is the initial plasma concentration (point A), and K_e is the first-order elimination rate constant for amiodarone. Because the initial amiodarone concentration $(C_p)_0$ was obtained following a bolus dose, it can be substituted by $\frac{F \cdot Dose}{V_d}$ based on the fundamental relationship between amount (dose), concentration, and volume, where F is the bioavailability (equal to 1 for an IV dose), and V_d is the amiodarone volume of distribution.

$$\text{Equation 2: } C_p = \frac{F \cdot Dose}{V_d} \times e^{-K_e t}$$

To calculate the portion of C_p that is attributed to the IV infusion for 6 hours, the following equation can be used:

$$\text{Equation 3: } C_p = \frac{R_0}{K_e V_d} (1 - e^{-K_e t})$$

where R_0 is the infusion rate constant (i.e., 1 mg/min for the first 6 hours). Hence, amiodarone C_p following both the IV bolus and IV infusion can be estimated using the combined equation:

$$\text{Equation 4: } C_p = \frac{R_0}{K_e V_d} (1 - e^{-K_e t}) + \left(\frac{F \cdot Dose}{V_d} \times e^{-K_e t} \right)$$

It is important to keep in mind that the utilization of this equation will give an estimate that is only as accurate as the variability in the underlying pharmacokinetic parameters. Population data will have to be used to estimate the pharmacokinetic parameters for amiodarone in this patient because no plasma concentrations have been clinically assessed. Amiodarone is characterized as having a large and variable V_d that ranges between 50 and 150 L/kg. This result is associated with a long half-life, which has been reported up to 120 days, with most of the patients in clinical studies demonstrating half-lives ranging from 40 to 50 days. Therefore, the inherent variability in the intersubject variability of amiodarone will reflect on the estimated C_p in this example. For the required calculation in this case, an average V_d of 100 L/kg and a half-life of 45 days will be used.

Using this patient's body weight, the volume of distribution is estimated as follows:

$$V_d = 100 \frac{L}{kg} \times \text{body wieght (kg)}$$

$$= 100 \times 50 = 5000 \text{ L}$$

K_e can be estimated from the half-life using the following equation:

$$K_e = \frac{0.693}{t_{1/2}}$$

$$= \frac{0.693}{45 \text{ days}} = 0.0154 \text{ days}^{-1}$$

and converted to hours by

$$= \frac{0.0154}{24} = 6.4 \times 10^{-4} \text{ h}^{-1}$$

The infusion rate R_0 (1 mg/min) is equivalent to 60 mg/h.

Given this information, the C_p after 6 hours can be estimated using equation 4:

$$= \frac{60}{6.4 \times 10^{-4} \times 5000} \times (1 - e^{-(6.4 \times 10^{-4} \times 6)}) + \left(\frac{150}{5000} \times e^{-(6.4 \times 10^{-4} \times 6)} \right)$$

$$= 0.072 + 0.030 = 0.102 \text{ mg/L}$$

Administration of a 150 mg IV-bolus followed by an IV-infusion of amiodarone 1 mg/min for 6 hours results in an estimated plasma concentration of 0.102 mg/L using average population data for V_d and half-life. Performing the same calculation and assuming the lower and upper limits of the reported V_d range of 50–150 L/kg yields C_p at 6 hours of 0.068 and 0.203 mg/L, respectively. Therefore, the administered IV-bolus and 6 hours infusion should yield C_p in the range of 0.068–0.203 mg/L in this patient.

QUESTION 2

Estimate MH's amiodarone plasma concentration at the end of the 36-hour infusion administered at a rate of 0.5 mg/min (i.e., following the 150 mg bolus, 6-hour 1 mg/min infusion and 36-hour 0.5 mg/min infusion).

Answer:

The 36-hour infusion of amiodarone at 0.5 mg/min followed the initial loading dose and 6-hour infusion at 1 mg/min. The total amiodarone administration time in this patient is equal to 42 hours, represented by point C in Figure 1-1. At the end of the 42 hours, the plasma concentration should reflect the following:

1. The remaining amount of amiodarone following the initial IV bolus and the previous infusion (1.0 mg/min for 6 hours), which was estimated to be 0.102 mg/L at 6 hours. This amount will decrease over the next 36 hours, as depicted in Figure 1-1 by a dashed line from point B over the 36 hours of the new infusion. The amount remaining can be estimated using a slightly modified version of equation 1.

$$C_p = (C_p)_0 e^{-K_e (t-T)}$$

where $(C_p)_0$ is the initial concentration that was estimated to be 0.102 mg/L in question 1 (Point B in Figure 1-1), while T is the infusion time of the initial IV infusion (i.e., 6 hours) and t is the total time of amiodarone administration (i.e., 42 hours).

2. The resulting amiodarone concentration from the second infusion (0.5 mg/min for 36 hours) can be estimated using equation 3.

$$C_p = \frac{R_0}{K_e V_d}(1 - e^{-K_e t})$$

Therefore, the estimated amiodarone C_p after 36 hours of 0.5-mg/min infusion $(C_p)_{42}$ is calculated by adding both components as follows in equation 5:

$$\text{Equation 5: } (C_p)_t = \frac{R_0}{K_e V_d}\left(1 - e^{-K_e T}\right) + (C_p)_0 e^{-K_e(t-T)}$$

$$R_0 = 0.5 \text{ mg/min} \times 60 = 30 \text{ mg/h}$$

Similar to question 1, average values of V_d and K_e will be used to perform the calculation.

$$(C_p)_{42} = \frac{30}{(6.4 \times 10^{-4})(5000)} \times (1 - e^{-6.4 \times 10^{-4} \times 36})$$
$$+ 0.102 \times (e^{-6.4 \times 10^{-4} \times (42 - 6)})$$
$$= 0.214 + 0.099 = 0.313 \text{ mg}$$

After changing the IV-infusion rate and continuing amiodarone administration for 36 more hours, the estimated plasma concentration is 0.313 mg/L. Performing the same calculation and assuming the lower and upper limits of the reported V_d range of 50–150 L/kg yield C_p of 0.208 and 0.626 mg/L, respectively. Therefore, the total intravenously administered amiodarone should achieve C_p in the range of 0.208–0.626 mg/L in this patient. This concentration range is below the reported therapeutic range of amiodarone (1.0–2.5 mg/L) that is targeted by the loading regimen before switching the patient to a maintenance regimen.

QUESTION 3

What is an appropriate oral regimen of amiodarone that MH should be administered to complete the loading dose phase?

Answer:

As described, amiodarone has a complex pharmacokinetic behavior given its extensive accumulation in body tissues. Thus, amiodarone has a large volume of distribution associated with a lengthened half-life and time to reach steady-steady plasma concentrations. Consequently, a loading dose of amiodarone is recommended in certain situations to expedite the time for amiodarone to exert its full therapeutic action. Amiodarone loading is achieved clinically by giving a maximum daily dose of 1,600 mg orally until reaching a total loading dose of 10 g before switching to a maintenance regimen. It is common for patients to be started on IV amiodarone to attain rapid electrophysiological effects before being switched to an oral regimen of 400 mg twice (BID) or three times (TID) daily. It should be noted that the bioavailability of amiodarone is highly variable between patients (usually 0.2–0.8). Therefore, clinically 10 g of total amiodarone is commonly targeted for total IV and oral doses. In order to switch MH to an oral regimen, the total amount administered intravenously should be calculated.

Amount already administered = 150 mg IV bolus
+ 1 mg/min for 6 h + 0.5 mg/min for 36 h
= 150 + (1 × 60 × 6) + (0.5 × 60 × 36)
= 1,590 mg

Amount remaining to be administered for the loading dose = 10,000 mg – 1,590 mg = 8,410 mg.

Given a dose of 400 mg TID (i.e., 1,200 mg per day):

The time to reach the total loading dose
$= \frac{8410}{1200} = 7$ days of 400 mg TID dosing.

Given a dose of 400 mg BID (i.e., 800 mg per day):

The time to reach the total loading dose
$= \frac{8410}{800} = 10.5$ days of 400 mg BID dosing.

When choosing the daily dose regimen of amiodarone, the risk-to-benefit ratio should be assessed for the individual patient. In this case, if MH had converted to normal sinus rhythm from the IV regimen alone, it would likely be beneficial to give her the lower daily dose to minimize adverse effects given her age and comorbid conditions. However, if MH had paroxysmal AF with hemodynamic instability, then the shorter period of higher dose loading may be preferred.

Following the loading phase, the recommended maintenance dose for AF is 200–400 mg/day.

QUESTION 4

MH was switched from IV amiodarone to 400 mg orally three times daily for 7 days to complete the loading dose phase. Estimate the amiodarone concentration postloading dose following the postinfusion oral regimen of amiodarone.

Answer:

Because amiodarone has a long elimination half-life, 7 days is not enough time to reach steady state, which theoretically requires five to seven half-lives. In such a case, one method to estimate amiodarone concentrations at the end of the loading period is to use multiple-dose kinetics represented by equation 6:

$$\text{Equation 6: } (C_p)_{N,max} = \frac{F \cdot \text{Dose}}{V_d} \times \frac{1 - e^{-NK_e \tau}}{1 - e^{-K_e \tau}}$$

where $(C_p)_{N,max}$ is the maximum plasma concentration after N administered doses, and τ is the dosing interval. This equation enables the estimation of the maximum plasma concentration after any number of doses before reaching steady state. When the oral regimen is postinfusion, the remaining IV amiodarone prior to starting the oral administration should be considered. Thus, in addition to the oral amiodarone accumulating and estimated by equation 6, postinfusion amiodarone is eliminated in the same time over the 7 days and can be estimated using the previously mentioned first-order elimination equation:

$$C_p = (C_p)_{42} e^{-K_e \times 7 \text{ days}}$$

where $(C_p)_{42}$ is concentration of amiodarone following the 42-hour IV regimen (estimated to be 0.313 mg/L in the answer to question 2). With oral and infusion regimens, amiodarone plasma concentration can be estimated at the end of the 7 days (168 hours) by adding both as represented in the following equation:

$$\text{Equation 7: } (C_p)_{N,max}$$
$$= \frac{F \cdot \text{Dose}}{V_d} \times \frac{1 - e^{-NK_e \tau}}{1 - e^{-K_e \tau}} + (C_p)_{42} e^{-(K_e)(7 \text{ days or 168 hours})}$$

MH was administered 400 mg TID for the oral loading phase, so the number of doses administered orally is

N = 3 doses × 7 days = 21 doses

τ = 8 hours

$$(C_p)_{N,max} = \frac{0.5 \times 400 \text{ mg}}{5000 \text{ L}} \times \frac{1 - e^{-(21 \times 6.4 \times 10^{-4} \times 8\,h)}}{1 - e^{-(6.4 \times 10^{-4} \times 8\,h)}}$$

$$+ 0.313 \times e^{-(6.4 \times 10^{-4} \times 168\,h)}$$

$$= 0.829 + 0.252 = 1.081 \text{ mg/L}$$

Therefore, considering elimination characterized by the long half-life reported for amiodarone, the plasma concentration is estimated to be 1.081 mg/L.

QUESTION 5

Estimate the amiodarone concentration after the entire loading phase (IV and oral), assuming **NO amiodarone elimination** *during the loading phase. Compare your answer to that estimated in question 4 and explain the similarities.*

Answer:

If amiodarone is theoretically not eliminated during the entire loading phase, the estimation of plasma concentrations is quite simple. All that needs to be done is to estimate the total amount of amiodarone that reaches the systemic circulation and divide by the volume of distribution to get an estimated concentration. In the loading phase, MH received 1,590 mg of amiodarone intravenously and 8,400 mg orally. Amiodarone has an oral bioavailability that can range from 20 percent to 80 percent or higher with an approximate average of 50 percent (F = 0.5). Therefore, F = 0.5 will be used for the calculation of amiodarone concentration following oral administration in this case. Theoretically, if no elimination occurred during this loading phase, amiodarone would accumulate in the body without elimination. First, the total amount of amiodarone administered that reached systemic circulation needs to be calculated:

The total amount administered was 1,590 mg IV and 8,400 mg orally (400 mg TID for one week). Therefore, the total amount to reach systemic circulation

= 1,590 mg + (8,400 mg × F)

= 1,590 mg + (8,400 mg × 0.5) = 5,790 mg

Second, amiodarone concentration can be estimated using the fundamental relationship between dose, volume, and plasma concentration as follows:

$$C_p = \frac{\text{Amount Reaching Systemic Circulation}}{V_d}$$

$$C_p = \frac{5790 \text{ mg}}{5000 \text{ L}}$$

$$= 1.158 \text{ mg/L}$$

Thus, assuming no elimination, the administered loading regimen is estimated to yield a plasma concentration of 1.158 mg/L assuming a 50 percent oral bioavailability. Therefore, if no elimination occurred, the estimated plasma concentration (1.158 mg/L) is only 7 percent higher than that estimated (1.081 mg/L) when considering elimination. The similarity is due to the long half-life for amiodarone, which is characterized by a slow elimination from the body. Theoretically, drugs with long half-lives will not have rapidly changing plasma concentrations due to slow elimination. This characteristic can be taken advantage of to make estimates of plasma concentrations following complex regimens as demonstrated by the similarities in the answers to questions 4 and 5.

CASE 2: CONVERTING A PATIENT FROM AMIODARONE TO DRONEDARONE THERAPY

SA is a 62-year-old man with mild left ventricular systolic dysfunction who has been receiving amiodarone 400 mg daily as maintenance therapy for atrial fibrillation for 3 years. He presents to the clinic for his routine appointment with complaints of hand tremors and heat intolerance. The physical exam indicates that he has lost approximately 15 kg since his last appointment and has a moderately enlarged thyroid gland. SA was diagnosed with amiodarone-induced thyrotoxicosis and will be transitioned to dronedarone therapy.

QUESTION 1

What considerations should be made to determine how long amiodarone should be washed out before dronedarone is initiated? What should be monitored closely?

Answer:

The decision whether or not and the length of time to washout a drug before switching to a similar therapeutic agent requires a combination of pharmacokinetic and pharmacodynamic considerations. In general, it is accepted that after five half-lives a drug is adequately eliminated from the body. By definition, 50 percent of any given drug that follows linear first-order kinetics is eliminated from the body after one half-life. After each additional half-life, 50 percent of the remaining amount of drug in the body is lost. Therefore, after two half-lives only 25 percent of the original amount administered would remain. Therefore, theoretically, 96.875 percent of a drug will be eliminated from the body after five half-lives as displayed in Table 1-4.

As mentioned, amiodarone has a complex pharmacokinetic profile due to its extensive accumulation in tissue, which corresponds to an unusually large volume of distribution. The half-life ($t_{1/2}$) of a drug is influenced by its elimination clearance (CL) and volume of distribution (Vd) as demonstrated in equation 8:

$$\text{Equation 8: } t_{1/2} \equiv \frac{V_d \bullet 0.693}{CL}$$

Therefore, drugs that are highly distributed to tissues and have large volumes of distribution will generally have a long half-life. For amiodarone, the half-life can be up to 100 days given its unusual accumulation in tissues. In this extreme case, it would require waiting 500 days (1.4 years) to fully wash out the drug from systemic circulation. This amount of washout time is clearly unrealistic. Therefore, pharmacokinetic principles do not provide a complete picture of the factors that need to be considered in switching a patient from amiodarone to dronedarone.

Even though amiodarone is detectable in the systemic circulation for a long period of time, it does not remain effective at arrhythmia suppression for this extended time interval. Therefore, consideration

TABLE 1-4	Theoretical Amount of Drug Remaining and Lost Based on Number of Half-Lives in the Body	
No. of Half Lives	Amount Remaining (%)	Amount Eliminated (%)
0	100	0
1	50	50
2	25	75
3	12.5	87.5
4	6.25	93.75
5	3.125	96.875

of pharmacodynamic parameters such as the time of effectiveness is necessary to consider for drugs with long half-lives. Amiodarone remains effective at suppressing arrhythmias for several days after discontinuation but may lose effectiveness as soon as 3 to 5 days after discontinuation. Therefore, the potential accentuating of amiodarone toxicity versus the risk of losing the effectiveness of arrhythmia suppression needs to be considered. In this case amiodarone is being used to maintain sinus rhythm in a patient with atrial fibrillation with a current toxicity of thyrotoxicosis. Dronedarone, in theory, should not accentuate the thyroid toxicity of amiodarone because it lacks an iodine group and has a significantly decreased propensity to cause thyroid-related problems in clinical trials. Furthermore, the administration of dronedarone or continued course of amiodarone therapy will not change the course of therapy to treat thyrotoxicosis, such as the administration of methimazole. However, by not administering one of these agents, it may decrease the effectiveness of treatment.

The most likely immediate concern related to toxicity of dronedarone and amiodarone would be associated with an excessive QT-interval prolongation and the increased risk for torsades de pointes. This consideration is important because both drugs have similar mechanisms related to ion channel function and Vaughn-Williams classification. Therefore, pharmacodynamic monitoring of ECG data becomes important in patients switching from amiodarone to dronedarone. Given a normal heart-rate corrected QTc-interval, maintenance of normal sinus rhythm, and absence of other amiodarone-related adverse effects, it would be reasonable to begin dronedarone after a 3- to 5-day washout in this patient.

The pharmacokinetic and pharmacodynamic (effectiveness and toxicity) considerations described are important to consider regarding the decision on an appropriate washout period. One additional consideration should be based on the literature and washout periods that were used in the clinical trials that evaluated dronedarone therapy. Two of the trials did not require a washout period when converting patients from amiodarone to dronedarone, although the largest trial had a 28-day washout. However, the rationale for the 28-day washout in the ATHENA trial was because the trial outcome was not related to the maintenance of sinus rhythm. In summary, it is not feasible to wait for five half-lives for amiodarone to be eliminated from this patient before beginning dronedarone given the intense amiodarone accumulation. Previous trials started dronedarone without a washout period, and if there are no current toxicities other than thyrotoxicosis, it would make the most sense to start dronedarone immediately to optimally avoid atrial fibrillation recurrence.

CASE 3: DRUG INTERACTIONS I

DN is a 64-year-old man who presented to the emergency department complaining of lightheadedness, palpitations, and one episode of syncope that made him decide to seek medical attention. Upon initial presentation his heart rate was 45 beats per minute and his electrocardiogram displayed first-degree heart block.

His past medical history includes hypertension, atrial fibrillation, hyperlipidemia, HIV, and depression. His medications include:

Lisinopril 20 mg daily

Metoprolol 25 mg twice daily

Atorvastatin 40 mg daily

Amiodarone 400 mg daily

Atazanavir 400 mg once daily

Ritonavir 600 mg twice daily

Truvada® (emtricitabine plus tenofovir)

Sertraline 100 mg daily

He has been taking all medications for several years other than the initiation of the antiretroviral therapy (ART) 6 months ago. DN states that he uses a pillbox and has been taking his medications as prescribed.

QUESTION 1

What may be possible drug interactions and mechanisms that are precipitating DN's symptoms?

Answer:

The occurrence of undesirable clinical manifestations following a change in a medication record may be an adverse event of the added medications or a result of drug-drug interaction. Coadministration of amiodarone and metoprolol could possibly cause bradycardia and dizziness as experienced by this patient. However, the patient was stabilized on both medications with no reported adverse events before he started taking the ART. Both atazanavir and ritonavir (protease inhibitors) are potent CYP3A4 inhibitors that can increase amiodarone plasma concentrations (CYP3A4 substrate) and should be carefully administered in patients receiving atorvastatin. Coadministration of these drugs leads to pharmacokinetic drug interactions due to the inhibition of CYP3A4 metabolizing enzyme that may result in elevated concentrations of its substrates (amiodarone and atorvastatin). This inhibition of CYP3A4 can be associated with an increased risk of developing adverse events from both drugs. Therefore, the most likely drug interaction would be due to amiodarone toxicity manifested by dizziness, bradycardia, and AV block. Amiodarone should be stopped in this patient immediately until symptoms are controlled, and alternative therapies should be considered. Atorvastatin toxicity is also a potential concern in this patient and dosing changes may be considered along with assessing liver function and myopathy.

QUESTION 2

DN had an amiodarone concentration of 2.2 mg/L 6 months ago before starting ART. Estimate the steady-state clearance of amiodarone for DN.

Answer:

Because the patient has been taking amiodarone for more than 6 months, the plasma concentration may be at or close to steady state. Steady-state amiodarone clearance, CL_{ss}, can be calculated using equation 9 or 10:

$$\text{Equation 9: } CL_{ss} \times (C_p)_{ss} = \frac{F \cdot Dose}{\tau}$$

where F is amiodarone bioavailability, $(C_p)_{ss}$ is the steady-state plasma concentration, and τ is the dosing interval. This equation represents the steady state in which the left-hand side of the equation represents the output rate of the drug and the right-hand side represents the input rate. By definition the rates of input and output are equal at steady state. Equation 9 can be rearranged to estimate CL_{ss} for amiodarone.

$$\text{Equation 10: } CL_{ss} = \frac{F \cdot Dose}{(C_p)_{ss} \times \tau}$$

As previously used, the F value of 50 percent (0.5) will be used to estimate amiodarone clearance.

$$CL_{ss} = \frac{0.5 \times 400 \text{ mg}}{2.2 \text{ mg} / L \times 24 \text{ h}}$$

$$= 3.79 \text{ L/h}$$

Therefore, the steady-state clearance of amiodarone by DN is approximately 3.79 L/h.

QUESTION 3

Given the reported adverse effects of DN, an amiodarone plasma concentration was ordered and determined to be 3.7 mg/L. Calculate the clearance of amiodarone, assuming no change in bioavailability.

Answer:

Similar to question 2, amiodarone steady-state clearance can again be calculated using the equation and the newly determined plasma concentration:

Equation 10: $CL_{ss} = \dfrac{F \bullet Dose}{(C_p)_{ss} \times \tau}$

$$= \frac{0.5 \times 400 \text{ mg}}{3.7 \text{ mg} / L \times 24 \text{ h}}$$

$$= 2.25 \text{ L/h}$$

Based on the observed amiodarone $(C_p)_{ss}$ and its calculated CL_{ss}, amiodarone clearance was estimated to be reduced from 3.79 to 2.25 L/h after initiation of the ART. The increased amiodarone concentration is a likely cause of the adverse events experienced by DN. The decreased amiodarone clearance may be attributed to a reduced elimination of amiodarone due to inhibition of CYP3A4 by atazanavir and ritonavir.

QUESTION 4

Based on the calculated clearance in answer 3, recommend a new maintenance dose to maintain amiodarone plasma concentration near 2.2 mg/L.

Answer:

A new dose to achieve the desired concentration can be calculated by rearranging equation 10 as follows:

Equation 11: $Dose = \dfrac{CL_{ss} \times (C_p)_{ss} \times \tau}{F}$

$$= \frac{2.25 \dfrac{L}{h} \times 2.2 \dfrac{mg}{L} \times 24 \text{ h}}{0.5}$$

$$= 237.6 \text{ mg}$$

Based on this estimation, DN requires only half of his regular daily amiodarone dose, which can be reduced from 400 mg daily to 200 mg daily once his symptoms are alleviated.

CASE 4: DRUG INTERACTIONS II

DK is a 59-year-old, 60-kg, female who just underwent a coronary artery bypass grafting surgery. After the surgery, DK experienced left-sided hemiplegia that may be a cardiovascular embolism associated with intermittent atrial fibrillation. Her inpatient medications included:

Aspirin 81 mg/day

Propranolol 25 mg BID

Furosemide 40 mg/day

Simvastatin 40 mg/day

A week later she was transferred to a rehabilitation facility without any changes in her medication order. Two days later, atrial fibrillation recurred. Oral anticoagulation and amiodarone were indicated.

QUESTION 1

Explain why amiodarone was selected for the treatment of DK and specify the proper dosing regimen.

Answer:

DK's atrial fibrillation is considered recurrent with a history of coronary artery disease (CAD). The 2011 update from the American College of Cardiology and American Heart Association on the management of AF recommends restoration of normal sinus rhythm (NSR).[19] Pharmacological cardioversion with amiodarone or dofetilide is recommended for restoration of NSR in patients with CAD or underlying structural heart disease. Dofetilide needs to be initiated in the hospital after administration of AV node blocking drugs to avoid a paradoxical increase of the ventricular response. Because DK has been already discharged, amiodarone is the best choice for pharmacological cardioversion. According to the aforementioned 2011 consensus guidelines, the recommended amiodarone dose for the conversion to NSR is 400 mg BID until a 10 gm total dose is achieved, followed by a 200 mg/day maintenance dose.

A dosing regimen can be calculated as follows:

The total number of doses required for loading $= \dfrac{\text{Total loading dose}}{\text{Single dose}}$

$$= \frac{10 \text{ gm}}{400 \text{ mg}} = \frac{10000 \text{ mg}}{400 \text{ mg}} = 25 \text{ doses}$$

Because the dosing calls for administering amiodarone twice daily in this patient, therapy should continue for 12.5 days (i.e., 25/2). Therefore, a potential regimen for this patient would be amiodarone 400 mg BID for 12.5 days as a loading regimen followed by a maintenance regimen of 200 mg daily.

QUESTION 2

Two weeks following the initiation of amiodarone, DK complained of generalized muscle weakness and severe muscle pain preventing her from leaving bed.

Laboratory results: INR 1.91, LDH 820 U/L, CK 17,923 U/L, and TSH 1.3 mU/L. What are the suspected causes of DK's myopathy and what do you recommend to manage it?

Answer:

Several possible causes may explain the myopathy experienced by DK. Hypothyroidism could be a possible cause of muscle weakness and pain; however, DK's lab results show her TSH is within the normal range, making this diagnosis unlikely. Another cause of myopathy could be related to simvastatin therapy. Amiodarone is a known inhibitor of CYP3A4, and simvastatin is predominantly metabolized by CYP3A4. Concomitant administration of both drugs may result in reduced simvastatin elimination; hence, elevated plasma concentrations of simvastatin may be precipitating myopathy. This adverse event may be reversible upon discontinuation of simvastatin. An alternative option for DK would be to switch to another HMG-CoA reductase inhibitor, pravastatin, which is not metabolized by the cytochrome P450 enzymatic system.

CASE 5: AMIODARONE IN ACLS

DM is a 68-year-old man (body weight = 83 kg) with a history of coronary artery disease, congestive heart failure (EF 15%), type II diabetes mellitus, hypertension, and hyperlipidemia, who presented to the emergency department with chest pain and dyspnea. Upon presentation, the patient was hypotensive and diaphoretic. Soon after arrival the patient suddenly became unresponsive and pulseless. CPR was initiated and a code was activated. The initial rhythm showed ventricular fibrillation (VF). The patient was defibrillated at 200 J and CPR was resumed. After 2 minutes of CPR the patient was still pulseless and ventricular fibrillation persisted. The patient was then defibrillated again at 200 J, CPR was resumed, and epinephrine 1 mg IV push was administered. After an additional two minutes of CPR the patient remained in ventricular fibrillation. As the code team prepared to defibrillate the patient for a third time, the physician leading the resuscitative effort requested antiarrhythmic therapy with amiodarone.

QUESTION 1

What initial dose would you recommend and when would you expect to see an effect of amiodarone administration?

Answer:

The 2010 American Heart Association Guidelines for Cardiopulmonary Resuscitation and Emergency Cardiovascular Care recommend amiodarone 300 mg IV or intraosseus (IO) first line for treatment of VF or pulseless ventricular tachycardia (VT) unresponsive to defibrillation, CPR, and a vasopressor.[62] Although amiodarone administered orally may have an onset of action up to 2 days to 3 weeks, the onset is much more rapid following IV administration. The rapid response following IV administration may be a result of enhanced delivery to the site of action with increased plasma concentrations and hence exposing cardiac tissue to greater amiodarone concentrations. Given the variability in the bioavailability of amiodarone, IV administration should be considered in life-threatening scenarios. Therefore, even though amiodarone has extensive tissue distribution and a long time to reach steady state, IV administration is effective for the treatment of patients with life-threatening ventricular arrhythmias.

QUESTION 2

Following 300 mg of IV amiodarone administration, DM is defibrillated again and CPR continues; however, ventricular fibrillation persists. Would it be appropriate to administer a second dose of amiodarone at this time and, if so, at what dose?

Answer:

It is not uncommon to need to administer a repeated dose of amiodarone when ventricular fibrillation persists especially in overweight or obese patients. The larger volume of distribution in these patients would result in lower concentrations of amiodarone immediately achieving the target tissue and hence potentially decreasing

efficacy at arrhythmia suppression. It has been reported that amiodarone dosed at 5 mg/kg is superior to lidocaine in patients with shock-resistant ventricular fibrillation followed by a repeat dose of 2.5 mg/kg if needed.[5] Using the initial dose of 300 mg IV as the guidelines recommend would only provide 5 mg/kg for patients with a body weight of 60 kg or less (5 mg/kg × 60 kg = 300 mg). Indeed, the 2010 American Heart Association Guidelines for Cardiopulmonary Resuscitation and Emergency Cardiovascular Care recommend a second dose of amiodarone 150 mg IV/IO if ventricular fibrillation persists after further defibrillation.[62] Therefore, it would be appropriate to redose amiodarone in this patient at the recommended dose of 150 mg IV/IO.

HOMEWORK QUESTIONS

QUESTION 1

A patient with bradycardia has an amiodarone concentration of 3.2 mg/L at steady state following a regimen of 400 mg daily. Estimate a dosing regimen to maintain a steady-state concentration of 2.0 mg/L while assuming 50 percent bioavailability for amiodarone.

Answer:

$$\text{Equation 10: } CL_{ss} = \frac{F \bullet Dose}{(C_p)_{ss} \times \tau}$$

$$CL_{ss} = \frac{0.5 \times 400 \text{ mg}}{3.2 \text{ mg}/L \times 24 \text{ h}}$$

$$CL_{ss} = 2.60 \text{ L/h}$$

$$\text{Equation 11: } Dose = \frac{CL_{ss} \times (C_p)_{ss} \times \tau}{F}$$

$$= \frac{2.60\frac{L}{h} \times 2.0 \frac{mg}{L} \times 24 \text{ h}}{0.5}$$

$$= 250 \text{ mg}$$

The recommended dose would be 200 mg daily.

QUESTION 2

A loading dose of amiodarone was administered to a patient (weight = 70 kg) as a 150 mg intravenous (IV) bolus. Estimate the amiodarone plasma concentration 3 hours after administration of the bolus dose assuming amiodarone's Vd is equal to 100 L/kg and the half-life is 45 days in this patient.

Answer:

$$V_d = 100\frac{L}{kg} \times \text{body wieght (kg)}$$

$$= 100 \times 70 = 7000 \text{ L}$$

K_e can be estimated from the half-life using the following equation:

$$K_e = \frac{0.693}{t_{1/2}}$$

$$= \frac{0.693}{45 \text{ days}} = 0.0154 \text{ days}^{-1}$$

and converted to hours by

$$= \frac{0.0154}{24} = 6.4 \times 10^{-4} \text{ h}^{-1}$$

Equation 2: $C_p = \frac{F \cdot Dose}{V_d} \times e^{-K_e t}$

$$C_p = \frac{150}{7000} \times e^{-(6.4 \times 10^{-4} \times 3)}$$

$$C_p = 0.021 \text{ mg/L}$$

The amiodarone plasma concentration after 3 hours is 0.021 mg/L.

QUESTION 3

A loading dose of amiodarone was administered to a patient and a serum amiodarone concentration of 0.05 mg/L was achieved. An amiodarone infusion was started at 1 mg/min for eight hours. Estimate the amiodarone plasma concentration following the 8-hour infusion of amiodarone assuming the V_d is equal to 10,000 L and the half-life is 45 days for amiodarone in this patient.

Answer:

To calculate the portion of C_p that is attributed to the IV infusion for 8 hours, the following equation can be used:

Equation 3: $C_p = Amt \text{ from bolus} + \frac{R_0}{K_e V_d}(1 - e^{-K_e t})$

where R_0 is the infusion rate constant (i.e., 1 mg/min for the first 6 hours). The infusion rate R_0 (1 mg/min) is equivalent to 60 mg/h.

Amount remaining from bolus can be calculated using the following equation:

$$C_p = 0.05 \frac{mg}{L} \times e^{-(6.4 \times 10^{-4} \times 8 \text{ hr})}$$

Given this information the C_p after 8 hours can be estimated:

$$= (0.05 \times e^{-(6.4 \times 10^{-4} \times 8)}) + \frac{60}{6.4 \times 10^{-4} \times 10,000} \times (1 - e^{-(6.4 \times 10^{-4} \times 8)})$$

$$= 0.049 + 0.048 = 0.097 \text{ mg/L}$$

The estimated plasma concentration is 0.097 mg/L.

REFERENCES

1. Singh BN, Vaughan Williams EM. The effect of amiodarone, a new antianginal drug, on cardiac muscle. *Br J Pharmacol.* Aug 1970;39(4):657–667.
2. Mason JW, Hondeghem LM, Katzung BG. Amiodarone blocks inactivated cardiac sodium channels. *Pflugers Arch.* Jan 1983;396(1):79–81.
3. Charlier R. Cardiac actions in the dog of a new antagonist of adrenergic excitation which does not produce competitive blockade of adrenoceptors. *Br J Pharmacol* Aug 1970;39(4):668–674.
4. Wheeler PJ, Puritz R, Ingram DV, Chamberlain DA. Amiodarone in the treatment of refractory supraventricular and ventricular arrhythmias. *Postgrad Med J.* Jan 1979;55(639):1–9.
5. Dorian P, Cass D, Schwartz B, Cooper R, Gelaznikas R, Barr A. Amiodarone as compared with lidocaine for shock-resistant ventricular fibrillation. *N Engl J Med.* Mar 2002;346(12):884–890.
6. Nademanee K, Singh BN, Hendrickson J, et al. Amiodarone in refractory life-threatening ventricular arrhythmias. *Ann Intern Med.* May 1983;98(5 Pt 1):577–584.
7. Intravenous amiodarone in atrial fibrillation complicating myocardial infarction. *Br Med J (Clin Res Ed).* Feb 1982;284(6314):506–507.
8. Sullivan M. Intravenous amiodarone in atrial fibrillation complicating myocardial infarction. *Br Med J (Clin Res Ed).* Jan 1982;284(6310):197.
9. Anastasiou-Nana M, Levis GM, Moulopoulos SD. Amiodarone—application and clinical pharmacology in atrial fibrillation and other arrhythmias. *Int J Clin Pharmacol Ther Toxicol.* May 1984;22(5):229–235.
10. Horowitz LN, Spielman SR, Greenspan AM, et al. Use of amiodarone in the treatment of persistent and paroxysmal atrial fibrillation resistant to quinidine therapy. *J Am Coll Cardiol.* Dec 1985;6(6):1402–1407.
11. Strasberg B, Arditti A, Sclarovsky S, Lewin RF, Buimovici B, Agmon J. Efficacy of intravenous amiodarone in the management of paroxysmal or new atrial fibrillation with fast ventricular response. *Int J Cardiol.* Jan 1985;7(1):47–58.
12. Cowan JC, Gardiner P, Reid DS, Newell DJ, Campbell RW. Amiodarone in the management of atrial fibrillation complicating myocardial infarction. *Br J Clin Pract Suppl.* Apr 1986;44:155–163.
13. Cowan JC, Gardiner P, Reid DS, Newell DJ, Campbell RW. A comparison of amiodarone and digoxin in the treatment of atrial fibrillation complicating suspected acute myocardial infarction. *J Cardiovasc Pharmacol.* Mar–Apr 1986;8(2):252–256.
14. Gold RL, Haffajee CI, Charos G, Sloan K, Baker S, Alpert JS. Amiodarone for refractory atrial fibrillation. *Am J Cardiol.* Jan 1986;57(1):124–127.
15. McCarthy ST, McCarthy GL, John S, Chadwick D, Wollner L. Amiodarone as a treatment for atrial fibrillation refractory to digoxin therapy. *Br J Clin Pract Suppl.* Apr 1986;44:49–51.
16. Strasberg B. Intravenous amiodarone for conversion of atrial fibrillation to sinus rhythm. *Am J Cardiol.* Feb 1991;67(4):325.
17. Gosselink AT, Crijns HJ, Van Gelder IC, Hillige H, Wiesfeld AC, Lie KI. Low-dose amiodarone for maintenance of sinus rhythm after cardioversion of atrial fibrillation or flutter. *JAMA.* Jun 1992;267(24):3289–3293.
18. Di Biasi P, Scrofani R, Paje A, Cappiello E, Mangini A, Santoli C. Intravenous amiodarone vs. propafenone for atrial fibrillation and flutter after cardiac operation. *Eur J Cardiothorac Surg.* 1995;9(10):587–591.
19. Howard PA. Amiodarone for the maintenance of sinus rhythm in patients with atrial fibrillation. *Ann Pharmacother.* Jun 1995;29(6):596–602.
20. Opolski G, Stanislawska J, Gorecki A, Swiecicka G, Torbicki A, Kraska T. Amiodarone in restoration and maintenance of sinus rhythm in patients with chronic atrial fibrillation after unsuccessful direct-current cardioversion. *Clin Cardiol.* Apr 1997;20(4):337–340.
21. Tieleman RG, Gosselink AT, Crijns HJ, et al. Efficacy, safety, and determinants of conversion of atrial fibrillation and flutter with oral amiodarone. *Am J Cardiol.* Jan 1997;79(1):53–57.
22. Hamer AW, Mandel WJ, Zaher CA, Karagueuzin HS, Peter T. The electrophysiologic basis for the use of amiodarone for treatment of cardiac arrhythmias. *Pacing Clin Electrophysiol.* Jul 1983;6(4):784–794.
23. Heger JJ, Prystowsky EN, Jackman WM, et al. Clinical efficacy and electrophysiology during long-term therapy for recurrent ventricular tachycardia or ventricular fibrillation. *N Engl J Med.* Sep 1981;305(10):539–545.
24. Mitchell LB, Wyse DG, Gillis AM, Duff HJ. Electropharmacology of amiodarone therapy initiation. Time courses of onset of electrophysiologic and antiarrhythmic effects. *Circulation.* Jul 1989;80(1):34–42.
25. Wann LS, Curtis AB, Ellenbogen KA, et al. 2011 ACCF/AHA/HRS focused update on the management of patients with atrial fibrillation (update on Dabigatran): a report of the American College of Cardiology Foundation/American Heart Association Task Force on practice guidelines. *Circulation.* Mar 2011;123(10):1144–1150.
26. Wann LS, Curtis AB, January CT, et al. 2011 ACCF/AHA/HRS focused update on the management of patients with atrial fibrillation (updating the 2006 guideline): a report of the American College of Cardiology Foundation/American Heart Association Task Force on Practice Guidelines. *Circulation.* Jan 2011;123(1):104–123.
27. Roy D, Talajic M, Dorian P, et al. Amiodarone to prevent recurrence of atrial fibrillation. Canadian Trial of Atrial Fibrillation Investigators. *N Engl J Med.* Mar 2000;342(13):913–920.
28. Sleilaty G, Madi-Jebara S, Yazigi A, et al. Postoperative oral amiodarone versus oral bisoprolol as prophylaxis against atrial fibrillation after coronary artery bypass graft surgery: a prospective randomized trial. *Int J Cardiol.* Oct 2009;137(2):116–122.
29. Solomon AJ, Greenberg MD, Kilborn MJ, Katz NM. Amiodarone versus a beta-blocker to prevent atrial fibrillation after cardiovascular surgery. *Am Heart J.* Nov 2001;142(5):811–815.

30. Stamou SC, Hill PC, Sample GA, et al. Prevention of atrial fibrillation after cardiac surgery: the significance of postoperative oral amiodarone. *Chest.* Dec 2001;120(6):1936–1941.

31. Tisdale JE, Wroblewski HA, Wall DS, et al. A randomized, controlled study of amiodarone for prevention of atrial fibrillation after transthoracic esophagectomy. *J Thorac Cardiovasc Surg.* Jul 2010;140(1):45–51.

32. Tokmakoglu H, Kandemir O, Gunaydin S, Catav Z, Yorgancioglu C, Zorlutuna Y. Amiodarone versus digoxin and metoprolol combination for the prevention of postcoronary bypass atrial fibrillation. *Eur J Cardiothorac Surg.* Mar 2002;21(3):401–405.

33. Turk T, Ata Y, Vural H, Ozkan H, Yavuz S, Ozyazicioglu A. Intravenous and oral amiodarone for the prevention of postoperative atrial fibrillation in patients undergoing off-pump coronary artery bypass surgery. *Heart Surg Forum.* 2007;10(4):E299–303.

34. van 't Hof AW, Mosterd A, Suttorp MJ. Amiodarone for prevention of atrial fibrillation. *Am J Cardiol.* Feb 1996;77(4):327.

35. Yagdi T, Nalbantgil S, Ayik F, et al. Amiodarone reduces the incidence of atrial fibrillation after coronary artery bypass grafting. *J Thorac Cardiovasc Surg.* Jun 2003;125(6):1420–1425.

36. Yazigi A, Rahbani P, Zeid HA, Madi-Jebara S, Haddad F, Hayek G. Postoperative oral amiodarone as prophylaxis against atrial fibrillation after coronary artery surgery. *J Cardiothorac Vasc Anesth.* Oct 2002;16(5):603–606.

37. Kojuri J, Mahmoodi Y, Jannati M, Shafa M, Ghazinoor M, Sharifkazemi MB. Ability of amiodarone and propranolol alone or in combination to prevent post-coronary bypass atrial fibrillation. *Cardiovasc Ther.* Winter 2009;27(4):253–258.

38. Connolly SJ. Evidence-based analysis of amiodarone efficacy and safety. *Circulation.* Nov 1999;100(19):2025–2034.

39. Dusman RE, Stanton MS, Miles WM, et al. Clinical features of amiodarone-induced pulmonary toxicity. *Circulation.* Jul 1990;82(1):51–59.

40. Rady MY, Ryan T, Starr NJ. Preoperative therapy with amiodarone and the incidence of acute organ dysfunction after cardiac surgery. *Anesth Analg.* Sep 1997;85(3):489–497.

41. Andreasen F, Agerbaek H, Bjerregaard P, Gotzsche H. Pharmacokinetics of amiodarone after intravenous and oral administration. *Eur J Clin Pharmacol.* Mar 1981;19(4):293–299.

42. Holt DW, Tucker GT, Jackson PR, Storey GC. Amiodarone pharmacokinetics. *Am Heart J.* Oct 1983;106(4 Pt 2):840–847.

43. Roden DM. Pharmacokinetics of amiodarone: implications for drug therapy. *Am J Cardiol.* Nov 1993;72(16):45F–50F.

44. Freedman MD, Somberg JC. Pharmacology and pharmacokinetics of amiodarone. *J Clin Pharmacol.* Nov 1991;31(11):1061–1069.

45. Fabre G, Julian B, Saint-Aubert B, Joyeux H, Berger Y. Evidence for CYP3A-mediated N-deethylation of amiodarone in human liver microsomal fractions. *Drug Metab Dispos.* Nov–Dec 1993;21(6):978–985.

46. Ohyama K, Nakajima M, Nakamura S, Shimada N, Yamazaki H, Yokoi T. A significant role of human cytochrome P450 2C8 in amiodarone N-deethylation: an approach to predict the contribution with relative activity factor. *Drug Metab Dispos.* Nov 2000;28(11):1303–1310.

47. Nattel S, Davies M, Quantz M. The antiarrhythmic efficacy of amiodarone and desethylamiodarone, alone and in combination, in dogs with acute myocardial infarction. *Circulation.* Jan 1988;77(1):200–208.

48. Riva E, Hearse DJ. Anti-arrhythmic effects of amiodarone and desethylamiodarone on malignant ventricular arrhythmias arising as a consequence of ischaemia and reperfusion in the anaesthetised rat. *Cardiovasc Res.* Apr 1989;23(4):331–339.

49. Mahmarian JJ, Smart FW, Moye LA, et al. Exploring the minimal dose of amiodarone with antiarrhythmic and hemodynamic activity. *Am J Cardiol.* Oct 1994;74(7):681–686.

50. Pollak PT. Clinical organ toxicity of antiarrhythmic compounds: ocular and pulmonary manifestations. *Am J Cardiol.* Nov 1999;84(9A):37R–45R.

51. Rotmensch HH, Belhassen B, Swanson BN, et al. Steady-state serum amiodarone concentrations: relationships with antiarrhythmic efficacy and toxicity. *Ann Intern Med.* Oct 1984;101(4):462–469.

52. Ohyama K, Nakajima M, Suzuki M, Shimada N, Yamazaki H, Yokoi T. Inhibitory effects of amiodarone and its N-deethylated metabolite on human cytochrome P450 activities: prediction of in vivo drug interactions. *Br J Clin Pharmacol.* Mar 2000;49(3):244–253.

53. Touboul P, Brugada J, Capucci A, Crijns HJ, Edvardsson N, Hohnloser SH. Dronedarone for prevention of atrial fibrillation: a dose-ranging study. *Eur Heart J.* Aug 2003;24(16):1481–1487.

54. Kathofer S, Thomas D, Karle CA. The novel antiarrhythmic drug dronedarone: comparison with amiodarone. *Cardiovasc Drug Rev.* Fall 2005;23(3):217–230.

55. Varro A, Takacs J, Nemeth M, et al. Electrophysiological effects of dronedarone (SR 33589), a noniodinated amiodarone derivative in the canine heart: comparison with amiodarone. *Br J Pharmacol.* Jul 2001;133(5):625–634.

56. Sun W, Sarma JS, Singh BN. Electrophysiological effects of dronedarone (SR33589), a noniodinated benzofuran derivative, in the rabbit heart : comparison with amiodarone. *Circulation.* Nov 1999;100(22):2276–2281.

57. Le Heuzey JY, De Ferrari GM, Radzik D, Santini M, Zhu J, Davy JM. A short-term, randomized, double-blind, parallel-group study to evaluate the efficacy and safety of dronedarone versus amiodarone in patients with persistent atrial fibrillation: the DIONYSOS study. *J Cardiovasc Electrophysiol.* Jun 2010;21(6):597–605.

58. Connolly SJ, Crijns HJ, Torp-Pedersen C, et al. Analysis of stroke in ATHENA: a placebo-controlled, double-blind, parallel-arm trial to assess the efficacy of dronedarone 400 mg BID for the prevention of cardiovascular hospitalization or death from any cause in patients with atrial fibrillation/atrial flutter. *Circulation.* Sep 29 2009;120(13):1174–1180.

59. Piccini JP, Hasselblad V, Peterson ED, Washam JB, Califf RM, Kong DF. Comparative efficacy of dronedarone and amiodarone for the maintenance of sinus rhythm in patients with atrial fibrillation. *J Am Coll Cardiol.* Sep 2009;54(12):1089–1095.

60. Davy JM, Herold M, Hoglund C, et al. Dronedarone for the control of ventricular rate in permanent atrial fibrillation: the Efficacy and safety of dRonedArone for the cOntrol of ventricular rate during atrial fibrillation (ERATO) study. *Am Heart J.* Sep 2008;156(3):527.

61. Cook GE, Sasich LD, Sukkari SR. Atrial fibrillation. DIONYSOS study comparing dronedarone with amiodarone. *BMJ.* 2010;340:c285.

62. Zipes DP, Camm AJ, Borggrefe M, et al. ACC/AHA/ESC 2006 guidelines for management of patients with ventricular arrhythmias and the prevention of sudden cardiac death: a report of the American College of Cardiology/American Heart Association Task Force and the European Society of Cardiology Committee for Practice Guidelines (writing committee to develop Guidelines for Management of Patients With Ventricular Arrhythmias and the Prevention of Sudden Cardiac Death): developed in collaboration with the European Heart Rhythm Association and the Heart Rhythm Society. *Circulation.* Sep 2006;114(10):e385–e484.

63. FDA. FDA Drug Safety Communication: Severe liver injury associated with the use of dronedarone (marketed as Multaq). 2011. Accessed April 11, 2011.

64. Sanofi-Aventis. Full prescribing information for Mutlaq. In: Sanofi-Aventis, ed. NJ2009.

65. Damy T, Pousset F, Caplain H, Hulot JS, Lechat P. Pharmacokinetic and pharmacodynamic interactions between metoprolol and dronedarone in extensive and poor CYP2D6 metabolizers healthy subjects. *Fundam Clin Pharmacol.* Feb 2004;18(1):113–123.

MANNY SALTIEL, PharmD, FASHP, FCCP
SERINA TART, PharmD
KELLY A. KILLIUS, PharmD, BCPS
TRACEY H. TRUESDALE, PharmD, BCPS
DANIELLE PERRODIN, PharmD
NICOLE D. VERKLEEREN, PharmD, BCPS
ERICA MACEIRA, PharmD, BCPS, CACP
CHRISTY VAUGHAN, PharmD, BCPS
ANGELA M. PLEWA, PharmD, BCPS

CHAPTER 2

Aminoglycoside Pharmacokinetics

INTRODUCTION

The aminoglycoside class of antibiotics represents the class of drugs whose pharmacokinetics has been studied more extensively than any other. Remarkably resilient, these antibiotics continue to provide valuable weapons in the fight against infectious disease. Yet their well-known toxicities prevent their more frequent use. Clinical pharmacists are expected to serve as experts on the pharmacokinetic dosing of these drugs, and yet complex issues still lead to misunderstandings in their optimal use. In this chapter, several aspects of dosing will be presented:

- Extended interval dosing versus conventional dosing
- Traditional dosing and peak optimization
- Aminoglycoside ADRs related to trough concentrations
- Aminoglycoside dosing in acute renal failure
- Rounding serum creatinine in the elderly
- Aminoglycoside dosing in the obese patient
- Aminoglycosides used in the treatment of gram-positive endocarditis
- Aminoglycosides pharmacokinetics in pediatrics patients with cystic fibrosis

EXTENDED-INTERVAL DOSING VERSUS CONVENTIONAL DOSING

CASE 1

TJ is a 25-year-old male transferred from an outside hospital after walking in front of a moving city snowplow. X-rays taken at the outside hospital show left open pelvic fracture and a right open tibula/fibula fracture. He was intubated prior to arrival for combativeness and airway protection. Medications received prior to arrival include cefazolin 1gm via intravenous piggyback (IVPB) and fentanyl 150 mcg slow IV push. The orthopedics team is consulted in the emergency department and wants to add gentamicin for additional coverage of the open fracture.

Height: 5'11''   Weight: 180 lbs

PMH: Schizophrenia, depression

Allergies: Depakote

Vital Signs:

Blood pressure: 162/92.   Heart rate: 102 beat/min.

Temperature: 98.0°F

Respiratory rate: 12 breath/min on vent   100% on vent

Labs:

Sodium: 140   Chloride: 109   Potassium: 4.4

Glucose: 122   Bicarbonate: 25

Blood Urea Nitrogen (BUN): 15   Serum Creatinine (SCr): 0.86

What is your recommendation for starting gentamicin?

The first step to approaching an aminoglycoside patient is to calculate the weight to be used for dosing. Convert the patient's actual body weight (ABW) from pounds (lb) to kilograms (kg) and determine the ideal body weight (IBW). Utilization of a calculated dosing weight may be necessary if the actual body weight is greater than 20 percent of the ideal body weight. This concept will be discussed in detail in another section.

$$ABW = 180 \text{ lbs}/2.2 = 81.8 \text{ kg}$$
$$IBW = 50 \ [45.5 \text{ for females}] + (2.3 \times \text{inches over 5 ft})$$
$$= 50 + (2.3 + 11) = 75.3 \text{ kg}$$

Because ABW <1.2(IBW), actual body weight will be used.

The next step is to determine the patient's renal function, which is most often done by estimating their creatinine clearance (CrCl), utilizing the Cockcroft-Gault equation.[1] Estimating CrCl will assist in determining whether the patient is a candidate for extended interval dosing versus conventional dosing and for selecting the appropriate dosing schedule.

$$CrCl = \frac{(140 - \text{Age}) \times IBW}{72 \times \text{SCr}} (\times 0.85 \text{ for female})$$
$$= \frac{(140 - 25) \times 75.3}{72 \times 0.86} = >100 \text{ mL/min}$$

Once the determination to use an aminoglycoside has been made, the pharmacist can assist with the selection of the regimen.

Three common methods are used in designing an effective and safe aminoglycoside regimen: conventional or traditional dosing (CD), individualized dosing, and extended interval dosing (EID). Conventional dosing involves giving the total daily dose of the aminoglycoside divided throughout the day, typically every 8 to 12 hours in patients with good renal function. Monitoring includes determination of peak and trough serum concentrations at steady state, which occurs after three to five half-lives of the drug. Once serum levels are available, the patient's pharmacokinetic parameters can be calculated and utilized for regimen adjustments. Individualized dosing determines patient-specific pharmacokinetic parameters to achieve the desired peak and trough concentrations. Similar to conventional dosing, this method requires obtaining steady-state peak and trough serum concentrations.

EID is also referred to as once-daily dosing, high dose, or nontraditional dosing. EID has become an accepted alternative method for dosing, based on favorable pharmacodynamic and pharmacokinetic features. It is recommended that EID be the term used, in order to avoid confusion with patients with renal dysfunction who may receive conventional dosing on a once-daily basis. EID is becoming the preferred method at many institutions based on comparable efficacy, potential reduction in toxicity, and decreased monitoring when compared with other dosing methods.[2]

Aminoglycosides exhibit concentration-dependent bactericidal activity, meaning the bactericidal activity increases as the concentration of aminoglycoside increases. Utilization of EID maximizes the concentration-dependent killing effect of aminoglycosides by providing the total daily dose as a single infusion. This approach produces an elevated peak and undetectable trough concentrations.[3] The significance of undetectable trough concentrations will be discussed later. For antimicrobials that exhibit concentration-dependent killing, a serum concentration 10 times the minimum inhibitory concentration (MIC) of the organism is necessary to achieve optimal bactericidal activity.[3,4] For example, a concentration of 20 mcg/mL is necessary for an organism with an MIC of 2.

As our knowledge of pharmacokinetic and pharmacodynamics of aminoglycosides has grown, so has the acceptance and implementation of EID. The recommended dosing for gentamicin and tobramycin is 5–7 mg/kg and amikacin is 15 mg/kg. The landmark trial supporting the use of EID was published by Nicolau and colleagues.[3] The authors described their experience utilizing 7 mg/kg of gentamicin/tobramycin or 15 mg/kg of amikacin. In phase one, they sought to determine the dose necessary to achieve a peak concentration of 20 mcg/mL (to provide 10 times an MIC of 2 for *Pseudomonas*) with at least a four-hour drug-free interval. They found EID to be clinically as effective with a lower incidence of nephrotoxicity as a historical group of patients receiving traditional dosing. In addition, serum concentrations obtained during therapy were used to construct a nomogram for regimen monitoring.[3] (See the following section on monitoring.)

Subsequent to Nicolau's pivotal trial, additional studies utilizing 5 mg/kg were conducted,[5,6] confirming similar results of comparative efficacy and reduced toxicity when compared with conventional dosing. A separate nomogram for assessing the regimen should be utilized when the lower dose is selected. A common mistake when using the 5 mg/kg EID regimen is to use the Nicolau (or "Hartford") nomogram and multiply the serum levels on the y-axis by 5/7ths. This strategy has not been validated. To help determine which dosing scheme should be selected, Wallace and colleagues[7] compared four available EID protocols. Based on patient-specific pharmacokinetic parameters, they determined the peak and trough concentrations and dosing interval based on each protocol. The 7 mg/kg protocol produced peak concentrations closer to the target when compared with the 5 mg/kg protocols. A limitation of this evaluation is that it was a simulation and therefore does not offer insight into clinical or microbiologic efficacy or toxicity related to achieving higher peak concentrations.[7] Knowing local resistance patterns and MIC of commonly encountered organisms can assist in the selection of a dosing regimen. For example, if the local strain of *Pseudomonas* has an MIC of 2, then a 7 mg/kg dose of gentamicin/tobramycin will be more appropriate, whereas a 5 mg/kg dose may be adequate if the MIC is <1. Based on the limited available evidence, 7 mg/kg of gentamicin/tobramycin or 15 mg/kg of amikacin is an appropriate starting dose for most patients.

One of the primary benefits of EID is that it results in a drug-free interval. For several hours per day, the serum concentration of the aminoglycoside falls well below the MIC of the organism, but bactericidal activity continues. This phenomenon of continued killing despite subtherapeutic concentrations is referred to as the "postantibiotic effect" (PAE).[8] The duration of PAE for conventional doses of aminoglycosides varies but is generally 2–7 hours depending on the organism, based on animal models.[8] EID potentially increases the duration of PAE because a higher single dose is administered. A trough concentration that is undetectable is acceptable because of PAE. The typical drug-free interval can be 4–6 hours for an aminoglycoside, which is why a serum concentration is obtained 6–14 hours after the dose for monitoring. The drug-free interval decreases the amount of time the aminoglycoside can accumulate in renal cortical tissues, thereby potentially reducing the risk of toxicity.

Adaptive resistance is the third pharmacodynamic characteristic exhibited with EID that may offer benefit over CD.[9] The organism is exposed to the antimicrobial and is initially susceptible to bactericidal action of the aminoglycoside or other antimicrobial. As the antimicrobial concentration decreases, the effectiveness of bactericidal action decreases due to a relative resistance of a subpopulation of the organism colony. For aminoglycosides, the administration of a larger dose exhibits more rapid bactericidal activity. In the following 2–4 hours, the organism starts to develop relative resistance to the aminoglycoside. Over the next 8–12 hours, bacterial susceptibility gradually returns to baseline. By 24 hours postdose, the majority of bacterial susceptibility is reestablished. With EID, the next dose of aminoglycoside would be due when minimal to no resistance is present. Subsequent doses with conventional dosing regimen will be scheduled during the 8–12-hour period when the bacteria are resistant or minimally susceptible, therefore not providing maximal bacterial killing.[9] The concept of adaptive resistance has been assessed in vitro and in vivo animal studies. However, human studies are lacking. The concept of adaptive resistance appears to be a favorable component in the effectiveness of EID.

The overall effectiveness of extended interval aminoglycoside dosing is likely due to the combination of maximizing the concentration-dependent killing, the postantibiotic effect, and adaptive resistance.[4] By achieving higher peak concentrations for rapid bactericidal activity followed by a drug-free interval with continued bactericidal activity during which some of the bacteria are exhibiting temporary resistance to the aminoglycoside all may play a role in the clinical effectiveness as well as potentially reducing the incidence of toxicity.

Aminoglycosides are often overlooked as an antimicrobial option because of the associated toxicities: nephrotoxicity and otovestibular toxicity. Nephrotoxicity occurs when the aminoglycoside accumulates within the cortical tissues of the proximal tubule. The result is cell lysis and resultant presentation of initial nonoliguric renal failure that can progress to oliguric renal failure. For most patients, this toxicity is reversible.[2,4] Nephrotoxicity is often associated with elevated trough concentrations in patients receiving conventional dosing regimens when the drug is allowed to accumulate. EID is thought to decrease the incidence of nephrotoxicity due to the drug-free interval, thereby decreasing the amount of time the kidney is exposed to the drug. Nicolau and Colleagues[3] found a prevalence of nephrotoxicity of 1.2 percent, defined as an elevation in SCr of 0.5 mg/dL or greater. This level was lower than their previous experience of 3–5 percent occurrence with multiple daily dosing. A meta-analysis found an absolute risk reduction of 0.6 percent when using EID, compared with conventional dosing, although this finding was not statistically significant.[5] The current evidence is inconsistent with the definition and reporting of aminoglycoside-induced nephrotoxicity. Based on the available literature, an increased risk of nephrotoxicity is not apparent and potentially a decreased risk was noted with EID.

The occurrence of otovestibular toxicity has not been extensively studied in patients receiving EID. In the limited number of trials using objective evaluation of otovestibular function, EID did not

TABLE 2-1	Dosing Interval Determination[3]
CrCl (mL/min)	**Dosing Interval**
≥60	Every 24 hours
40–59	Every 36 hours
20–39	Every 48 hours
<20	Use alternative dosing regimen

result in an increased incidence of toxicity when compared with conventional dosing regimens.[5,6] Similar to nephrotoxicity, oto-vestibular toxicity is likely the result of prolonged exposure of the tissue to the aminoglycoside. Extended interval dosing allows for a drug-free period to reduce potential accumulation.

Once the dose has been determined, the dosing interval for EID can be selected. The interval is based on the patient's current renal function, which is based on the Cockcroft-Gault equation for CrCl, calculated in Step 2. Although many institutions have implemented laboratory reporting of a modification of diet in renal disease (MDRD) equation as an estimate of GFR for staging of kidney disease, its application for determining aminoglycoside clearance has not been fully evaluated. Table 2-1 can be utilized in determining the dosing interval for the patient's aminoglycoside regimen.[3]

It should be noted that EID may not be appropriate for all patients, including those with increased clearance (e.g., burns involving >20% of the patient's body surface area, cystic fibrosis, pregnancy) or with variable pharmacokinetic parameters (i.e., pregnancy, neonates and pediatrics, ascites, hemodialysis). Patients with such contraindications to EID should be considered for alternative dosing strategies.

$$7 \text{ mg/kg} \times 81.8 \text{ kg} = 572.6 \text{ mg}$$

$$\text{Rounding to nearest 25 mg} = 575 \text{ mg}$$

Because CrCl was estimated as greater than 100 mL/min, the dosing interval is every 24 hours.

Final recommendations: 575 mg every 24 hours.

The final step involves monitoring the selected aminoglycoside regimen. One advantage of using aminoglycosides is the ability to obtain serum concentrations, calculate patient-specific pharmacokinetic parameters to adjust the regimen, and thereby potentially optimize efficacy and avoid toxicity. Conventional dosing regimens require the assessment of peak and trough serum concentrations, ideally once the patient has achieved steady state. With these measured values, the elimination rate constant, half-life, and volume of distribution can be calculated, and a new, patient-specific dosage regimen can be determined to achieve the desired concentrations, if the current regimen does not. This process can be time-consuming and tedious, especially when the peak and/or trough concentrations are not obtained at the scheduled times (e.g., when a patient is unavailable for blood draws due to the need to go to another area for therapy or diagnostic imaging). With EID, evaluation of just a single serum concentration after the first dose is all that is necessary to determine regimen appropriateness. The nomogram by Nicolau and Colleagues[3] (Figure 2-1) allows for determination of regimen appropriateness based on single serum concentration. (As stated previously, if a 5 mg/kg regimen is selected, a separate nomogram should be utilized for monitoring. See Figure 2-2.)[5] When the serum concentration obtained 6–14 hours after the dose is administered falls below the designated interval line, the regimen should be continued. If the level moves above the current dosing interval line, the interval should be extended. These same principles apply to amikacin (Figure 2-3). If the serum concentration cannot be plotted on the nomogram, clinical judgment should be used to determine an appropriate regimen, and is beyond the scope of this section.

Lastly, the operational attributes of EID include decreased time spent by nursing, pharmacy, and laboratory personnel on

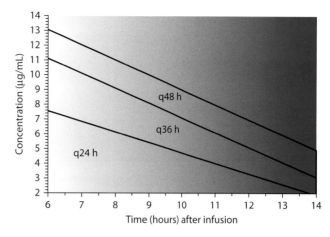

FIGURE 2-1. ODA nomogram for gentamicin and tobramycin at 7 mg/kg. Reproduced with permission from Nicolau DP, Freeman CD, Belliveau PP, Nightingale CH, Ross JW, Quintiliani R. Experience with a once-daily aminoglycoside program administered to 2,184 adult patients. *Antimicrob Agents Chemother.* 1995;39(3):650–655.

administration of doses and obtaining and evaluating serum aminoglycoside concentrations. A decrease in cost of therapy is related to intravenous tubing, infusion pumps, and laboratory samples as well.

CASE 2

KT is a 30-year-old male who fell 20 feet at a construction site with no loss of consciousness. He is brought into the emergency department by EMS with his right leg splinted for an open fracture of his tibia and fibula. He also complains of right arm pain, with no obvious deformity. He is currently able to protect his airway.

Orthopedics is evaluating the patient and requests 1gm of cefazolin and gentamicin per pharmacy.

Height: 5'7"	Weight: 165 lbs	VSS
PMH: denies	Allergy: NKA	
Labs:		
BUN 18	SCr 0.93	

QUESTIONS

1. *What are your initial recommendations for starting gentamicin?*

2. *If the 10-hour gentamicin level was 4.8, what would be your recommendation?*

3. *What would be your recommendation if an 8-hour level was 8.1?*

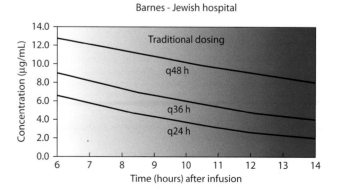

FIGURE 2-2. Extended-interval aminoglycoside nomogram for gentamicin and tobramycin at 5 mg/kg. Reproduced with permission from Bailey TC, Little JR, Littenberg B, Reichley RM, Dunagan WC. A metaanalysis of extended-interval dosing versus multiple daily dosing of aminoglycosides. *Clin Infect Dis.* 1997;24:786–795.

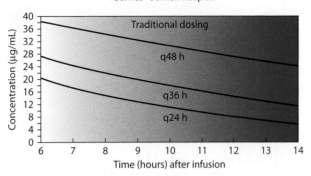

FIGURE 2-3. Extended-interval aminoglycoside nomogram for amikacin at 15 mg/kg. Reproduced with permission from Bailey TC, Little JR, Littenberg B, Reichley RM, Dunagan WC. A metaanalysis of extended-interval dosing versus multiple daily dosing of aminoglycosides. *Clin Infect Dis.* 1997;24:786–795.

Answers:

1. Calculate dosing weight.

$$165 \text{ lbs}/2.2 = 75 \text{ kg}$$

$$IBW = 50 + (2.3 \times 7) = 66.1 \text{ kg}$$

Calculate CrCl.

$$\frac{140 - 30(66.1)}{72 \times 0.93} = >100 \text{ mL/min}$$

Calculate gentamicin dose and determine interval.

$$7 \text{ mg/kg} \times 75 \text{ kg} = 525 \text{ mg}$$

Because CrCl is greater than 100 mL/min, a 24-hour dosing interval will be used.

Recommend serum gentamicin level be obtained 6–14 hours after the dose is administered.

2. The 10-hour gentamicin level is 4.8. Maintain continue current regimen of 525 mg every 24 hours (see Figure 2-1).

3. Extend the interval and change regimen to 525 mg every 36 hours. Also recommend obtaining a gentamicin level 6–14 hours after the regimen change.

TRADITIONAL DOSING AND PEAK OPTIMIZATION

CASE 1

LH, a 79-year-old female with a medical history significant for congestive heart failure, hypothyroidism, and hypercholesterolemia, presents to the emergency department from a nursing home with cough, shortness of breath, and altered mental status. She was admitted to the ICU with a diagnosis of bilateral pneumonia. Admission data include the following:

Height: 62 in   Weight 52 kg   SCr 1.4 mg/dL
WBC 18,000/mm³ with 85% neutrophils   Temperature of 101° F.

Sputum gram stain showed gram-negative rods. Cefepime and tobramycin are ordered for empiric coverage of health care–associated pneumonia. You are consulted to do maintenance dosing of tobramycin using traditional dosing due to the patient's age and renal function.

Desired Aminoglycoside Plasma Concentrations

The microbiologic activity of aminoglycosides is pH-dependent. Due to the low pH in the lung and bronchial secretions, especially in the presence of pneumonia,[10] the antimicrobial effectiveness of aminoglycosides may be reduced. The MICs of most gram-negative bacteria are usually less than 2 mcg/mL for gentamicin and tobramycin and 8 mcg/mL for amikacin. Aminoglycosides eradicate bacteria optimally when they achieve a peak/MIC ratio of at least 8 to 10 times greater than the MIC.[3,4,11] Whereas peak concentrations of 5–7 mcg/mL may be adequate for other infections, for gram-negative pneumonia or in patients who are critically ill due to a life-threatening gram-negative infection, peak concentrations of 8–10 mcg/mL should be targeted with traditional dosing.[12] Because the patient is elderly, she is at increased risk of aminoglycoside-induced nephrotoxicity.[13,14] Therefore, the trough level should be maintained at less than or equal to 1 mcg/mL. The relationship between aminoglycoside trough concentrations and adverse effects is discussed in the next section.

To solve this case, the following steps need to be taken:

1. Determine the CrCl.
2. Calculate population estimates for volume of distribution (Vd) and elimination rate constant (Ke).
3. Calculate the dosing interval, τ.
4. Determine maintenance dose (infusion time (t) will be assumed to be 1 hour), optimizing peak concentrations (Cmax desired = 9 mcg/mL) while keeping the trough below 1 mcg/ml (Cmin desired = 1 mcg/mL).
5. Calculate a loading dose.
6. Determine when to order peak and trough levels based on calculated half-life.

Step 1: Calculate CrCl.

Start by calculating the IBW for LH, in order to determine her CrCl.

$$IBW = 45.5 + 2.3 \text{ kg per inch over 60 inches (female)}$$

$$= 45.5 \text{ kg} + 2.3(2 \text{ inches over 5 ft}) = 50.1 \text{ kg}$$

Her IBW is less than actual body weight of 52 kg, and she does not weigh 20 percent over her IBW. Thus, IBW can be used for the CrCl calculation.

$$CrCl^1 = \frac{(140 - \text{Age})IBW}{72 \times SCr} \times 0.85 \text{ (woman)}$$

$$= \frac{(140 - 79) \times 50 \text{ kg}}{72 \times 1.4} \times 0.85 = 26 \text{ mL/min}$$

Step 2: Calculate population pharmacokinetic variables.

To calculate an initial maintenance dose and dosing interval for LH, population estimate equations for Ke[1] and Vd[15] need to be used:

$$Ke = 0.00293 \text{ (CrCl)} + 0.014 = 0.00293 (26) + 0.014 = 0.090 \text{ hr}^{-1}$$

$$Vd = 0.24 \text{ L/kg (IBW)} = 0.24 \times 50 \text{ kg} = 12 \text{ L}$$

Note: Because the clearance of aminoglycosides approximates CrCl,[16] some experts recommend using CrCl as the clearance of aminoglycosides and using the equation Cl = ke × Vd to calculate Ke.

Step 3: Calculate dosing interval.

$$\tau = 1/Ke \text{ (ln [Cmax desired/Cmin desired]) + t}$$

$$= 1/0.090 \text{ (ln[9/1])} + 1 = 25.4 \text{ hours}$$

To obtain the desired peak of 9 and trough of 1, a dosing interval of 25.4 hours was calculated, which can be rounded to 24 hours.

Step 4: Calculate maintenance dose (MD).

Next, the maintenance dose must be determined to be given at an interval of every 24 hours.

$$C_{max} = MD(1-e^{-ket})/(Vd \times Ke)(1-e^{-keT})$$
$$9\ mg/L = Ko(1-e^{-0.09(1\ hr)})/(0.09 \times 12)(1-e^{-0.9(24\ hr)})$$
$$= Ko(0.086)/(1.08)(0.885)$$
$$Ko(0.086/0.9558) = Ko(0.090)$$
$$Ko = 9\ mg/L/(0.090) = 100\ mg$$

Our maintenance dose for LH would be 100 mg tobramycin IV q24h.

Step 5: Calculate loading dose (LD).

Because LH has renal dysfunction, subtherapeutic concentrations may exists for 1–2 days of therapy until she reaches steady-state concentrations. Time to steady state cannot be shortened by giving a loading dose infusion; however, a loading dose can produce a plasma level that may approximate the steady-state concentration earlier in treatment.

$$LD = Cmax(Vd \times Ke)/(1-e^{-ket}) = 9(12 \times 0.09)/(1-e^{-0.09 \times 1\ hr})$$
$$= 9.72/0.086 = 113\ mg$$

The dose for aminoglycosides is generally rounded to the nearest 10 or 20 mg in practice. The loading dose of tobramycin for LH should be 110 mg given over 1 hour.

Step 6: Therapeutic drug monitoring.

With traditional aminoglycoside dosing, peak and trough serum concentrations need to be monitored in order to assure optimal dosing and to minimize the risk of toxicity (i.e., nephrotoxicity, ototoxicity).[17,18] Once steady-state conditions have been achieved, a trough level within 30 minutes prior to the next dose and a peak level timed to be drawn 30 minutes after the end of the infusion of the following dose need to ordered. (A peak level measured at least 30 minutes after the end of the infusion will avoid the distributive phase of tobramycin, thereby preventing an inaccurate level.)[19,20] As noted previously, goal peak concentrations for pneumonia are 8–10 mcg/mL for gentamicin or tobramycin.

$$\text{Calculate } t_{1/2} \text{ (half-life)} = 0.693/Ke = 0.693/0.090 = 7.7\ hours$$

Three half-lives (87.5% of steady state) will be reached at 23.1 hours, so steady-state concentrations should almost be obtained by the second dose. A trough concentration can be obtained then for close monitoring due to the patient's critical status and poor renal function. A peak will be obtained immediately following the dose to make sure it is adequate for maximum bactericidal activity.

CASE 2

DT is a 32-year-old male who comes into the emergency department with coughing and productive sputum. He admits to drinking alcohol daily and was admitted two weeks ago with a five-day stay in the ICU for severe alcohol withdrawal symptoms. Admission data include the following:

Height: 74 in Weight: 80 kg BUN 12 mg/dL
SCr 0.7 mg/dL Oral temp 101.5° F WBC 16,000/mm³
and infiltrate is seen in left lower lobe on chest X-ray.

DT is diagnosed with pneumonia and started on piperacillin/tazobactam 4.5 grams q6h and gentamicin 140 mg load. Physician requests consult. What will DT's initial maintenance dose be to obtain a peak of 8 mcg/mL and trough of 1 mcg/mL, using an infusion time of 0.5 hours?

1. Estimated IBW.
2. Estimated CrCl.

3. Estimate the elimination rate constant, Ke.
4. Estimate T½.
5. Estimate Vd.
6. Calculate dosing interval (T).
7. Calculate a maintenance dose (MD).
8. Calculate the predicted peak and trough levels at steady state.
9. Provide a final recommendation.

Answers:

1. Estimated IBW = 50 kg + (2.3 × 14) = 82.2 kg
2. Estimated CrCl = [(14 – Age) × IBW] / 72 × SCr
   = [(140 – 32) × 80] / 72 × 0.7
   Note: Used ABW because ABW <IBW.
3. Estimated Ke = 0.00293 (CrCl) + 0.014 = hr−1
4. Estimated T$_{1/2}$ = Ln(2)/ Ke = hours
5. Estimated Vd: BUN/SCr = 17 (assume normal hydration)

   Vd = 0.24 L/kg × 80 kg = 19.2 liters

6. Calculate dosing interval (T):

   Quick method: T = 3 × T$_{1/2}$ = 3 × 2.44 = 7.3 hours
   (Interval = 8 hours)

   Longer method: T = Ln (Cmax/Cmin) / Ke + ti
   = Ln (8/1)/+0.5 = hrs (Interval = 8 hours)

7. Maintenance dose (MD):

   $$MD = [(Ke) \times (Vd) \times (ti) \times (Cpeak\ desired) \times (1-e^{-kT})] / (1-e^{-kti})$$

8. Calculated predicted peak and trough at steady state.

   $$Cmax = [Dose \times 1-e^{-kti}] / (Ke)(Vd)(ti)1-e^{-kT}$$
   $$Cmin = Cmax \times e^{-k(T-ti)}$$
   $$Cmax = [140\ mg \times 1-e^{-(0.284 \times 0.5)}] / [0.284 \times 17.5 \times 0.5 \times 1-e^{-(0.284 \times 8hr)}]$$
   $$= 8.3\ mcg/mL\ (Expected\ peak)$$
   $$Cmin = Cmax \times e^{-ke(T-ti)} = 8.3 \times e^{-0.284(8-0.5)} = 0.99 = \sim 1.0$$

   Regimen is therefore appropriate.

9. Recommendation: Give gentamicin 140 mg IVPB q8h. Infuse over 30 minutes. Estimated Cpeak = 8–8.5 mcg/mL. Ctrough ~ 1 mcg/mL.

AMINOGLYCOSIDE ADRs RELATED TO TROUGH CONCENTRATIONS

CASE 1

CB is a 59-year-old female who presents to the emergency room with chills, fever, and cough. Her past medical history is significant for COPD, diabetes, and hypertension. She was hospitalized for pneumonia two months ago. She states that she has had increased shortness of breath over the past few weeks. She visited her doctor and received a course of levofloxacin two weeks prior to this current admission. However, she only took five days of her antibiotic course because she began to feel better.

Height: 62 in. Weight: 111 kg BP: 150/90
RR: 25 Temperature: 38°C

Allergies: Penicillins (reaction – anaphylaxis)

Labs:

WBC 18.2 (76% segs)   SCr 2.2 mg/dL   BUN 37 mg/dL

Gram stain of sputum and bronchoalveolar lavage reveals gram-negative rods.

CT pulmonary angiography is negative for pulmonary embolism.

Given her recent (<90 days prior to current admission) hospitalization and antibiotic use, the concern is that CB is at risk for multidrug-resistant pneumonia. The physician wishes to start a broad-spectrum antibiotic regimen. Given her poor renal function and her penicillin allergy history, you suggest aztreonam, tobramycin, and linezolid. The team agrees, and you calculate a tobramycin dose of 140 mg IVPB every 24 hours. (You are unable to use high-dose [7 mg/kg] extended-interval dosing due to the patient's renal function.) Four days later, you remind the team that tobramycin levels need to be drawn to properly assess the dose and risk of toxicity. The resident is reluctant to order levels, stating that the urine output has been adequate despite the IV fluids having been stopped two days ago. You persist, and he orders the levels, which return as follows:

Tobramycin trough 3.2 mg/L Tobramycin peak 7.9 mg/L
(SCr now 2.9)

QUESTION 1

Which of these levels, if any, are most concerning and may lead to an adverse reaction?

    a. trough level

    b. peak level

    c. neither trough nor peak level

    d. both trough and peak level

QUESTION 2

Which of the following statements is false?

    a. Volume depletion may increase the risk of nephrotoxicity with aminoglycosides.

    b. The contrast given for the CT four days ago has been eliminated and therefore cannot be correlated to the increase in SCr nor the risk of nephrotoxicity in this patient.

    c. Typically nephrotoxicity seen with aminoglycosides occurs as a delayed reaction with continued therapy.

    d. The presence of diabetes or hypotension and the use of other nephrotoxic drugs and iodinated contrast are all considered independent risk factors for the development of aminoglycoside-associated nephrotoxicity.

Discussion

Despite having been used since the 1940s, aminoglycosides remain active against a broad range of gram-negative pathogens and are therefore a viable choice for the treatment of serious gram-negative systemic infections. Their association with nephrotoxicity and ototoxicity may have prevented overuse of this class of medications.[21]

Nephrotoxicity associated with aminoglycosides has been clinically correlated to an elevated trough level concentration (>2 mg/L), but more recent studies show that the overall incidence of nephrotoxicity is highly dependent on the duration of therapy (most often if greater than or equal to 14 days). Typically, aminoglycoside nephrotoxicity presents without a decrease in urine output (nonoliguric renal failure) and with a slow rise in SCr that develops after 4–5 days of therapy.[22,23] Although the reported incidence of nephrotoxicity varies substantially between studies, averaging 6 percent to 10 percent, the nephrotoxicity rates do not vary significantly among the different aminoglycosides. Most common risk factors that have been associated with nephrotoxicity include duration of treatment, increasing age, compromised baseline renal function, volume depletion, elevated peak and trough levels, concurrent nephrotoxic drugs (e.g., vancomycin, amphotericin, NSAIDs, iodinated IV contrast, etc.), diabetes, and previous exposure to aminoglycosides.[22-24] In this patient case, the peak level is within range but the trough is elevated (>2 mg/L). The patient has multiple risk factors predisposing her to acute kidney injury with tobramycin, including volume depletion, diabetes, and recent iodinated contrast exposure.

Aminoglycoside-associated nephrotoxicity results from renal cortical accumulation resulting in proximal tubular cell necrosis. Examination of urine sediment may reveal dark-brown, fine, or granulated casts consistent with acute tubular necrosis but not specific for aminoglycoside renal toxicity. Although SCr levels are frequently monitored during aminoglycoside use, an elevation of SCr is more likely to reflect glomerular damage rather than tubular damage. In most clinical trials of aminoglycosides, however, nephrotoxicity has been defined by an elevation of SCr. Periodic monitoring of SCr concentrations—as well as peak and trough drug levels—may alert the clinician to renal toxicity. Treatment of aminoglycoside-induced nephrotoxicity is supportive. The aminoglycoside and any other nephrotoxic agents should be discontinued while maintaining the fluid and electrolyte balance.[21-24,25,26]

Unlike nephrotoxicity, the vestibular and/or auditory ototoxicity caused by aminoglycosides is often permanent. Overt otoxicity occurs in 0.5 percent to 7 percent of patients treated with aminoglycosides.[27,28] Originally, ototoxicity was thought to be the result of high peak serum concentrations that led to high concentrations of the drug in the inner ear. Later studies concluded that aminoglycoside accumulation in the ear is dose-dependent but saturable.[29,30,31,32] Recently, investigators demonstrated that audiometry testing was significantly better than monitoring symptoms in identifying early aminoglycoside auditory toxicity in patients prescribed aminoglycosides for more than 21 days.[33]

Factors associated with otoxicity include increasing age, duration of therapy, elevated peak and trough levels, concurrent ototoxic medications (e.g., loop diuretics, vancomycin), underlying disease states, and previous exposure to aminoglycosides.[33]

Vestibulotoxicity is difficult to diagnose, and no reliable monitoring process is available. Recent studies indicate a genetic predisposition to aminoglycoside auditory ototoxicity due to a mutation of mitochondrial DNA. However, this genetic component does not appear to influence aminoglycoside vestibular ototoxicity. Gentamicin toxicity is the most common single known cause of bilateral vestibulopathy, accounting for 15–50 percent of all cases.[31,32,34]

For gentamicin, tobramycin, and netilmicin, the risk of ototoxicity and nephrotoxicity is increased if peak levels are consistently maintained above 12–14 mcg/mL or trough levels consistently exceed 2 mcg/mL. For amikacin, peak levels above 32–34 mcg/mL or trough levels greater than 10 mcg/mL have been associated with a higher risk of ototoxicity and nephrotoxicity.[32,34,35]

CASE 2

CP is a 67-year-old male with HIV/AIDS admitted to the ICU with respiratory failure. Other significant past medical history includes CHF for which the patient takes furosemide 40 mg PO b.i.d. at home. Current antibiotic regimen consists of trimethoprim/sulfamethoxazole IV, piperacillin/tazobactam 3.375 gm IVPB q6h, and azithromycin 500 mg IV q24h. Sputum culture reveals 4+ enterobacter cloacae.

Based on the culture, the physician decides to discontinue piperacillin/ tazobactam and azithromycin, and start levofloxacin 750 mg IVPB q24h and gentamicin. On admission, a chest x-ray (CXR) reveals bilateral infiltrates and fluid accumulation.

Height: 61 in   Weight: 140 lbs   BP: 125/70

RR: 23   Temp 39°C NKDA

Labs:

WBC: 8.2 (66% segs)   SCr: 1.0 mg/dL   BUN: 15 mg/dL
(CrCl ~ 53 mL/min)

Due to fluid overload, the patient's furosemide is changed to 60 mg IV push q12h.

QUESTION 3

How many risk factors for aminoglycoside-induced nephrotoxicity does CP have at this time?

Answer:

The patient is elderly and is starting gentamicin concomitantly with a diuretic (furosemide).

AMINOGLYCOSIDE DOSING IN ACUTE RENAL FAILURE

Aminoglycoside dosing in patients with renal failure can be difficult. Significant changes in the pharmacokinetic profiles of these drugs and lack of consistent data provide little guidance for the clinician. Because aminoglycosides are excreted largely as unchanged drug in the urine (95%), their clearance is directly proportional to the patient's glomerular filtration rate (GFR).[16] The elimination half-life of aminoglycosides is approximately 1.5–3 hours in patients with normal renal function, but it is extended to as long as 20–60 hours in patients with end-stage renal disease (ESRD).[16,36,37] Also, a slower tissue distribution rate of aminoglycosides in patients with renal failure delays the time to peak concentration.[38] These factors in turn may significantly affect pharmacokinetic calculations if not taken into account. For example, a falsely low volume of distribution (Vd) may be calculated as a result of drawing peak serum concentrations too soon (30–60 minutes after infusion end time).[38,39] Patients with ESRD may also require hemodialysis. which adds to the variability of drug clearance. Characteristic behaviors of aminoglycosides with concurrent hemodialysis treatment have been determined to include increased elimination and shortened half-lives during the actual session, a rebound phenomenon in plasma serum concentrations immediately after the session has ended (plasma rebound), and a delayed post-dose distribution. Aminoglycoside clearance is determined by the type of dialyzer used, length and frequency of dialysis sessions, blood flow rates, as well as other factors.[38,39,40,41,42,43,44] In fact, reported differences in serum concentrations during plasma rebound and postdistribution vary widely, especially when looking at different types of dialysis schedules, such as intermittent (IHD) and slow daily home hemodialysis (SDH).[36,41] It is therefore recommended that predialysis levels be used to assess the need for supplemental aminoglycoside dosing.[43] The variability observed in patients with renal failure in both Vd and clearance is too large to rely on a standard dosing approach. Serum level monitoring must be done in order to achieve desired therapeutic outcomes of efficacy and safety, especially if therapy is to be continued for more than a few days. Reported peak concentration ranges of 7–10 mg/L and troughs (prehemodialysis) of 3.5–5 mg/L have been shown to improve outcomes in this population.[41]

CASE 1

EC is a 68-year-old male (height = 6′2″, ABW = 155 lbs, IBW = 81 kg) with a history of Type II DM and HTN who was started on cefepime plus gentamicin 500 mg IVPB every 24 hours for health care–associated pneumonia on February 4. On admission, he underwent chest CT with contrast to rule out a pulmonary embolism. His SCr and BUN have increased from 0.9 to 1.5 mg/dl and 15.1 to 30.6, respectively, within the last 24 hours, and his urine output over the last 6 hours has been zero. You have made a recommendation to the physician to switch to an alternative antibiotic, given the patient's worsening renal function. The physician denied your request, stating that he believes that the decrease in renal function is not due to the aminoglycoside and that the patient has a multidrug-resistant Pseudomonas in the sputum. He thus believes the benefit is much greater than the risk of further renal damage.

2/5, Day #2

Vital Signs:

BP: 100/72   HR: 92   RR: 16   Temp: 100.3° F

Labs:

WBC: 22   SCr: 1.5   BUN: 30.6

I/Os:

Input: 2682 mL   Output: 661 mL   Urine Output (U/O): 0 mL/hr

ASSIGNMENT I

Determine EC's CrCl, and develop a plan for his gentamicin therapy.

Answer:

EC has an estimated CrCl of <10 mL/min.[1]

U/O: 0 mL/hr   WBC: 22   Temp: 99°F

Plan

Stop EC's gentamicin maintenance dose and check a gentamicin random level in the AM. Check SCr and BUN daily and monitor for ototoxicity. Redose gentamicin 1 mg/kg once levels are decreased to below 2.5 mg/L.

Rationale

Cockcroft-Gault equation[1] for CrCl

$$= \frac{(140 - Age) \times (Wt. \text{ in kg}) \times (0.85 \text{ if Female})}{72 \times SCr}$$

(Use IBW unless ABW is less.)

ABW = 155/2.2 = 70 kg

EC's Calculated CrCl $= \frac{(140 - 70) \times (70.5)}{72 \times 1.5} = 46$ mL/min

Using the Cockcroft-Gault equation for EC's CrCl estimation yields a value of 46 mL/min; however, the problem with using equations to calculate GFR is that they use a snapshot in time of the patient's renal function, and they assume stable renal function (or steady state). The

[1]Note that the Brater equation can be used to more accurately estimate the patients creatinine clearance in a situation of changing renal function: CrCl (mL/min/70 kg) = [[293 – (2.03 × age)] × [1.035 – 0.01685 × (SCr^1 + SCr^2)]] / (SCr^1 + SCr^2) + [49 × (SCr^1 – SCr^2)] / (SCr^1 + SCr^2) × (Time difference in days). For females: Male value × 0.86. Brater DC. Drug Use In Renal Disease. *ADIS Health Science Press*, Balgowlah, Australia 1983;22–56.

results will be unreliable if the SCr is changing (such as in acute kidney failure) and thus not a true indicator of the patient's renal function. An increasing SCr will overestimate CrCl, and a decreasing SCr will underestimate CrCl until steady state is reached. Because this patient's SCr is rising and not at steady state, it may be assumed that his CrCl is less than the value calculated by standard equations. His lack of urine output confirms the concern that he is in acute renal failure.[45] A common mistake made by clinicians is to rely too heavily on computer calculations, not taking the entire clinical picture into consideration prior to making conclusions. EC was positive approximately two liters yesterday, and he is not excreting any urine. Given the fact that he is a diabetic and he has recently received IV contrast, he is at high risk of developing acute renal failure. Another risk factor may be hypoperfusion to the kidneys, caused by hypotension.[22-24]

2/6, Day #3

Vital Signs:

BP: 110/75   HR: 89   RR: 15   Temp: 99°F

Labs:

WBC: 16   SCr: 2.2   BUN: 36.8   Gent R: 3.6 mg/L

I/Os:

Input: 1550 mL   Output: 0 mL   U/O: 0 mL/hr

The physician has ordered a 4-hour dialysis session for today.

ASSIGNMENT II

Develop an assessment and plan for EC's gentamicin therapy today.

Answer:

EC has an estimated CrCl of <10 mL/min. U/O = 0 mL/hr. WBC = 16. T = 99° F. Gentamicin random level = 3.6 mg/L. Intermittent hemodialysis is to begin today.

Plan

Give gentamicin 1 mg/kg (or 70 mg) today at the end of the dialysis session and repeat random level prior to the next dialysis session. Redose as needed when the predicted gentamicin level <2.5 mg/L. Check SCr and BUN daily and monitor for ototoxicity.

Rationale

$$ABW = 155/2.2 = 70 \text{ kg}$$

$$\text{Supplemental dose} = 1 \text{ mg/kg} \times 70 \text{ kg} = 70 \text{ mg}$$

$$(\text{Use IBW unless ABW is less.})$$

A 4-hour intermittent dialysis session removes approximately 50 percent of aminoglycoside concentrations.[40] Several known factors may contribute to a lesser degree of removal, including dialysis session characteristics (e.g., shorter session duration, ultrafiltration only, or use of less permeable dialyzers) and patient characteristics (e.g., volume overload or reduced blood flow).[41] Current practice recommendations for aminoglycoside dosing in adults with ESRD on hemodialysis are to administer one-half of the full dose after each session.[16] However, as mentioned previously, therapeutic drug monitoring is required to ensure that sufficient excretion of drug has occurred and that troughs are below toxic levels. An additional dose of 1–1.8 mg/kg (depending on time lapsed from the dose, the specific dialysis prescription, and the patient's presentation) should be given at the end or after dialysis.[40,41] For severe infections or cases requiring prolonged treatment, as in the case of osteomyelitis and endocarditis, it may be desirable to calculate the patient's half-life

off of dialysis. This calculation may be done by obtaining a peak concentration 2–3 hours after the dose and a second level just before the next dialysis session.

CASE

JF is a 62-year-old female (Height = 5'6'', ABW = 131 lbs, IBW = 60 kg) with a history of recurrent UTIs who has been admitted to the hospital for multidrug-resistant Klebsiella *in the urine, which is only sensitive to tobramycin (MIC = 2 mcg/mL) and started on tobramycin 400 mg IVPB every 24 hours. On the fourth day of therapy, her SCr and BUN have increased to 2.2 mg/dL and 39 mg/dL, respectively, from baseline of 1.1 mg/dL and 17.1 mg/dL. She is currently anuric and the physician has consulted nephrology, who has now ordered a 6-hour intermittent hemodialysis session to begin tomorrow morning.*

3/31, Day #4

Vital Signs:

BP: 92/57   HR: 89   RR: 12   Temp: 99.1°F

Labs:

WBC: 12   SCr: 2.2 mg/dL   BUN: 39 mg/dL

I/Os:

Input: 3250 mL   Output: 220 mL   U/O: 0 mL/hr

QUESTION

Determine JF's CrCl and develop a plan for her tobramycin therapy.

Answer.

JF has an estimated CrCl of <10 mL/min.

U/O: 0 mL/hr   I/O: +2 liters   WBC: 12   Temp: 99.1°F

Plan

Stop JF's tobramycin maintenance dose and check a tobramycin random level in the AM, prior to dialysis. Redose with tobramycin 1 mg/kg when predicted level <2.5 mg/L. Check SCr and BUN daily and monitor for ototoxicity.

4/1, Day #5

Vital Signs:

BP: 98/60   HR: 87   RR: 14   Temp: 99.2°F

Labs:

WBC: 11.7   SCr: 3.4 mg/dL   BUN: 42 mg/dL
Tobra trough level: 3.8 mg/L

I/Os:

Input: 2117 mL   Output: 0 mL   U/O: 0 mL/hr

Develop an Assessment and Plan for JF's tobramycin therapy today.

Answer:

JF has an estimated CrCl of <10 mL/min.

U/O = 0 mL/hr I/O = +2 L WBC = 16 T = 99°F

Tobramycin random level = 3.8 mg/L. Intermittent hemodialysis is to begin today.

Plan

Give tobramycin 1 mg/kg (60 mg) today at the end of the dialysis session and repeat random level prior to the next dialysis session. Redose as needed when the predicted tobramycin level ≤2.5 mg/L. Check SCr and BUN daily and monitor for ototoxicity.

ROUNDING SERUM CREATININE IN THE ELDERLY

As previously noted, aminoglycosides are eliminated by the kidneys, and a decline in renal function affects the dosage interval that is used. However, the effect of renal dysfunction on individual doses is minor.[46,47] Serum concentrations of creatinine, a by-product of muscle metabolism, are reduced in patients who are malnourished or have advanced liver disease. SCr is also affected by a person's muscle mass. Geriatric patients have relatively less muscle mass than younger persons, and as a result their SCr values are often low.[48] Despite the frequent finding that elderly patients have normal SCr values, they often have slowly declining renal function.[49,50]

Using the standard equations to calculate CrCl with the low SCr values often seen in the elderly can lead to a significant overestimation of GFR and as a result an inappropriate dosing interval with aminoglycosides, possibly resulting in nephrotoxicity. In a study investigating drug dosing in elderly hospitalized patients, the Cockcroft-Gault equation was less predictive of the correct dose in patients with a SCr of less than 1 mg/dL than those with higher SCr values.[51] For this reason, clinicians often round low SCr values up to a higher value, 1 mg/dL. However, data to support this practice is limited. In elderly patients, rounding the SCr to 1 mg/dL can lead to an underestimate of the CrCl when using the Cockcroft-Gault equation.[52,53,54] Thus, some clinicians round SCr to 0.8 mg/dL. In one study, rounding up to a SCr of 0.8 mg/dL actual improved the predictive ability of Cockcroft-Gault equation in patients with a GFR ≤100 mL/min.[55]

In all patients, but in especially in the elderly, avoiding aminoglycoside-associated nephrotoxicity and ototoxicity is an important part of therapy. Calculating CrCl by rounding low SCr to a higher value allows clinicians to better calculate an empiric dosing interval for aminoglycosides until levels can be drawn.

CASE 1

VM, a 93-year-old female resident of a local nursing home, presents to the emergency department (ED) accompanied by her daughter, who states that the patient has had recent mental status changes. Upon presentation to the ED, she is febrile with a temperature of 101.9 F. She is 5'1'' and 98 pounds. Recent labs show WBC 21.2, Bands 36%, and SCr 0.3. She has no known drug allergies. Cultures are drawn, and VM is to be started on piperacillin/ tazobactam, linezolid, and amikacin. The ED attending calls to request pharmacy dosing of the amikacin.

1. Calculating the IBW.
$$IBW = 45.5 + (2.3 \times 1) = 45.5 + 2.3 = 47.8 \text{ kg}$$

2. Calculate CrCl.
$$CrCl = \frac{(140 - Age) \times IBW}{SCr \times 72} \times 0.85 \text{ (female)}$$
$$CrCl = \frac{(140 - 93) \times 47.8 \times 0.85}{0.8^a \times 72} = 33 \text{ mL/min}$$

[a]Note that the patient's SCr of 0.3 has been rounded up to 0.8, as discussed earlier.

3. Determine loading dose.
$$Dose = 20 \text{ mg/kg}$$
$$= 20 \text{ mg} \times 44.6 \text{ kg} = 890 \text{ mg}.$$
Round to 900 mg.

4. Estimated Ke.[46]
$$Ke = (0.0024 \times CrCl)^b + 0.01$$
$$= (0.0024 \times 33) + 0.01 = 0.09 \text{ hour}^{-1}$$

[b]Note that a different formula to calculate the elimination rate constant has been used here than was used in Section 2 in order to illustrate that both have been validated and either can be used.

5. Estimating half-life ($t_{1/2}$).
$$t_{1/2} = 0.693/Ke = 0.693/ 0.09 = 7.7 \text{ hours}$$

6. Calculate dosing interval.[56,57]
$$Dosing\ interval = 3 \times t_{1/2} = 3 \times 7.7 = 23 \text{ hours}$$

OR

Dosing Interval[57]	
CrCl (mL/min)	**Dosing Interval**
≥60	Administer every 8 hours
40–60	Administer every 12 hours
20–40	Administer every 24 hours
<20	Loading dose, then monitor levels

Answer:

Recommended dosing regimen would be amikacin 900 mg IVPB every 24 hours. A 1-hour postdose level (peak) and 10-hour level (random) are ordered for appropriate dose adjustments.

CASE 2

RS, an 89-year-old male, is admitted to the hospital for a persistent cough that has gotten worse over the last several days despite being on amoxicillin/clavulanic acid 875 mg b.i.d. and azithromycin for 4 days. He is febrile with a temperature of 100.9 F. He is 5'10'' and 180 pounds. Recent labs show WBC 17.9 and SCr 0.3. His only allergy is to statins, which he reports cause muscle pain. RS is being started on cefepime and gentamicin. The resident calls and requests dosing recommendations for gentamicin.

1. Calculate the IBW.
2. Calculate CrCl.
3. Determine loading dose.
4. Estimate the elimination rate constant, Ke.
5. Estimate the half-life ($t_{1/2}$).
6. Calculate a dosing interval.

Answers:

1. $IBW = 50 + (2.3 \times 8) = 50 + 18.4 = 68.4 \text{ kg}$

2. $CrCl = \dfrac{(140 - Age) \times IBW}{SCr \times 72} = \dfrac{(140 - 89) \times 68}{0.8 \times 72} = 60 \text{ mL/min}$

3. Loading dose = 7 mg/kg = 7 mg × 81.8 kg = 572.6 mg
   Round to 570 mg.

4. Estimated Ke = (0.0024 × CrCl) + 0.01 = (0.0024 × 60) + 0.01 = 0.15

5. $t_{1/2} = 0.693/Ke = 0.693/0.15 = 4.6 \text{ hours}$

6. Dosing interval = 3 × $t_{1/2}$ = 3 × 4.6 = 14 hours

OR

Dosing Interval	
CrCl (mL/min)	**Dosing Interval**
≥60	Administer every 8 hours
40–60	Administer every 12 hours
20–40	Administer every 24 hours
<20	Loading dose, then monitor levels

Recommended dosing regimen would be gentamicin 570 mg IV q12h plus checking a 1-hour level (peak) and 10-hour level (random) for appropriate dose adjustments.

AMINOGLYCOSIDE DOSING IN THE OBESE PATIENT

CASE 1

AM is a 67-year-old male (5'10", 283 pounds) who was transferred to the ICU from a general surgical floor with severe, acute abdominal pain, fever (39.2°C), and hypotension (92/58 mm Hg). He is post-op day #2; status is post laparoscopic ventral hernia repair and extensive lysis of adhesions. On exam, his abdomen is tender and firm, and the intensivist, suspecting a bowel perforation, wants to start broad-spectrum antibiotics while awaiting surgical intervention. The team chooses cefepime, metronidazole, and gentamicin and asks for you to recommend an extended-interval dosing regimen for gentamicin. Labs drawn earlier today reveal a stable SCr of 1.2 mg/dL. PMH is significant only for DM and COPD. Surgical history reveals a previous cholecystectomy and an amputation of his left forearm due to a fireworks accident five years ago.

Discussion

Drug dosing in obese patients is a challenge for clinical pharmacists in all settings and for virtually all drugs, due to the paucity of obese patients in clinical trials. Two independent issues come into play when dosing aminoglycoside in overweight patients: (1) adjustment of the dose to account for the increased Vd, and (2) estimation of renal function in this population via formulas that utilize weight as one of the independent variables.

Many of the physiologic changes that occur in obesity influence aminoglycoside dosing. Obese patients have an increased body mass compared to their normal-weight counterparts due to an increase in both lean and adipose tissue. Organ hypertrophy and increased blood volume also contribute to the increase in total body weight (TBW). Aminoglycosides are hydrophilic drugs primarily distributed into the extracellular fluid space. Because blood flow to adipose tissue accounts for less than 5 percent of total cardiac output and its water content is roughly 30 percent that of other body tissues, aminoglycoside kinetics are affected less by excess adipose tissue than are more hydrophobic drugs. Therefore, dosing based on TBW is not warranted and is likely to result in supratherapeutic drug concentrations.[58,59] Fortunately, aminoglycosides are likely the most pharmacokinetically studied antimicrobials in obesity, and numerous studies have been conducted in overweight patients in order to determine the dosing weight conversion factor (DWCF) that can be used to appropriately estimate dosing weight for patients receiving aminoglycosides. The DWCF is intended to account for the increase in lean body mass seen in obese patients that is not reflected by calculated IBW. Published studies have classified patients into various, somewhat arbitrary categories, ranging from "overweight" to "morbidly obese" and have suggested DWCFs ranging from 0.38 to 0.58.[60-67] Overall, literature supports employing a DWCF of 0.4 for overweight patients defined as those weighing 125 percent or more of their calculated IBW to determine a dosing weight for aminoglycosides.

When calculating IBW for AM, his forearm amputation must also be taken into consideration. This is accomplished by reducing the calculated IBW by a percentage that estimates what portion of IBW the missing body part (or parts) normally contributes to total body weight. (See Table 2-2.)

The average body weight distribution for each body part can be used to approximate an adjustment to the calculated IBW for

TABLE 2-2	Average Body Weight Distribution by Anatomic Location
Body Part	**Percent of Total Body Weight**
Hand	0.6
Forearm and hand	2.2
Upper arm	2.7
Total arm	4.9
Foot	1.4
Lower leg (including knee) and foot	6.0
Thigh	9.7
Total leg	15.6

Data from Smith LK, Weiss EL, Lehmkuhl LD. *Brunnstrom's Clinical Kinesiology*, 5th ed. Philadelphia: F. A. Davis Company, 1996, pp. 20–68.

amputees. For example, when accounting for the amputated limb in a patient with an above-knee amputation at midthigh:

$$6.0\% \text{ (for knee, lower leg, and foot)}$$
$$+ 4.8\% \text{ (estimating half of thigh)} = 10.8\%$$

Step 1: Calculate the patient's IBW.

For patient AM, first calculate what his IBW would be without a forearm amputation:

$$\text{For men, IBW (kg)} = 50 + 2.3 \text{ (inches over 5 ft tall)}$$
$$= 50 + 2.3(10) = 73 \text{ kg}$$

Now subtract the appropriate amount to account for his forearm amputation:

$$\% \text{ of BW for amputated body part} \times \text{IBW}$$
$$= \text{kg to be subtracted from IBW}$$
$$= 2.2\% \times 73 \text{ kg} = 1.6 \text{ kg}$$

$$\text{IBW} - \text{adjustment for amputation}$$
$$= \text{IBW for AM considering his amputation}$$
$$= 73 \text{ kg} - 1.6 \text{ kg} = 71.4 \text{ kg}$$

(Be sure to use this IBW, which accounts for his amputation, in all future calculations.)

Step 2: Determine whether a DW should be calculated for the patient.

Calculate what percentage of IBW is AM's TBW:

$$\text{TBW} = 283 \text{ lbs, or } 129 \text{ kg}$$
$$\text{TBW/IBW} = 129 \text{ kg}/71.4 \text{ kg} = 1.81 \text{ or } 181\%$$

AM's TBW is 181 percent of his calculated IBW. Because he weighs more than 125 percent of his IBW, a DW should be calculated:

$$\text{DW} = \text{IBW} + \text{DWCF(TBW} - \text{IBW)}$$
$$= 71.4 \text{ kg} + 0.4 (129 \text{ kg} - 71.4 \text{ kg}) = 94.4 \text{ kg}$$

Step 3: Use DW to calculate the dose of gentamicin.

$$7 \text{ mg/kg} \times 94.4 \text{ kg} = 660.8 \text{ mg}$$

Round the dose to 660 mg for ease of preparation.

The second issue to consider when dosing aminoglycosides in obese patients is how to most accurately estimate renal function. As noted previously in this chapter, the gold standard for estimating renal function for drug dosing considerations is the Cockcroft-Gault (CG) equation:

$$\text{CrCl} = [(140 - \text{Age}) \times \text{Wt.}]/(72 \times \text{SCr}) \times (0.85 \text{ if female})$$

where CrCl is estimated creatinine clearance in mL/min, age is in years, weight is in kilograms, and SCr is serum creatinine concentration in mg/dL. Cockcroft and Gault derived this formula from a group of male patients with stable renal function, all of whom were within 10 percent of their ideal body weight (IBW).[1] Naturally, the validity of this method in different patient populations, including those who are overweight, has been questioned. The original CG equation is not adjusted for body surface area (BSA), and it has been shown to grossly overestimate renal function when used in obese patients.[60–74] Various attempts have been made to validate the CG equation in obese patients by substituting IBW,[60,69,72,75–77] fat-free weight (FFW),[69,76] lean body weight (LBW),[69,76,78,79] predicted normal weight (PNWT),[76,80] or adjusted body weight (ABW)[60,69,76] for TBW in the formula. Although not unanimous, most studies have found that the use of LBW as the weight descriptor in the CG equation leads to the most accurate estimation of CrCl when compared to measured values obtained by 24-hour urine collections.[69,78,79] Erroneously, the assumption has been made that LBW is the same as IBW, which has led to the widespread adoption by clinicians of the use of IBW in the CG equation for patients of all sizes, except those whose actual body weight is less than IBW. Multiple studies, however, have demonstrated that use of IBW in the CG equation consistently underestimates renal function.[60,69,72,75–77] Even though the literature cannot give clear direction on which weight descriptor performs best for estimating renal function with the CG equation, the assumption might be made that a descriptor that is less than TBW (which overestimates CrCl) and greater than IBW (which underestimates CrCl) is likely most accurate. This assumption is supported in a study by Leader and colleagues that determined use of dosing weight (DW) as a replacement for TBW in the CG equation was best at predicting gentamicin clearance in obese patients.[60]

An alternative method of estimating CrCl in obese patients was developed by Salazar and Corcoran:

$$\text{CrCl (male)} = \frac{(137 - \text{Age}) \times [(0.285 \times \text{TBW}) + (12.1 \times \text{Ht}^2)]}{51 \times \text{SCr}}$$

$$\text{CrCl (female)} = \frac{(146 - \text{Age}) \times [(0.287 \times \text{TBW}) + (9.74 \times \text{Ht}^2)]}{60 \times \text{SCr}}$$

where CrCl is estimated creatinine clearance in mL/min, age is in years, TBW is in kilograms, height is in meters, and SCr is in mg/dL.[81] The Salazar-Corcoran (S-C) equation was developed using an obese rat model and then validated using patient data. Some studies have been able to further validate the S-C method in obese patients as the most accurate of available equations for estimating renal function from SCr,[77] but others have not been able to draw the same conclusion.[60,69,82] The S-C equation is not widely used by clinicians, perhaps because it is a more complicated equation to remember and compute.

The Modification of Diet in Renal Disease (MDRD) Study equation for estimation of glomerular filtration rate (GFR) was derived from data from men and women with chronic kidney disease and has been validated for accuracy of GFR estimation in many studies.[73,74,83–86] The four-variable MDRD equation has been most widely accepted and reexpressed for use with the standardized creatinine assay:

$$\text{GFR} = 175 \times (\text{SCr})^{-1.154} \times (\text{Age})^{-0.203} \times 0.742 \text{ if female}$$
$$\times 1.212 \text{ if African American}$$

where GFR is expressed in mL/min/1.73m², SCr is in mg/dL, and age is in years.[87] Initially there was reluctance to use this method for estimating renal function for drug dosage adjustments because the FDA's Guidance for Industry requiring study and publication of renal dose adjustments in drug labeling recommends use of measured CrCl or estimated CrCl using the CG equation, and it was not known whether the MDRD calculation would correlate to the breakpoints established with these methods.[88] Recently, Stevens and colleagues conducted a large simulation study looking at dosage adjustments determined via the MDRD method, CG equation

using TBW, or CG equation using IBW (or adjusted body weight for overweight individuals) and found that the MDRD equation has a high rate of concordance with established breakpoints and drug dosage recommendations.[72] These findings led to revision of the National Kidney Disease Education Program recommendations for estimation of kidney function for prescription medication dosage in adults to include the use of the four-variable MDRD equation adjusted for the patient's actual BSA or the CG equation utilizing TBW.[89] Additionally, a draft revision to the FDA's Guidance for Industry includes both the CG and MDRD equations as acceptable methods for describing renal function for dose adjustments in drug labeling.[90] The MDRD equation is less reliable in patients whose estimated GFR is >60 mL/min/m²; therefore, it is not the best choice for calculating drug doses in patients with near normal renal function.[74,86,91] The MDRD equation would therefore seem to be attractive for use in obese patients because it is normalized for an average body surface area (BSA) and can be adjusted according to a patient's actual BSA by multiplying by the patient's calculated BSA. However, several studies have shown the MDRD to be less accurate when applied to overweight patients. In the Stevens simulation study previously described, the MDRD equation underestimated renal function in the portion of the study population weighing more than 90 kg.[72] These findings are consistent with other studies that show the MDRD to be accurate for the population overall, but somewhat less accurate and likely to underestimate renal function in overweight patients.[73,74] Based on current evidence, the MDRD should not be used to estimate renal function for drug dosing in obese patients.

It is important to recognize the limitations of any SCr-based estimate of renal function and that these limitations may be more pronounced in obese patients. Twenty-four-hour urine collections for obese patients have been suggested.[82] However, this process is time-consuming and fraught with error in the not-unlikely event that a patient may forget and urinate without monitoring the volume. Additionally, it is not feasible when quantification of renal function is needed to start a drug right away. When estimating renal function for dosing aminoglycosides, particularly in obese patients, the appropriate use of therapeutic drug monitoring becomes even more important to assure efficacy and prevent toxicity. Because no single method of estimating renal function in obesity has been shown to be superior, use of either the S-C equation, which has been validated for use in obese patients, or the CG equation utilizing dosing weight, which has been shown to be accurate for estimating gentamicin clearance, is acceptable for determining an initial dosage interval for aminoglycosides. However, it is imperative that drug concentration levels are utilized to dictate continued dosing.

Step 4: Estimate the patient's renal function.

Cockcroft-Gault equation using dosing weight:

$$\begin{aligned}
\text{CrCl}_r &= [(140 - \text{Age}) \times \text{DW}]/(72 \times \text{SCr}) \\
&= [(140 - 67) \times 94.4 \text{ kg}]/(72 \times 1.2 \text{ mg/dL}) \\
&= 80 \text{ mL/min}
\end{aligned}$$

Salazar-Corcoran equation:

$$\begin{aligned}
\text{CrCl (male)} &= \frac{(137 - \text{Age}) \times [(0.285 \times \text{TBW}) + (12.1 \times \text{Ht}^2)]}{51 \times \text{SCr}} \\
&= \frac{(137 - 67) \times [(0.285 \times 129 \text{ kg}) + (12.1 \times 1.78 \text{ m}^2)]}{51 \times 1.2 \text{ mg/dl}} \\
&= 86 \text{ mL/min}
\end{aligned}$$

Step 5: Use estimated CrCl to determine appropriate dosage interval and complete dose and monitoring recommendation (see Section 1).

Recommended dose: 660 mg IV every 24 hours

Check level 10 hours after first dose is finished infusing and follow nomogram for adjustment.

CASE 2

LP is a 48-year-old female (5′6″, 207 pounds) admitted yesterday morning with pyelonephritis. She was initially started on ceftriaxone, but today continues to worsen clinically and blood cultures from admission are showing gram-negative rods on gram stain. The physician wants to add tobramycin to the antibiotic regimen until definitive culture results are back. LP's PMH is significant only for HTN (poorly controlled). SCr = 1.6 mg/dL on today's labs. Outpatient blood work from one month ago showed SCr = 1.6 mg/dL at that time. Recommend a dose and monitoring plan for tobramycin for LP.

Answers:

Step 1: Calculate the patient's IBW.

Women: IBW (kg) = 45.5 + 2.3(inches over 5 ft tall)
= 45.5 + 2.3(6) = 54 kg

Step 2: Determine whether a DW should be calculated for the patient.

Calculate what percentage of IBW is LP's TBW:

TBW = 207 lbs, or 94 kg

TBW/IBW = 94 kg/54 kg = 1.74, or 174%

Because she weighs more than 125 percent of her IBW, a DW should be calculated:

DW = IBW + DWCF(TBW − IBW)
= 54 kg + 0.4(94 kg − 54 kg) = 70 kg

Step 3: Use DW to calculate the dose of tobramycin.

7 mg/kg × 70 kg = 490 mg

Round the dose to 500 mg.

Step 4: Estimate the patient's renal function.

Cockcroft-Gault equation:

$CrCl_r$ = [(140 − Age) × DW]/(72 × SCr) × 0.85 (for female)
= [(140 − 48) × 70 kg]/(72 × 1.6 mg/dL) = 48 mL/min

Salazar-Corcoran equation:

$$ClCr(female) = \frac{(146 - Age) \times [(0.287 \times TBW) + (9.74 \times Ht^2)]}{60 \times SCr}$$

$$= \frac{(146 - 48) \times [(0.287 \times 94\ kg) + (9.74 \times 1.68\ m^2)]}{60 \times 1.6\ mg/dl} = 56\ mL/min$$

Step 5: Use estimated CrCl to determine dosage interval and dose.

Recommended dose: 500 mg IV every 36 hours.

Check level 10 hours after first dose is finished infusing; follow nomogram for adjustment.

AMINOGLYCOSIDES USED IN THE TREATMENT OF GRAM-POSITIVE ENDOCARDITIS

Infective endocarditis can be associated with significant morbidity and mortality. Choosing appropriate antimicrobial therapy is essential, but has been made more challenging with the emergence of resistant pathogens. The 2005 American Heart Association recommendations for the treatment of infective endocarditis include antibiotic selections for the most common pathogens. In some settings, the recommendations utilize synergy with aminoglycosides.[92]

CASE 1

A 29-year-old man presents to the trauma bay after suffering blunt trauma by multiple assailants. Workup is negative for traumatic head bleeding, fractures, or dislocations. Upon questioning, the patient complains of fever and chills for the last three days and admits to illicit intravenous drug use (IVDU) as noted by multiple skin tracks on both upper extremities. Imaging studies reveal pulmonary cavitary lesions. He subsequently undergoes transthoracic echocardiography (TTE) with a finding of definitive tricuspid valve vegetation (2 cm) with moderate regurgitation. Two sets of peripheral blood cultures are drawn by the bedside nurse; gram stain returns with gram-positive cocci on all four with culture pending.

Height: 6′1″ Weight: 70 kg SCr: 0.9 Allergies: NKDA

Blood culture × 4 pending

While ruling out other differential diagnoses, the attending physician asks his resident to initiate antibiotic therapy for what he believes to be cavitary lesions due to septic emboli secondary to infective endocarditis (based on Modified Duke Criteria).[92]

The resident remembers learning that streptococcus is a common pathogen associated with endocarditis but that staphylococcus should also be considered due to patient's history of IVDU. He writes an order for ceftriaxone 2 gm IV every 24 hours, vancomycin 15 mg/kg every 12 hours, and gentamicin "pharmacy to dose."

Case Analysis

Per the current AHA guidelines, the usual synergy dose of gentamicin is 3 mg/kg per day divided into three doses, adjusted for renal dysfunction.[92]

1. Calculate the initial dose (based on the guidelines) and frequency of gentamicin therapy in this patient based on the information given.

   3 mg/kg/day in three divided doses = 3 mg × 70 kg
   = 210 mg/day
   = 70 mg q 8 hrs

2. Use population-based pharmacokinetic parameters to calculate the initial gentamicin dose.

   a. Determine IBW[93] = 50 + (2.3 × inches over 5 feet)
   [50 + 2.3(13)] = 80 kg

   b. Using the Cockcroft-Gault equation[1], calculate the patient's CrCl.

   $$CrCl = \frac{(140 - Age)(Wt)^c}{72(SCr)} = \frac{(140 - 29)(70)}{72(0.9)} = 109\ mL/min$$

   Note: [c]Because the patient weighs less than his IBW, his actual weight can be used.

   c. Calculate Ke.

   Ke = 0.00293 × CrCl + 0.014 = 0.00293 (109) + 0.014 = 0.33

   d. Calculate half-life.

   $t_{1/2}$ = 0.693/Ke = 0.693/0.33337 = 2.1 hours

   e. Calculate the Vd.

   Vd = 0.25 L/kg = 0.25 L/kg × 70 kg = 17.5 L

   f. Calculate dosing interval[15] (τ).

   $$\tau = \frac{\ln (Cpk/Ctr)}{Ke} + t + T$$

where t = infusion time (30 min = 0.5 hr), Cpk and Ctr are the peak and trough concentrations, respectively. T = time difference of when Cpk drawn and time at end of infusion (30 min = 0.5 hr) [i.e., Infusion ends at 9:00 and Cpk level is drawn at 9:30, then T = 9:30 – 9:00 = 30 min = 0.5 hr].

$$\tau = \frac{\ln(4/0.25)}{0.33337} + 0.5 + 0.5 = 8.3 \text{ hours}$$

Round to 8 hours.

g. Calculate the maintenance dose rate (Ko).[15]

$$Ko = \frac{(Cpk[ss])(Vd)(K)(1-e^{-K\tau})}{(1-e^{-Kt})(e^{-KT})}$$

where Cpk[ss] is the desired steady-state peak concentration. Ko is measured as mg/hr and dose must be adjusted for 0.5-hour infusion.

$$Ko = 168 \text{ mg/hr, or } 82 \text{ mg/0.5 hr}$$

Round to 80 mg IVPB over 30 minutes.

3. The next day, speciation of blood cultures is in process. As the clinical pharmacist caring for the patient, you request peak and trough gentamicin levels to be drawn. The physician accepts your recommendations to initiate gentamicin as follows:

80 mg IVPB every 8 hours at exactly 1:00 AM, 9:00 AM, and 5:00 PM.

Use the following serum concentration data to determine individualized patient pharmacokinetic parameters: trough: 0.4 mcg/mL (drawn at 08:30 AM), and peak: 4.6 mcg/mL (drawn at 10:00 AM, 30 minutes after completion of IV infusion).

Dosages should be adjusted to achieve a peak serum concentration of 3–4 mcg/mL and trough serum concentration of 1 mcg/mL.[92]

a. Calculate the patient's elimination rate constant, Ke.

$$Ke = \frac{\ln(Cpk[ss])/Ctr[ss]}{T'} = \frac{\ln(4.6/0.4)}{8-1.5} = \frac{2.4}{6.5} = 0.375$$

where T' = τ (interval) minus the time difference between Cpk and Ctr (in hours).

b. Calculate $t_{1/2}$.

$$t_{1/2} = \frac{0.693}{Ke} = \frac{0.693}{0.375} = 1.85 \text{ hours}$$

c. Calculate Vd.

$$Vd = Ko(1-e^{-Kt})(e^{-KT}) = 80(0.17)(0.83) = 11.28 = 13.1 \text{ L}$$
$$Cpk[ss] \ (K)(1-e^{-K\tau}) \ 4.6(0.375)(0.5) \ 0.933$$

It is possible that errors in administration, sampling, and documentation may have altered the interpretation of the measured serum levels. Therefore, it is important to note the exact times of infusion as well as level sampling.[19]

d. Calculate the new dosing interval (τ).

$$\tau = \frac{\ln(Cpk/Ctr)}{K} + t + T = 8.4 \text{ hours}$$

e. Calculate the new dosing rate (Ko).

$$Ko = \frac{(Cpk[ss])(Vd)(K)(1-e^{-K\tau})}{(1-e^{-Kt})(e^{-KT})} = 132 \text{ mg/hr, or } 66 \text{ mg/0.5 hr}$$
$$= 60 \text{ mg dose infused over 30 minutes}$$

f. Recalculate the actual Cpk.

$$\text{Actual Cpk} = \text{Desired Cpk} \times \frac{\text{Actual (rounded) dose}}{\text{Calculated dose}}$$
$$= 4 \text{ mcg/mL} \times 60 \text{ mg/66 mg} = 3.64 \text{ mcg/mL}$$

CASE 2

JR is a 45-year-old woman (5′6″, 155 lbs) with a history of prosthetic mitral valve replacement, presenting with a temperature 102.5°F. A large vegetation is seen on TTE and the patient is taken to surgery to avoid embolization. The patient's urine output decreases significantly postoperatively and her SCr remains mildly elevated at 1.2. The diagnosis of acute renal failure (ARF) secondary to extended time on cardiopulmonary bypass is made. Blood cultures return showing streptococcus species with minimum inhibitory concentration (MIC) 0.12–0.5 g/mL (relatively resistant) to penicillin.[86] Therefore, the physician would like to proceed with ceftriaxone and gentamicin. The cardiothoracic surgeon seeks your assistance in adjusting all the patient's medication doses.

1. Calculate an appropriate starting dose of gentamicin (to achieve peaks of 3–4 mcg/mL and troughs of <1 mcg/mL) using population-based pharmacokinetic parameters of gentamicin.

    a. Determine ideal body weight (IBW).

    b. Using the Cockcroft-Gault equation, calculate the patient's CrCl.

    c. Estimate Ke (elimination rate constant).

    d. Estimate $t_{1/2}$ (half-life).

    e. Calculate the volume of distribution (Vd).

    f. Calculate dosing interval (τ).

    g. Calculate the maintenance dose rate (Ko).

2. Use the following serum concentration data to determine individualized patient pharmacokinetic parameters:

Dose: 80 mg IVPB every 18 hours
Trough: 0.6 mcg/mL (drawn 30 minutes before the third dose)
Peak: 4.8 mcg/mL (drawn 30 minutes after completion of IV infusion)

    a. Calculate Ke.

    b. Calculate $t_{1/2}$.

    c. Calculate Vd.

    d. Calculate the new dosing interval (τ).

    e. Calculate the new dosing rate (Ko).

    f. Recalculate the actual Cpk.

Answers:

1. Calculate an appropriate starting dose of gentamicin (to achieve peaks of 3–4 mcg/mL and troughs of <1 mcg/mL) using population-based pharmacokinetic parameters of gentamicin.

    a. Determine ideal body weight (IBW).

      IBW (kg) = 50 (kg) + (2.3[kg] × every inch over 5 feet [height]) male

      IBW (kg) = 45.5 (kg) + (2.3[kg] × every inch over 5 feet [height]) female

      = 45.5 + 2.3(6) = 59.3

    b. Using the Cockcroft-Gault equation, calculate the patient's CrCl.

$$\frac{(140 - \text{Age})(\text{IBW})(0.85)}{72(\text{SCr})} = \frac{(140 - 45)(59.3) \times 0.85}{72(1.2)}$$
$$= 55 \text{ mL/min}$$

    c. Estimate Ke (elimination rate constant).

$$Ke = 0.00293(\text{CrCl}) + 0.014 = 0.00293(55) + 0.014 = 0.17515$$

d. Estimate $t_{1/2}$ (half-life).

$$t_{1/2} = 0.693/Ke = 0.693/0.17515 = 3.96 \text{ hours}$$

e. Calculate the volume of distribution (Vd).

$$Vd = 0.25 \text{ L/kg} = 0.25 \text{ L/kg} \times 70 \text{ kg} = 17.5 \text{ L}$$

f. Calculate dosing interval (τ).

$$\tau = \frac{\ln (Cpk/Ctr)}{Ke} + t + T = \frac{\ln (4/0.25)}{0.17515} + 0.5 + 0.5 = 16.8 \text{ hour}$$

g. Calculate the maintenance dose rate (Ko).

$$Ko = \frac{(Cpk[ss])(Vd)(K)(1-e^{-K\tau})}{(1-e^{-Kt})(e^{-KT})} = 151 \text{ mg/hr, or } 75.5 \text{ mg/0.5 hr}$$

Consider 80 mg dose infused over 30 minutes.

2. Individualized patient pharmacokinetic parameters.

a. Calculate Ke.

$$Ke = \frac{\ln (Cpk[ss])/ Ctr[ss]}{T'} = \frac{\ln (4.8 \text{ mcg/mL}/ 0.6 \text{ mcg/mL})}{18 - 1.5}$$

$$= \frac{2.1}{16.5} = 0.127$$

b. Calculate $t_{1/2}$.

$$t_{1/2} = \frac{0.693}{Ke} = \frac{0.693}{0.127} = 5.46 \text{ hours}$$

c. Calculate Vd.

$$Vd = \frac{Ko(1-e^{-Kt})(e^{-KT})}{Cpk[ss](K)(1-e^{-K\tau})} = \frac{80(0.06)(0.94)}{4.8(0.127)(0.9)} = \frac{4.512}{0.547} = 8.2 \text{ L}$$

d. Calculate the new dosing interval (τ):

$$\tau = \frac{\ln (Cpk/Ctr)}{Ke} + t + T = 22.8 \text{ hours (round to 24 hours)}$$

e. Calculate the new dosing rate (Ko):

$$Ko = \frac{(Cpk[ss])(Vd)(K)(1-e^{-K\tau})}{(1-e^{-Kt})(e^{-KT})}$$

$$= 70 \text{ mg/hr, or } 35 \text{ mg/0.5 hour}$$

$$= 40 \text{ mg dose infused over 30 minutes}$$

f. Recalculate the actual Cpk

$$\text{Desired Cpk} \times \frac{\text{Actual (rounded) dose}}{\text{Calculated dose}} = \text{Actual Cpk}$$

$$4 \text{ mcg/mL} \times (35 \text{ mg}/40 \text{ mg}) = 3.5 \text{ mcg/mL}$$

AMINOGLYCOSIDES PHARMACOKINETICS IN PEDIATRICS PATIENTS WITH CYSTIC FIBROSIS

As described previously, EID of aminoglycosides maximizes their bactericidal activity by utilizing a higher peak concentration to MIC ratio and maximizing the postantibiotic effect. Several studies have evaluated extended-interval aminoglycoside administration in pediatric patients with cystic fibrosis (CF). EID was found to be equally efficacious in improving pulmonary function (change in FEV_1, the forced expiratory volume in one second) and was associated with a lower risk of nephrotoxicity.[94,95] The CF Foundation guidelines support the use of EID in patients with normal renal function. For CF patients with renal dysfunction, traditional dosing methods should be used.[96] Nomograms for EID have been developed to simplify dosing, but they should not be used in patients who have altered pharmacokinetics, including those with CF. A nomogram has been developed for use specifically in pediatric CF patients based on a tobramycin dose of 12 mg/kg once daily, but lacks supporting data.[97]

Higher doses of antibiotics are often required in CF patients due to higher volumes of distribution and increased clearance. Because of the considerable interpatient variability in clearance rates, it is important to monitor serum concentrations soon after initiation of aminoglycoside therapy. Serum concentrations should be monitored 2 hours after the start of the infusion, to account for distribution time, and a second random level 10 hours after the start of the infusion. One-compartment kinetics can then be used to determine the volume of distribution and clearance. The peak level can be calculated with a target of 20 to 30 mcg/mL (or 10 times the MIC if known) and can be extrapolated forward to ensure a 6-hour period when the serum level will be below 1.5 mcg/mL. Serum trough concentrations should be below the detectable range; therefore, they are not useful.[98]

Barclay and colleagues described another method to assess dosing. These investigators calculated the 24-hour AUC (area under the curve). EID should give the same level of drug exposure as conventional multiple daily dosing regimens (AUC_{24} 70 to 100 mg·hr/L).[99]

CASE 1

AK, a 10-year-old female with cystic fibrosis (CF), presents to the clinic with a 4-day history of shortness of breath, increasing cough, and sputum production, which is green and foul smelling. AK has an oral temperature of 100.6°F. Her current height is 4'8'' and weight is 75 lbs.

AK has had previous sputum cultures positive for Pseudomonas aeruginosa. *Other pertinent lab findings include: WBC 18,000, BUN 7, SCr 0.5. A new pulmonary infiltrate is noted on chest X-ray. Due to her acute exacerbation of CF, AK is admitted to the hospital for IV antibiotics, respiratory treatments, and aggressive chest percussion to improve airway clearance. It is likely she is again infected with* Pseudomonas, *since the organism is rarely eradicated in patients with CF. The physician orders ceftazidime 50 mg/kg IV q8h and tobramycin to be dosed by pharmacy.*

Estimate of CrCl using the Schwartz's equation for pediatric patients:

$$CrCl = K \times L/SCr \text{ (in mL/minute/1.73 m}^2)$$

K = constant of proportionality that is age-specific:

Age	K
Preterm infants up to 1 year	0.33
Full-term infants up to 1 year	0.45
2–12 years	0.55
13–21 years, female	0.55
13–21 years, male	0.7

L = Length or height in cm

SCr = Serum creatinine concentration in mg/dL

Thus, for AK, CrCl = 0.55×140 cm/0.5 mg/dL = 154 mL/min. AK has normal renal function and EID would be appropriate. Tobramycin 10 mg/kg IVPB every 24h (340 mg IVPB q24h) is ordered.

Tobramycin 340mg IV infused over 30 minutes at 1400 hours

Cmax (C1) drawn at 1600 hours = 20.1

Random level (C2) drawn at 2300 hours = 1.3

Calculate the volume of distribution (Vd) and elimination rate constant (Ke) for AK using × the tobramycin levels. The time interval between 1600 hours and 2300 hours is 7 hours and can be used to determine the elimination rate constant.

$$Ke = \ln (C1/C2)/\Delta t = \ln (20.1/1.3)/7 \text{ hours} = 0.39 \text{ hour}^{-1}$$

$$Vd = \frac{Dose/C1}{(1-e^{-kt})} \times e^{-k\tau} = \frac{340 \text{ mg}/20.1}{1-e^{-0.39 \text{ hr}^{-1} (24 \text{ hr})}} \times e^{-0.39 \text{ hr}^{-1} (2 \text{ hr})} = 7.8 \text{ L}$$

The clearance of the drug can then be calculated using the volume of distribution and elimination rate constant.

$$CL = (Ke)(Vd) = 0.39 \text{ hr}^{-1}(7.8 \text{ L}) = 3.04 \text{ L/hr}$$

The elimination rate constant can be used to calculate the expected plasma concentration at 1500 hours (or one hour before the observed peak of 22.6) and the expected trough concentration (30 minutes prior to the next dose). In the following equations, t represents the time difference from the measured plasma concentration.

$$Cpeak = \frac{C1}{e^{-kt}} = \frac{20.1}{e^{-0.39 \text{ hr}-1(1)}} = 29.7 \text{ mg/L}$$

$$Ctrough = C1 \times e^{-kt} = 20.1 \times e^{-0.39(21.5)} = 0.0046 \text{ mg/L}$$

Another method to assess dosing would be to calculate the AUC_{24} (target 70–100 mg·h/L).

$$AUC_{24} = \frac{Dose \text{ (mg)}}{CL \text{ (L/hr)}} = \frac{340 \text{ mg}}{3.04 \text{ L/hr}} = 111.8 \text{ mg·hr/L}$$

Although AUC slightly is slightly above the target range, the peak is within the target range and AK is clearing the drug. The dose of tobramycin 340 mg IV q24h would be appropriate.

CASE 2

GJ is a 6-year-old boy admitted to the hospital with a CF exacerbation. GJ weighs 42 lbs and is 4′ tall; his SCr is 0.4. GJ was recently hospitalized for IV antibiotics to treat a respiratory infection with positive sputum cultures for methicillin-resistant Staphylococcus aureus and Pseudomonas. Along with vancomycin, GJ has an order for tobramycin to be dosed by pharmacy. The pharmacist orders tobramycin 200 mg IVPB q24h, based on the dose used during his previous admission. Serum levels were drawn to assess dosing:

Tobramycin 200 mg IV infused over 30 minutes at 0900 hours

Cmax (C1) drawn at 1130 hours = 17.2

Random level (C2) drawn at 1800 hours = 1.4

Based on the tobramycin concentrations obtained for GJ, estimate his elimination rate constant (K), clearance (Cl), and volume of distributions (Vd) to assess the dose. Thereafter, using the calculated pharmacokinetic parameters for GJ, calculate the expected peak, trough, and AUC_{24} for the current dose.

Answers:

$$K = \ln(C1/C2)/\Delta t = \ln(17.2/1.4)/6.5 \text{ hours} = 0.39 \text{ hr}^{-1}$$

$$Vd = \frac{Dose/C1}{(1-e^{-kt})} \times e^{-k\tau} = \frac{200 \text{ mg}/17.2}{1-e^{-0.39 \text{ hr}-1 (24 \text{ hr})}} \times e^{-0.39 \text{ hr}-1(2.5 \text{ hr})} = 4.4 \text{ L}$$

$$CL = (K)(Vd) = 0.39 \text{ hr}^{-1} (4.4 \text{ L}) = 1.7 \text{ L/hr}$$

$$Cpeak = \frac{C1}{e^{-kt}} = \frac{17.2}{1-e^{-0.39 \text{ hr}-1(24 \text{ hr})}} = 30.9 \text{ mg/L}$$

$$Ctrough = C1 \times e^{-kt} = 17.2 \times e^{-0.39 \text{ hr}-1(21 \text{ hr})} = 0.0048 \text{ mg/L}$$

$$AUC_{24} = \frac{Dose \text{ (mg)}}{CL \text{ (L/hr)}} = \frac{200 \text{ mg}}{1.7 \text{ L/hr}} = 117.6 \text{ mg·hr/L}$$

REFERENCES

1. Cockcroft DW, Gault MH. Prediction of creatinine clearance from serum creatinine. *Nephron.* 1976;16(1):31–41.
2. Chambers HF. Chapter 45. Aminoglycosides. In: Brunton LL, Lazo JS, Parker KL. *Goodman & Gilman's The Pharmacological Basis of Therapeutics*, 11th ed.. Available at: http://www.accessmedicine.com/content.aspx?aID=949068.
3. Nicolau DP, Freeman CD, Belliveau PP, Nightingale CH, Ross JW, Quintiliani R. Experience with a once-daily aminoglycoside program administered to 2,184 adult patients. *Antimicrob Agents Chemother.* 1995;39(3):650–655.
4. Maglio D, Nightingale C, Nicolau D. Extended interval aminoglycoside dosing: From concept to clinic. *Int J Antimicrob.* 2002;19:341–348.
5. Bailey TC, Little JR, Littenberg B, Reichley RM, Dunagan WC. A meta-analysis of extended-interval dosing versus multiple daily dosing of aminoglycosides. *Clin Infect Dis.* 1997;24:786–795.
6. Gilbert DN, Lee BL, Dworkin RJ, et al. A randomized comparison of the safety and efficacy of once-daily gentamicin or thrice-daily gentamicin in combination with ticarcillin-clavulanate. *Am J Med.* 1998;105:182–191.
7. Wallace AW, Jones M, Bertino JS. Evaluation of four once-daily aminoglycoside dosing nomograms. *Pharmacotherapy.* 2002;22(9):1077–1083.
8. Spivey JM. The postantibiotic effect. *Clin Pharm.* 1992;11:865–875.
9. Barclay ML, Begg EJ. Aminoglycoside adaptive resistance: Importance for effective dosage regimens. *Drugs.* 2001;61(6):713–721.
10. Bodem CR, Lampton LM, Miller DP, et al. Endobronchial pH. Relevance of aminoglycoside activity in gram-negative bacillary pneumonia. *Am Rev Respir Dis.* 1983;127(1):39–41.
11. Moore Rd, Leitman P, Smith CR. Clinical response to aminoglycoside therapy: Importance of the ratio of peak concentration to minimum inhibitory concentration. *J Infect Dis.* 1987;155:93–97.
12. Moore RD, Smith CR, Lietman PS. Association of aminoglycoside plasma levels with therapeutic outcome in gram-negative pneumonia. *Am J Med.* 1984;77:657–662.
13. Bertino JS, Booker LA, Franck PA, et al. Incidence of and significant risk factors for aminoglycoside-associated nephrotoxicity in patients dosed by using individualized pharmacokinetic monitoring. *Infect Dis.* 1993;167(1):173–179.
14. Leehey DJ, Braun BI, Tholl DA, et al. Can pharmacokinetic dosing decrease nephrotoxicity associated with aminoglycoside therapy? *J Amer Soc Neph.* 1993;4(1):81–90.
15. Evans WE, Schentag JJ, Jusko WJ (Eds.). *Applied Pharmacokinetic Principles of Therapeutic Drug Monitoring*, 2nd ed. Spokane, WA: Applied Therapeutics, 1986.
16. Aronoff G, Bennett W, et al. *Drug Prescribing in Renal Failure: Dosing Guidelines for Adults and Children*, 5th ed. Philadelphia: American College of Physicians, 2007.
17. Radigan EA, Gilchrist NA, Miller MA. Management of aminoglycosides in the intensive care unit. *J Intensive Care Med.* 2010;25:327–342.
18. McCormack JP, Jewesson PJ. A critical reevaluation of the "therapeutic range" of aminoglycosides. *Clin Infect Dis.* 1992;14(1): 320–339.
19. Demczar DJ, Nafziger AN, Bertino JS Jr. Pharmacokinetics of gentamicin at traditional versus high doses: Implications for once-daily aminoglycoside dosing. *Antimicrob Agents Chemother.* 1997;41:1115–1119.
20. McNamara DR, Nafziger AN, Menhinick AM, Bertino JS Jr. A dose-ranging study of gentamicin pharmacokinetics: Implications for extended interval aminoglycoside therapy. *J Clin Pharmacol.* 2001;41:374–7.
21. Gonzalez LS, Spencer JP Aminoglycosides: A practical review. *Am Assoc Fam Pract.* 1998;58(8):1811–1820.
22. Lopez-Novoa J, Quiros Y, Vicente L, et al. New insights into the mechanism of aminoglycoside nephrotoxicity: An integrative point of view. *Kidney Int.* 2011;79:33–45.
23. Oliveira J, Silva C, Barbieri C, et al. Prevalence and risk factors for aminoglycoside nephrotoxicity in intensive care units. *Antimicrob Agents Chemother.* 2009;53(7):2887–2891.
24. Leehey D, Braun B, Tholl D, et al. Can pharmacokinetic dosing decrease nephrotoxicity associated with aminoglycoside therapy? *J Am Soc Nephrol.* 1993;4:81–90.
25. Sandhu J, Sehgal A, Gupta O, et al. Aminoglycoside nephrotoxicity revisited. *JIACM.* 2007;8(4):331–333.
26. Nayak-Rao S. Aminoglycoside use in renal failure. *Ind J Nephrol.* 2010;20(3):121–124.
27. Munckhof WJ, Grayson ML, Turnidge JD. A meta-analysis of studies on the safety and efficacy of aminoglycosides given either once daily or as divided doses. *J Antimicrob Chemother.* 1996;37:645–663.
28. Jackson GG, Arcieri G. Ototoxicity of gentamicin in man: A survey and controlled analysis of clinical experience in the United States. *J Infect Dis.* 1971;124(suppl):S130–S137.

29. Tran P, Deffrennes D. Aminoglycoside ototoxicity: Influence of dosage regimen on drug uptake and correlation between membrane binding and some clinical features. *Acta Otolaryngol.* 1988;105:511–15.

30. Cosgrove S, Vigliani G, Campion M, et al. Initial low-dose gentamicin for staphylococcus aureus bacteremia and endocarditis is nephrotoxic. *Clin Infect Dis.* 2009;48:713–721.

31. Balakumar P, Rohilla A, Thangathirupathi A. Gentamicin-induced nephrotoxicity: Do we have a promising therapeutic approach to blunt it? *Pharmacol Res.* 2010;62:179–186.

32. Guan M, Fischel-Ghodsian N, Giuseppe A. A biochemical basis for the inherited susceptibility to aminoglycoside ototoxicity. *Human Mol Genet.* 2000;9(12):1787–1793.

33. Palmay L, Walker SAN, Walker SE, Simor AE. Symptom reporting compared with audiometry for the detection of cochleotoxicity in patients on long-term aminoglycoside therapy. *Ann Pharmacother.* 2011. Published online ahead of print, 10.1345/aph.1P729: http://www.theannals.com/cgi/content/abstract/aph.1P729v1.

34. Cortopassi G, Hutchin T. A molecular and cellular hypothesis for aminoglycoside-induced deafness. *Hearing Res.* 1994;78:27–30.

35. Mulheran M, Degg C, Burr S, et al. Occurrence and risk of cochleotoxicity in cystic fibrosis patients receiving repeated high-dose aminoglycoside therapy. *Antimicrob Agents Chemother.* 2001;45(9):2502–2509.

36. Sowinski KM, Magner SJ, Lucksiri A, et al. Influence of hemodialysis on gentamicin pharmacokinetics, removal during hemodialysis and recommended dosing. *Clin J AM Soc Nephrol.* 2008;3:355–361.

37. Zaske D. Aminoglycosides. In: Evans W, Shentag J, Jusko W (Eds.). *Applied Pharmacokinetic Principles of Therapeutic Drug Monitoring,* 3rd ed.; also *Appl Ther.* 2006; 1:331–381.

38. Halstenson CE, Berkseth RO, Mann HJ, Matzke GR. Aminoglycoside redistribution and tobramycin. *Int J Clin Pharmacol Ther Toxicol.* 1987;25:50–55.

39. Manley HJ, Bailie GR, McClaran ML, Bender WL. Gentamicin pharmacokinetics during slow daily home hemodialysis. *Kidney Int.* 2003;63:1072–1078.

40. Dager W, King J. Aminoglycosides in intermittent hemodialysis: Pharmacokinetics with individual dosing. *Ann Pharmacother.* 2005;40(1):9–14.

41. Matze GR, Halstenson CE, Keane WF. Hemodialysis elimination rates and clearance of gentamicin and tobramycin. *Antimicrob Agents Chemother.* 1984;25:128–130.

42. Catolico M, Campbell J, Jones W, et al. Time course of gentamicin serum concentration rebound following hemodialysis. *Drug Intell Clin Pharm.* 1987;21:46–49.

43. Amin N, Padhi I, et al. Characterization of gentamicin pharmacokinetics in patients hemodialyzed with high-flux polysulfone membranes. *Am J Kidney Dis.* 1999;34:222–227.

44. Argawal R, Cronin R. Heterogeneity in gentamicin clearance between high-efficiency hemodialyzers. *Am J Kidney Dis.* 1994;23(1):47–51.

45. Manjunath G, Sarnak M, Levey A. Estimating the glomerular filtration rate: Do's and Don'ts for assessing kidney function. *Post Grad Med.* 2001;110(6):55–62.

46. Murphy John E. Aminoglycosides (AHFS 8;12.02). *Clinical Pharmacokinetics,* 4th ed. American Society of Health-System Pharmacists, Inc., 2008.

47. Giannelli SV, Patel KV, Windham G et al. Magnitude of unascertainment of impaired kidney function in older adults with normal serum creatinine. *J Am Geriatr Soc.* 2007;55(6):816–823.

48. Chan P. Pharmacokinetic and pharmacodynamic considerations in geriatrics. *Calif J of Health-System Pharm.* 2010;22:5–12. Available at: www.cshp.org/uploads/file/CJHP/CJHP%20SepOct%202010.pdf (accessed May 8, 2011).

49. Laroche ML, Charmes JP, Marcheix A, Bouthier F, Merle L. Estimation of glomerular filtration rate in the elderly: Cockcroft-Gault formula versus modification of diet in renal disease formula. *Pharmacotherapy.* 2006;26(7):1041–1046.

50. Gral T, Young M. Measured versus estimated creatinine clearance in the elderly as an index of renal function. *J Am Geriatr Soc.* 1980;28:492–496.

51. O'Connell MB, Dwindell AM, Bannick-Mohrland SB. Predictive performance of equations to estimate creatinine clearance in hospitalized elderly patients. *Ann Pharmacother.* 1992;26:627–635.

52. Smythe M, Hoffman J, Kizy K, Dmuchowski C. Estimating creatinine clearance in elderly patients with low serum creatinine concentrations. *Am J Hosp Pharm.* 1994;51:198–204.

53. Bertino JS Jr. Measured versus estimated creatinine clearance in patients with low serum creatinine values. *Ann Pharmacother.* 1993;27:1439–1442.

54. Reichley RM, Ritchie DJ, Bailey TC. Analysis of various creatinine clearance formulas in predicting gentamicin elimination in patients with low serum creatinine. *Pharmacotherapy.* 1995;15(5):625–630.

55. Dooley MJ, Sungh S, and Rischin D. Rounding of low serum creatinine values and the consequent impact on accuracy of bedside estimates of renal function in cancer patients. *Br J Cancer.* 2004;90:911–915.

56. McAuley, David F. Pharmacokinetic dosing. Aminoglycoside-vancomycin dosing. GlobalRPH.com. Available at: http://www.globalrph.com/aminoglycosides.htm (accessed March 4, 2011)

57. Adberg JA, Goldman MP, Gray LD, Long JK. *Infectious Disease Handbook,* 6th ed. Lexi-Comp, Inc., 2006.

58. Wurtz R, Itokazu G, Rodvold K. Antimicrobial dosing in obese patients. *Clin Infect Dis.* 1997;25:112–118.

59. Pai MP, Bearden DT. Antimicrobial dosing considerations in obese adult patients. *Pharmacotherapy.* 2007;27(8):1081–1091.

60. Leader WG, Tsubaki T, Chandler MH. Creatinine-clearance estimates for predicting gentamicin pharmacokinetic values in obese patients. *Am J Hosp Pharm.* 1994;51:2125–2130.

61. Traynor AM, Nafziger AN, Bertino JS. Aminoglycoside dosing weight correction factors for patients of various body sizes. *Antimicrob Agents Chemother.* 1995;39:545–548.

62. Sketris I, Lesar T, Zaske DE, et al. Effect of obesity on gentamicin pharmacokinetics. *J Clin Pharmacol.* 1982;21:288–293.

63. Korsager S. Administration of gentamicin to obese patients. *Int J Clin Pharmacol Ther Toxicol.* 1980;18:549–553.

64. Schwartz SN, Pazin GJ, Lyon JA, et al. A controlled investigation of the pharmacokinetics of gentamicin and tobramycin in obese subjects. *J Infect Dis.* 1978;138:499–505.

65. Bauer LA, Blouin RA, Griffen WO, et al. Amikacin pharmacokinetics in morbidly obese patients. *Am J Hosp Pharm.* 1980;37:519–522.

66. Bauer LA, Edwards WA, Dellinger EP, et al. Influence of weight on aminoglycoside pharmocokinetics in normal weight and morbidly obese patients. *Eur J Clin Pharmacol.* 1983;24:643–647.

67. Blouin RA, Mann HJ, Griffen WO, et al. Tobramycin pharmacokinetics in morbidly obese patients. *Clin Pharmcol Ther.* 1979;26:508–512.

68. Smith LK, Weiss EL, Lehmkuhl LD. *Brunnstom's Clinical Kinesiology,* 5th ed. Philadelphia: F. A. Davis Company, 1996, pp. 20–68.

69. Demirovic JA, Pai AB, Pai MP. Estimation of creatinine clearance in morbidly obese patients. *Am J Health-Syst Pharm.* 2009;66:642–648.

70. Dionne RE, Bauer LA, Gibson GA, et al. Estimating creatinine clearance in morbidly obese patients. *Am J Hosp Pharm.* 1981;38:841–844.

71. Verhave JC, Fesler P, Ribstein J, et al. Estimation of renal function in subjects with normal serum creatinine levels: Influence of age and body mass index. *Am J Kidney Dis.* 2005;46(2):233–241.

72. Stevens LA, Nolin TD, Richardson MM, et al. Comparison of drug dosing recommendations based on measured GFR and kidney function estimating equations. *Am J Kidney Dis.* 2009;54(1):233–242.

73. Froissart M, Rossert J, Jacquot C, et al. Predictive performance of the modification of diet in renal disease and Cockcroft-Gault equations for estimating renal function. *J Am Soc Nephrol.* 2005;16(3): 8763–8773.

74. Cirillo M, Anastasio P, DeSanto NG. Relationship of gender, age, and body mass index to errors in predicted kidney function. *Nephrol Dial Transplant.* 2005;20:1791–1798.

75. Hermsen ED, Maiefski M, Florescu MC, et al. Comparison of the modification of diet in renal disease and Cockcroft-Gault equations for dosing antimicrobials. *Pharmacotherapy.* 2009;29(6):649–655.

76. Green B, Duffull SB. What is the best size descriptor to use for pharmacokinetic studies in the obese? *Br J Clin Pharmacol.* 2004;58(2):119–133.

77. Spinler SA, Nawarskas JJ, Boyce EG, et al. Predictive performance of ten equations for estimating creatinine clearance in cardiac patients. *Ann Pharmacother.* 1998;32:1275–1283.

78. Janmahasatian S, Duffull SB, Chagnac A, et al. Lean body mass normalizes the effect of obesity on renal function. *Br J Clin Pharmacol.* 2008;65:964–965.

79. Ozmen S, Kaplan MA, Kaya H, et al. Role of lean body mass for estimation of glomerular filtration rate in patients with chronic kidney disease with various body mass indices. *Scand J Urol Nephrol.* 2009;43:171–176.

80. Duffull S, Dooley M, Green B, et al. A standard weight descriptor for dose adjustment in the obese patient. *Clin Pharmacokinet.* 2004;43(15):1167–1178.

81. Salazar DE, Corcoran GB. Predicting creatinine clearance and renal drug clearance in obese patients from estimated fat-free body mass. *Am J Med.* 1988;84:1053–1060.

82. Snider RD, Kruse JA, Bander JJ, et al. Accuracy of estimated creatinine clearance in obese patients with stable renal function in the intensive care unit. *Pharmacotherapy* 1995;15(6):747–753.

83. Levey AS, Bosch JP, Lewis JB, et al. A more accurate method to estimate glomerular filtration rate from serum creatinine: A new prediction equation. Modification of Diet in Renal Disease Study Group. *Ann Intern Med.* 1999;130(6):461–70.

84. Lewis JB, Agodoba L, Cheek D, et al. Comparison of cross-sectional renal function measurements in African-Americans with hypertensive nephrosclerosis and of primary formulas to estimate glomerular filtration rate. *Am J Kidney Dis.* 2001;38(4):744–753.

85. Rule AD, Larson TS, Bergstralh EJ, et al. Using serum creatinine to estimate glomerular filtration rate: Accuracy in good health and in chronic kidney disease. *Ann Intern Med.* 2004;141(12):929–937.

86. Poggio ED, Wang X, Greene T, et al. Performance of the modification of diet in renal disease and Cockcroft-Gault equations in the estimation of GFR in health and in chronic kidney disease. *J Am Soc Nephrol.* 2005;16(2):459–466.

87. Levey AS, Coresh J, Greene T, et al. Using standardized serum creatinine values in the modification of diet in renal disease study equation for estimating glomerular filtration rate. *Ann Intern Med.* 2006;145(4): 247–254.

88. Food and Drug Administration. Guidance for industry: Pharmacokinetics in patients with impaired renal function-study design, data analysis, and the impact on dosing. Rockville, MD, U.S. Department of Health and Human Services, May 1998. Available at: www.fda.gov/downloads/Drugs/GuidanceComplianceRegulatoryInformation/Guidances/ucm072127.pdf (accessed March 1, 2011).

89. National Kidney Disease Education Program. CKD and drug dosing: Information for providers. Available at: http://www.nkdep.nih.gov/professionals/drug-dosing-information.htm (accessed February 28, 2011).

90. Food and Drug Administration. Guidance for industry: Pharmacokinetics in patients with impaired renal function-study design, data analysis, and the impact on dosing. Draft Guidance. Rockville, MD, US Department of Health and Human Services, March 2010. Available at: www.fda.gov/downloads/Drugs/GuidanceComplianceRegulatoryInformation/Guidances/UCM204959.pdf (accessed March 13, 2011).

91. Levey AS, Stevens LA, Schmid CH, et al. A new equation to estimate glomerular filtration rate. *Ann Intern Med.* 2009;150:604–612.

92. Baddour LM, Wilson WR, Bayer AS, et al. Infective endocarditis: Diagnosis, antimicrobial therapy and management of complications: A statement from the committee on rheumatic fever, endocarditis and Kawasaki disease. *Circulation.* 2005;111:e394–e434.

93. Pai MP, Paloucek FP. The origin of the "ideal" body weight equations. *Ann Pharmacother.* 2000;34:1066–1069.

94. Smyth A, Tan K, Hyman-Taylor P, et al. Once versus three times daily regimens of tobramycin treatment for pulmonary exacerbations of cystic fibrosis—the TOPIC study: A randomized controlled trial. *Lancet.* 2005;365:573–578.

95. Smyth AR, Bhatt J. Once daily versus multiple daily dosing with intravenous aminoglycosides for cystic fibrosis. *Cochrane Database Syst Rev.* 2010:CD002009. DOI: 10.1002/14651858.CD002009.pub3.

96. Flume PA, Mogayzel PJ, Robinson KA, et al. Cystic fibrosis pulmonary guidelines: Treatment of pulmonary exacerbations. *Am J Respir Crit Care Med.* 2009;180:802–808.

97. Massie J, Cranswick N. Pharmacokinetic profile of once daily intravenous tobramycin in children with cystic fibrosis. *J Paediatr Child Health.* 2006;42(10):601–605.

98. Prayle A, Smyth AR. Aminoglycoside use in cystic fibrosis: Therapeutic strategies and toxicity. *Curr Opin Pulm Me.d* 2010;16(6):604–610.

99. Barclay M, Duffull SB, Begg EJ, et al. Experience of once-daily aminoglycoside dosing using a target area under the concentration-time curve. *Aust NZ J Med* 1995;25:230–235.

CHAPTER 3

Continuous and Intermittent Infusion Beta-Lactam Antibiotics

DORA E. WISKIRCHEN, PharmD, BCPS
REBECCA A. KEEL-JAYAKUMAR, PharmD
DAVID P. NICOLAU, PharmD, FCCP, FIDSA

DRUG OVERVIEW

As a class, beta-lactam antibiotics are a mainstay of therapy and are recommended for nearly all infection types in clinical practice guidelines[1-6], often as first-line agents. Overall, they are a broad class of antibiotics and consist of penicillins, cephalosporins, monobactams, and carbapenems. Beta-lactams exhibit bactericidal activity by binding to penicillin-binding proteins and, ultimately, inhibiting cell wall synthesis. Since the discovery of penicillin, it has been known that prolonging the infusion duration (originally done as a continuous infusion) or more frequent dosing resulted in improved outcomes[7-8]; however, the utilization of prolonged or continuous infusion has remained a matter of debate and much research has been undertaken to understand and justify these dosing strategies.

THERAPEUTIC CONCENTRATIONS

With increasing antimicrobial resistance and limited novel antimicrobials on the horizon, a resurgence of interest in optimizing currently available treatment options has occurred. The potency of an antimicrobial is measured as the lowest concentration that inhibits visible bacterial growth, also known as the minimum inhibitory concentration (MIC). While *in vitro* potency is relatively straightforward, *in vivo* potency is much more complex and is described using pharmacodynamics. The pharmacodynamic parameter for beta-lactams that best correlates with efficacy is the percentage of the dosing interval that free drug concentration remains above the MIC (f T>MIC)[9]. Thus, the optimization of beta-lactam therapy relies on the duration of exposure (i.e., time-dependent) to maximize f T>MIC (Figure 3-1).

Three factors affect the clinical outcome of the patient: the patient, the bug, and the drug. Of these factors, the drug is the only one that is easily modified, and the various methods to achieve maximal f T>MIC include administering doses more frequently, administering higher doses, or changing the infusion duration. Dose escalation strategies add little additional benefit in optimizing the drug exposures and are not cost effective when the overall drug cost is often doubled. However, decreasing the dosing interval or increasing the length of infusion can have a considerable impact on f T>MIC (Figure 3-2). When designing dosing regimens to optimize beta-lactam therapy, it is important to consider what f T>MIC are required to maximize antibacterial activity, and these targets vary by class of beta-lactam. In general, maximal efficacy, often denoted as a 2-log decrease in bacterial density, requires a f T>MIC of 40 percent for carbapenems, 50 percent for penicillins, and 50–70 percent for cephalosporins; whereas, the f T>MIC for stasis (i.e., no bacterial killing or growth) is 20 percent for carbapenems, 30 percent for penicillins, and 40 percent for cephalosporins.[10-12]

This efficacy has been associated with serum concentrations, and it is unknown whether the same exposures are needed in tissue at the site of infection.

TOXIC CONCENTRATIONS

Beta-lactams have a wide therapeutic index, therefore, toxic concentrations are rare. When toxicities do occur, they are typically observed with high peak concentrations. Because extending the infusion duration results in lower peak concentrations when administrating the same dose (as evident in Figure 3-2), prolonged and continuous infusions have a low propensity for attaining toxic concentrations.

MONITORING DRUG LEVELS

The potential for toxicity is rare; therefore, routine serum concentration monitoring is not performed. Additionally, assays for drug monitoring are not widely available and have historically only been used for research purposes. Likewise, population pharmacokinetic parameter estimates are often used for dosing calculations.

BIOAVAILABILITY (F)

A number of β-lactam antibiotics have good bioavailability and are available in oral formulations. However, for oral drug administration, it is clearly not possible to alter the infusion time. For the purposes of this chapter, we will only focus on selected intravenous agents that are commonly administered over a prolonged period of time in order to achieve a higher amount of time in which free drug concentration remains above the MIC of the offending pathogen.

VOLUME OF DISTRIBUTION (V)

The volume of distribution for the β-lactam antibiotics discussed herein is generally low, as depicted in Table 3-1. In addition, these particular agents typically also demonstrate relatively low protein binding.

CLEARANCE (CL)

The rate of clearance for the β-lactam antibiotics that are often administered as prolonged or continuous infusions are presented in Table 3-1. It is important to note that these values come from patients with normal renal function. These antibiotics are largely excreted by the kidneys through glomerular filtration and tubular secretion. Therefore, renal function can have a significant impact on the rate of clearance for most of these drugs, requiring dose

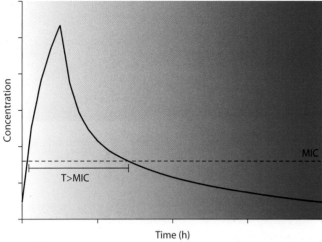

FIGURE 3-1. Beta-lactam in vivo efficacy is best predicted by the percentage of the dosing interval that free drug concentrations remains above the MIC (fT>MIC).

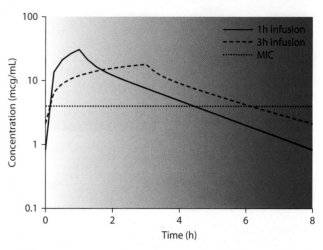

FIGURE 3-2. Comparison of administrating the same dose as a traditional infusion (1 hour) with prolonged infusion (3 hours). The prolonged infusion increases the percentage of the dosing interval that the drug concentration is above the MIC.

adjustments in the face of severe renal dysfunction. Additionally, many β-lactam antibiotics are removed with hemodialysis and supplemental doses following dialysis may be required.

ELIMINATION HALF-LIFE (T½)

The elimination half-lives for these agents are rather short and, therefore, must be administered more frequently, typically multiple times per day in patients with normal renal function. Half-lives for β-lactam antibiotics commonly administered as prolonged infusions are also listed in Table 3-1.

THERAPEUTIC MONITORING

As mentioned previously, assays for monitoring therapeutic drug levels are not readily available and utilized in the clinical setting. Rather, response to therapy should be monitored by observing improvement in the signs and symptoms of the infection.

MONTE CARLO SIMULATION

Monte Carlo simulation can be used to predict the ability to various dosing regimens to achieve the required pharmacodynamic target or exposures (fT>MIC for β-lactams) within a large simulated population. The simulation is performed with the aid of a computer software program and utilizes a semirandom number generator along with known population pharmacokinetic parameter estimates and corresponding statistical distributions to generate pharmacokinetic parameter values that are then used to construct

concentration-time profiles for each simulated patient within the simulated population. These profiles are then analyzed against the susceptibility or MIC profile for a given set of organisms. Using these data, the likelihood of achieving the pharmacodynamic target, also known as probability of target attainment (PTA), can be calculated for the entire simulated population.[27,28] Data generated from Monte Carlo simulation have been used in guiding empiric dose selection for the development of clinical treatment pathways and protocols.

DRUG STABILITY

Drug stability at room temperature is dependent on the particular antimicrobial agent as well as the diluent utilized to reconstitute. Stability issues can limit what type of infusion can be initiated (i.e., prolonged vs. continuous infusion). When determining what infusion duration to utilize, the duration of time needed to prepare, store, and deliver the medication must be taken into account in addition to the infusion duration. Normally, the package insert for the antimicrobial contains the most conservative estimate of stability, while other research studies may report an extended stability profile for the agent (Table 3-1).

CASE 1: PIPERACILLIN/TAZOBACTAM LOADING DOSE

WR has cystic fibrosis and is admitted to the hospital with an acute exacerbation. He has a history of respiratory Pseudomonas

TABLE 3-1	Pharmacokinetic Parameters of Select β-Lactam Antibiotics					
β-lactam Antibiotic	Volume of Distribution (L/kg)	Clearance (mL/min/1.73 m²)	Elimination Half-Life (h)	Protein Binding (%)	Stability (hours)	References
Penicillin:						
Piperacillin/tazobactam	0.15	180	0.8	25–35	24–48	13,14,15
Cephalosporins:						
Cefepime	0.16	75	2.1	10–20	24	16,17,18
Carbapenems:						
Meropenem	0.27	240	0.9	2–15	4–12	19,20,21,22
Doripenem	0.22	205	1	8	12–24	2, 3, 7

aeruginosa with a piperacillin/tazobactam MIC of 32 mcg/mL. Calculate a loading dose that achieves a free serum concentration of at least 32 mcg/mL. WR is 5 foot, 9 inches and weighs 59 kg.

$$\text{Equation: LD} = (V)(C)/(S)(F)$$

Step 1: Calculate V.

Because the population pharmacokinetic value for volume of distribution in Table 3-1 is normalized for weight (in L/kg), this value will need to be multiplied by the patient's weight (in kg) in order to calculate their volume of distribution.

$$V = (0.15 \text{ L/kg})(59 \text{ kg})$$
$$V = 8.85 \text{ L}$$

Step 2: Calculate C_{total}.

Free drug concentration is calculated by multiplying the total desired concentration by the fraction of unbound drug (f_u), where $f_u = (100 - \%$ protein binding$)/100$.

$$C_{free} = C_{total} \times f_u$$

This equation can be rearranged to determine the total concentration needed to attain a specific free concentration.

$$C_{total} = C_{free}/f_u$$
$$C_{total} = (32 \text{ mcg/mL})/ [(100 - 30)/100]$$
$$C_{total} = 45.71 \text{ mcg/mL}$$

Step 3: Calculate LD.

$$LD = (V)(C)/(S)(F)$$

Both S and F are assumed to be 1.

$$LD = (8.85 \text{ L})(45.71 \text{ mcg/mL})$$

Convert L to mL and mcg to mg.

$$LD = (8.85)(1,000/1)(45.71)(1 \text{ mg}/1,000)$$
$$LD = 404.53 \text{ mg}$$

Convert this dose to g, as piperacillin/tazobactam is dosed in g.

$$LD = 404.53 (1 \text{ g}/1,000)$$
$$LD = 0.405 \text{ g}$$

Administering a loading dose followed by a maintenance dose (continuous infusion) allows for the desired steady-state concentration to be achieved much earlier in treatment. The loading dose for WR would be rounded up to 2.25 g piperacillin/tazobactam, which is only commercially available in fixed dosage concentrations (1:8 ratio of piperacillin/tazobactam) that include 2 g piperacillin/0.25 g tazobactam, 3 g piperacillin/0.375 g tazobactam, and 4 g piperacillin/0.5 g tazobactam. (The dose is reported as the combination of the two components thus 2 g piperacillin/0.25 g tazobactam = 2.25 g piperacillin/tazobactam.) Due to these dosage restrictions, our answer must be rounded up the closest commercially available dose of 2.25 g piperacillin/tazobactam.

CASE 2: PIPERACILLIN/TAZOBACTAM MAINTENANCE DOSE

What continuous infusion dose would WR need to maintain an average free concentration of 32 mcg/mL?

$$\text{Equation: MD} = (Cl)(C_{ss\,ave})(f_u)(\text{infusion duration})/(S)(F)$$

Step 1: Calculate Cl.

Because the population pharmacokinetic value for clearance provided in Table 3-1 is normalized for body surface area (BSA, in mL/

min/1.73 m²), this value will need to be multiplied by the patient's BSA (in m²) in order to calculate their clearance.

$$BSA = (\text{weight}/70 \text{ kg})^{0.7}(1.73 \text{ m}^2)$$
$$BSA = (59 \text{ kg}/ 70 \text{ kg})^{0.7}(1.73 \text{ m}^2)$$
$$BSA = 1.54 \text{ m}^2$$
$$Cl = (180 \text{ mL/min}/1.73)(1.54)$$
$$Cl = 160.23 \text{ ml/min}$$

Step 2: Calculate MD.

$$MD = (Cl)(C_{total})(\text{infusion duration})/(S)(F)$$

Both S and F are assumed to be 1.

$$MD = (160.23 \text{ mL/min})(45.71 \text{ mcg/mL})(24 \text{ h})$$

Convert min to h.

$$MD = (160.23)(60/1)(45.71 \text{ mcg})(24 \text{ h})$$
$$MD = 10546723.15 \text{ mcg}$$

Convert mcg to g.

$$MD = 10546723.15 (1 \text{ g}/1,000,000)$$
$$MD = 10.55 \text{ g}$$

This maintenance dose can be calculated and rounded up in a number of ways. The easiest and most cost effective would be to reconstitute three vials of 4.5 g piperacillin/tazobactam to equate a total of 13.5 g. Another option would be to give four vials of 3.375 g piperacillin/tazobactam to also equate 13.5 g. This dose should be infused over the entire 24 hours to maintain the piperacillin/tazobactam free concentration above 32 mcg/mL.

CASE 3: DRUG INTERACTIONS

BA is a 57-year-old woman who developed VAP while intubated in the ICU. She is being treated with piperacillin/tazobactam 3.35 g IV q8h over 4h. Her other medications are as follows:

Propofol 10 mcg/kg/min IV

Enoxaparin 40 mg IV daily

Famotidine 20 mg IV q12h

KCL 40 mEq IV prn per protocol

Sliding scale insulin

Does piperacillin/tazobactam interact with any of her concurrent medications? If so, what adjustments need to be made?

Piperacillin/tazobactam does not interact with any of BA's concurrent medications. Few medications interact with the beta-lactam antibiotics that are typically administered as continuous or prolonged infusions. Probenecid is the only medication to date that has the ability to affect plasma concentrations of beta-lactams, because probenecid competes with these agents for active tubular secretion, thus increasing the elimination half-life and plasma or serum concentrations of beta-lactam antibiotics.

CASE 4: MEROPENEM DOSING IN RENAL FAILURE

NJ, a 67-year-old female (5′3″, 55 kg) was receiving meropenem 1 g every 8 hours as a 3-hour infusion for an intra-abdominal infection. Escherichia coli with a meropenem MIC of 4 mcg/mL has been isolated and identified from an abdominal wash. When she was initiated on this regimen, her serum creatinine (SCr) was 0.8 mg/dL; however, her condition has worsened and her serum creatinine has increased to

1.5 mg/dL. Subsequently, her meropenem dose was changed to 500 mg every 12 hours, but the debate is whether a traditional infusion (1 hour) or an extended infusion of 3 hours should be utilized. What percentage of the dosing interval exceeds the MIC (4 mcg/mL) for each of these infusion durations and which infusion duration would you recommend?

Equations:

1. $C = [((S)(F)(Dose/t_{in}))/(Cl)](1-e^{-kt1})$
2. $C = [((S)(F)(Dose/t_{in}))/(Cl)](1-e^{-ktin})(e^{-kt2})$
3. $t = (infusion\ duration - t1) + t2$
4. $\%T{>}MIC = t/dosing\ interval \times 100$

The first equation allows you to solve for t1, which is the time it takes to reach the MIC during infusion. This value (t1) is subtracted from the infusion duration to determine the actual time that concentrations remain above the MIC during the infusion. The second equation allows you to solve for t2, which is the time it takes after the infusion stops for the concentration to return to the MIC due to drug elimination. The third equation adds t1 to t2, resulting in the total time that concentrations remain above the MIC during infusion. Finally, the fourth equation is used to determine the %T>MIC, by dividing the total time above the MIC by the dosing interval, multiplied by 100.

Step 1: Calculate Cl using population pharmacokinetic values.

$$BSA = (weight/70\ kg)^{0.7}(1.73\ m^2)$$
$$BSA = (55\ kg/70\ kg)^{0.7}(1.73\ m^2)$$
$$BSA = 1.46\ m^2$$
$$Cl = (240\ mL/min/1.73)(1.46)$$
$$Cl = 202.54\ ml/min$$

Convert to L/hr.

$$Cl = (202.54)(1\ L/1,000)(60/1\ h)$$
$$Cl = 12.15\ L/h$$

Step 2: Calculate a revised Cl based on renal function.

The clearance calculated from the population pharmacokinetic parameters must be adjusted to reflect NJ's reduced renal function. In order to calculate a revised CL, a correction factor is determined from the following equation:

$$Cl_{adjusted} = (CLm) + [(Clr)(fraction\ of\ normal\ renal\ function\ remaining)]$$
$$Cl_{adjusted} = (CLm) + [(Clr)(current\ SCr/baseline\ SCr)]$$

Meropenem has one inactive metabolite, and 70 percent of the drug is recovered in urine unchanged. Thus, the fraction of metabolic clearance is 0.3, whereas the fraction of renal clearance is 0.7.

Correction factor = (0.3) + [(0.7)(0.8 mg/dL /1.5 mg/dL)]

Correction factor = 0.67

Therefore, NJ's clearance should be 67 percent of the clearance calculated using population pharmacokinetic parameters.

$$Cl_{adjusted} = (Cl)(correction\ factor)$$
$$Cl_{adjusted} = (12.15\ L/h)(0.67)$$
$$Cl_{adjusted} = 8.14\ L/hr$$

Step 3: Calculate elimination rate constant (K).

$$K = Cl/V$$
$$K = (8.14\ L/h)/[(0.27\ L/kg)(55\ kg)]$$
$$K = 0.55\ h^{-1}$$

Step 4: Calculate the %*f* T>MIC for a 1-hour infusion.

a. Because the pharmacodynamic parameter for beta-lactams that best correlates with efficacy is the percentage of the dosing interval that free drug concentration remains above the MIC, the total drug concentration corresponding to a <u>free</u> drug concentration of 4 mcg/mL (the MIC) must be calculated for use in subsequent equations. The range of % protein binding given in Table 3-1 is 2 to 15 percent; we will use 15 percent in these calculations in order to produce the most conservative estimate, or worst-case scenario, of %*f* T>MIC with each infusion.

$$C_{total} = C_{free}/f_u$$
$$C_{total} = (4\ mcg/mL)/[(100 - 15)/100]$$
$$C_{total} = 4.71\ mcg/mL$$

b. Determine the time that the free drug concentration remains above the MIC during the infusion by solving the following equation for t1. Since we determined that the MIC of 4 mcg/mL corresponds to a total drug concentration of 4.71 mcg/mL, we will use this value for C. Again, S and F are both assumed to equal 1.

$$C = [((S)(F)(Dose/t_{in}))/(Cl)](1-e^{-kt1})$$
$$4.71\ mg/L = [(500\ mg/1\ h)/8.14\ L/h)](1-e^{-0.55\ h^{-1} \times t1})$$
$$4.71 = 61.43(1-e^{-0.55\ h^{-1} \times t1})$$
$$0.08 = 1-e^{-0.55\ h^{-1} \times t1}$$
$$0.92 = e^{-0.55\ h^{-1} \times t1}$$
$$ln\ (0.92) = -0.55\ h^{-1} \times t1$$
$$-0.08 = -0.55\ h^{-1} \times t1$$
$$t1 = 0.15\ h$$

c. Determine the time that the free drug concentration remains above the MIC after the infusion has ended by solving the following equation for t2.

$$C = [((S)(F)(Dose/t_{in}))/(Cl)](1-e^{-ktin})(e^{-kt2})$$
$$4.71\ mg/L = [(500\ mg/1)/8.14\ L](1-e^{-0.55\ h^{-1} \times 1\ h})(e^{-0.55\ h^{-1} \times t2})$$
$$4.71 = 61.43(1-e^{-0.55})(e^{-0.55\ h^{-1} \times t2})$$
$$0.08 = (0.43)(e^{-0.55\ h^{-1} \times t2})$$
$$0.19 = (e^{-0.55\ h^{-1} \times t2})$$
$$ln\ (0.19) = ln\ (e^{-0.55\ h^{-1} \times t2})$$
$$-1.66 = -0.55\ h^{-1} \times t2$$
$$t2 = 3.02\ h$$

d. Calculate the total time in hours that concentration remains above the MIC.

$$t = (infusion\ duration - t1) + t2$$
$$t = (1 - 0.15\ h) + 3.02\ h$$
$$t = 3.87\ h$$

e. Calculate the %*f* T>MIC.

$$\%f\ T{>}MIC = t/dosing\ interval \times 100$$
$$\%f\ T{>}MIC = 3.87\ h/12\ h \times 100$$
$$\%f\ T{>}MIC = 32.3\ \%\ of\ the\ dosing\ interval$$

Step 5. Calculate the %*f* T>MIC for a 3-hour infusion.

a. Determine the time that the free drug concentration remains above the MIC during the infusion by solving the following equation for t1.

$$C = [((S)(F)(Dose/t_{in}))/(Cl)](1-e^{-kt1})$$
$$4.71\ mg/L = [(500\ mg/3\ h)/8.14\ L/h](1-e^{-0.55\ h^{-1} \times t1})$$
$$4.71 = 20.48(1-e^{-0.55\ h^{-1} \times t1})$$

$$0.23 = 1 - e^{-0.55 \text{ h}^{-1} \times t1}$$
$$0.77 = e^{-0.55 \text{ h}^{-1} \times t1}$$
$$\ln(0.77) = -0.55 \text{ h}^{-1} \times t1$$
$$-0.26 = -0.55 \text{ h}^{-1} \times t1$$
$$t1 = 0.47 \text{ h}$$

b. Determine the time that the free drug concentration remains above the MIC after the infusion has ended by solving the following equation for t2.

$$C = [((S)(F)(Dose/t_{in}))/(Cl)](1-e^{-ktin})(e^{-kt2})$$
$$4.71 \text{ mg/L} = [(500 \text{ mg}/3)/8.14 \text{ L})](1-e^{-0.55 \text{ h}^{-1} \times 3 \text{ h}})(e^{-0.55 \text{ h}^{-1} \times t2})$$
$$4.71 = 20.48(1-e^{-1.65})(e^{-0.55 \text{ h}^{-1} \times t2})$$
$$0.23 = (0.81)(e^{-0.55 \text{ h}^{-1} \times t2})$$
$$0.28 = (e^{-0.55 \text{ h}^{-1} \times t2})$$
$$\ln(0.28) = \ln(e^{-0.55 \text{ h}^{-1} \times t2})$$
$$-1.27 = -0.55 \text{ h}^{-1} \times t2$$
$$t2 = 2.31 \text{ h}$$

c. Calculate the total time in hours that concentration remains above the MIC.

$$t = (\text{infusion duration} - t1) + t2$$
$$t = (3 - 0.47 \text{ h}) + 2.31 \text{ h}$$
$$t = 4.84 \text{ h}$$

d. Calculate the %fT>MIC.

$$\%fT\text{>MIC} = t/\text{dosing interval} \times 100$$
$$\%fT\text{>MIC} = 4.84 \text{ h}/12 \text{ h} \times 100$$
$$\%fT\text{>MIC} = 40.33 \% \text{ of the dosing interval}$$

Because meropenem belongs to the carbapenem class of beta-lactams, a %fT>MIC of 40 percent is needed for maximal bacterial activity, thus the most appropriate regimen for NJ is meropenem 500 mg every 12 hours as a 3-hour infusion.

CASE 5: CEFEPIME DOSING IN HEMODIALYSIS

FT is a 68-year-old, 50 kg woman with end-stage renal disease and a serum creatinine of 8 mg/dL. She normally undergoes hemodialysis treatments three times a week, and her last treatment was 3 days ago. She has suspected urosepsis and one dose of cefepime 1,000 mg intravenously was administered 24 hours ago. Calculate an appropriate replacement dose for FT of cefepime after dialysis, which is schedule for later today.

Equation: $Dose = (V)(\Delta C)/(S)(F)$

Step 1. Determine the maximum concentration (C_{max}) for the previous dose.

Cefepime is primarily excreted by the kidneys, and therefore, those with renal dysfunction, especially end-stage renal disease, have prolonged half-lives. An average half-life ($t_{1/2}$) in patients requiring hemodialysis is 13.5 hours, and 19 hours in those requiring continuous peritoneal dialysis. Also, it is recommended that on hemodialysis days, cefepime should be administered after completion of hemodialysis. Approximately 68 percent of the total cefepime present in the body at the start of hemodialysis will be removed during a 3-hour dialysis period. To determine how much is lost during dialysis, we first need to determine the C_{max} after one dose followed by the predialysis concentration in order to determine the postdialysis concentration. Again, S and F are equal to 1.

$$C_0 = (S)(F)(\text{Loading dose})/V$$
$$C_0 = (1,000 \text{ mg})/(0.16 \text{ L/kg} \times 50 \text{ kg})$$
$$C_0 = 125 \text{ mg/L}$$

Step 2. Determine the predialysis concentration ($C_{predialysis}$).

The initial concentration after the dose can be used to determine the concentration prior to initiating dialysis.

$$C_{predialysis} = C_0(e^{-kt})$$

a. Calculate K for use in the preceding equation.

$$K = 0.693/t_{1/2}$$
$$K = 0.693/13.5 \text{ h}$$
$$K = 0.051 \text{ h}^{-1}$$

b. Solve for $C_{predialysis}$.

$$C_{predialysis} = 125 \text{ mg/L}(e^{-0.051 \text{ h}^{-1} \times 24 \text{ h}})$$
$$C_{predialysis} = 125 \text{ mg/L}(0.294)$$
$$C_{predialysis} = 36.8 \text{ mg/L}$$

Step 3. Determine the postdialysis concentration ($C_{postdialysis}$).

If the plasma concentration declines by approximately 68 percent due to hemodialysis, the postdialysis concentration will be 32 percent of the predialysis concentration.

$$C_{postdialysis} = (36.8 \text{ mg/L})(0.32)$$
$$C_{postdialysis} = 11.8 \text{ mg/L}$$

Step 4. Calculate a replacement dose.

If a replacement dose is desired at this point, the dose can be calculated by using the following equation:

$$Dose = (V)(\Delta C)/(S)(F)$$
$$Dose = (0.16 \text{ L/kg} \times 50 \text{ kg})(125 \text{ mg/L} - 11.8 \text{ mg/L})$$
$$Dose = (8 \text{ L})(113.2 \text{ mg})$$
$$Dose = 905.6 \text{ mg}$$

Because 905.6 mg is not a standard dose available for cefepime, this amount can be rounded up to 1,000 mg. Additionally, because the patient is receiving hemodialysis every two days, this dose could be divided by two and given daily (on hemodialysis days, administer after hemodialysis is completed). Cefepime 500 mg once daily is consistent with the current prescribing information recommendations for those undergoing hemodialysis. (You can double-check the resultant maximum concentration and minimum concentration without dialysis by the preceding equations). A similar approach can be used to determine the dosing needs on any particular day and dialysis schedule. The actual amount of drug loss will depend on the individual patient intrinsic clearance, volume, time since last dose, duration of hemodialysis, and efficiency of the dialysis treatment.

CASE 6: CEFEPIME DOSING IN CONTINUOUS RENAL REPLACEMENT THERAPY (CRRT)

FT is now hemodynamically unstable and hemodialysis has been discontinued. She is to be initiated on CRRT with an ultrafiltration rate of 1.5 L/hr. How should her cefepime dose be changed to result in the same average concentration as when she was on hemodialysis?

Equation: $\text{Maintenance Dose} = (Cl)(C_{ss \text{ ave}})(\text{dosing interval})/(S)(F)$

Step 1. Calculate the average concentration ($C_{ss \text{ ave}}$) that resulted from her last dose.

First, we need to calculate the average concentration that resulted from her cefepime 500 mg once daily dose during hemodialysis. This calculation is made with the following equation:

$$C_{ss \text{ ave}} = (S)(F)(\text{Dose/dosing interval})/Cl$$

S and F can be assumed to be 1 and Cl = (K)(V).

$$C_{ss\,ave} = (Dose/dosing\ interval)/(k)(V)$$
$$C_{ss\,ave} = (500\ mg/24\ h)/(0.051\ h^{-1})(0.16\ L/kg)(50\ kg)$$
$$C_{ss\,ave} = 51.05\ mg/L$$

Step 2. Determine the rate of cefepime clearance from CRRT.

Using an unbound fraction of 0.8 (from Table 3-1), we can estimate the CRRT clearance.

$$Cl_{CRRT}\ Maximum = (f_u)(CRRT\ flow\ rate)$$
$$Cl_{CRRT}\ Maximum = (0.8)(1.5\ L/h)$$
$$Cl_{CRRT}\ Maximum = 1.2\ L/h$$

Step 3. Determine her total cefepime clearance.

The total cefepime clearance would be the sum of the clearance by CRRT and the estimated intrinsic clearance.

$$Cl = Cl_{CRRT} + Clpat;\ where\ Clpat = K(V)$$
$$Clpat = (0.051\ h^{-1})(0.16\ L/kg)(50\ kg)$$
$$Clpat = 0.41\ L/h$$
$$Cl = 1.2\ L/h + 0.41\ L/h$$
$$Cl = 1.61\ L/h$$

Step 4. Calculate her elimination rate constant and half-life while on CRRT.

$$K = Cl/V$$
$$K = 1.61\ L/h/8\ L$$
$$K = 0.20\ h^{-1}$$
$$t_{1/2} = 0.693/K$$
$$t_{1/2} = 0.693/0.20\ h^{-1}$$
$$t_{1/2} = 3.46\ h$$

This calculation of a half-life of 3.5 hours is slightly higher than the population average of 2.1 hours, but much less than the average half-life for those receiving hemodialysis. Based on this information, we can use the following equations to determine an appropriate dosing regimen.

Step 5. Calculate her new dose.

$$MD = (Cl)(C_{ss\,ave})(dosing\ interval)/(S)(F)$$

Both S and F can be assumed to be 1. Additionally, because her half-life on CRRT is similar to those with normal kidney function, we can determine the dose to be given using either an 8-hour or 12-hour dosing interval.

a. Calculate a q8h dose.

$$MD = (1.61\ L/h)(51.05\ mg/L)(8\ h)$$
$$MD = 657.52\ mg$$

This dose would be rounded to 750 mg every 8 hours. Now let's see what the maintenance dose would be if it was to be administered every 12 hours.

b. Calculate a q12h dose.

$$MD = (1.61\ L/h)(51.05\ mg/L)(12\ h)$$
$$MD = 986.29\ mg$$

This dose would be rounded to 1,000 mg every 12 hours. Either of these dosing intervals would be appropriate; however, 1,000 mg every 12 hours involves less rounding of the dose to maintain the same average steady-state concentrations of cefepime.

CASE 7: DOSING CONSIDERATIONS IN THE CRITICALLY ILL

SH is a 67-year-old male who was transferred to the ICU five days ago and has been on mechanical ventilation since the day of his ICU admission. He was recently diagnosed with VAP and has become septic. He weighs 81 kg as of this morning, and his renal function was normal. His most recent sputum culture grew P. aeruginosa. Sensitivity data are not yet available, but your institution has recently seen a number of P. aeruginosa infections with higher MICs. The attending physician just wrote an order for cefepime 2 g every 12 hours at a standard 30-minute infusion. Will this regimen cover P. aeruginosa up to an MIC of 16 mcg/mL? Should the infusion time be extended to 3 hours?

Before calculating the %f T>MIC to determine whether either of these doses can achieve the appropriate pharmacodynamic target, the effect that critical illness can have on beta-lactam pharmacokinetics must be considered. Critically ill patients often have altered volumes of distribution. An increase in volume of distribution is most common and occurs as a result of extravascular fluid shifts secondary to sepsis, but can also be observed with other disease states such as congestive heart failure, renal failure, and severe burns. We know that SH is septic and likely has an increased volume of distribution. The volume of distribution for cefepime from a population pharmacokinetic study conducted in critically ill patients was 0.26 L/kg, which is much higher than the value reported in healthy volunteers, 0.16 L/kg.[29] The following equations will be utilized to calculate %f T>MIC for each regimen.

Step 1: Calculate Cl using population pharmacokinetic values.

$$BSA = (weight/70\ kg)^{0.7}(1.73\ m^2)$$
$$BSA = (81\ kg/70\ kg)^{0.7}(1.73\ m^2)$$
$$BSA = 1.92\ m^2$$
$$Cl = (75\ mL/min/1.73)(1.92)$$
$$Cl = 83.24\ ml/min$$

Convert to L/hr.

$$Cl = (83.24)(1\ L/1,000\ mL)(60\ min/1\ h)$$
$$Cl = 4.99\ L/h$$

Step 2: Calculate volume of distribution (V).

$$V = (0.26\ L/kg)(81\ kg)$$
$$V = 21.06\ kg$$

Step 3: Calculate elimination rate constant (K).

$$K = Cl/V$$
$$K = (4.99\ L/h)/(21.06\ L)$$
$$K = 0.24\ h^{-1}$$

Step 4: Calculate the %f T>MIC for the 30-minute infusion.

a. Calculate the total drug concentration corresponding to a free drug concentration of 32 mcg/mL (the MIC of interest) for use in subsequent equations. The protein binding of cefepime (20%) is given in Table 3-1.

$$C_{total} = C_{free}/f_u$$
$$C_{total} = (16\ mcg/mL)/[(100 - 20)/100]$$
$$C_{total} = 20\ mcg/mL$$

b. Determine the time that the free drug concentration remains above the MIC during the infusion by solving the following equation for t1. S and F are both assumed to equal 1.

$$C = [((S)(F)(Dose/t_{in}))/(Cl)](1-e^{-kt1})$$

$$20\ mg/L = [(2{,}000\ mg/0.5\ h)/4.99\ L/h)](1-e^{-0.24\ h^{-1} \times t1})$$

$$20 = 801.60(1-e^{-0.24\ h^{-1} \times t1})$$

$$0.025 = 1-e^{-0.24\ h^{-1} \times t1}$$

$$0.975 = e^{-0.24\ h^{-1} \times t1}$$

$$\ln (0.975) = -0.24\ h^{-1} \times t1$$

$$-0.025 = -0.24\ h^{-1} \times t1$$

$$t1 = 0.11\ h$$

c. Determine the time that the free drug concentration remains above the MIC after the infusion has ended by solving the following equation for t2.

$$C = [((S)(F)(Dose/t_{in}))/(Cl)](1-e^{-ktin})(e^{-kt2})$$

$$20\ mg/L = [(2{,}000\ mg/0.5)/(4.99\ L)]$$
$$(1-e^{-0.24\ h^{-1} \times 0.5\ h})(e^{-0.24\ h^{-1} \times t2})$$

$$20 = 801.60(1-e^{-0.12})(e^{-0.24\ h^{-1} \times t2})$$

$$0.025 = (0.11)(e^{-0.24\ h^{-1} \times t2})$$

$$0.23 = (e^{-0.24\ h^{-1} \times t2})$$

$$\ln (0.23) = \ln (e^{-0.24\ h^{-1} \times t2})$$

$$-1.47 = -0.24\ h^{-1} \times t2$$

$$t2 = 6.13\ h$$

d. Determine the total amount of time that free drug concentrations remain above the MIC.

$$t = (\text{infusion duration} - t1) + t2$$

$$t = (0.5 - 0.11\ h) + 6.13\ h$$

$$t = 6.52\ h$$

e. Calculate the %fT>MIC.

$$\%f\,T{>}MIC = t/\text{dosing interval} \times 100$$

$$\%f\,T{>}MIC = 6.52\ h/12\ h \times 100$$

$$\%f\,T{>}MIC = 54.33\%\ \text{of the dosing interval}$$

Step 5: Calculate the %fT>MIC for the 3-hour infusion.

a. Determine the time that the free drug concentration remains above the MIC during the infusion by solving the following equation for t1. S and F are both assumed to equal 1.

$$C = [((S)(F)(Dose/t_{in}))/(Cl)](1-e^{-kt1})$$

$$20\ mg/L = [(2{,}000\ mg/3\ h)/4.99\ L/h)](1-e^{-0.24\ h^{-1} \times t1})$$

$$20 = 133.60(1-e^{-0.24\ h^{-1} \times t1})$$

$$0.15 = 1-e^{-0.24\ h^{-1} \times t1}$$

$$0.85 = e^{-0.24\ h^{-1} \times t1}$$

$$\ln (0.85) = -0.24\ h^{-1} \times t1$$

$$-0.16 = -0.24\ h^{-1} \times t1$$

$$t1 = 0.67\ h$$

b. Determine the time that the free drug concentration remains above the MIC after the infusion has ended by solving the following equation for t2.

$$C = [((S)(F)(Dose/t_{in}))/(Cl)](1-e^{-ktin})(e^{-kt2})$$

$$20\ mg/L = [(2{,}000\ mg/3)/(4.99\ L)](1-e^{-0.24\ h^{-1} \times 3\ h})(e^{-0.24\ h^{-1} \times t2})$$

$$20 = 133.60(1-e^{-0.72})(e^{-0.24\ h^{-1} \times t2})$$

$$0.15 = (0.51)(e^{-0.24\ h^{-1} \times t2})$$

$$0.29 = (e^{-0.24\ h^{-1} \times t2})$$

$$\ln (0.29) = \ln (e^{-0.24\ h^{-1} \times t2})$$

$$-1.24 = -0.24\ h^{-1} \times t2$$

$$T2 = 5.17\ h$$

c. Determine the total amount of time that free drug concentrations remain above the MIC.

$$t = (\text{infusion duration} - t1) + t2$$

$$t = (3 - 0.67\ h) + 5.17\ h$$

$$t = 7.5\ h$$

d. Calculate the %fT>MIC.

$$\%f\,T{>}MIC = t/\text{dosing interval} \times 100$$

$$\%f\,T{>}MIC = 7.5\ h/12\ h \times 100$$

$$\%f\,T{>}MIC = 62.5\%\ \text{of the dosing interval}$$

Because cefepime is a cephalosporin, a %fT>MIC of 50–70 percent is needed for maximal antibacterial activity. Both regimens result in a %fT>MIC that is within this range, however, the 3-hour infusion has a slightly higher %fT>MIC and would be the better option.

CASE 8: DOSING IN OBESE OR UNDERWEIGHT PATIENTS

ND, a 52-year-old morbidly obese male, weighing 171 kg, was admitted to the hospital for IV antibiotics and management of a recurrent diabetic foot infection on his right great toe. The wound was cultured in the operating room upon admission and initial surgical debridement, which grew P. aeruginosa with a piperacillin/tazobactam MIC of 16 mcg/mL. Additionally, an X-ray of the limb shows possible osteomyelitis. He is currently receiving piperacillin/tazobactam 4.5 g IV q8h, which is being given as a 30-minute infusion. Is this dose adequate? Would decreasing the dosing interval to q6h help? How about extending the infusion time to 4 hours?

The pharmacokinetics of the beta-lactam agents that are often given as prolonged or continuous infusions have not been widely studied in obese patients. Several older cephalosporin agents that are no longer commonly used have been studied in obese patients, where increases in both volume of distribution and clearance were observed, necessitating larger doses in this patient population.[30-31] To date, one case report has been published describing the alterations in piperacillin/tazobactam pharmacokinetics observed in one obese patient.[32] The 39-year-old, 167 kg, obese male had an increased volume of distribution (0.33 L/kg based on total body weight) and a longer elimination half-life (1.4 hours). Likewise, meropenem pharmacokinetics have been studied in nine obese patients, where a 38 percent increase in volume of distribution and a 28 percent increase in clearance were noted over corresponding values in normal weight controls.[33]

Step 1: Calculate Cl using population pharmacokinetic values.

Despite the fact that the pharmacokinetics of piperacillin/tazobactam have only been described in one obese subject to date, no data describe obesity-related alterations in clearance. Therefore, we will calculate the Cl using the values derived from normal weight subjects in Table 3-1.

$$BSA = (\text{weight}/70\ kg)^{0.7}(1.73\ m^2)$$

$$BSA = (171\ kg/70\ kg)^{0.7}(1.73\ m^2)$$

$$BSA = 3.23\ m^2$$

$$Cl = (180\ mL/min/1.73)(3.23)$$

$$Cl = 336.07\ ml/min$$

Convert to L/hr.

$$Cl = (336.07)(1\ L/1{,}000)(60/1\ h)$$
$$Cl = 20.16\ L/h$$

It is also important to note that this clearance is similar to the clearance reported in the case study described above (26.57/h).

Step 2: Calculate volume of distribution (V).

We will calculate volume of distribution using the value listed in Table 3-1 from normal weight patients, as well as the value from the case report in an obese patient for comparison.

From Table 3-1:

$$V = (0.15\ L/kg)(171\ kg)$$
$$V = 25.65\ kg$$

From obesity case report:

$$V = (0.33\ L/kg)(171\ kg)$$
$$V = 56.43\ L$$

We will use a value of 56.43 L moving forward for this patient, because of the evidence that suggests an increased volume of distribution in obese patients for piperacillin/tazobactam, as well as a number of other beta-lactams.

Step 3: Calculate elimination rate constant (K).

$$K = Cl/V$$
$$K = (20.16\ L/h)/(56.43\ L)$$
$$K = 0.36\ h^{-1}$$

Step 4: Calculate the %fT>MIC for the 30-minute infusion.

a. Calculate the total drug concentration corresponding to a free drug concentration of 16 mcg/mL (the MIC of interest) for use in subsequent equations. The protein binding of piperacillin/tazobactam (35%) is given in Table 3-1.

$$C_{total} = C_{free}/f_u$$
$$C_{total} = (16\ mcg/mL\ )/[(100 - 35)/100]$$
$$C_{total} = 24.62\ mcg/mL$$

b. Determine the time that the free drug concentration remains above the MIC during the infusion by solving the following equation for t1. S and F are both assumed to equal 1.

$$C = [((S)(F)(Dose/t_{in}))/(Cl)](1 - e^{-kt1})$$
$$24.62\ mg/L = [(4500\ mg/0.5\ h)/20.16\ L/h](1 - e^{-0.36\ h^{-1} \times t1})$$
$$24.62 = 446.43(1 - e^{-0.36\ h^{-1} \times t1})$$
$$0.055 = 1 - e^{-0.36\ h^{-1} \times t1}$$
$$0.94 = e^{-0.36\ h^{-1} \times t1}$$
$$\ln(0.94) = -0.36\ h^{-1} \times t1$$
$$-0.062 = -0.36\ h^{-1} \times t1$$
$$t1 = 0.17\ h$$

c. Determine the time that the free drug concentration remains above the MIC after the infusion has ended by solving the following equation for t2.

$$C = [((S)(F)(Dose/t_{in}))/(Cl)](1 - e^{-ktin})(e^{-kt2})$$
$$24.62\ mg/L = [(4500\ mg/0.5)/20.16\ L](1 - e^{-0.36\ h^{-1} \times 0.5\ h})$$
$$(e^{-0.36\ h^{-1} \times t2})$$
$$24.62 = 446.43(1 - e^{-0.18})(e^{-0.36\ h^{-1} \times t2})$$
$$0.055 = (0.16)(e^{-0.36\ h^{-1} \times t2})$$
$$0.34 = (e^{-0.36\ h^{-1} \times t2})$$

$$\ln(0.34) = \ln(e^{-0.36\ h^{-1} \times t2})$$
$$-1.08 = -0.24\ h^{-1} \times t2$$
$$t2 = 3\ h$$

d. Determine the total amount of time that free drug concentrations remain above the MIC.

$$t = (\text{infusion duration} - t1) + t2$$
$$t = (0.5 - 0.17\ h) + 3\ h$$
$$t = 3.33\ h$$

e. Calculate the %fT>MIC.

$$\%f\text{T>MIC} = t/\text{dosing interval} \times 100$$
$$\%f\text{T>MIC} = 3.33\ h/8\ h \times 100$$
$$\%f\text{T>MIC} = 41.6\%\ \text{of the dosing interval}$$

A fT>MIC of 41.6 percent is less than the target need for maximal antibacterial activity of 50 percent. Therefore, a dose of 4.5 g q8h administered as 30-minute infusion is not adequate for this patient.

Step 5. Calculate the % fT>MIC for a 4.5 g q6h regimen.

Because we know that the amount of time that the free drug concentration remains above the MIC following a 4.5 g dose in this patient is 3.33 hours, we can simply divide this value by the new dosing interval (6 hours) to obtain % fT>MIC.

$$\%f\text{T>MIC} = t/\text{dosing interval} \times 100$$
$$\%f\text{T>MIC} = 3.33\ h/6\ h \times 100$$
$$\%f\text{T>MIC} = 55.5\%\ \text{of the dosing interval}$$

A regimen of 4.5 g IV q6h as a 30-minute infusion would be appropriate as the %fT>MIC target of 50 percent.

Step 6. Calculate the % fT>MIC for a 4.5 g q8h regimen, administered as a 4-hour infusion.

a.
$$C = [((S)(F)(Dose/t_{in}))/(Cl)](1 - e^{-kt1})$$
$$24.62\ mg/L = [(4500\ mg/4\ h)/(20.16\ L/h)](1 - e^{-0.36\ h^{-1} \times t1})$$
$$24.62 = 55.80(1 - e^{-0.36\ h^{-1} \times t1})$$
$$0.44 = 1 - e^{-0.36\ h^{-1} \times t1}$$
$$0.56 = e^{-0.36\ h^{-1} \times t1}$$
$$\ln(0.56) = -0.36\ h^{-1} \times t1$$
$$-0.58 = -0.36\ h^{-1} \times t1$$
$$t1 = 1.61\ h$$

b.
$$C = [((S)(F)(Dose/t_{in}))/(Cl)](1 - e^{-ktin})(e^{-kt2})$$
$$24.62\ mg/L = [(4500\ mg/4)/20.16\ L]$$
$$(1 - e^{-0.36\ h^{-1} \times 4\ h})(e^{-0.36\ h^{-1} \times t2})$$
$$24.62 = 55.80(1 - e^{-1.44})(e^{-0.36\ h^{-1} \times t2})$$
$$0.44 = (0.76)(e^{-0.36\ h^{-1} \times t2})$$
$$0.58 = (e^{-0.36\ h^{-1} \times t2})$$
$$\ln(0.58) = \ln(e^{-0.36\ h^{-1} \times t2})$$
$$-0.54 = -0.36\ h^{-1} \times t2$$
$$t2 = 1.50\ h$$

c.
$$t = (\text{infusion duration} - t1) + t2$$
$$t = (4\ h - 1.61\ h) + 1.50\ h$$
$$t = 3.89\ h$$

d.

$\%f\,\text{T>MIC} = \text{t/dosing interval} \times 100$

$\%f\,\text{T>MIC} = 3.89\ \text{h/8 h} \times 100$

$\%f\,\text{T>MIC} = 48.6\%$ of the dosing interval

While prolonging the infusion time from 30 minutes to 4 hours increased the $f\,\text{T>MIC}$ from 41.6 percent to 48.6 percent, it was not sufficient to achieve the target of 50 percent. The best regimen for this patient would be to shorten the dosing interval to 4.5 g IV q6h or less. An adequate prolonged infusion dose could also be calculated.

CASE 9: DORIPENEM DOSING AND DETERMINING NEED FOR PROLONGED INFUSION

AS is 44-year-old female with a complicated urinary tract infection. Her last urine culture grew Klebsiella pneumoniae with a doripenem MIC of 4 mcg/mL. She is currently receiving doripenem 500 mg IV q8h. She weighs 80 kg and has good renal function. Calculate the %f T>MIC achieved with this regimen and determine whether this dose is adequate for the treatment of her infection.

$\text{BSA} = (\text{weight/70 kg})^{0.7}(1.73\ \text{m}^2)$

$\text{BSA} = (80\ \text{kg/70 kg})^{0.7}(1.73\ \text{m}^2)$

$\text{BSA} = 1.9\ \text{m}^2$

$\text{Cl} = (205\ \text{mL/min/1.73})(1.9)$

$\text{Cl} = 225.14\ \text{ml/min}$

Convert to L/hr.

$\text{Cl} = (225.14)(1\ \text{L/1,000 mL})(60/1\ \text{h})$

$\text{Cl} = 13.51\ \text{L/h}$

$V = (0.22\ \text{L/kg})(80\ \text{kg})$

$V = 17.6\ \text{L}$

$K = \text{Cl/V}$

$K = (13.51\ \text{L/h})/(17.6\ \text{L})$

$K = 0.77\ \text{h}^{-1}$

$C_{\text{total}} = C_{\text{free}}/f_u$

$C_{\text{total}} = (4\ \text{mcg/mL})/[(100 - 8)/100]$

$C_{\text{total}} = 4.35\ \text{mcg/mL}$

$C = [((S)(F)(\text{Dose/t}_{\text{in}}))/(Cl)](1-e^{-kt1})$

$4.35\ \text{mg/L} = [(500\ \text{mg/1 h})/(13.51\ \text{L/h})](1-e^{-0.77\ \text{h}^{-1} \times t1})$

$4.35 = 37.01(1-e^{-0.77\ \text{h}^{-1} \times t1})$

$0.12 = 1-e^{-0.77\ \text{h}^{-1} \times t1}$

$0.88 = e^{-0.77\ \text{h}^{-1} \times t1}$

$\ln(0.88) = -0.77\ \text{h}^{-1} \times t1$

$-0.13 = -0.77\ \text{h}^{-1} \times t1$

$t1 = 0.17\ \text{h}$

$C = [((S)(F)(\text{Dose/t}_{\text{in}}))/(Cl)](1-e^{-ktin})(e^{-kt2})$

$4.35\ \text{mg/L} = [(500\ \text{mg/1})/(13.51\ \text{L})](1-e^{-0.77\ \text{h}^{-1} \times 1\ \text{h}})(e^{-0.77\ \text{h}^{-1} \times t2})$

$4.35 = 37.01(1-e^{-0.77})(e^{-0.77\ \text{h}^{-1} \times t2})$

$0.12 = (0.54)(e^{-0.77\ \text{h}^{-1} \times t2})$

$0.22 = (e^{-0.77\ \text{h}^{-1} \times t2})$

$\ln(0.22) = \ln(e^{-0.77\ \text{h}^{-1} \times t2})$

$-1.51 = -0.77\ \text{h}^{-1} \times t2$

$t2 = 1.97\ \text{h}$

$t = (\text{infusion duration} - t1) + t2$

$t = (1 - 0.17\ \text{h}) + 1.97\ \text{h}$

$t = 2.8\ \text{h}$

Calculate the $\%f\,\text{T>MIC}$.

$\%f\,\text{T>MIC} = \text{t/dosing interval} \times 100$

$\%f\,\text{T>MIC} = 2.8\ \text{h/8 h} \times 100$

$\%f\,\text{T>MIC} = 35\%$ of the dosing interval

A $f\,\text{T>MIC}$ of 35 percent is less than the target need for maximal antibacterial activity with a carbapenem of 40 percent. A prolonged high-dose infusion would likely be needed in order to achieve this target.

CASE 10: PIPERACILLIN/TAZOBACTAM CONTINUOUS INFUSION DOSING

PJ, a 90 kg, 5′6″ male who was initiated on 2.25 g piperacillin/tazobactam loading dose followed by a 9 g continuous infusion over 24 hours for the treatment of sepsis caused by P. aeruginosa with a piperacillin/tazobactam MIC of 32 mcg/mL. What concentration will these doses attain at 20 hours and will this concentration be sufficient for free concentrations to be above the MIC during the entire infusion? If not, what dose will be needed?

$C_{20} = [((S)(F)(LD)/(V))(e^{-kt})] + [((S)(F)(\text{Dose/infusion duration})/(Cl))(1-e^{-kt})]$

This equation adds the amount of drug remaining at 20 hours from the loading dose to the steady-state concentration (at 20 hours) from the continuous infusion. Again S and F can be assumed to be 1. At 20 hours, little to no concentration is expected to remain from the loading dose, thus this portion of the equation can be removed. It has been calculated here for confirmation that it does not contribute to the concentration at 20 hours.

$C_{20} = [(2250\ \text{mg})/((0.15\ \text{L/kg})(90\ \text{kg}))(e^{-0.866\ \text{h}^{-1} \times 20\ \text{h}})]$

$C_{20} = [((166.67\ \text{mg/L})(e^{-17.3})]$

$C_{20} = 0.000005\ \text{mg/L}$

As expected, this result did not contribute any sizable portion to the overall concentration at 20 hours. Only the concentration that remains from the continuous infusion will need to be determined.

$C_{20} = (S)(F)(\text{Dose/infusion duration})/(Cl)(1-e^{-kt})$

Because $K = 0.693/t_{1/2}$, K can be calculated using the parameters from Table 3-1.

$K = 0.693/0.8\ \text{h}$

$K = 0.866\ \text{h}^{-1}$

$C_{20} = ((9,000\ \text{mg/24 h})/(214)(60/\text{h})(1\ \text{L/1,000}))(1-e^{-0.866\cdot1 \times 20})$

$C_{20} = ((375\ \text{mg})/(12.8\ \text{L}))(1-e^{-17.3})$

$C_{20} = (29.2\ \text{mg/L})(1)$

$C_{20} = 29.2\ \text{mg/L}$

To determine the free concentration, the fraction unbound needs to be multiplied by this concentration.

$C_{20\text{free}} = 29.2\ \text{mg/L} \times 0.7$

$C_{20\text{free}} = 20.4\ \text{mg/L}$

Because 20.4 mg/L (mcg/mL) is not sufficient to treat this organism with an MIC of 32 mcg/mL, a larger dose will be needed. To determine what dose, the following equation can be used to calculate the maintenance dose needed.

$\text{MD} = (Cl)(C_{\text{ss ave}})(f_u)(\text{infusion duration})/(S)(F)$

If you remember from case #2, the equation can be rearranged so $C_{ss\,ave} \times f_u$ equals C_{total}, and the total drug needed to attain a free concentration of 32 mg/L can be calculated. Also, his BSA needs to be calculated.

$$C_{free} = C_{total} \times F_u$$
$$C_{total} = C_{free}/f_u$$
$$C_{total} = 32\ mcg/mL \times 0.7$$
$$C_{total} = 45.7\ mcg/mL$$

$$BSA = (weight/70\ kg)^{0.7}(1.73\ m^2)$$
$$BSA = (90\ kg/70\ kg)^{0.7}(1.73\ m^2)$$
$$BSA = (1.29)^{0.7}(1.73\ m^2)$$
$$BSA = (1.19)(1.73\ m^2)$$
$$BSA = 2.06\ m^2$$

$$MD = (180\ mL/min/1.73)(2.06\ m^2)(60\ min/1\ h)$$
$$(1\ L/1{,}000\ mL)(45.7\ mg/L)(24\ h)$$
$$MD = 12.86\ L/h(45.7\ mg/L)(24\ h)$$
$$MD = 14104.8\ mg(1\ g/1{,}000\ mg)$$
$$MD = 14.1\ g$$

This dose should be rounded up to 18 g (four vials of the 4.5 g piperacillin/tazobactam) and be infused over 24 hours.

CASE 11: MEROPENEM PROLONGED INFUSION DOSING

CB is a 27-year-old female with cystic fibrosis and Acinetobacter baumannii pneumonia with a meropenem MIC of 16. Her team of physicians just asked you to assist with dosing her meropenem. They know she will need a prolonged infusion regimen, but are unsure as to what dose to give. Half of the team wants to give 1 g q8h and the rest want to give 2 g q8h. She is 5′10″ and weighs 59 kg. Which regimen would be the most appropriate?

Calculate her BSA, clearance, and volume of distribution.

$$BSA = (weight/70\ kg)^{0.7}(1.73\ m^2)$$
$$BSA = (59\ kg/70\ kg)^{0.7}(1.73\ m^2)$$
$$BSA = 1.53\ m^2$$
$$Cl = (240\ mL/min/1.73)(1.53)$$
$$Cl = 212.25\ ml/min$$

Convert to L/hr.

$$Cl = (212.25\ mL/min)(1\ L/1{,}000\ mL)(60\ min/1\ h)$$
$$Cl = 12.74\ L/h$$
$$V = (0.27\ L/kg)(62\ kg)$$
$$V = 16.74\ L$$
$$K = Cl/V$$
$$K = (12.74\ L/h)/(16.74\ L)$$
$$K = 0.76\ h^{-1}$$

Calculate the total drug concentration corresponding to the MIC.

$$C_{total} = C_{free}/f_u$$
$$C_{total} = (16\ mcg/mL\ )/[(100-15)/100]$$
$$C_{total} = 18.82\ mcg/mL$$

Calculate the %*f* T>MIC for the 1 g q8h regimen as a 3-hour infusion.

$$C = [((S)(F)(Dose/t_{in}))/(Cl)](1-e^{-kt1})$$

$$18.82\ mg/L = [(1{,}000\ mg/3\ h)/12.74\ L/h)](1-e^{-0.76\ h^{-1} \times t1})$$
$$18.82 = 26.16(1-e^{-0.76\ h^{-1} \times t1})$$
$$0.72 = 1-e^{-0.76\ h^{-1} \times t1}$$
$$0.28 = e^{-0.76\ h^{-1} \times t1}$$
$$\ln(0.28) = -0.76\ h^{-1} \times t1$$
$$-1.27 = -0.76\ h^{-1} \times t1$$
$$t1 = 1.67\ h$$

$$C = [((S)(F)(Dose/t_{in}))/(Cl)](1-e^{-ktin})(e^{-kt2})$$
$$18.82\ mg/L = [(1{,}000\ mg/3)/12.74\ L](1-e^{-0.76\ h^{-1} \times 3\ h})(e^{-0.76\ h^{-1} \times t2})$$
$$18.82 = 26.16(1-e^{-2.28})(e^{-0.76\ h^{-1} \times t2})$$
$$0.72 = (0.90)(e^{-0.76\ h^{-1} \times t2})$$
$$0.80 = (e^{-0.76\ h^{-1} \times t2})$$
$$\ln(0.80) = \ln(e^{-0.76\ h^{-1} \times t2})$$
$$-0.22 = -0.76\ h^{-1} \times t2$$
$$t2 = 0.29\ h$$

$$t = (infusion\ duration - t1) + t2$$
$$t = (3 - 1.67\ h) + 0.29\ h$$
$$t = 1.62\ h$$

$$\%f\ T{>}MIC = t/dosing\ interval \times 100$$
$$\%f\ T{>}MIC = 1.62\ h/8\ h \times 100$$
$$\%f\ T{>}MIC = 20.25\%\ of\ the\ dosing\ interval$$

Calculate the %*f* T>MIC for the 2 g q8h regimen as a 3-hour infusion.

$$C = [((S)(F)(Dose/t_{in}))/(Cl)](1-e^{-kt1})$$
$$18.82\ mg/L = [(2{,}000\ mg/3\ h)/12.74\ L/h)](1-e^{-0.76\ h^{-1} \times t1})$$
$$18.82 = 52.33(1-e^{-0.76\ h^{-1} \times t1})$$
$$0.36 = 1-e^{-0.76\ h^{-1} \times t1}$$
$$0.64 = e^{-0.76\ h^{-1} \times t1}$$
$$\ln(0.64) = -0.76\ h^{-1} \times t1$$
$$-0.45 = -0.76\ h^{-1} \times t1$$
$$t1 = 0.59\ h$$

$$C = [((S)(F)(Dose/t_{in}))/(Cl)](1-e^{-ktin})(e^{-kt2})$$
$$18.82\ mg/L = [(2{,}000\ mg/3)/12.74\ L](1-e^{-0.76\ h^{-1} \times 3\ h})(e^{-0.76\ h^{-1} \times t2})$$
$$18.82 = 52.33(1-e^{-2.28})(e^{-0.76\ h^{-1} \times t2})$$
$$0.36 = (0.90)(e^{-0.76\ h^{-1} \times t2})$$
$$0.40 = (e^{-0.76\ h^{-1} \times t2})$$
$$\ln(0.40) = \ln(e^{-0.76\ h^{-1} \times t2})$$
$$-0.92 = -0.76\ h^{-1} \times t2$$
$$t2 = 1.21\ h$$

$$t = (infusion\ duration - t1) + t2$$
$$t = (3 - 0.59\ h) + 1.21\ h$$
$$t = 3.62\ h$$

$$\%f\ T{>}MIC = t/dosing\ interval \times 100$$
$$\%f\ T{>}MIC = 3.62\ h/8\ h \times 100$$
$$\%f\ T{>}MIC = 45.25\%\ of\ the\ dosing\ interval$$

Only the 2 g dose q8h as a 3-hour infusion exceeds the 40% *f* T>MIC target needed for maximal antibacterial activity for carbapenems, therefore, this dose would be correct.

REFERENCES

1. Gupta K, Hooton TM, Naber KG, et al. International clinical practice guidelines for the treatment of acute uncomplicated cystitis and pyelonephritis in women: A 2010 update by the Infectious Diseases Society of America and the European Society for Microbiology and Infectious Diseases. *Clin Infect Dis.* 2011;52:e103–e120.

2. Solomkin JS, Mazuski JE, Bradley JS, et al. Diagnosis and management of complicated intra-abdominal infection in adults and children: Guidelines by the Surgical Infection Society and the Infectious Disease Society of America. *Clin Infect Dis.* 2010;50:133–164.

3. Mandell LA, Wunderink RG, Anzueto A, et al. Infectious Diseases Society of America/American Thoracic Society consensus guidelines on the management of community-acquired pneumonia in adults. *Clin Infect Dis.* 2007;44:S27–S72.

4. Lipsky BA, Berendt AR, Deery HG, et al. Diagnosis and treatment of diabetic foot infections. *Clin Infect Dis.* 2004;39:885–910.

5. Stevens Dl, Bisno AL, Chambers HF, et al. Practice guidelines for the diagnosis and management of skin and soft tissue infections. *Clin Infect Dis.* 2005;41:1373–1406.

6. American Thoracic Society. Guidelines for the management of adults with hospital-acquired, ventilator-associated, and healthcare-associated pneumonia. *Am J Respir Crit Care Med.* 2005;171:388–416.

7. Eagle H, Fleischman R, Levy M. Continuous vs. discontinuous therapy with penicillin; the effect of the interval between injection on therapeutic efficacy. *N Engl J Med.* 1953;248:481–488.

8. Eagle H, Fleischman R, Musselman AD. Effect of schedule of administration on the therapeutic efficacy of penicillin; importance of the aggregate time penicillin remains at effectively bactericidal levels. *Am J Med.* 1950;9:280–299.

9. Fluckiger U, Segessenmann C, Gerber AU. Integration of pharmacokinetics and pharmacodynamics of imipenem in a human-adapted mouse model. *Antimicrob Agents Chemother.* 1991;35:1905–1910.

10. Drusano GL. Antimicrobial pharmacodynamics: critical interactions of "bug and drug." *Nat Rev Microbiol.* 2004;2:289–300.

11. Crandon JL, Bulik CC, Kuti JL, et al. Clinical pharmacodynamics of cefepime in patients infected with *Pseudomonas aeruginosa*. *Antimicrob Agents Chemother.* 2010;54:1111–1116.

12. Turnidge JD. The pharmacodynamics of beta-lactams. *Clin Infect Dis.* 1998;27:10–22.

13. Occhipinti, DJ, Pendland SL, Schoonover LL, et al. Pharmacokinetics and pharmacodynamics of two multiple-dose piperacillin-tazobactam regimens. *Antimicrob Agents Chemother.* 1997;41:2511–2517.

14. Zosyn (piperacillin and tazobactam) package insert. Wyeth Pharmaceuticals, Inc., Philadelphia, PA. 2009.

15. Mathew M, Das Gupta V, Bethea C. Stability of piperacillin sodium in the presence of tazobactam sodium in 5% dextrose and normal saline injections. *J Clin Pharm Ther.* 1994;19:397–399.

16. Nye, KJ, Shi YG, Andrews JM, et al. Pharmacokinetics and tissue penetration of cefepime. *J. Antimicrob Chemother.* 1989;24:23–28.

17. Fubara JO, Notari RE. Influence of pH, temperature and buffers on cefepime degradation kinetics and stability predictions in aqueous solutions. *J Pharm. Sci.* 1998;87:1572–1576.

18. Maxipime (cefepime) package insert. Elan Pharmaceuticals, Inc., South San Francisco, CA. 2009.

19. Moon YS, Chung KC, Gill MA. Pharmacokinetics of meropenem in animals, healthy volunteers, and patients. *Clin Infect Dis.* 1997;24(Suppl 2): S249–S255.

20. Dreetz, M, Hammacher J, Eller J, et al. Serum bactericidal activities and comparative pharmacokinetics of meropenem and imipenem-cilastatin. *Antimicrob Agents and Chemother.* 1996;40:105–109.

21. Merrem (meropenem) package insert. AstraZeneca Pharmaceuticals LP, Wilmington, DE. 2009.

22. Berthoin K, Le Duff CS, Marchand-Brynaert J, et al. Stability of meropenem and doripenem solutions for administration by continuous infusion. *J Antimicrob Chemother.* 2010;65:1073–1075.

23. Paterson DL, Depestel DD. Doripenem. *Clin Infect Dis.* 2009;49:291–298.

24. Doribax (doripenem) package insert. Ortho-McNeil-Janssen Pharmaceutical, Inc., Raritan, NJ. 2009.

25. Cirillo, I, Vacarro N, Turner K. Pharmacokinetics, safety, and tolerability of doripenem after 0.5-, 1-, and 4-hour infusions in healthy volunteers. *J Clin Pharmacol.* 2009;49:798–806.

26. Crandon JL, Sutherland CA, Nicolau DP. Stability of doripenem in polyvinyl chloride bags and elastomeric pumps. *Am J Health Syst Pharm.* 2010;67:1539–1544.

27. Crandon JL, Nicolau DP. Pharmacodynamic approaches to optimizing beta-lactam therapy. *Crit Care Clin.* 2011;27:77–93.

28. Roberts JA, Kirkpatrick CM, Lipman J. Monte Carlo simulations; maximizing pharmacokinetic data to optimize clinical practice for critically ill patients. *J Antimicrob Chemother.* 2011;66:227–231.

29. Nicasio AM, Ariano RE, Zelenitsky SA, et al. Population pharmacokinetics of high-dose, prolonged-infusion cefepime in adult critically ill patients with ventilator-associated pneumonia. *Antimicrob Agents Chemother.* 2009;53:1476–1481.

30. Pai MP, Bearden DT. Antimicrobial dosing considerations in obese adult patients. *Pharmacother.* 2007;27:1081–1091.

31. Bearden DT, Rodvold KA. Dosage adjustments for antibacterials in obese patients: Applying clinical pharmacokinetics. *Clin Pharmacokinet.* 2000;38:415–426.

32. Newman D, Scheetz MH, Adeyemi OA, et al. Serum piperacillin/tazobactam pharmacokinetics in a morbidly obese individual. *Ann Pharmacother.* 2007;41:1734–1739.

33. Bearden DT, Earle SB, McConnell DB, et al. Pharmacokinetics of meropenem in extreme obesity [abstract]. In program and abstracts of the 45th Interscience Conference on Antimicrobial Agents and Chemotherapy. Washington, DC, American Society for Microbiology, 2005:2.

CHAPTER 4

Antiepileptic Drugs: Second-Generation/Newer Agents

KERI S. KIM, PharmD, MS CTS, BCPS
JEFFREY J. MUCKSAVAGE, PharmD, BCPS
GRETCHEN M. BROPHY, PharmD, BCPS, FCCP, FCCM, FNCS

REVIEW OF SECOND-GENERATION/ NEWER AGENTS

PLACE IN THERAPY

The advent of the second-generation antiepileptic drugs ushered in a period of improved management of patients with epilepsy. The introduction of these agents began in 1993 and greatly expanded the available epilepsy treatment options. Currently, 11 second-generation antiepileptic drugs (AEDs) are approved for use in the United States. Table 4-1 provides a summary of the available second-generation AEDs. Due to the regulations of the Food and Drug Administration (FDA) with respect to studying AEDs in the United States, many of these agents are initially approved as adjunctive agents. In essence, they are added to an established therapeutic regimen of patients being managed primarily with a first-generation AED (i.e., carbamazepine, phenobarbital, phenytoin, or valproic acid). Most of them are approved for use as adjunctive therapy in the management of partial seizures with or without secondary generalization, primary generalized tonic-clonic seizures, or myoclonic seizures. As more data emerge, monotherapy approval for these agents may be pursued and the use of these agents will inevitably be expanded in clinical practice. At times, these agents may also be used for nonepileptic purposes. For example, gabapentin and pregabalin, while initially used for seizure management, are used almost exclusively today for the management of neuropathic pain and other pain syndromes.

ADVANTAGES/DISADVANTAGES

Prior to the approval of the second-generation AEDs and for most of the twentieth century, the management of epilepsy was limited to only a few AEDs. Although the first-generation AEDs are undoubtedly efficacious, clinically, these drugs are problematic from both prescriber and patient points of view. The management of patients with these agents (i.e., carbamazepine, phenobarbital, phenytoin, and valproic acid) continues to be fraught with challenges due to their toxicity, the complex nature of their kinetic profiles, adverse effects, the need for therapeutic drug monitoring, and the cross-reactivity of hypersensitivity reactions.[1] The second-generation AEDs generally tends to be more predictable from a kinetic standpoint and have a cleaner adverse event profile compared to their first-generation counterparts, making them an attractive advantageous therapeutic option.

Globally, the second-generation AEDs offer a number of specific pharmacokinetic advantages when compared with the first-generation AEDs. First, oral absorption of the second-generation agents tends to be complete (with the exception of gabapentin), which is in contrast with the saturable absorption properties of phenytoin that at times may complicate a patient's oral regimen. In addition, concomitant administration with food appears to slow the oral absorption of the majority of the second-generation AEDs delaying the time to the maximum concentration (Cmax), but has little to no effect on extent of absorption (i.e., bioavailability).[2] This aspect is noteworthy from a patient counseling perspective and may be advantageous from a medication adherence perspective as well.

The issue of plasma protein binding also plays a less prominent role in the management of the second-generation AEDs. A number of the first-generation agents are significantly bound to plasma protein, namely albumin, which can lead to difficulties in interpreting total concentrations. Significant drug interactions or potential toxicities may occur when other highly protein-bound medications are added to a patient's regimen secondary to displacement. The relatively low degree of plasma protein binding of the second-generations AEDs decreases the risk of significant protein binding interactions, simplifying the use of these agents with other highly protein-bound medications. Tiagabine is the sole exception to the low protein binding characteristic. More details describing the individual agents can be found in Table 4-2.

Second-generation AEDs have significantly fewer drug-drug interactions because they have little to no effect on the activity of hepatic metabolic enzymes except for felbamate, topiramate, and oxcarbazepine, which mildly inhibit CYP450 2C19 and induce 3A4 isoenzymes (see Table 4-3) In addition, lamotrigine monotherapy is the only second-generation AED that is known to autoinduce its own metabolism. In contrast, many of the first-generation AEDs affect the hepatic metabolism of other AEDs as well as non-AED medications in a patient's regimen. For example, phenytoin, phenobarbital, and carbamazepine induce specific isoenzymes of the P450 system that can alter the concentrations of second-generation AEDs and non-AED substrates. This effect is particularly important for drugs with a narrow therapeutic index, such as proteases inhibitors, oral contraceptives, and antirejection agents (i.e., cyclosporine and tacrolimus), to name a few. Thus, the potential for drug-drug interactions via metabolic pathways is minimized, which is an advantage when selecting second-generation AED for a patient currently on non-AED medications that are substrates of the cytochrome P450 system. Routine therapeutic drug monitoring is not recommended for second-generation AEDs because clinical trials to date have not been able to determine an actual therapeutic range. However, therapeutic drug monitoring may be of particular benefit in unique settings including in the management of toxicity, drug-drug interaction, and patient compliance. Without well-established correlations between drug concentrations and clinical efficacy or toxicity, concentrations must be interpreted with caution and correlated with the patient's clinical condition if therapeutic drug monitoring is conducted.

From an elimination perspective, some second-generation AEDs have renal elimination as a major pathway for elimination

TABLE 4-1 Summary of Second-Generation Antiepileptic Drugs

	Felbamate Felbatol[68] 1993	Gabapentin Neurontin[12] 1994	Lamotrigine Lamictal[69] 1994	Topiramate Topamax[70] 1996	Tiagabine Gabitril[26] 1997	Levetiracetam Keppra[28,29] 1999	Oxcarbazepine Trileptal[39] 2000	Zonisamide Zonegran[51] 2000	Pregabalin Lyrica[11] 2004	Lacosamide Vimpat[61] 2008	Ezogabine Potiga[71] 2011
AED/Year of FDA Approval											
FDA Indication	Alternative agent as monotherapy or adjunctive therapy for partial seizure with and without secondary generalization in adults (>14 yrs)

Alternative agent as adjunctive therapy for partial and generalized seizures associated with Lennox-Gastaut syndrome in children (2–14 yrs) | Adjunctive therapy for partial seizures with and without secondary generalization (>12 yrs)

Adjunctive therapy for partial seizures in children (3–12 yrs) | Adjunctive therapy for partial seizures, primary generalized TC seizures, generalized seizures of Lennox-Gastaut syndrome (>2 yrs)

Monotherapy for partial seizures (conversion to monotherapy from CBZ, PB, PHT, VPA, PRM (>16 yrs) | Monotherapy (>10 yrs) or adjunctive (2–16 yrs) for partial onset or primary generalized TC seizures Lennox-Gastaut syndrome (>2 yrs) | Adjunctive therapy for partial seizures in adults and children (>12 yrs) | Adjunctive therapy for partial onset seizures (>4 yrs), myoclonic seizures (>12 yrs), primary generalized TC seizures (>6 yrs) | Monotherapy or adjunctive therapy for partial seizures in adults

Monotherapy for partial seizures in children (>4 yrs)

Adjunctive therapy for partial seizures (>2 yrs) | Adjunctive therapy for partial seizures in adults (>16 yrs) | Adjunctive therapy for partial onset seizures in adults | Adjunctive therapy for partial-onset seizures (>17 yrs) | Add-on treatment for partial onset seizures (>18 yrs) |
| **Mechanism of Action** | Antagonist, strychnine-insensitive glycine recognition site of the NMDA receptor-ionophore complex | Binds to alpha2-delta site (auxiliary subunit of voltage-gated Ca channels)[9] | Inhibits voltage-sensitive Na channels | Blocks voltage-dependent Na channels, augment sactivity of the GABA at some subtypes of GABA-A receptor Antagonizes AMPA/kainate subtype of the glutamate receptor Inhibits carbonic anhydrase enzyme –isozymes II, IV | Enhances GABA activity by blocking GABA uptake into presynaptic neurons (via GABA transporter, GAT-1)[21] | Binds to synaptic vesicle protein (SV2A) Indirectly modulates GABA inhibition[72] | Blocks voltage-sensitive Na channels, increases K conductance and modulation of high-voltage activated Ca channels | Binds to inactive Na channel and increases action potential threshold[49] Reduces voltage-dependent, transient inward currents (t-type Ca²⁺ currents) Carbonic anhydrase inhibitor | Binds to alpha2-delta site (auxiliary subunit of voltage-gated Ca channels) | Selectively enhances slow inactivation of voltage-gated Na channels; Binds to collapsing response mediator protein-2 (CRMP-2) | Opens/activates neuronal voltage-gated K channels (KCNQ2/3, KCN Q3/5); Enhances GABA-mediated inhibition |
| **Dose (Adults)** | 1200–3600 mg daily (divide into 3–4 doses) ⌃Titrate by 1200 mg weekly | 900–3600 mg daily (divide into 3 doses) ⌃Titrate by 50% weekly | *See Table 4-4 | 25–400 mg daily (divide into 2 doses) ⌃Titrate by 25–50 mg weekly | Without AED inhibitor/inducer: 4–32 mg daily monotherapy (divide into 2–4 doses) With AED inducer (CBZ, PB, PHT, PRM): 4–56 mg/day with (divide into 2–4 doses) ⌃Titrate by 4–8 mg weekly | 500–3000 mg daily (divide into 2 doses) ⌃Titrate by 1000 mg every 2 weeks | 600–2400 mg daily (divide into 2 doses) ⌃Titrate by 600 mg weekly | 100–600 mg daily ⌃Titrate by 100 mg every 2 weeks | 150–600 mg daily (divide into 2–3 doses) ⌃Titrate by 150 mg weekly | 100–400 mg daily (divide into 2 doses) ⌃Titrate by 100 mg weekly | 300–1200 mg daily (divide into 3 doses) ⌃Titrate by 150 mg weekly[66] |

TABLE 4-1 Summary of Second-Generation Antiepileptic Drugs (Continued)

Dose (Children)	15–45 mg/kg/day (divide into 3–4 doses)	10–35 mg/kg/day for age >5 yrs (divide into 3 doses) 10–40 mg/kg/day for ages 3–4 yrs (divide into 3 doses)	*See Table 4-4	2–16 yrs: 1–3 mg/kg/day, max 5–9 mg/kg/day (divide into 2 doses) ∧Titrate by 1–3 mg/kg/day every 1–2 weeks	Monotherapy & AED inducer for 12–18 yrs: 4–32 mg/day (divide into 2–4 doses) ∧Titrate by 4–8 mg weekly	4 to <16 yrs & 20.1–40 kg: 500–1500 mg/day, max dose 60 mg/kg/day (divide into 2 doses) >40 kg: 1000–3000 mg/day, max dose 60 mg/kg/day (divide into 2 doses) ∧Titrate by 10–20 mg/kg every 2 weeks	2–16 yrs: 8–10 mg/kg, max 600 mg/day (divide into 2 doses) <20 kg: 16–20 mg/kg/day (divide into 2 doses) 20–29 kg: 900 mg/day 29.1–39 kg: 1200 mg/day >39 kg: 1800 mg/day	NA	NA
Pregnancy Category	C	C	C	D	C	C	C	C	C
Lactation (excreted in human milk)	Yes	Yes	Yes	Yes	Unknown	Yes	Yes	Unknown	Unknown
Drug Levels at Therapeutic Doses[2]	30–60 mcg/mL	12–20 mcg/mL	2.5–15 mcg/mL	0.5–250 mcg/mL	20–100 ng/mL	8–26 mcg/mL	12–35 mcg/mL licarbazepine	2.8–9.2 mcg/mL	10–38 mcg/mL
Dose Adjustments for Organ Dysfunction	Renal impairment 50% dosage reduction	Renal impairment Cl_{cr} 30–59 mL/min: 400–1400 mg/day Cl_{cr} 15–29 mL/min: 200–700 mg/day Cl_{cr} 7–15 mL/min: 100–300 mg/day Cl_{cr} <7 mL/min: 50–150 mg/day ESRD on HD: MD as supplemental dose	Liver impairment Moderate-severe without ascites: decrease dose by 25% Severe with ascites: decrease dose by 50%	Renal impairment Cl_{cr} <70 mL/min: 50% dosage reduction ESRD on HD: supplemental dose may be required	Hepatic impairment Child-Pugh Class B: 60% dose reduction	Renal impairment Cl_{cr} 50–80 mL/min: 500–1000 mg/day Cl_{cr} 30–50 mL/min: 250–750 mg/day Cl_{cr} <30 mL/min: 250–500 mg/day ESRD on HD: 500–1000 mg/day with 50% of MD as supplemental dose	Renal impairment Cl_{cr} <30 mL/min: 50% dose reduction Liver impairment consider dose reduction	Renal impairment Cl_{cr} 30–60 mL/min: 75–300 mg/day (divide into 2–3 doses) Cl_{cr} 15–30 mL/min: 25–150 mg/day (divide into 1–2 doses) Cl_{cr} <15 mL/min: 25–75 mg/day ESRD on HD: MD 25 mg/day with 25 or 50 mg as supplemental dose MD 25–50 mg/day with 50 or 75 mg as supplemental dose MD 50–75 mg/day with 75 or 100 mg as supplemental dose MD 75 mg/day with 100 or 150 mg as supplemental dose	Renal impairment Cl_{cr} <30 mL/min: max 300 mg/day ESRD on HD: 300 mg/day with 50% MD as supplement dose Hepatic impairment Mild-moderate: 300 mg/day

(Continued)

TABLE 4-1 Summary of Second-Generation Antiepileptic Drugs *(Continued)*

AED/Year of FDA Approval	Felbamate Felbatol® 1993	Gabapentin Neurontin®[12] 1994	Lamotrigine Lamictal®[69] 1994	Topiramate Topamax®[70] 1996	Tiagabine Gabitril®[26] 1997	Levetiracetam Keppra®[28,29] 1999	Oxcarbazepine Trileptal®[39] 2000	Zonisamide Zonegran®[51] 2000	Pregabalin Lyrica®[11] 2004	Lacosamide Vimpat®[61] 2008	Ezogabine Potiga® 2011
Common Side Effects[68]	Anorexia Dizziness Headache Insomnia Nausea Somnolence Vomiting	Ataxia Dizziness Emotional lability Fatigue Hostility Hyperkinesia Nystagmus Somnolence	Blurred vision Diplopia Dizziness Headache Insomnia Skin rash	Anorexia Ataxia Difficulty with concentration Drowsiness Metabolic acidosis Nephrolithiasis Oligohydrosis Paresthesias Weight loss Word-finding difficulty	Abdominal pain Asthenia Difficulty with concentration Dizziness Nausea Nervousness Somnolence Tremor	Dizziness Fatigue Irritability Mood swings Somnolence	Abdominal pain Ataxia Blurred vision Difficulty with concentration Diplopia Dizziness Dyspepsia Fatigue Headache Hyponatremia Nausea Psychomotor slowing Somnolence Tremor Vomiting	Anorexia Ataxia Difficulty with concentration Drowsiness Nephrolithiasis Oligohydrosis Somnolence Weight loss	Ataxia Difficulty with concentration Diplopia Dizziness Edema Fatigue Somnolence Weight gain	Diplopia Dizziness Headache Nausea Nystagmus Somnolence	Ataxia Blurred vision Confusion Dizziness Fatigue Headache Speech disorder Somnolence Tremor Urinary retention Weight gain[66,67]
Serious Side Effects[68]	Aplastic anemia Acute hepatic failure	None reported	Hepatic failure SJS TEN	Acute close angle glaucoma Heat stroke	None reported	Psychosis	Anaphylaxis Angioedema SJS TEN	Anxiety Aplastic anemia Depression Heat stroke Rash SJS TEN	None reported	PR interval prolongation Atrial fibrillation/flutter Multiorgan hypersensitivity	None reported
Formulation	Tablet: 400 mg 600 mg Suspension: 600 mg/5mL	Capsule: 100 mg 300 mg 400 mg Tablet: 100 mg 300 mg 400 mg Tablet, film-coated: 600 mg 800 mg Oral solution: 250 mg/5mL	Tablet: 25 mg 100 mg 150 mg 200 mg Tablet 24-hr: 25 mg 50 mg 100 mg 200 mg Chewable dispersible tablet: 2 mg 5 mg 25 mg ODT: 25 mg 50 mg 100 mg 200 mg Starter kit (tablet or ODT): Blue kit (VPA) Green kit (CBZ, PHT, PB, PRM & no VPA) Orange kit (no CBZ, FHT, PB, PRM, VPA)	Capsule, sprinkles: 15 mg 25 mg Tablet: 25 mg 50 mg 100 mg 200 mg	Tablet: 2 mg 4 mg 12 mg 16 mg	Tablet: 250 mg 500 mg 750 mg 1000 mg XR Tablet 24-hr: 500 mg Oral solution: 100 mg/mL Injection: 500 mg/5mL	Tablet film-coated: 150 mg 300 mg 600 mg Oral suspension: 300 mg/5mL	Capsule: 25 mg 100 mg	Capsule: 25 mg 50 mg 75 mg 100 mg 150 mg 200 mg 225 mg 300 mg Oral solution: 20 mg/mL	Tablet: 50 mg 100 mg 150 mg 200 mg Oral solution: 10 mg/mL Injection: 200 mg/20mL	

AED, antiepileptic drug; FDA, Food and Drug Administration; NMDA, N-methyl-D-aspartate; GABA, gamma aminobutyric acid; CBZ, carbamazepine; PB, phenobarbital; PHT, phenytoin; VPA, valproic acid; PRM, primidone; TC, tonic-clonic; yrs, years; HD, hemodialysis; CI_{cr}, creatinine clearance; SJS, Stevens-Johnson syndrome; TEN, toxic epidermal necrolysis; MD, maintenance dose; ESRD, end-stage renal disease; ODT, orally disintegrating tablet; NA, not applicable.

TABLE 4-2 Pharmacokinetic Parameters of Second-Generation Antiepileptic Drugs

AED and Year of FDA Approval	Felbamate Felbatol[68] 1993	Gabapentin Neurontin[812] 1994	Lamotrigine Lamictal[669] 1994	Topiramate Topamax[670] 1996	Tiagabine Gabitril[026] 1997	Levetiracetam Keppra[28,29] 1999	Oxcarbazepine Trileptal[839] 2000	Zonisamide Zonegran[651] 2000	Pregabalin Lyrica[811] 2004	Lacosamide Vimpat[661] 2008	Ezogabine[71] Potiga® 2011
Absorption	Well-absorbed	Saturable	Complete		Complete	Complete	Complete	Well-absorbed	Well-absorbed	Complete	
Bioavailability (F)	90%	27–60% Dose proportional decrease in F	98%	80%	90%	100%	100%	95%	>90%	100%	60%
Volume of Distribution (Vd)	0.7 L/kg	0.8 L/kg[9]	0.9–1.3 L/kg	0.6–0.8 L/kg[32]		0.7 L/kg	0.3–0.8 L/kg[15] (MHD)	1.45 L/kg	0.5 L/kg	0.6 L/kg	7.3 L/kg
Protein Binding	22–25% (albumin)	<3%	55%	15–41%	96%	<10%	40% (MHD)	40%	None	<15%	<80%[74]
Metabolism	CYP 2E1, 3A4[75]: Parahydroxyfelbamate (pOHF), 2-hydroxyfelbamate (2-OHF), felbamate monocarbamate (MCF)[69]	N-methylation[9]	Glucuronic acid conjugation: 2-N-glucuronide, 5-N-glucuronide, 2-N-methyl metabolite; Autoinduction (25% decrease in $t_{1/2}$) when monotherapy	Hydroxylation, hydrolysis, glucuronidation: 6 metabolites (none account for 5% of total dose)	3A substrate: 5-oxo-tiagabine Glucuronidation	Hydrolysis: 24% of dose as carboxylic acid metabolite (UCB L057), 2% of dose as 2-oxo-pyrrolidine ring, 1% of dose as opening of 2-oxo-pyrrolidine ring in position 5	Keto-reduction: 10-monohydroxy metabolite (MHD) → conjugated with glucuronic acid OR oxidation to 10,11-trans-dihydroxy metabolite (DHD)[15]	Acetylation: N-acetyl zonisamide, Reduction via CYP3A4: 2-sulfamoylacetyl phenol (SMAP)	N-methylation[9]	2C19: 0-desmethyl-lacosamide	Glucuronidation to N-glucuronide metabolite; acetylation to mono-acetylated metabolite
Active Metabolite	No	NA	No	No	No	No	Yes (MHD) No (DHD)		No	No	
Time to Peak Serum Concentration (Tmax)		3 hrs[76]	1.4–4.8 hrs	2 hrs	45 min (fasting) 2.5 hrs (high-fat meal)	1 hr	MHD: 4.5 hrs median (tablet) vs. 6 hrs median (suspension)	2–6 hrs (delayed at 4–6 hrs with food)	1.5 hrs (no food) 3 hrs (with food)	1–4 hrs	0.9–2.1 hrs
Elimination Half-Life ($t_{1/2}$), hrs	20–23	5–7	25	21	7–9	6–8	2 (OXC) 9 (MHD)	63 (105 in RBC)	6	13	7.4–9.2
Time to Reach Steady-State Concentration[2] (Tss)	3–5 days	2 days		4 days	2 days	2 days	2–3 days	14 days	1–2 days	3 days	
Elimination via Kidney	40–50% unchanged, 40% metabolites and conjugates	99% unchanged, <1% N-methyl metabolite[9]	90% metabolites, 10% unchanged	70% unchanged	25% metabolites, 2% unchanged (63% metabolites via feces)	66% unchanged, 24% metabolites (via glomerular filtration with partial tubular reabsorption)	49% glucuronides of MHD, 27% unchanged MHD, 3% DHD, <1% OXC	31% glucuronide of SMAP, 22% unchanged, 9% N-acetyl zonisamide	90% unchanged, 0.9% N-methylated derivative	40% unchanged, 30% 0-desmethyl-lacosamide, 20% unknown polar fraction	Ezogabine metabolites

AED, antiepileptic drug; FDA, Food and Drug Administration.

Antiepileptic Drugs: Second-Generation/Newer Agents

TABLE 4-3 Pharmacokinetic Parameters of Second-Generation Antiepileptic Drugs

AED and Year of FDA Approval	Felbamate Felbatol[68] 1993		Gabapentin Neurontin[12] 1994		Lamotrigine Lamictal[69] 1994		Topiramate Topamax[70] 1996		Tiagabine Gabitril[26] 1997		Levetiracetam Keppra[28,29] 1999		Oxcarbazepine Trileptal[39] 2000		Zonisamide Zonegran[51] 2000		Pregabalin Lyrica[11] 2004		Lacosamide Vimpat[61] 2008		Ezogabine Potiga[70] 2011	
Drug Interaction with First-Generation AEDs	Yes		No		Yes		Yes; mild CYP2C19 inhibitor, mild CYP3A4 inducer		Yes		None		Yes, Inhibit CYP2C19, Induce CYP 3A4/5; ↓ [MHD]		Yes		None		Yes		Yes	
aEffect on AEDs Based on AED Generation	**2nd**	**1st**	**2nd**	**1st**	**2nd**	**1st**	**2nd**	**1st**	**2nd**	**1st**	**2nd**	**1st**	**2nd**	**1st**	**2nd**	**1st**	**2nd**	**1st**	**2nd**	**1st**	**2nd**	**1st**
CBZ	CBZ ↓ epoxide ↑	→	None		None	↓40%	None	↓40%	None	↓60%	None	↓[31]	↓13%[40]	↓40%	None	→	None		None	↓15–20%	None	→
PB	↑	→	None		None	↓40%	None	↓[20]	None	↓60%	None	↓[31]	↑15%[40]	↓25%	NA	→	None		None	↓15–20%	None	None
PHT	↑	→	None		None	↓40%	↔ or ↑25% if BID PHT	↓48%	None	↓60%	None	↓[31]	↑40%[40]	↓30%	None	→	None		None	↓15–20%	None	→
VPA	↑	↔	None		↓25%	↑ >2×	↓11%	↓14%	↑10%	None	None	None	None	↓18%	None	↔→[77]	None		None	↔	None	None

AED, antiepileptic drug; FDA, Food and Drug Administration; CBZ, carbamazepine; PB, phenobarbital; PHT, phenytoin; VPA, valproic acid; PRM, primidone; MHD, monohydroxy metabolite

aEffect of second-generation AED on first-generation AEDs' drug serum concentrations; Column 2: Effect of first-generation AED on second-generation AED's drug serum concentration (i.e., gabapentin, pregabalin, levetiracetam, topiramate, and lacosamide), which is a major difference from first-generation AEDs that are almost exclusively hepatically metabolized. In addition, except for gabapentin and zonisamide at higher doses, the elimination kinetic profile of the second-generation AEDs are linear, or first order, compared with the nonlinear profile observed with phenytoin. This linear profile offers improved dose-response predictability and ease of dosing. More details describing the metabolism and elimination of the specific agents can be found in Table 4-2.

DRUG OVERVIEW

Felbamate

Felbamate was one of the first second-generation AEDs to gain FDA approval. However, the serious side effect profile documented with the use of this agent prevented its routine use. Clinically, it is reserved for patients with seizures refractory to other agents when other treatment options have been exhausted. Patients treated with felbamate have been reported to develop aplastic anemia and acute liver failure, with its risk reported at 1 in 4,800–37,000 and 1 in 18,500–25,000, respectively.[3] Patient deaths due to these adverse effects have also been reported. When choosing to initiate therapy with felbamate, clinicians must carefully evaluate the risk versus the benefits of the agent. Patients must be warned about the potential for serious adverse effects and informed consent must be documented. Blood counts and hepatic function should be monitored and felbamate should be discontinued at the first sign of these adverse effects.

Important pharmacokinetic interactions with felbamate should be noted. The addition of felbamate to an established regimen of first-generation AEDs may increase the concentrations of the first-generation AEDs and require subsequent dosage reduction by at least 20–25 percent.[4-8] This interaction is caused by felbamate's ability to inhibit the metabolism of these agents by various mechanisms. Felbamate can inhibit the beta-oxidation of valproic acid,[4] inhibit the parahydroxylation of phenobarbital that is partly due to the inhibition of CYP450 2C19,[5] decrease in phenytoin hydroxylation via inhibition of CYP450 2C19,[6] and enhance conversion of carbamazepine to epoxide via induction of P450 system with inhibition or saturation of epoxide clearance via inhibition of epoxide hydrolase.[7,8]

Gabapentin/Pregabalin

Gabapentin and pregabalin are structurally related agents that resemble γ-aminobutyric acid (GABA).[9] However, neither agent possesses GABA-like activity. Instead, they bind to $\alpha_2\delta$ protein, a subunit of the voltage-gated calcium channel. This bonding is presumed to be responsible for their antiepileptic activity. Pregabalin possesses superior antiepileptic activity and an improved pharmacokinetic profile when compared to gabapentin.[9,10] The improved pharmacokinetic profile of pregabalin compared to gabapentin is thought to be due entirely to the saturable absorption of gabapentin. The absorption of gabapentin occurs primarily in the small intestine via the intestinal system-L amino acid transporter 1 (LAT1).[9] Pregabalin is absorbed through this same mechanism, but is also absorbed via an additional unidentified pathway. Thus, pregabalin is more completely absorbed when compared to gabapentin. Clinically, then, as the dose of gabapentin is increased, the percentage absorbed decreases. For example, the bioavailability of gabapentin at the 300 mg/day dose is approximately 80 percent. Due to saturable absorption, the bioavailability decreases to approximately 27 percent when doses of 4,800 mg/day are administered. In contrast, pregablin's absorption is not saturable and does not decrease with increasing doses. This translates clinically into

improved efficacy. For example, the bioavailability of pregabalin is >90 percent from small doses of 75 mg/day to large doses of 900 mg/day. Food delays the rate of absorption of both gabapentin and pregabalin, but will not affect the extent of absorption. Thus, they can be given without regard to food. In terms of distribution, gabapentin and pregabalin exhibit a similar brain to whole-blood concentration ratio.

The major pathway for elimination of gabapentin and pregabalin is renal. Gabapentin elimination is dependent on creatinine clearance (Cl_{Cr}), and is inversely related to age. Thus, higher doses per kg are required for children 3-4 years of age compared to 5 years of age. Doses should be adjusted according to Cl_{Cr} among elderly patients. Patients with renal impairment defined as Cl_{Cr} <60 mL/min must have their doses adjusted due to the potential for accumulation.[11,12] In patients with chronic kidney disease, supplemental doses should be administered after every 4-hour hemodialysis session since a 50 percent decrease in plasma concentration has been observed postdialysis.

Clinical studies report euphoria with pregabalin therapy and potential withdrawal symptoms upon its discontinuation. Thus, pregabalin is marketed as a Schedule V controlled substance.[11]

Lamotrigine

The most common serious adverse reaction reported with monotherapy or add-on therapy with lamotrigine is rash.[13] It usually occurs during the titration period (within 8 weeks of therapy) and the risk is highest with a rapid titration and at the higher lamotrigine titration dose. Concomitant therapy with valproic acid also increases the risk of rash with lamotrigine. Both the rates of AED discontinuation and the risk for hospitalization due to rash with lamotrigine therapy are similar when compared to carbamazepine or phenytoin monotherapy. However, the morbilliform rash that may present during lamotrigine therapy rarely develops into Stevens-Johnson syndrome (SJS) or toxic epidermal necrolysis (TEN).

Lamotrigine has clinically significant drug interactions with first-generation AEDs that are known to induce or inhibit glucuronidation. Carbamazepine, phenytoin, phenobarbital, and primidone will induce metabolism of lamotrigine by 40 percent. Thus, when used in combination with these agents, lamotrigine should be initiated and titrated at a higher dose than typically recommended in order to achieve a therapeutic effect. On the other hand, valproic acid will inhibit lamotrigine's metabolism by 25 percent; thus lamotrigine should be initiated and titrated at a lower dose than recommended when used with this agent (see Table 4-4). Currently, commercially available lamotrigine starter kits help to simplify the complicated titration schedule based on the type of drug interactions anticipated.

TABLE 4-4	Lamotrigine Dosing Recommendations with Other Antiepileptic Drugs	
Concomitant AED	Adults	Pediatrics
Without AED inhibitor/inducer	25–375 mg/day (divide into 2 doses) ^Titrate by 50 mg every 1–2 weeks	0.3–7.5 mg/kg/day, max 300 mg/day (divide into 2 doses)
With AED inhibitor: valproic acid	25 mg every other day to 200 mg/day (divide into 2 doses) ^Titrate by 25–50 mg every 1–2 weeks	0.15–5 mg/kg/day, max 200 mg/day (divide into 1–2 doses)
With AED inducer: carbamazepine phenobarbital phenytoin primidone	50–500 mg/day (divide into 2 doses) ^Titrate by 100 mg every 1–2 weeks	0.6–15 mg/kg/day, max 400 mg/day (divide into 2 doses)

AED, antiepileptic drug.

Source: Lamictal [package insert]. Greenville, NC: *GlaxoSmithKline*, 2010.

Topiramate

Topiramate is associated with a high incidence of central nervous system (CNS) adverse reactions (e.g., headache, somnolence, fatigue, dizziness) and especially severe cognitive impairment that is not typically noted or is not as severe with other AEDs.[14,15] Cognitive impairment includes psychomotor slowing, difficulty with memory, difficulty with concentration/attention, and confusion. These adverse effects are primarily dose related and occur with rapid upward titration of topiramate.[16] Therefore, topiramate should be titrated weekly by 25–50 mg/day to a recommended dose of 200–400 mg/day. Another adverse reaction unique to topiramate therapy is metabolic acidosis due to the inhibition of HCO_3^- production from carbon dioxide. The sulfamate compound found within topiramate's structure is responsible for inhibiting carbonic anhydrase enzymes that are widely distributed in erythrocytes, gastrointestinal tract, eyes, bone, kidneys, lungs, and brain.[17] Inhibition of carbonic anhydrase isozymes II and IV in the proximal and distal renal tubules have been implicated for increasing the risk for calcium phosphate stone formation due to increase in urinary pH and decrease in urinary citrate excretion.[18] On the other hand, its potent inhibition of carbonic anhydrase isozymes II, VB, VII, and XII in the brain is believed to have minor contribution to topiramate's overall anticonvulsant activity.[19]

Although topiramate is primarily eliminated renally as unchanged drug, 30 percent will undergo hydroxylation, hydrolysis, and glucuronidation. Topiramate concentrations are significantly reduced when used concomitantly with phenytoin, carbamazepine, and phenobarbital; therefore, dosing adjustments may be necessary.[20]

Tiagabine

Tiagabine enhances γ-aminobutyric acid (GABA) activity by preventing reuptake of GABA into neurons and glial cells via GABA transporter, GAT-1.[21] As a result, GABA concentrations in the synapse are increased and inhibit neuroexcitation. Tiagabine is associated with CNS-adverse events (e.g., dizziness, asthenia, headache, somnolence, depression, confusion, and diplopia).[22] Tiagabine is associated with cognitive adverse events; however, these events appear to be dose related and are no more frequent than those seen with placebo therapy.[23-25] One major disadvantage of tiagabine is its short half-life, which necessitates administration three to four times daily, especially in the presence of CYP3A enzyme–inducing AEDs, such as carbamazepine, phenobarbital, and phenytoin. Patients receiving concomitant therapy with enzyme-inducing AEDs should have their dose titrated to clinical effect, up to a maximum daily dose of 56 mg/day.[26] Tiagabine was shown to reduce valproic acid concentrations by 10 percent; however, this reduction may not be clinically significant secondary to the broad therapeutic range of valproic acid.[27]

Levetiracetam

The exact mechanism of action of levetiracetam is still yet to be determined. It is apparent that it does not exhibit its antiepileptic properties via the more traditional targets of other AEDs (i.e., inhibition of voltage-gated sodium channels, alterations in GABAergic neurotransmission, etc.).[28,29] It is known to bind to synaptic vesicle protein 2A (SV2A), which is thought to play a role in its efficacy.[29] Levetiracetam is readily distributed in the cerebrospinal fluid (CSF), and its CSF concentration is similar to that of the plasma concentration. Of note, the elimination half-life of levetiracetam is three times longer in the CSF than the plasma.[30] This quality leads to a longer duration of action at the desired site of action and allows for twice daily administration. Levetiracetam is exclusively eliminated extrahepatically. Approximately two-thirds of levetiracetam is eliminated unchanged renally, and one-third is hydrolyzed in the blood to three inactive metabolites. Dose adjustments are thus required in moderate-to-severe renal impairment, including elderly patients and patients requiring hemodialysis. Currently, no dosing recommendations are made for its use in continuous renal replacement therapy due to a lack of pharmacokinetic data. Although levetiracetam is devoid of hepatic metabolism, concomitant administration with enzyme-inducing AEDs (phenobarbital, phenytoin, and carbamazepine) has shown to increase levetiracetam clearance.[31] The clinical significance of these data is yet to be determined, and no dosing adjustment of levetiracetam is currently recommended.

In addition to enteral dosage forms, levetiracetam is also available as an intravenous solution that provides another therapeutic option for critically ill patients, especially those in status epilepticus. Intravenous levetiracetam should be diluted in 100 mL NaCl, Lactated Ringer, or dextrose 5%, and infused over 15 minutes.[32] Various loading doses of levetiracetam have been instituted for the management of status epilepticus in infants, children, and adults. The loading doses ranged from 1,000 mg to 2,500 mg followed by maintenance doses of 2,000–3,000 mg/day in two divided doses.[33,34] Termination of status epilepticus was observed in at least 70 percent of patients receiving levetiracetam within 2 to 24 hours of initiation.[33,35] A loading dose provides faster achievement (within 24 hours) of plasma concentrations comparable to those concentrations seen with maintenance therapy.[30,36] For example, a levetiracetam loading dose of 1,000 mg achieves a similar levetiracetam concentration as compared to a levetiracetam maintenance dose of 500 mg every 12 hours. Adverse events associated with levetiracetam loading doses were mild and included somnolence, confusion, and disorientation.[35,37] Levetiracetam's role and optimal loading dose for status epilepticus is currently unknown because associations between levetiracetam concentrations and its clinical efficacy have not been established. Meanwhile, as the success rate with levetiracetam therapy in status epilepticus may depend on the duration of status epilepticus and the use of other AEDs, levetiracetam should be introduced early as a second- or third-line AED.[37]

Oxcarbazepine

Oxcarbazepine is rapidly reduced by arylketone reductase to its main active metabolite, 10-hydroxycarbazepine or licarbazepine (MHD), which is responsible for its antiepileptic activity.[38] Oxcarbazepine is structurally related to carbamazepine, but unlike its predecessor, oxcarbazepine's metabolism is devoid of producing the carbamazepine epoxide metabolite. This difference improves the pharmacokinetic and side effect profile of oxcarbazepine. For instance, MHD does not undergo autoinduction of its own metabolism. Instead, MHD undergoes glucuronidation to produce inactive metabolites. This step is enhanced by the presence of enzyme-inducing AEDs such as carbamazepine, phenobarbital, and phenytoin; and clinically significant increases in MHD metabolism by 25-40% have been observed.[39] Oxcarbazepine dose may need to be titrated to clinical effect when it is used concomitantly with enzyme-inducing AEDs. Valproic acid does not have a clinically significant effect on oxcarbazepine's metabolism, and no dosing adjustment is recommended. On the other hand, oxcarbazepine doses greater than 1,200 mg/day have been shown to increase phenytoin concentrations by 40 percent.[40] Phenytoin concentrations should be monitored and doses may need to be adjusted to avoid concentrations above the patient's target range and toxicity.

Adverse reactions with oxcarbazepine therapy are similar to that of carbamazepine therapy but with decreased frequency and severity.[41,42] The most notable adverse reactions include dizziness, sedation, fatigue, nausea, drug rash, and hyponatremia.[43,44] Neurological adverse reactions were most commonly noted with high-dose, fast up-titration, or during conversion to oxcarbazepine monotherapy.[45,46] High cross-reactivity of skin rash is observed in patients who are switched from phenytoin or carbamazepine to oxcarbazepine therapy, notably in 25–30 percent of patients with history of previous carbamazepine therapy.[39,41,47,48]

Zonisamide

Zonisamide has a number of potential mechanisms by which it exerts its beneficial effects in the management of epilepsy. It is thought that the effects are primarily due to the alteration in sodium and low-threshold T-type calcium channel activity.[49] Zonisamide has other modes of antiepileptic activities whereby it influences various cycles of neurotransmitter metabolism, but these contributions are minor. The neurotransmitters affected include glutamate, GABA, dopamine, serotonin, and acetylcholine. Zonisamide contains a nonarylamine sulfonamide group and should be used with caution in patients with history of antibiotic/nonantibiotic sulfonamide hypersensitivity.[50] The sulfamoyl group of zonisamide is a weak carbonic anhydrase inhibitor that provides little antiepileptic activity at therapeutic doses.[19] Instead, it has been associated with adverse events such as metabolic acidosis and renal stones. Zonisamide exhibits first-order distribution kinetics at therapeutic doses. However, at supratherapeutic doses of ≥800 mg/day distribution of this agent is greatly altered due to the saturable binding property of zonisamide. At supratherapeutic doses, erythrocytes become saturated with zonisamide and the area under-the-curve (AUC) and maximum concentrations (Cmax) increase disproportionately compared to therapeutic doses.[51] Zonisamide is a substrate of the CYP3A4 isoenzyme but does not induce or inhibit its activity. It is only susceptible to drug interactions with enzyme-inducing AEDs (i.e., carbamazepine, phenobarbital, and phenytoin), whereby the clearance of zonisamide will be enhanced with a subsequent decrease in its half-life.[52] This results in a decreased time to reach steady-state concentrations, allowing for a faster (i.e., less than 2-week) titration schedule and evaluation of efficacy.

Common adverse events associated with zonisamide are primarily dose-related CNS effects, which are manifested when it is titrated too rapidly or when it is initiated at the same time as other AED therapy.[53-56] Oligohidrosis, hyperthermia, and heat stroke have been rarely observed but are more commonly observed in pediatric patients.[57,58] Currently, the safety and efficacy data in the pediatric population in the United States are not well established, so zonisamide's use is limited to adults.[51]

Lacosamide

Lacosamide is a novel agent that selectively enhances slow inactivation of voltage-dependent sodium channels without affecting fast inactivation sodium channels.[59] This novel mechanism elevates resting membrane potential threshold and decreases hyperresponsiveness to neuroexcitation. Lacosamide also binds to collapsin-response mediator protein 2 (CRMP-2), which has been shown to prevent neuronal outgrowth and neuronal cell excitotoxicity and apoptosis.

Adverse events associated with lacosamide therapy are often dose related and include the CNS and gastrointestinal systems.[60] Lacosamide has been associated with a dose-dependent increase in PR interval due to its ability to inhibit cardiac sodium channels. It must be used with caution in patients with underlying heart disease due to this effect.[59-61] Lacosamide is primarily eliminated unchanged renally, but it is partly metabolized via the CYP 2C19 isoenzyme, which produces an inactive O-desmethyl metabolite.[61] Thus, the plasma concentration of lacosamide may be decreased when used concomitantly with enzyme-inducing AEDs (carbamazepine, phenobarbital, and phenytoin). Thus, a dose adjustment of lacosamide may be necessary based on clinical effect. Lacosamide should be adjusted to a maximum dose of 300 mg/day in hepatic and renal

impairment defined as Child-Pugh B and Cl_Cr ≤30 mL/min, respectively. In patients with chronic kidney disease on hemodialysis, a supplemental dose of up to 50 percent after a 4-hour hemodialysis treatment should be considered.

Lacosamide is available in multiple dosage forms, including intravenous solution, which makes it an ideal agent in critically ill and status epilepticus patients.[62] Intravenous lacosamide is well tolerated without serious adverse effects and may be administered undiluted over 15, 30, or 60 minutes.[63] Adverse events associated with intravenous formulations are mild and include injection site discomfort, irritation, and erythema.[61,63] Common adverse events associated with lacosamide therapy are dose-related CNS symptoms that are mild to moderate in severity.[63]

No safety or efficacy studies evaluate the use of lacosamide in children.[61] Due to its effect on neuronal growth via CRMP-2 binding capacity, it has the potential to cause detrimental effects on neuronal development as demonstrated in animal studies. Case reports support its efficacy as an adjunctive therapy for refractory seizures of various types in pediatric patients, but the long-term safety of lacosamide in children still remains to be elucidated.[64,65]

Ezogabine

Ezogabine was recently approved as an add-on treatment for partial onset seizures in the United States on June 14, 2011. It is considered a controlled substance but is yet to be classified. Detailed pharmacokinetic information is yet to be revealed. Most common adverse events associated with ezogabine therapy are dose-related CNS symptoms.[66,67]

CASES

CASE 1: LAMOTRIGINE

Loading Dose

A 50-year-old male, with a history of hypertension, diabetes mellitus type 2, hyperlipidemia, and kidney transplantation five years ago, is recently diagnosed with partial seizure. His medications include tacrolimus, cyclosporine, metoprolol, atorvastatin, and insulin glargine with aspart. The plan was to initiate an AED as monotherapy that does not have significant drug interaction with his antirejection medications. The team decided to initiate lamotrigine. What is the best recommendation for initiation of lamotrigine?

A loading dose of lamotrigine is not recommended as high-dose and fast up-titration has been associated with increased risk for drug rash. Thus, lamotrigine should be titrated over 8 weeks to a maintenance dose of 300 mg/day (see Table 4-4).

Week 1–2: 25 mg/day

Week 3–4: 25 mg every 12 hours (= 50 mg/day)

Week 5: 50 mg every 12 hours (= 100 mg/day)

Week 6: 50 mg every morning and 100 mg every evening (= 150 mg/day)

Week 7: 100 mg every 12 hours (= 200 mg/day)

Week 8: 100 mg every morning and 150 mg every evening (= 250 mg/day)

Week 9: 150 mg every 12 hours (= 300 mg/day)

Drug Interaction That Decreases Levels

A 45-year-old female with a history of partial seizure presents to the epilepsy clinic with complaints of difficulty walking straight, sleepiness, and vision changes. The patient also complains of driving about an hour every month to get her phenytoin concentration checked.

Today, the phenytoin concentration is 27 mcg/mL. Upon further discussion, the plan is to transition her to lamotrigine, because it has reliable absorption, fewer adverse reactions, and does not require therapeutic drug monitoring. What is your dosing recommendation for the titration phase of lamotrigine therapy while the patient remains on phenytoin?

Because phenytoin will increase the metabolism of lamotrigine by approximately 40 percent by inducing glucuronidation, it is recommended to start lamotrigine at a higher dose than what is currently recommended as monotherapy. Thus, lamotrigine should be titrated up by 100 mg weekly over 6 weeks to a maintenance dose of 400 mg/day (see Table 4-4).

Week 1–2: 50 mg/day

Week 3–4: 50 mg every 12 hours (= 100 mg/day)

Week 5: 100 mg every 12 hours (= 200 mg/day)

Week 6: 150 mg every 12 hours (= 300 mg/day)

Week 7: 200 mg every 12 hours (= 400 mg/day)

Once her lamotrigine maintenance dose is achieved, she can begin her phenytoin taper. After the phenytoin is discontinued, a slow decrease in the lamotrigine dose to 300 mg/day over the following 1–2 weeks may be considered.

Drug Interaction That Increases Levels

A 30-year-old female was recently diagnosed with partial seizures. Her past medical history is significant for bipolar disorder, and she is currently being treated with valproic acid. Lamotrigine is to be initiated for the treatment of her seizure disorder. What initial and maintenance lamotrigine doses would you recommended for this patient?

Because valproic acid will inhibit lamotrigine's metabolism by approximately 25 percent, the current recommendation is to decrease the overall dose of lamotrigine by 50 percent and to titrate up by 25–50 mg weekly to a maintenance dose of 200 mg/day (see Table 4-4).

Week 1–2: 25 mg every other day

Week 3–4: 25 mg/day

Week 5: 25 mg every 12 hours (= 50 mg/day)

Week 6: 50 mg every 12 hours (= 100 mg/day)

Week 7: 50 mg every morning and 100 mg every evening (= 150 mg/day)

Week 8: 100 mg every 12 hours (= 200 mg/day)

Dosing in Renal Dysfunction

A 58-year-old female (weight: 65 kg, height 5'5") with history of hypertension, partial seizure, diabetes mellitus type 2, and chronic kidney disease (baseline serum creatinine (SCr) 1.5 mg/dL) presents with severe chest pain and is being evaluated for myocardial infarction. The patient received iodinated contrast in order to undergo a left-heart catheterization to visualize the cardiac vessels. In the next 24 hours, her urine output decreased from 100 mL/hr to 20 mL/hr and her SCr increased to 2.7 mg/dL. Her medications include metoprolol 100 mg every 12 hours, lamotrigine 150 mg every 12 hours, and insulin glargine 25 units every night at bedtime. How would you adjust the lamotrigine dose for reduced renal function?

Lamotrigine is primarily converted to inactive metabolites by glucuronidation and only 10 percent of lamotrigine is eliminated unchanged. Although the half-life of lamotrigine is increased in patients with reduced creatinine clearance, its clinical significance is minimal and overall lamotrigine plasma concentrations are not greatly affected. Thus, dosing adjustments are not required in patients with reduced renal function (see Table 4-1).

Continue lamotrigine 150 mg every 12 hours.

Dosing in Hemodialysis

A 45-year-old male with history of hypertension, diabetes, chronic kidney disease, congestive heart failure, dyslipidemia, panic disorder, and partial seizures recently was placed on the kidney transplantation list and was initiated on hemodialysis (every Monday, Wednesday, and Friday). One of his medications is lamotrigine 150 mg every 12 hours for seizure management. What is your recommendation for lamotrigine dosing adjustment in this patient undergoing hemodialysis?

Hemodialysis removes approximately 20 percent of the plasma concentration of lamotrigine. However, it is not clinically significant, and routine administration of a supplemental dose after hemodialysis is not required at this time (see Table 4-1).

Continue lamotrigine 150 mg every 12 hours.

Dosing in Hepatic Dysfunction

A 50-year-old male with history of alcoholic cirrhosis with ascites is admitted to the medical intensive care unit service with altered mental status including dizziness and blurry vision. Upon further evaluation, the patient reports he is taking lamotrigine 150 mg every 12 hours for partial seizures. What is your recommendation for adjusting his lamotrigine dose?

Due to decreased lamotrigine metabolism in patients with hepatic dysfunction, the dose should be decreased by 25 percent in moderate-to-severe liver impairment without ascites and by 50 percent in severe liver impairment with ascites (see Table 4-1).

Lamotrigine dose should be decreased to 75 mg every 12 hours.

CASE 2: LEVETIRACETAM

Loading Dose

A 60-year-old male with a witnessed generalized tonic-clonic seizure was transferred from a local community hospital for the management of a large subdural hematoma and seizure. The patient was loaded with phenytoin 1,000 mg IV at the community hospital. Upon arrival, the patient was immediately taken to the operating room for evacuation of the hematoma. On post-op day 1, the patient was noted to have twitching of his left cheek rhythmically and EEG was ordered to evaluate for seizures. The patient received two 4 mg doses of lorazepam IV within the next 15 minutes without successful termination of seizure activity on EEG. A total phenytoin level was drawn and reported to be 19 mcg/mL. The plan was to initiate a second antiepileptic agent, and levetiracetam was chosen due to its benign adverse reaction profile, low potential for drug interactions, and the availability of multiple formulations including an intravenous solution. The patient weighs 85 kg. What would be the best dosing recommendation for levetiracetam in this patient?

Levetiracetam loading doses of 1,000 mg to 3,000 mg have been used in status epilepticus with minimal complications. However, no well-controlled trials currently support one levetiracetam loading dose over another for termination of status epilepticus. As the patient is in status epilepticus, intravenous levetiracetam should be used to achieve a therapeutic concentration immediately. Therefore, a loading dose of 1,000–3,000 mg IV over 15 minutes would be a reasonable recommendation.

Maintenance dose using population pharmacokinetics

As this patient is in status epilepticus, the maximum established maintenance dose of 1,500 mg every 12 hours should be initiated.

Drug Interaction That Decreases Levels

The patient is already receiving phenytoin, which is a known enzyme-inducing AED. Does the levetiracetam dose need to be adjusted?

No, levetiracetam is primarily eliminated renally as unchanged drug and does not undergo any hepatic metabolism. Thus, no drug interaction occurs and no adjustments need to be made.

Dosing in Renal Dysfunction

HL, an 85-year-old female with a large left subdural hematoma and acute renal failure (SCr 2 mg/dL), was admitted to the neuroscience intensive care unit for further observation. No neurosurgical intervention is planned for the patient. Of note, the patient's past medical history includes congestive heart failure, hypertension, coronary artery disease, depression, dementia, and emphysema. She weighs 60 kg. Due to her multiple medical conditions and age, levetiracetam was initiated for seizure prophylaxis. What is the best dosing recommendation for HL?

Levetiracetam is primarily eliminated renally and should be adjusted in renally impaired patients, especially in elderly patients, to avoid unwanted CNS adverse effects. Because this patient's Cl_{Cr} is 19 mL/min, a levetiracetam dose of 250 mg tablet by mouth every 12 hours would be recommended.

Dosing in Hemodialysis

The patient, HL, is showing signs and symptoms of progressive renal dysfunction and is now anuric, with shortness of breath and crackles in both lungs, and is started on 4 L supplemental oxygen. Her chest X-ray shows pulmonary edema due to fluid overload. The renal service is consulted for an emergent hemodialysis session. Does the levetiracetam dose need to be adjusted for hemodialysis?

The clearance of levetiracetam is reduced by 70 percent in anuric patients, but 50 percent of it is removed during 4-hour hemodialysis. Thus, her dose of levetiracetam would need to be adjusted. Initiate 500 mg administered every 24 hours with a supplemental dose of 250 mg given after each hemodialysis session.

Dosing in Hepatic Dysfunction

A 45-year-old male with an extensive alcohol history is admitted with a traumatic intracerebral hemorrhage. The patient has signs of hepatic dysfunction including jaundice, a platelet count of 89,000, and an INR of 3. Levetiracetam is to be initiated for seizure prophylaxis over the next seven days. What dose should be recommended?

Levetiracetam does not undergo liver metabolism, but approximately 30 percent is hydrolyzed to inactive metabolites. Thus, levetiracetam does not need to be reduced in hepatic dysfunction unless the patient also has compromised renal function. A levetiracetam dose of 500 mg every 12 hours is reasonable for short-term seizure prophylaxis.

CASE 3: TOPIRAMATE

Loading dose

A 30-year-old female with history of migraines was initiated on topiramate 25 mg every night at bedtime for migraine prophylaxis. She was involved in a motor vehicle crash and sustained a head trauma. Approximately 10 months after the crash, the patient developed seizures. Topiramate will be continued for the management of migraines and seizures. What new maintenance dose would you recommend for this patient?

A topiramate loading dose is not recommended due to dose-related CNS adverse reactions, including cognitive impairment.

Maintenance Dose Using Population Pharmacokinetics

In order to minimize adverse CNS effects, topiramate should be titrated slowly over 6 weeks to a maintenance dose of up to 400 mg/day.

Week 1: 25 mg every 12 hours

Week 2: 50 mg every 12 hours

Week 3: 75 mg every 12 hours

Week 4: 100 mg every 12 hours

Week 5: 150 mg every 12 hours

Week 6 and after: 200 mg every 12 hours

Drug Interaction That Decreases Levels

After three months of topiramate therapy, RV presents to the neurology clinic with complains of five seizures per week. Phenytoin is added as a second AED for further seizure control. Does the topiramate dose need to be adjusted?

Phenytoin is known to induce the hepatic metabolism of topiramate and decrease its plasma concentration by approximately 48 percent. Therefore, the dose of topiramate should be increased empirically over the next few weeks up to 400 mg every 12 hours and further titrated based on clinical effect.

Drug Interaction That Increases Levels

If RV was started on valproic acid instead of phenytoin as concomitant therapy with topiramate, would the topiramate dose need to be adjusted?

Valproic acid has been reported to decrease topiramate concentrations by 10–15 percent but without any clinical significance. Therefore, topiramate dose does not need to be adjusted and topiramate can be continued at 200 mg every 12 hours.

Dosing in Renal Dysfunction (No Hemodialysis)

JM, a 40-year-old female with chronic kidney disease (baseline SCr 1.5 mg/dL) and hypertension, is newly diagnosed with partial seizures, and topiramate was recommended by a neurologist. She weighs 65 kg. What is the dose recommendation for topiramate in this patient with Cl_{Cr} of 51 mL/min?

The majority (70%) of topiramate is eliminated renally as unchanged drug, and its clearance is reduced by 42 percent in patients with moderate renal impairment (Cl_{Cr} 30–69 mL/min) and 54 percent in patients with severe renal impairment (Cl_{Cr} <30 mL/min). Thus, it is recommended to reduce the dose by 50 percent in patients with renal impairment with Cl_{Cr} <70 mL/min.

Week 1: 25 mg every daily

Week 2: 25 mg every 12 hours

Week 3: 50 mg every 12 hours

Week 4: 75 mg every 12 hours

Week 5 and after: 100 mg every 12 hours

Dosing in Hemodialysis

How would you adjust the dose if JM's renal function progressively worsened requiring three times weekly hemodialysis?

Topiramate is removed by hemodialysis and its plasma concentration is reduced by 50 percent. Therefore, a supplemental dose of 100 mg is recommended after each hemodialysis session for this patient.

REFERENCES

1. Asconape JJ. The selection of antiepileptic drugs for the treatment of epilepsy in children and adults. *Neurol Clin.* 2010;28:843–852.
2. Johannessen SI, Tomson T. Pharmacokinetic variability of newer antiepileptic drugs: When is monitoring needed? *Clin Pharmacokinet.* 2006;45:1061–1075.

3. Dieckhaus CM, Thompson CD, Roller SG, Macdonald TL. Mechanisms of idiosyncratic drug reactions: The case of felbamate. *Chem Biol Interact.* 2002;142:99–117.

4. Hooper WD, Franklin ME, Glue P, et al. Effect of felbamate on valproic acid disposition in healthy volunteers: Inhibition of beta-oxidation. *Epilepsia.* 1996;37:91–97.

5. Reidenberg P, Glue P, Banfield CR, et al. Effects of felbamate on the pharmacokinetics of phenobarbital. *Clin Pharmacol Ther.* 1995;58:279–287.

6. Sachdeo R, Wagner ML, Sachdeo S, et al. Coadministration of phenytoin and felbamate: Evidence of additional phenytoin dose-reduction requirements based on pharmacokinetics and tolerability with increasing doses of felbamate. *Epilepsia.* 1999;40:1122–1128.

7. Wagner ML, Remmel RP, Graves NM, Leppik IE. Effect of felbamate on carbamazepine and its major metabolites. *Clin Pharmacol Ther.* 1993;53:536–543.

8. Albani F, Theodore WH, Washington P, et al. Effect of felbamate on plasma levels of carbamazepine and its metabolites. *Epilepsia.* 1991;32:130–132.

9. Bockbrader HN, Wesche D, Miller R, Chapel S, Janiczek N, Burger P. A comparison of the pharmacokinetics and pharmacodynamics of pregabalin and gabapentin. *Clin Pharmacokinet.* 2010;49:661–669.

10. Delahoy P, Thompson S, Marschner IC. Pregabalin versus gabapentin in partial epilepsy: A meta-analysis of dose-response relationships. *BMC Neurol.* 2010;10:104.

11. Lyrica [package insert]. New York: Pfizer, Inc., 2009.

12. Neurontin [package insert]. New York: Parke-Davis Division of Pfizer Inc., 2010.

13. Messenheimer J, Mullens EL, Giorgi L, Young F. Safety review of adult clinical trial experience with lamotrigine. *Drug Saf.* 1998;18:281–296.

14. Bootsma HP, Ricker L, Hekster YA, et al. The impact of side effects on long-term retention in three new antiepileptic drugs. *Seizure.* 2009;18:327–331.

15. Kennedy GM, Lhatoo SD. CNS adverse events associated with antiepileptic drugs. *CNS Drugs.* 2008;22:739–760.

16. Ben-Menachem E, Henriksen O, Dam M, et al. Double-blind, placebo-controlled trial of topiramate as add-on therapy in patients with refractory partial seizures. *Epilepsia.* 1996;37:539–543.

17. Supuran CT. Carbonic anhydrases: An overview. *Curr Pharm Des.* 2008;14:603–614.

18. Welch BJ, Graybeal D, Moe OW, Maalouf NM, Sakhaee K. Biochemical and stone-risk profiles with topiramate treatment. *Am J Kidney Dis.* 2006;48:555–563.

19. Thiry A, Dogne JM, Supuran CT, Masereel B. Anticonvulsant sulfonamides/sulfamates/sulfamides with carbonic anhydrase inhibitory activity: Drug design and mechanism of action. *Curr Pharm Des.* 2008;14:661–671.

20. May TW, Rambeck B, Jurgens U. Serum concentrations of topiramate in patients with epilepsy: Influence of dose, age, and comedication. *Ther Drug Monit.* 2002;24:366–374.

21. Adkins JC, Noble S. Tiagabine. A review of its pharmacodynamic and pharmacokinetic properties and therapeutic potential in the management of epilepsy. *Drugs.* 1998;55:437–460.

22. Kalviainen R. Long-term safety of tiagabine. *Epilepsia.* 2001;42(Suppl 3):46–48.

23. Uthman BM, Rowan AJ, Ahmann PA, et al. Tiagabine for complex partial seizures: A randomized, add-on, dose-response trial. *Arch Neurol.* 1998;55:56–62.

24. Aikia M, Jutila L, Salmenpera T, Mervaala E, Kalviainen R. Comparison of the cognitive effects of tiagabine and carbamazepine as monotherapy in newly diagnosed adult patients with partial epilepsy: Pooled analysis of two long-term, randomized, follow-up studies. *Epilepsia.* 2006;47:1121–1127.

25. Kalviainen R, Aikia M, Mervaala E, Saukkonen AM, Pitkanen A, Riekkinen PJ, Sr. Long-term cognitive and EEG effects of tiagabine in drug-resistant partial epilepsy. *Epilepsy Res.* 1996;25:291–297.

26. Gabitril [package insert]. Frazer, PA: Cephalon, Inc., 2010.

27. Gustavson LE, Sommerville KW, Boellner SW, Witt GF, Guenther HJ, Granneman GR. Lack of a clinically significant pharmacokinetic drug interaction between tiagabine and valproate. *Am J Ther.* 1998;5:73–79.

28. Keppra oral [package insert]. Smyrna, GA: UBC, Inc., 2009.

29. Keppra IV [package insert]. Smyrna, GA: UCB, Inc., 2010.

30. Meehan AL, Yang X, McAdams BD, Yuan L, Rothman SM. A new mechanism for antiepileptic drug action: Vesicular entry may mediate the effects of levetiracetam. *J Neurophysiol.* 2011;106:1227–1239.

31. Patsalos PN. Clinical pharmacokinetics of levetiracetam. *Clin Pharmacokinet.* 2004;43:707–724.

32. Hirsch LJ, Arif H, Buchsbaum R, et al. Effect of age and comedication on levetiracetam pharmacokinetics and tolerability. *Epilepsia.* 2007;48:1351–1359.

33. Gamez-Leyva G, Aristin JL, Fernandez E, Pascual J. Experience with intravenous levetiracetam in status epilepticus: A retrospective case series. *CNS Drugs.* 2009;23:983–987.

34. Fattouch J, Di Bonaventura C, Casciato S, et al. Intravenous levetiracetam as first-line treatment of status epilepticus in the elderly. *Acta Neurol Scand.* 2010;121:418–421.

35. Uges JW, van Huizen MD, Engelsman J, et al. Safety and pharmacokinetics of intravenous levetiracetam infusion as add-on in status epilepticus. *Epilepsia.* 2009;50:415–421.

36. Wheless JW, Clarke D, Hovinga CA, et al. Rapid infusion of a loading dose of intravenous levetiracetam with minimal dilution: A safety study. *J Child Neurol.* 2009;24:946–951.

37. Aiguabella M, Falip M, Villanueva V, et al. Efficacy of intravenous levetiracetam as an add-on treatment in status epilepticus: A multicentric observational study. *Seizure.* 2011;20:60–64.

38. May TW, Korn-Merker E, Rambeck B. Clinical pharmacokinetics of oxcarbazepine. *Clin Pharmacokinet.* 2003;42:1023–1042.

39. Trileptal [package insert]. East Hanover, NJ: Novartis Pharmaceuticals Corporation, 2011.

40. Barcs G, Walker EB, Elger CE, et al. Oxcarbazepine placebo-controlled, dose-ranging trial in refractory partial epilepsy. *Epilepsia.* 2000;41:1597–1607.

41. Marson AG, Al-Kharusi AM, Alwaidh M, et al. The SANAD study of effectiveness of carbamazepine, gabapentin, lamotrigine, oxcarbazepine, or topiramate for treatment of partial epilepsy: An unblinded randomised controlled trial. *Lancet.* 2007;369:1000–1015.

42. Koch MW, Polman SK. Oxcarbazepine versus carbamazepine monotherapy for partial onset seizures. *Cochrane Database Syst Rev.* 2009:CD006453.

43. Friis ML, Kristensen O, Boas J, et al. Therapeutic experiences with 947 epileptic outpatients in oxcarbazepine treatment. *Acta Neurol Scand.* 1993;87:224–227.

44. Buggy Y, Layton D, Fogg C, Shakir SA. Safety profile of oxcarbazepine: Results from a prescription-event monitoring study. *Epilepsia.* 2010;51:818–829.

45. Martinez W, Ingenito A, Blakeslee M, Barkley GL, McCague K, D'Souza J. Efficacy, safety, and tolerability of oxcarbazepine monotherapy. *Epilepsy Behav.* 2006;9:448–456.

46. Schachter SC, Vazquez B, Fisher RS, et al. Oxcarbazepine: Double-blind, randomized, placebo-control, monotherapy trial for partial seizures. *Neurology.* 1999;52:732–737.

47. Alvestad S, Lydersen S, Brodtkorb E. Cross-reactivity pattern of rash from current aromatic antiepileptic drugs. *Epilepsy Res.* 2008;80:194–200.

48. Hirsch LJ, Arif H, Nahm EA, Buchsbaum R, Resor SR, Jr., Bazil CW. Cross-sensitivity of skin rashes with antiepileptic drug use. *Neurology.* 2008;71:1527–1534.

49. Biton V. Clinical pharmacology and mechanism of action of zonisamide. *Clin Neuropharmacol.* 2007;30:230–240.

50. Baulac M. Introduction to zonisamide. *Epilepsy Res.* 2006;68(Suppl 2):S3–S9.

51. Zonegran [package insert]. Woodcliff Lake, NJ: Eisai Inc., 2010.

52. Sills G, Brodie M. Pharmacokinetics and drug interactions with zonisamide. *Epilepsia.* 2007;48:435–441.

53. Sackellares JC, Ramsay RE, Wilder BJ, Browne TR, Shellenberger MK. Randomized, controlled clinical trial of zonisamide as adjunctive treatment for refractory partial seizures. *Epilepsia.* 2004;45:610–617.

54. Brodie MJ, Duncan R, Vespignani H, Solyom A, Bitenskyy V, Lucas C. Dose-dependent safety and efficacy of zonisamide: A randomized, double-blind, placebo-controlled study in patients with refractory partial seizures. *Epilepsia.* 2005;46:31–41.

55. Zaccara G, Gangemi PF, Cincotta M. Central nervous system adverse effects of new antiepileptic drugs. A meta-analysis of placebo-controlled studies. *Seizure.* 2008;17:405–421.

56. Ohtahara S, Yamatogi Y. Safety of zonisamide therapy: Prospective follow-up survey. *Seizure.* 2004;13(Suppl 1):S50–55; discussion S6.

57. Ohtahara S. Zonisamide in the management of epilepsy—Japanese experience. *Epilepsy Res.* 2006;68(Suppl 2):S25–S33.

58. Knudsen JF, Thambi LR, Kapcala LP, Racoosin JA. Oligohydrosis and fever in pediatric patients treated with zonisamide. *Pediatr Neurol.* 2003;28:184–189.

59. Beyreuther BK, Freitag J, Heers C, Krebsfanger N, Scharfenecker U, Stohr T. Lacosamide: A review of preclinical properties. *CNS Drug Rev.* 2007;13:21–42.

60. Ben-Menachem E, Biton V, Jatuzis D, Abou-Khalil B, Doty P, Rudd GD. Efficacy and safety of oral lacosamide as adjunctive therapy in adults with partial-onset seizures. *Epilepsia.* 2007;48:1308–1317.

61. Vimpat [package insert]. Smyrna, GA: UCB, Inc., 2010.

62. Kellinghaus C, Berning S, Immisch I, et al. Intravenous lacosamide for treatment of status epilepticus. *Acta Neurol Scand.* 2011;123: 137–141.

63. Krauss G, Ben-Menachem E, Mameniskiene R, et al. Intravenous lacosamide as short-term replacement for oral lacosamide in partial-onset seizures. *Epilepsia.* 2010;51:951–957.

64. Shiloh-Malawsky Y, Fan Z, Greenwood R, Tennison M. Successful treatment of childhood prolonged refractory status epilepticus with lacosamide. *Seizure.* 2011;7:586–588.

65. Guilhoto LM, Loddenkemper T, Gooty VD, et al. Experience with lacosamide in a series of children with drug-resistant focal epilepsy. *Pediatr Neurol.* 2011;44:414–419.

66. French JA, Abou-Khalil BW, Leroy RF, et al. Randomized, double-blind, placebo-controlled trial of ezogabine (retigabine) in partial epilepsy. *Neurology.* 2011;76:1555–1563.

67. Brodie MJ, Lerche H, Gil-Nagel A, et al. Efficacy and safety of adjunctive ezogabine (retigabine) in refractory partial epilepsy. *Neurology.* 2010;75:1817–1824.

68. Felbatol [package insert]. Somerset, NJ: MEDA Pharmaceuticals, 2008.

69. Lamictal [package insert]. Greenville, NC: GlaxoSmithKline, 2010.

70. Topamax [package insert]. Titusville, NJ: Ortho-McNeil-Janssen Pharmaceuticals, Inc., 2009.

71. Plosker GL, Scott LJ. Retigabine: In partial seizures. *CNS Drugs.* 2006;20:601–608; discussion 9–10.

72. Abou-Khalil B. Benefit-risk assessment of levetiracetam in the treatment of partial seizures. *Drug Saf.* 2005;28:871–890.

73. Garnett WR. Clinical pharmacology of topiramate: *Chem Biol Interact.* A review. *Epilepsia.* 2000;41(Suppl 1):S61–65.

74. Johannessen Landmark C, Johannessen SI. Pharmacological management of epilepsy: Recent advances and future prospects. *Drugs.* 2008; 68:1925–1939.

75. Glue P, Banfield CR, Perhach JL, Mather GG, Racha JK, Levy RH. Pharmacokinetic interactions with felbamate. In vitro-in vivo correlation. *Clin Pharmacokinet.* 1997;33:214–224.

76. Gidal BE, Radulovic LL, Kruger S, Rutecki P, Pitterle M, Bockbrader HN. Inter- and intra-subject variability in gabapentin absorption and absolute bioavailability. *Epilepsy Res.* 2000;40:123–127.

77. Ragueneau-Majlessi I, Levy RH, Brodie M, Smith D, Shah J, Grundy JS. Lack of pharmacokinetic interactions between steady-state zonisamide and valproic acid in patients with epilepsy. *Clin Pharmacokinet.* 2005;44: 517–523.

CHAPTER 5

Carbamazepine

HENRY COHEN, MS, PharmD, FCCM, BCPP, CGP

Carbamazepine was first indicated and marketed for trigeminal neuralgia and was later found to be an effective antiepileptic.[1] Carbamazepine is a broad-spectrum antiepileptic drug (AED) and is indicated for partial seizures with complex symptomatology (psychomotor, temporal lobe), generalized tonic-clonic seizures (grand mal), and mixed seizure patterns.[2,3] Extended-release carbamazepine is also indicated alone or in combination with other antipsychotic agents for acute manic or mixed episodes associated with bipolar 1 disorder either as treatment or prevention.[4] Carbamazepine may be used as an adjunct for the symptomatic management of the acute phase of schizophrenia in patients who are refractory to antipsychotics.[4] Carbamazepine has also been used for the management of restless leg syndrome, peripheral neuropathy, diabetic peripheral neuropathy, and posttraumatic stress disorders.[3,4]

THERAPEUTIC AND TOXIC PLASMA CONCENTRATIONS

The therapeutic serum level for carbamazepine is 4–12 mg/L. Central nervous system (CNS) adverse effects such as drowsiness, dizziness, and headaches, increase when levels are greater than 8 mg/L.[5] Carbamazepine exhibits concentration related toxicity, serum levels of 11–15 mg/L are associated with somnolence, nystagmus, and ataxia; levels of 15–25 mg/L are associated with combativeness, hallucinations, and chorea; and levels greater than 25 mg/L are associated with seizures and coma. In order to minimize carbamazepine CNS adverse effects, clinicians may target a therapeutic serum level of 4–8 mg/L.[6]

ADVERSE EFFECTS

Carbamazepine causes gastrointestinal adverse effects such as nausea, vomiting, and anorexia.[4] Carbamazepine has mild anticholinergic properties and occasionally can cause xerostomia.[4] Carbamazepine may cause bradycardia in the elderly, and patients over 50 years of age should have a baseline electrocardiogram completed prior to use.[8-10] Conversely, in young patients, toxic carbamazepine levels will manifest with tachycardia.[8-10] Carbamazepine may cause osteoporosis and elevated alkaline phosphatases are common with its use.[11] Carbamazepine is hepatotoxic, and liver enzyme tests and liver function tests should be monitored at baseline and periodically.[3,4]

Carbamazepine is known to cause blood dyscrasias including aplastic anemia, agranulocytosis, leukopenia, thrombocytopenia, anemias, and pancytopenia.[4] A boxed warning for carbamazepine-induced aplastic anemia and agranulocytosis exists due to a risk five to eight times greater than in the general population. However, the risk of these reactions in the general population is low, approximately six patients per 1 million population per year for agranulocytosis and two patients per 1 million population per year for aplastic anemia.[7] Carbamazepine should be discontinued when the white blood cell count is less than 2,500/mm³ or the absolute neutrophil count is less than 1,000/mm.[3,7] Most patients who develop leukopenia do not progress to aplastic anemia or agranulocytosis.

Carbamazepine has been known to cause the antiepileptic drug (AED) hypersensitivity syndrome and is contraindicated due to cross-reactivity with other aromatic anticonvulsant agents that may also cause the AED hypersensitivity syndrome such oxcarbazepine, phenytoin, phenobarbital, zonisamide, lamotrigine, lacosamide, and felbamate.[12,13] Carbamazepine-induced Steven Johnson syndrome (SJS) and toxic epidermal necrolysis syndrome (TENS) occur in 1–6 per 100,000 in Caucasians, but the incidence increases to 10-fold higher in Asians. A lymphocyte toxicity assay can be used to determine patients at high risk of carbamazepine-induced SJS/TENS or the AED hypersensitivity syndrome.[7] Asians and South Asian Indians are at high risk of developing SJS/TENS because they have the human leukocyte antigen (HLA) allele. HLA-B*1502 genotype screening should be completed prior to carbamazepine administration, and only after a negative test should carbamazepine be administered. Patients from any ethnicity who have been on carbamazepine for several months without developing skin reactions are at low risk of developing SJS/TENS.[7]

Carbamazepine is known to cause hyponatremia and the syndrome of inappropriate diuretic hormone (SIADH).[14] SIADH may present with nausea and vomiting, depression, confusion, lethargy, and seizures. Because carbamazepine is indicated for the treatment of bipolar disorders and seizures, patients with an acute exacerbations of depression, psychosis, or seizures should have their serum sodium analyzed. SIADH presents with serum hyponatremia and hypoosmolality and urinary hypernatremia and hyperosmolality.[15] Many patients can be maintained on carbamazepine with mild hyponatremia. These patients are asymptomatic with serum sodium levels above 130 mEq/L.

CARBAMAZEPINE-10,11-EPOXIDE

Carbamazepine-10,11-epoxide (CBZE) is the active metabolite of carbamazepine is both antiepileptic and neurotoxic.[16,17] Carbamazepine-10,11-epoxide is 50 percent plasma protein bound.[18] The carbamazepine to CBZE ratios for patients on monotherapy defined as not receiving any other cytochrome (CYP)-450 hepatic enzyme inducing AEDs is 0.1–0.25 and increases with polytherapy defined as receiving a CYP-450 hepatic enzyme inducing AED to 0.25–0.5.[19] Hence, with carbamazepine monotherapy, a patient with a carbamazepine serum level of 10 mg/L would have a CBZE serum level between 0.1–0.25 mg/L. A patient with a carbamazepine serum level of 10 mg/L while on polytherapy (e.g., phenytoin) would have a CBZE serum level of 2.5–5 mg/L. Carbamazepine-epoxide neurotoxicity has been noted with carbamazepine to CBZE ratios exceeding 0.35 and CBZE serum levels greater than 2 mg/L.[16-17,19] Patients exhibiting carbamazepine toxicity but have normal carbamazepine serum levels should have their CBZE serum level assessed for causality.

BIOAVAILABILITY

The bioavailability of carbamazepine immediate-release tablets, chewable tablets, oral suspension, and extended-release tablets is 80–90 percent.[3,4] In order to determine carbamazepine dosing regimens, 80 percent (F = 0.8) is used as the bioavailability of carbamazepine. The bioavailability of the extended-release Tegretol®-XR when comparing it to the bioavailability of carbamazepine suspension is 89 percent.[3] Hence, 100 mg of the carbamazepine suspension is equal to 112 mg carbamazepine XR. When switching from carbamazepine suspension to carbamazepine extended-release, the bioavailability factor is 0.71 (F = 0.71). No bioavailability data compares carbamazepine tablets to the XR dosage form; hence, the 80 percent is the bioavailability that should be used (F = 0.8). The salt factors for all carbamazepine dosage forms are 1.

VOLUME OF DISTRIBUTION

The volume of distribution of carbamazepine is 1.4 L/kg based on actual body weight, but can range from 0.8–2.0 L/kg.[20] In order to dose carbamazepine accurately, the volume of distribution of carbamazepine should be adjusted in hypovolemic or hypervolemic states. The T_{max} for the immediate-release tablets is 4–5 hours, for the suspension 1–2 hours, for the extended-release tablets is 3–12 hours, and for the extended-release capsules is 4–8 hours.[4] Carbamazepine is 70–80 percent plasma protein bound primarily to albumin and to a lesser extent to alpha-1 acid glycoproteins.[18] Albumin concentrations may decrease with age and in diabetes mellitus, leading to higher free carbamazepine serum levels. Alpha-1 acid glycoproteins are acute phase reactant proteins that increase during stress scenarios such as inflammation and myocardial infarction—leading to lower free carbamazepine serum levels. Carbamazepine undergoes diurnal fluctuations which may be caused by alterations in protein binding.[21]

HALF-LIFE ($T_{1/2}$)

The initial half-life of carbamazepine is 25–30 hours, and its clearance is 0.02 L/kg/hr.[22] Carbamazepine induces its own metabolism and undergoes the phenomenon of *auto-induction*.[23,24] Carbamazepine autoinduction is illustrated by the reduction in carbamazepine half-life from 25–30 hours at single doses to 12 hours at steady state. The carbamazepine half-life with *polytherapy* is reduced even further to 6–8 hours.[23,25] The carbamazepine clearance in monotherapy is 0.064 L/hr/kg and in polytherapy it is 0.1 L/hr/kg.[18,23]

CLEARANCE

Carbamazepine is metabolized predominantly via CYP3A4 and to a lesser extent via CYP2C8 to the active and neurotoxic metabolite carbamazepine-10,11-epoxide.[18] Carbamazepine-10,11-epoxide is metabolized by epoxide hydrolase to the inactive metabolite carbamazepine diol.[23] The CYP450 inhibitors will inhibit hepatic metabolism of carbamazepine and increase carbamazepine serum concentrations. A list of CYP3A4 inhibitors is depicted in Table 5-1. The CYP3A4 inducers will increase hepatic metabolism of carbamazepine and decrease carbamazepine serum concentrations. A list of CYP450 and CYP3A4 inducers is depicted in Table 5-2.

DIURNAL FLUCTUATIONS

Diurnal fluctuations generally occur in 40 percent of patients receiving carbamazepine with dosing three times a day, and the fluctuations increase to 75 percent with polytherapy.[21] Diurnal fluctuations may be due to changes in carbamazepine protein binding, changes in metabolism, and carbamazepine's mild anticholinergic effects that decrease absorption from the gastrointestinal tract. Carbamazepine may undergo Michaelis-Menten pharmacokinetic absorption. Due to the diurnal fluctuations the carbamazepine

TABLE 5-1	List of CYP3A4 Inhibitors
1. Grapefruit juice, red wine	
2. Quinine, tonic water (weak)	
3. Amiodarone	
4. Dronedarone	
5. Diltiazem	
6. Verapamil	
7. Clarithromycin	
8. Erythromycin	
9. Troleandomycin	
10. Fluconazole	
11. Ketoconazole	
12. Itraconazole	
13. Voriconazole	
14. Miconazole IV	
15. Metronidazole (weak)	
16. Fluoxetine	
17. Fluvoxamine	
18. Nefazodone	
19. Sertraline (weak)	
20. Indinavir	
21. Tipranavir	
22. Nelfinavir	
23. Fosamprenavir	
24. Ritonavir	
25. Atazanavir	
26. Saquinavir	
27. Darunavir	
28. Cimetidine	
29. Omeprazole (weak)	
30. Zafirlukast (weak)	
31. Isoniazid (weak)	

TABLE 5-2	List of CYP450 Inducers	
Universal Inducers (1A2, 2C9, 2C19, 3A4)		**Specific CYP3A4 Inducers**
1. Phenytoin		1. Dexamethasone
2. Carbamazepine		2. Nevirapine (Viramune)
3. Phenobarbital		
4. Primidone		**Weak–Moderate CYP3A4 Inducers**
5. Rifampin		1. Etravirine (Intelence®)
6. Rifabutin		2. Modafinil (Provigil®)
7. St. John's wort		3. Pioglitazone (Actos®)
		4. Topiramate
		5. Bosentan (Tracleer®)
		6. Dexamethasone

serum levels accompanied by CNS toxicity may increase gradually throughout the day. In order to minimize the effects of diurnal fluctuations, consider administering the highest doses of carbamazepine at bedtime or use a longer dosing interval prior to the evening dose, or use an extended-release dosage form. When monitoring for toxicity, diurnal fluctuations may limit the clinician's ability to rely on one single level that is not taken at the time of toxic manifestations.

DOSING

The approved dosing for carbamazepine prompt or extended-release in adults and children over 12 years of age is 200 mg twice daily or 100 mg four times a day as suspension.[7] The carbamazepine dose should be increased up to 200 mg/day at weekly intervals to a usual dose of 800–1,200 mg/day.[4] The immediate-release tablets are dosed three to four times a day. The usual dose for bipolar disorders is up to 1,600 mg/day. The usual dose for neuropathic pain is 400–800 mg/day.[3]

LOADING DOSES

Traditionally, carbamazepine was not loaded due to significant gastrointestinal and CNS adverse effects. However, a comprehensive review of loading dose studies yields either no adverse effects, only gastrointestinal side effects or only CNS adverse effects, and in many cases the adverse effects were tolerable.[1,26-29] Rapid carbamazepine loading can be achieved with the suspension dosage form, and a "therapeutic" serum level of 4 mg/dl can be achieved within 1–2 hours; the serum level will continue to rise over the next 4–8 hours. Carbamazepine can be loaded with 8 mg/kg in monotherapy followed by the maintenance dose in 12 hours and a higher dose of 10 mg/kg with polytherapy followed by the maintenance dose in 8 hours.[30] Loading doses of carbamazepine allow for the fastest oral loading of any AED including phenytoin (6–10 hours) and valproate (1–2 days).[31]

CARBAMAZEPINE DOSAGE FORMS

Carbamazepine is not available as an intravenous or parenteral dosage form; it can only be administered enterally. Carbamazepine is available as an immediate-release dosage form in 100 mg chewable tablets and 200 mg scored tablets that can be divided in half.[4] The immediate-release dosage form is designed to be administered two times a day when initiating therapy and

three or four times a day for maintenance doses. Moisture significantly reduces the potency of carbamazepine tablets; hence carbamazepine must be stored in tightly closed or sealed vials and bottles.[32] Carbamazepine suspension achieves a higher C_{max} and faster T_{max} than the tablets.[4] The carbamazepine suspension allows for more reliable and smoother absorption than the carbamazepine tablets. Carbamazepine suspension may be administered via feeding tubes. Enteral nutrition feeds may decrease the absorption of carbamazepine by 20 percent. The suspension is dosed with a greater frequency than the tablets and should be administered four times a day.[4]

Carbamazepine is available as an extended-release dosage form that is dosed every 12 hours.[7] The extended-release dosage forms are bioequivalent to the immediate-release tablets. The total daily dose of the immediate-release tablets can be administered twice daily with the extended-release tablets. A patient using 200 mg four times a day of immediate-release carbamazepine can be switched to carbamazepine extended-release 400 mg twice a day every 12 hours. The Tegretol-XR dosage form uses an osmotic-release delivery system—a single opening drilled on one side of the tablet is for drug release.[33] Patients should be counseled that the tablet will increase in size and the casing will be excreted in the feces. In order to ensure the integrity of the osmotic delivery system, pharmacy personnel should examine for chips and cracks on the extended-release tablets. The extended release carbamazepine tablets cannot be crushed or chewed.

The extended-release capsules, Carbatrol, are indicated for epilepsy and are administered every 12 hours.[3] The Carbatrol capsules use the microtol delivery system and contain three types of beads: immediate-release, extended-release, and enteric-release.[33-34] Although the beads in the capsules cannot be chewed or crushed, they can be opened and sprinkled in food. Additionally, the Carbatrol capsules may be opened and mixed with 30 mL of diluent and quickly administered through a feeding tube larger than 12 French. The recommended diluent is either normal saline or apple juice; D5W or sterile water should not be used with Carbatrol due to the mixture's propensity to clog the feeding tube. Both Carbatrol and Tegretol-XR are bioequivalent; however, Carbatrol has less variability in the rate of absorption than Tegretol-XR. Carbatrol and Tegretol-XR are indicated for epilepsy, while Equetro is a mood stabilizer indicated for the treatment of acute manic or mixed episodes associated with bipolar I disorder. Equetro is a two-piece hard gelatin capsule that should not be crushed or chewed, but may be opened and the beads sprinkled over food.[34] The carbamazepine dosage forms, product names, strengths, and generic availability is depicted in Table 5-3.

TABLE 5-3 Carbamazepine Dosage Forms

Dosage Form	Product	Strength	Generic Availability	Comments
Oral immediate-release tablets	Tegretol, Epitol	200 mg	Yes	Scored.
Oral immediate-release chewable tablets	Tegretol	100 mg	Yes	May be chewed or swallowed whole.
Oral suspension	Tegretol	100 mg	Yes	For four times a day dosing. Cannot mix with thioridazine or chlorpromazine liquids due to the formation of a nonabsorbable precipitate.
Extended-release tablets	Tegretol-XR	100 mg 200 mg 400 mg	Yes	Indicated for epilepsy and trigeminal neuralgia.
Extended-release capsules	Carbatrol	100 mg 200 mg 300 mg	Yes	Indicated for epilepsy and trigeminal neuralgia.
Extended-release capsules	Equetro	100 mg 200 mg 300 mg	Yes	Indicated for acute manic or mixed episodes associated with bipolar 1 disorder.

CARBAMAZEPINE BLOOD SAMPLING

The time to carbamazepine steady state depends on the carbamazepine half-life and the completion of autoinduction, hence the true carbamazepine half-life is difficult to ascertain. Additionally, carbamazepine absorption may occur throughout the dosing interval. Carbamazepine levels are most accurate after autoinduction is complete. As with all AEDs, trough levels are recommended to ensure that the serum levels are always above the lower end of the therapeutic range, in the case of carbamazepine the trough serum level should not be less than 4 mg/L. Carbamazepine levels may be measured weekly while titrating to the desired maintenance dose. Stable patients may be monitored every 3–6 months. When a loading dose with carbamazepine suspension is administered, a serum level may be taken after 2 hours to ensure that the carbamazepine level is therapeutic.

CASES

CASE 1: DIURNAL FLUCTUATIONS

ES is a 55-year-old white female on carbamazepine 200 mg every 6 hours (qid) for partial seizures. She is experiencing evening CNS adverse effects. A carbamazepine serum level at 12 noon is 4 mg/L and is within the target range; hence the medical team does not suspect carbamazepine toxicity. Is this patient undergoing carbamazepine CNS toxicity?

Answer:

Because carbamazepine undergoes diurnal fluctuations presenting with carbamazepine serum levels that gradually increase throughout the day, the 12 noon carbamazepine trough level may not reflect the patient's carbamazepine trough level in the evening. One can confirm that the carbamazepine is causing the patient's CNS toxicity by checking evening serum levels of carbamazepine or by simply adjusting the carbamazepine dose so that the lowest dose of the day is during the evening hours and monitoring for improvement of symptomatology. In this case serial carbamazepine trough levels were checked and are denoted in the following table:

Carbamazepine Dose	Time	Carbamazepine Trough	Adverse Effects
200 mg	6 a.m.	4 mg/L	
200 mg	12 noon	4 mg/L	
200 mg	6 p.m.	6 mg/L	Worsening dizziness, headaches, confusion, and drowsiness, between 7–9 M
200 mg	12 midnight	4 mg/L	

In ES, a new carbamazepine dosing regimen with the same total daily dose, but a lower evening dose will minimize the impact of diurnal fluctuations and the evening CNS adverse effects. Alternatively, switching from four times a day dosing to three times a day dosing, such that the 6 p.m. dose is skipped and a larger dose is administered at bedtime will also minimize the impact of diurnal fluctuations and the evening CNS adverse effects. A new recommended dosing regimen for this patient is carbamazepine 200 mg bid at 8 a.m. and 2 p.m. and 400 mg HS.

CASE 2: EMPIRIC CARBAMAZEPINE LOADING DOSE

TG is a 50-year-old, 70 kg male, with new onset generalized tonic-clonic seizures. Calculate an empiric carbamazepine loading dose for this patient. When should the maintenance dose be started?

Answer:

Loading dose = 8 mg/kg actual body weight
of carbamazepine suspension
70 kg (8 mg/kg) = 560 mg carbamazepine suspension

Administer carbamazepine suspension (100 mg/5 mL) 560 mg = 28 mL p.o. as one dose.

Because the patient is not hepatically induced, begin the carbamazepine maintenance dose in 12 hours.

CASE 3: EMPIRIC CARBAMAZEPINE LOADING DOSE AND MAINTENANCE DOSE

AJ is a 61-year-old, 100 kg male to be placed on carbamazepine for new onset clonic seizures. The neurologist would like AJ to receive a loading dose and then to be placed on a maintenance dose of 800 mg daily. Calculate an empiric carbamazepine loading dose for AJ. When should the maintenance dose be started?

Answer:

Loading dose = 8 mg/kg actual body weight
of carbamazepine suspension
100 kg (8 mg/kg) = 800 mg carbamazepine suspension

Administer carbamazepine suspension (100 mg/5 mL) 800 mg = 40 mL p.o. as one dose.

Because the patient is not hepatically induced, begin the carbamazepine maintenance dose in 12 hours.

Due to carbamazepine autoinduction it will take three weeks to achieve the maintenance dose of 800 mg/day. The carbamazepine dose should be increased by 200 mg weekly until autoinduction is complete, generally within 21–28 days. The following regimen should be recommended:

Carbamazepine 200 mg tablets:

Week 1: 200 mg bid

Week 2: 200 mg tid

Week 3: 200 mg qid

CASE 4: EMPIRIC CARBAMAZEPINE LOADING DOSE AND MAINTENANCE DOSE

DP is a 50-year-old, 100 kg white male, on carbamazepine 200 mg qid and HS for generalized tonic-clonic seizures. DP was noncompliant over the weekend and is having withdrawal seizures—his carbamazepine level is zero. Calculate an empiric carbamazepine loading dose for DP and restart his maintenance dose. When should the maintenance dose be started?

Answer:

Loading dose = 10 mg/kg actual body weight of
carbamazepine suspension for patients who
are on polytherapy and hepatically induced
100 kg (10 mg/kg) = 1,000 mg suspension

Administer carbamazepine suspension 1,000 mg = 50 mL (100 mg/5 mL) p.o. as one dose.

Begin the carbamazepine maintenance dose in 8 hours.

The maintenance dose is carbamazepine 200 mg p.o. qid and HS.

Generally the hepatic induction effects of carbamazepine will persist for 7–10 days. Although DP has not been receiving carbamazepine for 2–3 days, he is still hepatically induced and will require more aggressive carbamazepine loading doses, the start of an earlier maintenance dose, and will not require any weekly titrations of carbamazepine. After completing the loading dose, DP should be placed on his usual carbamazepine dose of 200 mg qid and HS.

CASE 5: EMPIRIC CARBAMAZEPINE LOADING DOSE AND MAINTENANCE DOSE

RS is a 40-year-old, 60 kg white female on carbamazepine 200 mg qid and phenytoin 100 mg tid for generalized tonic-clonic epilepsy. RS was noncompliant with her carbamazepine for the past 10 days and is having breakthrough seizures. Stat serum AED levels are phenytoin 12 mg/L and carbamazepine 0 mg/L. Calculate an empiric carbamazepine loading dose for RS and restart her maintenance dose. When should the maintenance dose be started?

Answer:

Loading dose = 10 mg/kg actual body weight of carbamazepine suspension for patients who are on polytherapy and hepatically induced

60 kg (10 mg/kg) = 600 mg carbamazepine suspension

Administer carbamazepine suspension (100 mg/5 mL) 600 mg = 30 mL p.o. as one dose.

Begin the carbamazepine maintenance dose in 8 hours at 200 mg p.o. qid.

Because this patient is on polytherapy and hepatically induced with phenytoin, accounting for carbamazepine autoinduction is not warranted and weekly carbamazepine dose titration should not be used in order to avoid subtherapeutic serum levels.

CASE 6: LOADING DOSE AND MAINTENANCE DOSE

AA is an 80-year-old African American male to be placed on carbamazepine for partial seizures with complex symptomatology. He is on no other medications. The medical team would like you to calculate a carbamazepine loading dose to achieve a target level of 10 mg/L and a maintenance dose to achieve a target level of 8 mg/L. When should the maintenance dose be started?

Height: 6 foot
Weight: 80 kg

Answer:

$$LD = \frac{(C_{pp})(Vd)}{(S)(F)}$$

$$LD = \frac{(10 \text{ mg/L})[(1.4 \text{ L/kg})(80 \text{ kg})]}{(1)(0.8)}$$

Loading dose = 1,400 mg

Administer carbamazepine suspension (100 mg/5 mL)1,400 mg = 70 mL p.o. as one dose.

Begin the maintenance dose in 12 hours.

Answer:

$$MD = \frac{(Cl \text{ in L/hr})(C_{pss\,AVG})(\tau[hr/day])}{(S)(F)}$$

$$MD = \frac{(0.064 \text{ L/hour}) (80 \text{ kg}) (8 \text{ mg/L}) (24 \text{ hours})}{(1) (0.8)}$$

$$MD = \frac{983}{0.8}$$

$$MD = 1,228 \text{ mg}$$

The maintenance dose may be rounded down to 1,200 mg or 400 mg tid. Because the patient is naïve to carbamazepine and is not on any enzyme inducers, the pharmacist will have to account for carbamazepine autoinduction, and carbamazepine should be titrated weekly to the full dose. The following carbamazepine regimen should be used:

Week 1: Carbamazepine 200 mg bid
Week 2: Carbamazepine 200 mg tid
Week 3: Carbamazepine 200 mg qid
Week 4: Carbamazepine 400 mg tid

CASE 7: LOADING DOSE AND MAINTENANCE DOSE

JM is a 60-year-old Hispanic male is to be placed on carbamazepine for partial seizures. He is on phenobarbital 30 mg bid. The medical team would like you to calculate a carbamazepine loading dose to achieve a target of 10 mg/L and a maintenance dose to achieve a target level of 9 mg/L. When should the maintenance dose be started?

Height: 6 feet
Weight: 90 kg

Answer:

$$\text{Loading dose} = \frac{(C_{pp})(Vd)}{(S)(F)}$$

$$LD = \frac{(10 \text{ mg/L})[(1.4 \text{ L/kg})(90 \text{ kg})]}{(1)(0.8)}$$

Loading dose = 1,575 mg

The loading dose may be rounded upward to 1,600 mg. Administer carbamazepine suspension (100 mg/5 mL) 1,600 mg = 80 mL p.o. as one dose.

The maintenance dose should begin in 8 hours.

$$\text{Maintenance dose} = \frac{(Cl \text{ in L/hr})(C_{pss\,AVG})(\tau[hr/day])}{(S)(F)}$$

$$MD = \frac{(0.1 \text{ L/hr})(90 \text{ kg})(9 \text{ mg/L})(24 \text{ hr})}{(1)(0.8)}$$

$$MD = 2,430 \text{ mg}$$

The maintenance dose may be rounded down to 2,400 mg daily. Because the patient is on concomitant phenobarbital a potent hepatic inducer of carbamazepine, carbamazepine autoinduction will not occur and is inconsequential. The following three carbamazepine regimens may be used:

1. Carbamazepine 600 mg qid, or
2. Tegretol-XR 1,200 mg q12h, or
3. Carbatrol 1,200 mg q12h (bid)

CASE 8: LOADING DOSE AND MAINTENANCE DOSE

WM is a 47-year-old white male who is to be placed on carbamazepine for partial seizures. He is on phenytoin 330 mg HS and Topiramate 200 mg bid but still has three seizures weekly. The medical team would like you to calculate a carbamazepine loading dose to achieve a target of 8 mg/L and a maintenance dose to achieve a target of target 6 mg/L. When should the maintenance dose be started?

Height: 5′10″

Weight: 60 kg

Answer:

$$\text{Loading dose} = \frac{(C_{pp})(Vd)}{(S)(F)}$$

$$LD = \frac{(8 \text{ mg/L})[(1.4 \text{ L/kg})(60 \text{ kg})]}{(1)(0.8)}$$

$$LD = 840 \text{ mg}$$

Administer carbamazepine suspension (100 mg/5 mL) 840 mg = 42 mL p.o. as one dose.

Because the patient is on phenytoin a potent CYP3A4 inducer and topiramate a mild-to-moderate CYP3A4 inducer, the maintenance dose should begin in 8 hours.

Answer:

$$\text{Maintenance dose} = \frac{(Cl \text{ in L/hr})(C_{pss\,AVG})(\tau[\text{hr/day}])}{(S)(F)}$$

$$MD = \frac{(0.1 \text{ L/hr})(60 \text{ kg})(6 \text{ mg/L})(24 \text{ hr})}{(1)(0.8)}$$

$$MD = 1,080 \text{ mg}$$

Because the patient is on concomitant phenytoin and topiramate both induce CYP3A4, no further autoinduction with carbamazepine will occur. Initially, the carbamazepine dose can be rounded down to 1 g daily. The following four carbamazepine regimens may be used:

1. Carbamazepine 200 mg qid & HS
2. Carbamazepine 300 mg qid
3. Tegretol-XR 500 mg q12h (bid) or 600 mg q12h (bid)
4. Carbatrol 500 mg q12h (bid) or 600 mg q12h (bid)

CASE 9: INCREMENTAL LOADING DOSE

HN is a 39-year-old white female who has been on carbamazepine XR 300 mg BID. She is having breakthrough seizures. A stat carbamazepine level is 2 mg/L. Calculate a carbamazepine loading dose to achieve a target serum level of 9 mg/L. When should the maintenance dose be started?

Height: 5′7″

Weight: 55 kg

Answer:

$$LD = \frac{(C_{pp})(Vd)}{(S)(F)}$$

$$C_{pp\,Target} = (\text{Carbamazepine target}) - (\text{Carbamazepine Level})$$

$$C_{pp\,Target} = (9 \text{ mg/L}) - (2 \text{ mg/L})$$

$$C_{pp\,Target} = 7 \text{ mg/L}$$

$$LD = \frac{(7 \text{ mg/L})[(1.4 \text{ L/kg})(55 \text{ kg})]}{(1)(0.8)}$$

Loading dose = 674 mg

The loading dose may be rounded off to 680 mg. Administer carbamazepine suspension (100 mg/5 mL) 60 mg = 34 mL p.o. as one dose.

Begin maintenance dose in 8 hours.

CASE 10: LOADING DOSE AND MAINTENANCE DOSE

LT is a 45-year-old white male who is to be placed on carbamazepine for refractory complex partial seizures. He is on gabapentin and levetiracetam. He completed a regimen of isoniazid, rifampin, ethambutol, and pyrazinamide 2 weeks ago. Calculate a carbamazepine loading dose to achieve a target serum level of 10 mg/L, and a maintenance dose to achieve a steady state carbamazepine level of 7 mg/L. When should the maintenance dose be started?

Height: 6 feet

Weight: 85 kg

Answer:

$$\text{Loading dose} = \frac{(C_{pp})(Vd)}{(S)(F)}$$

$$LD = \frac{(10 \text{ mg/L})[(1.4 \text{ L/kg})(85 \text{ kg})]}{(1)(0.8)}$$

$$LD = 1,488 \text{ mg}$$

The loading dose may be rounded to 1,500 mg. Administer carbamazepine suspension (100 mg/5 mL) 1,500 mg = 75 mL p.o. as one dose.

Answer:

$$\text{Maintenance dose} = \frac{(Cl \text{ in L/hr})(C_{pss\,AVG})(\tau[\text{hr/day}])}{(S)(F)}$$

$$MD = \frac{(0.064 \text{ L/hr})(85 \text{ kg})(7 \text{ mg/L})(24 \text{ hr})}{(1)(0.8)}$$

$$MD = 1,142 \text{ mg}$$

The carbamazepine maintenance dose may be rounded up to 1,200 daily.

The patient is on rifampin, a potent CYP3A4 enzyme inducer that increases hepatic clearance of carbamazepine; the enzyme induction effects may persist for up to 7–10 days. Because rifampin was discontinued 14 days ago, he is no longer enzyme-induced, and carbamazepine autoinduction should be accounted for with weekly dose titration.

The following carbamazepine dosing regimen should be used:

Week 1: Carbamazepine 200 mg bid

Week 2: Carbamazepine 200 mg tid

Week 3: Carbamazepine 200 mg qid

Week 4: Carbamazepine 400 mg tid

CASE 11: INCREMENTAL LOADING DOSE WITH HYPERVOLEMIA

CR is a 55-year-old male, a critically ill septic patient who is having breakthrough generalized tonic-clonic seizures. He has a history of epilepsy maintained on Tegretol-XR 600 mg bid. He received 6 L of intravenous fluid, is third spacing, and his current weight is 75 kg. He has been placed on a nasogastric tube. A stat carbamazepine level is

1 mg/L. Calculate a carbamazepine loading dose to achieve a target serum level of 8 mg/L.

Height: 5′10″

Weight: 73 kg

Answer:

$$\text{Loading dose} = \frac{(C_{pp})(V_d)}{(S)(F)}$$

$C_{pp\ Target}$ = Carbamazepine target – Carbamazepine level

$C_{pp\ Target}$ = 8 mg/L – 1 mg/L

$C_{pp\ Target}$ = 7 mg/L

Because the patient is third spacing, has received 6 L of fluid, and his weight has increased to 75 kg, the carbamazepine Vd to calculate his loading dose should be increased. The population Vd is 1.4 L/kg; however, in critically ill patients the Vd is higher and may be as high as 2 L/kg. In this case, the clinician may estimate the Vd to be 1.8 L/kg to calculate the loading dose.

$$\text{Loading dose} = \frac{(7\ \text{mg/L})[(1.8\ \text{L/kg})(75\ \text{kg})]}{(1)(0.8)}$$

$$\text{LD} = 1,181\ \text{mg}$$

The loading dose may be rounded off to 1,200 mg. Administer carbamazepine suspension (100 mg/5 mL)1,200 mg = 60 mL p.o. as one dose.

Begin the maintenance dose in 8 hours.

Because this patient has been placed on a nasogastric tube, he may be switched to immediate-release carbamazepine suspension or extended-release Carbatrol. Tegretol-XR cannot be crushed and administered via a feeding tube. Carbatrol may be opened and mixed with either normal saline or apple juice and administered through the adult feeding tube. CR may be placed on Carbatrol 600 mg bid.

REFERENCES

1. Kiluk KI, Knighton RS, Newman JD. The treatment of trigeminal neuralgia and other facial pain with carbamazepine. *Mich Med.* 1968;67:1066–1069.

2. Ramsey EG, Wilder BJ, Berger JR, et al. A double-blind study comparing carbamazepine with phenytoin as initial seizure therapy in adults. *Neurology.* 1983;33:904–910.

3. Lexi-Comp, Inc. Carbamazepine drug information. In Rose, BD (Ed.). *UpToDate.* Wellesley, MA, 2014.

4. McEvoy GK, Snow ED, (Eds.). *AHFS: Drug Information.* Bethesda, MD: American Society of Health-System Pharmacists, 2012:2266–2273.

5. Bialer M, Levy RH, Perucca E. Does carbamazepine have a narrow therapeutic plasma concentration range? *Ther Drug Monit.* 1998;20:56–59.

6. Höpener RJ, Kuyer A, Meijer JWA, Hulsman J. Correlation between the daily fluctuations of carbamazepine serum level and intermittent side effects. *Epilepsia.* 1980;21:341–350.

7. *Physicians' Desk Reference,* 68th ed. Montvale, NJ: Thomson PDR, 2014.

8. Hewetson KA, Ritch AE, Watson RD. Sick sinus syndrome aggravated by carbamazepine therapy for epilepsy. *Postgraduate Medical Journal.* 1986;62:497–498.

9. Kennebäck G, Bergfeldt L, Vallin H, Tomson T, Edhag O. Electrophysiologic effects and clinical hazards of carbamazepine treatment for neurologic disorders in patients with abnormalities of the cardiac conduction system. *Am Heart J.* 1991;121(5):1421–429.

10. Kennebäck G, Bergfeldt L, Tomson T, Spina E, Edhag O. Carbamazepine induced bradycardia—A problem in general or only in susceptible patients? A 24-hr long-term electrocardiogram study. *Epilepsy Res.* 1992;13(2):141–145.

11. Feldkamp J, Becker A, Witte OW, Scharff D, Scherbaum WA. Long-term anticonvulsant therapy leads to low bone mineral density—Evidence for direct drug effects of phenytoin and carbamazepine on human osteoblast-like cells. *Exp Clin Endocrinol Diabetes.* 2000;108(1):37–43.

12. De Vriese AS, Philippe J, Van Renterghem DM, De Cuyper CA, Hindryckx PH, Matthys EG, Louagie A. Carbamazepine hypersensitivity syndrome: Report of 4 cases and review of the literature. *Medicine* (Baltimore). 1995;74(3):144–151.

13. Seitz CS, Pfeuffer P, Raith P, Bröcker EB, Trautmann A. Anticonvulsant hypersensitivity syndrome: Cross-reactivity with tricyclic antidepressant agents. *Ann Allergy Asthma Immunol.* 2006;97(5):698–702.

14. Singh AN. Fluid retention during treatment with carbamazepine. *Can Med Assoc J.* 1978;118:24–28.

15. de Braganca AC, Mayses ZP, Magaldi AJ. Magaldi. Carbamazepine affects water and electrolyte homoeostasis in rat—similarities and differences to vasopressin antagonism. *Nephrol Dial Transplant.* 2012;27(10):3790–3798.

16. Tomson T, Almkvist O, Nilsson BY. Carbamazepine-10,11-epoxide in epilepsy: A pilot study. *Arch Neurol.* 1990;47:888–892.

17. Tomson T, Bertilsson L. Potent therapeutic effect of carbamazepine-10,11-epoxide in trigeminal neuralgia. *Arch Neurol.* 1984;41:598–601.

18. Levy RH, Bradley MK. Clinical pharmacokinetics of carbamazepine. *J Clin Psychiat.* 1988; 49(Suppl 4):58–61.

19. Brodie MJ, Forrest G, Rapeport WG. Carbamazepine-10,11-epoxide concentrations in epileptics on carbamazepine alone and in combination with other anticonvulsants. *Br J Clin Pharmacol.* 1983;16:747–750.

20. Bertilsson L, Tomson T. Clinical pharmacokinetics and pharmacological effects of carbamazepine-10,11-epoxide. An update. *Clin Pharmacokinet.* 1986;11(3):177–198.

21. Riva R, Albani F, Ambrosetto G, Contin M, Cortelli P, Perucca E, Baruzzi A. Diurnal fluctuations in free and total plasma concentrations of carbamazepine at steady state and correlation with intermittent side effects in epileptic patients. *Clin Pharmacokin.* 1984;9(1 Suppl):93–94.

22. Tomson T, Tybring G, Bertilsson L. Single-dose kinetics and metabolism of carbamazepine-10,11-epoxide. *Clin Pharmacol Ther.* 1983;33(1):58–65.

23. Bertilsson L. Clinical Pharmacokinetics of Carbamazepine. *Clin Pharmacokin.* 1978;3(2):128–143.

24. Kudriakova TB, Sirota LA, Rozova GI, Gorkov V. Autoinduction and steady-state pharmacokinetics of carbamazepine and its major metabolites. *Br J Clin Pharmac.* 1992;33:611–615.

25. Macphee GJA and Brodie MJ. Carbamazepine substitution in severe partial epilepsy: implication of autoinduction of metabolism. *Postgrad Med J.* 1985;61:779–783.

26. Porter RJ. How to initiate and maintain carbamazepine therapy in children and adults. *Epilepsia.* 1987;28(Suppl 3):S59–S63.

27. Blom S. Tic douloureux treated with new anticonvulsant experiences with G32883. *Arch Neurol.* 1963;9:285–290.

28. Gamstorp I. Treatment with carbamazepine: Children. *Adv Neurol.* 1975;11:237–248.

29. Cereghino JJ, Brock JT, VanMeter JC, Penry JK, Smith LD, White BG. Carbamazepine for epilepsy: A controlled prospective evaluation. *Neurology.* 1974;24:401–411.

30. Cohen H, Howland MA, Luciano DJ, Rubin RN, Kutt H, Hoffman RS, Leung LKH, Devinsky O, Goldfrank LR. Feasibility and pharmacokinetics of carbamazepine oral loading doses. *Am J Health-Syst Pharm.* 1998;55:1134–1140

31. Osborn HH, Zisfein J, Sparano R. Single-dose oral phenytoin loading. *Ann Emerg Med.* 1987;16:407–412.

32. Bell WL, Crawford IL, Shiu GK. Reduced bioavailability of moisture-exposed carbamazepine resulting in status epilepticus. *Epilepsia.* 1993;34(6):1102–1104.

33. Wheless JW, Venkataraman V. New formulations of drugs in epilepsy. *Expert Opin Pharmacother.* 1999;1:49–60.

34. El-Mallakh RS, Salem MR, Chopra A, Mickus GJ, Penagaluri P, Movva R. A blinded, randomized comparison of immediate-release and extended-release carbamazepine capsules in manic and depressed bipolar subjects. *Ann Clin Psychiat.* 2010;22(1):3–8.

CHAPTER 6

Digoxin

JOHN NOVIASKY, PharmD, BCPS
WILLIAM DARKO, BPharm, MPSG, PharmD
DAROWAN AKAJABOR, PharmD, BCPS
ARKADIY MAKARON, PharmD, BCPS
CHRISTOPHER MILLER, PharmD, BCPS, AAHIVP
DEIRDRE P. PIERCE PharmD, BCPS, CGP
ROBERT SEABURY, PharmD
KAREN WHALEN, BS, Pharm, BCPS

Digitalis is the oldest cardiovascular compound still in use today.[1] More than 200 years ago, Sir William Withering observed that foxglove flower derivative (digitalis purpura) could be used for "cardiac dropsy."[2] Since that time, the positive hemodynamic, neurohormonal, and electrophysiologic effects of digoxin have been well explored.[1]

The pharmacodynamic effects of digoxin include increased cardiac output, decreased pulmonary capillary wedge pressure, and increased ejection fraction. The neurohormonal effects of digoxin include improved baroreceptor sensitivity, decreased norepinephrine concentration, decreased renin-angiotensin activations, sympathoinhibitory effect, and increase release of atrial natriuretic peptide and brain natriuretic peptide. The electrophysiological effects are primarily mediated through the interaction of digoxin with the sodium-potassium-ATPase pump.[1,2]

Digoxin increases contractility by inhibiting the sodium-potassium exchange in the sodium-potassium-ATPase pump leading to an increase of sodium in the myocytes. This increase results in decreased outflow of calcium from the myocyte and greater contractile force of the myocardium.[1,2]

Digoxin also has electrophysiological effects. It has the ability to slow conduction through the AV node and it can slow the sinus rate via the S-A node. It is these effects that allow it to be used for atrial fibrillation.[3]

PHARMACOKINETIC PARAMETERS

The bioavailability of digoxin can range from 70 percent to nearly 100 percent, depending on the type of oral formulation. The elixir and tablet formulations are approximately 80 percent and 70 percent bioavailable, respectively.[4] Encapsulated digoxin solution is close to 100 percent bioavailable, but no longer manufactured. The bioavailability of intravenous digoxin is always complete. The estimated elimination half-life of digoxin can take as long as 48 hours.[5]

Digoxin is roughly 30 percent protein bound in the plasma and has a large volume of distribution (VD) of nearly 7 L/kg in healthy adults.[5,6] It follows a two-compartment kinetic model with an initial distribution phase into the central compartment consisting primarily of plasma and highly perfused tissues, such as the liver. A second, slower distribution phase soon occurs and moves the drug out of the central compartment and into the peripheral, deep tissue compartment.[5] The target site, the myocardium, is affected by drug concentration in the peripheral compartment and, therefore, clinical effect may not be seen until sufficient drug has accumulated at that site, which may take several hours after a loading dose. Serum drug concentrations early after a loading dose may not represent the true drug concentration at the site of action and may lead to inappropriate dosage adjustments.

The VD in obese patients best correlates with ideal body weight, rather than actual body weight.[7] Due to digoxin's hydrophilic nature, it does not significantly distribute into adipose tissue. However, actual body weight should be used in underweight patients, whose ideal body weight is greater than their actual body weight. Pediatric patients have a higher percentage of total body water and, therefore, would have an increased volume of distribution relative to their adult counterparts.

METABOLISM AND ELIMINATION

Digoxin is primarily eliminated via renal excretion as unchanged drug but does undergo hepatic metabolism to a small extent.[5,8] Roughly 15–20 percent of the drug is metabolized, with digoxigenin bisdigitoxoside and digoxigenin monodigitoxoside being the primary metabolites. The metabolic pathway for digoxin includes sequential hydrolysis followed by conjugation and oxidation into polar metabolites.[5,9] The cytochrome P450 isoenzyme system is responsible for some of digoxin's metabolism, but only to a minor extent. As such, drug interactions with agents that inhibit or induce CYP450 are minimal. Digoxin's metabolites have limited cardioactive properties when compared to the parent compound and these metabolites primarily undergo renal elimination.[9]

Roughly 80 percent of a digoxin dose is eliminated as unchanged drug by the kidneys. Renal elimination of digoxin occurs through a mixture of glomerular filtration and active tubular secretion.[5,8-10] Tubular secretion is mediated primarily by the P-glycoprotein transporter and is subject to drug interaction risks. For patients, dosing and safety concerns are highly dependent upon renal function. Patients with severe renal dysfunction may encounter drug accumulation and toxicity. Monitoring of renal function is necessary for patients receiving digoxin therapy, and creatinine clearance estimates remain the most important clinical tool to ensure appropriate dosing. Specific dosing adjustments are recommended for patients with decreased creatinine clearance.[11] Due to its high volume of distribution, digoxin is removed negligibly by hemodialysis, and clinical data have indicated higher mortality rates for digoxin-treated patients who require hemodialysis.[12,13] Extreme caution, and possibly alternative therapy, is required for these patients.

THERAPEUTIC CONCENTRATIONS

CHRONIC HEART FAILURE (CHF)

Historically, higher concentrations and wider targets were accepted for patients on digoxin, but contemporary literature suggests a more conservative approach in patients with heart failure. The new desired therapeutic range is lower and narrower at 0.5–0.9 ng/mL or less than 1 ng/mL.[14] Recent studies suggest that in addition to the positive inotropic effects of digoxin, neurohormonal modulation through inhibition of Na-K ATPase is evident at low digoxin concentrations. Further decreases in norepinephrine concentrations are not observed as the concentration of digoxin increases. In other words, digoxin serum concentrations between 0.7 ng/mL and 1.2 ng/mL attain therapeutic benefit while decreasing risk of toxicity in patients with CHF.[15,16]

ATRIAL FIBRILLATION (AF)

In patients with atrial fibrillation, the traditionally accepted range of digoxin serum concentration is 0.5–2 ng/mL, but achieving rate control may require targeting higher serum concentrations. In some patients, concentrations >2 ng/mL may be required to adequately control ventricular rate. However, higher levels are more often associated with toxicity (See DIGOXIN TOXICITY Section).

In general, the routine measurement of digoxin serum concentrations is not always necessary. Digoxin toxicity and explaining poor response to therapy are the main indications for measurement of serum digoxin concentrations. Clinical response to therapy should always be considered first.[11,17]

SAMPLING

Following a loading dose, serum digoxin concentration should be obtained at approximately 6–8 hours following the loading dose. Levels obtained earlier may be falsely elevated due to the slow distribution phase. Once steady state has been achieved, which usually occurs in about 7 to 14 days after a maintenance regimen is initiated or changed, routine samples for digoxin monitoring should be drawn just before the next dose is due.[4,11]

DOSING

LOADING DOSE

Loading doses are generally unnecessary and not required when digoxin is used to treat CHF. In this patient population, digoxin is used for its positive inotropic effects and neurohormonal modulation. It should be initiated at a maintenance dose dependent on factors such as age, lean body weight, and renal function.[16] In atrial fibrillation, digoxin loading dose may be administered at the onset of therapy to achieve a rapid attainment of target concentration. The advantage of giving a loading dose must be weighed against the disadvantage of exposing a patient to an abrupt toxic concentration of digoxin. To achieve adequate response and avoid toxicity, prescribers must account for patient-specific dosing characteristics such as lean body weight, age, renal function, and concomitant medications. These factors will vary from patient to patient.[1,3,18]

If a loading dose is used, it should be given in divided dosing to decrease the occurrence of toxic concentrations. Intravenous doses can be given in 2- to 4-hour intervals while oral formulations can be given in 6- to 8-hour intervals. For example, a 1 mg digoxin oral loading dose can be given as a 0.5 mg dose followed by a 0.25 mg dose every 6 hours for 2 doses with careful monitoring of the patient for efficacy and toxicity.

A loading dose can be calculated using the following equation:

$$LD = (VD)(C \text{ in ng/mL})/(F)$$

where VD is the volume of distribution, C is the desired concentration, and F is the bioavailability of the formulation.

Example I

MS is a 47-year-old female to be initiated on intravenous digoxin for atrial fibrillation. Her weight is 60 kg and height is 65 inches. Her CrCl is estimated to be at 95 mL/min. Calculate her digoxin loading dose for a desired plasma concentration of 1 ng/mL.

$$\text{Loading dose} = (VD)(C)/(F)$$

First calculate VD (using the Jusko equation).

$$
\begin{aligned}
VD &= 226 + [298(CrCl)/(29.1 + CrCl)] \\
&= 226 + [298(95 \text{ mL/min})/(29.1 + 95 \text{ mL/min})] \\
&= 454 \text{ L}
\end{aligned}
$$

$$
\begin{aligned}
\text{Loading dose} &= (VD)(C)/(F) \\
&= (454 \text{ L})(1 \text{ ng/mL})/(1) \\
&= 454 \text{ mcg} \sim 0.5 \text{ mg}
\end{aligned}
$$

MAINTENANCE DOSE

Most patients with CHF will achieve the target serum digoxin concentration of 0.5 to 1.0 ng/mL with doses of 0.125 to 0.25 mg daily. The dosing nomogram designed by Bauman and colleagues and the dosing formula by Koup and Jusko have been found to be the best methods of estimating digoxin dose in this modern era of new therapeutic range of digoxin in heart failure patients.[18,19] The new dosing nomogram for digoxin in patients with heart failure (see Figure 6-1) also takes into account ideal body weight in kilograms, creatinine clearance in mL/min, and height in inches to estimate the dose of digoxin.[18]

The maintenance dose equation takes into account age, gender, and renal function, which are known variables that can alter digoxin concentrations. The maintenance dose can be calculated using the maintenance dose equation: Maintenance dose = (CL)(Css)(T)/(F), where CL is the clearance of digoxin, Css is the steady state concentration, T is the dosing interval in days and F is the bioavailability of the formulation.

Example II

Calculate a maintenance dose (oral tablets) for MS in Example 1.

$$\text{Maintenance dose} = (CL)(Css)(T)/(F)$$

First calculate CL.

CL = 1.303 CrCl (mL/min) + CL_m, CL_m = 40 mL/min.
(Where Cl_m is non-renal clearance and Cl_m = 20 mL/min for patients with heart failure and 40 mL/min for patients without heart failure)

$$= 1.303 \times 95 \text{ mL/min} + 40$$

$$= 163.8 \text{ mL/min}$$

Converting to L/day = [(163.8 mL/min)(1,440 min/day)]/1,000 mL/L
$$= 235.9 \text{ L/day}$$

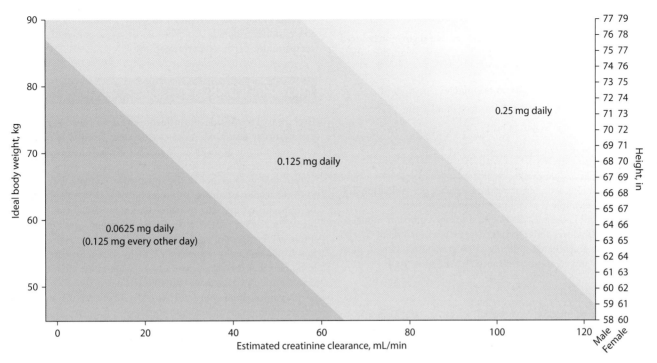

FIGURE 6-1. Dosing nomogram for digoxin in patients with heart failure. (Used with permission from Bauman LJ, DiDomenico JR, Viana M, et al. A method of determining the dose of digoxin for heart failure in the modern era. *Arch Intern Med.* 2006;166:2539–2545). *Note:* To select an appropriate digoxin maintenance dose, plot a patient's creatinine clearance (x-axis) (to convert creatinine clearance to milliliter per second, multiply by 0.01667) and ideal body weight (y-axis). The point at which these lines intersect is the recommended digoxin dose. If ideal body weight has not or cannot be calculated, an appropriate digoxin maintenance dose can be determined by plotting a patient's creatinine clearance (x-axis) and height (z-axis), depending on patient sex. In the 0.25 mg daily area of the nomogram, one may also consider a digoxin maintenance dose of 0.125 mg, alternating with 0.25 mg every other day (average daily dose of 0.1875 mg/day) as represented by the gradual shading of this area.

$$\text{Maintenance dose} = (CL)(Css)(T)/(F)$$
$$= [(235.9 \text{ L/day})(1 \text{ ng/mL})(1 \text{ day})]/(0.7)$$
$$= 337 \text{ mcg} \sim 375 \text{ mcg, or } 0.375 \text{ mg}$$

MS can be initiated on 0.25mg (1 tablet) or 0.375 mg (1½ tablets) daily.

MAINTENANCE DOSE BASED ON SERUM DIGOXIN CONCENTRATION

A more patient-specific maintenance dose can be determined using the patient's dosing history and the observed digoxin concentrations to derive a patient-specific drug clearance.

The equation for maintenance dose, MD = (CL)(Css)(T)/(F), can be rearranged to derive CL.

$$CL = (MD)(F)/(Css)(T)$$

Example III

Assuming MS (from Example II) was initiated on 0.375 mg tablets daily and in 14 days a steady-state serum digoxin concentration was obtained right before the next scheduled dose. The Css was measured to be 2.8 ng/mL. Calculate her true CL and a new dosing regimen to attain a new desired Css of 1.5 ng/mL.

First calculate CL.

$$CL = (375 \text{ mcg})(0.7)/(2.8 \text{ ng/mL})(1 \text{ day})$$
$$= 93.8 \text{ L/day (Note: Her true CL is significantly}$$
different from the estimated 229.3 L/day.)

$$\text{New MD} = (93.8 \text{ L/day})(1.5 \text{ ng/mL})(1\text{day})/(0.7)$$
$$= 201 \text{ mcg/day (rounded up to 250 mcg}$$
or 0.25 mg tabs daily)

PHARMACOKINETIC MODIFICATIONS FOR DISEASE STATES

Renal Disease

Due to extensive elimination by the kidney, any reduction in renal function will result in decreased elimination and potential accumulation of this narrow therapeutic index drug. Renal clearance of digoxin has been shown to be similar to creatinine clearance in patients with normal and impaired renal function.[20]

Patients with renal disease have a lower VD.[21] Although this pharmacokinetic change occurs, evidence indicates that myocardial and serum drug concentrations are still an acceptable estimate of digoxin efficacy and toxicity.[22] Decreases in VD and elimination by the kidney substantiate the need for lower digoxin loading and maintenance doses, and consideration to dosage interval extension. Because of the large volume of distribution of digoxin, removal by hemodialysis and peritoneal dialysis is minimal and not of benefit as a treatment for toxicity.[11,23]

Geriatrics

As aging occurs, renal excretion decreases as the number of effective nephrons is reduced and renal blood flow diminishes. Glomerular filtration rate declines 25–50 percent between the ages of 20 and 90.[24] In the patient without identified kidney disease, renal elimination of digoxin will still decrease with age. Consequently, the elderly patient should be managed as though they have recognized renal disease.[25]

Digoxin is largely distributed into skeletal muscle. Older patients experience a 10–20 percent decrease in volume of distribution of digoxin, attributed to loss of lean muscle mass. Additionally, age-related reduction in renal function will contribute to lower VD.[24] As a result, lower loading and maintenance doses and careful interval assessment are recommended.

Heart Failure

As compared to healthy adults, the clearance of digoxin is reduced 50 percent in those patients with heart failure as defined by these equations[26]:

$$CL = \text{clearance in mL/min}$$
$$CrCl = \text{creatinine clearance in mL/min}$$
$$Wt = \text{weight in kg}$$

$$CL \text{ (non HF)} = (0.8 \text{ mL/kg/min} \times Wt) + CrCl$$
$$CL \text{ (HF)} = (0.33 \text{ mL/kg/min} \times Wt) + 0.9(CrCl)$$

These equations are alternatives for clearance determination first illustrated in example II of Maintenance Dose section.

Bauman and colleagues developed a linear regression model to predict digoxin doses and intervals to target a serum level of 0.7 and subsequently constructed a dosing nomogram using height, ideal body weight, and creatinine clearance.[18] (See Figure 6-1.)

Hyperthyroidism

In hyperthyroid disease, myocardial sensitivity and response to digoxin are reduced.[20] Additionally, pharmacokinetics can change as VD is increased, which generally supports use of higher loading doses.[27] Enhanced elimination of digoxin occurs due to increases in creatinine clearance seen with these patients.[28]

Hypothyroidism

Conversely, VD of digoxin is reduced in hypothyroidism, suggesting that lower loading doses may be prudent. Clearance is also lower, which is attributed to reduced creatinine clearance evident in that disease state.[28]

Liver Disease

Adjustment of digoxin dosing is not required in liver disease patients. Pharmacokinetic parameters are not significantly changed.[29]

DRUG INTERACTIONS

Digoxin has multiple clinically significant drug interactions that alter clearance and result in supratherapeutic or subtherapeutic serum concentrations (Table 6-1). The mechanism of clearance changes is a result of interaction with the P-glycoprotein transporter system.[30-31] P-glycoprotein is normally located at the blood-brain barrier, liver, pancreas, placenta, testis, kidney, colon, and jejunum. It is suggested that the purpose of P-glycoprotein is protection against toxic compounds by excretion into urine, bile, and intestinal lumen.[30] When this transport system is inhibited or induced, substrates such as digoxin will not be excreted at the same rate, and serum concentrations will increase or decrease respectively.

Specific P-glycoprotein inhibitors that are expected to increase digoxin exposure by more than 25 percent include amiodarone, captopril, carvedilol, clarithromycin, conivaptan, cyclosporine, diltiazem, dronedarone, felodipine, itraconazole, lopinavir and ritonavir, quinidine, ranolazine, ticagrelor, and verapamil. Conversely, those agents that induce p-glycoprotein enzyme and decrease digoxin area under the curve by greater than 20 percent are phenytoin, rifampin, St. John's wort, and tipranavir/ritonavir.[32-47]

A pronounced interaction is seen when quinidine is added to a patient stabilized on digoxin, resulting in decreased volume of distribution and decreased clearance of digoxin. As a result, digoxin serum concentration increases rapidly and in a sustained fashion. Clinically, a reasonable plan is to decrease digoxin dose by 50 percent.[33] More commonly, cardiovascular drugs that will be used along with digoxin, and with potential to alter serum concentration, include amiodarone, dronedarone, diltiazem, and verapamil for rhythm and rate control.

DIGOXIN TOXICITY

Over the past few decades the incidence and severity of digoxin toxicity has drastically decreased. A prospective study from 1971 noted toxic manifestations in as many as 24 percent of digoxin treated patients, with fatal outcomes in 41 percent of toxicity cases.[48] More recent data suggest that 4–5 percent of digoxin treated patients develop toxicity, with fatality occurring in 9 percent of toxicity cases.[49] Authors have speculated that this reduction in the incidence and severity of digoxin toxicity is related to decreasing utilization, lower dosing, and improved therapeutic drug monitoring.[50] Despite these improvements toxicity and mortality secondary to toxicity still occurs. Therefore, it is important that clinical pharmacists understand the etiology, clinical manifestations, and management of digoxin toxicity.

A serum digoxin concentration (SDC) between 0.5 and 2.0 ng/mL is traditionally considered a therapeutic value, though some evidence suggests that lower levels may be equally as effective and reduce the risk of toxicity.[50] Concentrations greater than 2.0 ng/mL are potentially toxic, with one review noting toxic manifestations in 60 percent of patients with a postdistribution SDC greater than 2.0 ng/mL.[49] This finding illustrates that digoxin toxicity is at least in part concentration dependent and situations that precipitate an increase in concentration could also precipitate toxicity.

Digoxin is widely distributed and has an average VD of approximately 7 L/kg.[5] Reductions in digoxin's VD have been noted with renal disease and reductions in lean body mass.[5,25] A number of factors, including renal disease and drug interactions, can decrease digoxin clearance (CL).[5,25,50] Digoxin is mostly eliminated unchanged in the urine.[5,25] Renal insufficiency reduces the elimination of digoxin and can significantly prolong digoxin's half-life.[5,50] A number of medications, including amiodarone, quinidine, and verapamil, reduce digoxin elimination via inhibition of the p-glycoprotein efflux pump.[50] Reductions in CL will increase the apparent half-life with resulting drug accumulation with repeated dosing. Reductions in VD and CL will reciprocally increase SDCs and may lead to toxicity. Geriatric patients often are prescribed digoxin and are at greater risk for chronic poisoning.[25] Reductions in lean body mass and declining renal function commonly occur with the natural aging course.[25] These patients are also more commonly on multiple medications, putting them at an increased risk for toxicity secondary to drug interactions.

Clinical manifestations of digoxin toxicity are listed in Table 6-2. These signs and symptoms can be classified as gastrointestinal, neurologic, or cardiac manifestations, with cardiac manifestations being the primary cause of morbidity and mortality. Symptom evolution is dependent on the chronicity of exposure.[51] Nausea and vomiting are prominent with acute exposures and are typically the first symptom.[51] Neurologic symptoms such as weakness, confusion, and lethargy can be observed.[52] With chronic exposures, such as a patient with reduced digoxin CL due to a physiologic change, symptoms can be nonspecific and more difficult to diagnose.[51] Malaise and weakness are predominant features, along with visual disturbances, such as blurred vision.[51-52] Patients may have complaints of anorexia, while nausea and vomiting are thought to occur less commonly than acute ingestions.

Digoxin's cardiotoxicity is multifaceted and can be seen with both acute and chronic toxicity. At toxic levels digoxin increases intracellular calcium concentrations escalating excitability and automaticity in the atria and ventricles, which can lead to extrasystoles and tachydysrhythmias.[50-51] Additionally, digoxin reduces nodal conduction velocity and can induce bradydysrhythmias and

TABLE 6-1 Digoxin Drug Interactions: Summary of Studies

Drug Studied with Digoxin	Study Description	Study Subjects	N	PK Variables	Results	Reference
Amiodarone	Stable on po digoxin; amiodarone po 600 mg/day added	Patients with atrial fibrillation	7	Serum digoxin concentration (SDC) after 5 days	SDC increased from 1.17 to 1.98 ng/mL.	34
	Stable on po digoxin and amiodarone po 200 mg/day; amiodarone po increase to 600 mg/day	Patients with atrial fibrillation	2	Serum digoxin concentration (SDC) after 5 days	SDC increased from 0.4 to 0.7 ng/mL.	34
	Intravenous digoxin 1 mg given before and after amiodarone po 400 mg/day × 3 weeks	Healthy subjects	10	Digoxin renal and nonrenal CL • Digoxin half-life	CL reduced from 234 ± 72 mL/min to 172 ± 33 mL/min. Half-life increased from 34 ± 13 hours to 40 ± 16 hours.	35
	Stable (>2 weeks) on digoxin po 0.25 ± 0.05 mg/day; amiodarone po 600 mg to 1600 mg/day added	Heart failure (14), atrial fibrillation (9), both (5)	28	SDC after 16 days	SDC increase 104% from 0.97 ± 0.48 to 1.98 ± 0.84 ng/mL.	36
	Stable (>2 weeks) on digoxin po 0.25 ± 0.05 mg/day; amiodarone po 600 mg to 1600 mg/day added	Patients with atrial fibrillation	5	Amiodarone serum concentrations • Digoxin and amiodarone steady state • Correlation between SDC and amiodarone serum concentration	Amiodarone concentration average increase from 0 to about 3.5 mcg/mL over 16 days. Steady state was not obtained after 16 days coadministration of digoxin and amiodarone. SDC increase was parallel with serum amiodarone concentrations (no statistics mentioned).	36
	Intravenous digoxin 1 mg given before and after 2 weeks of oral amiodarone at 1600 mg/day	Patients with atrial fibrillation	6	Digoxin total body CL • Digoxin elimination half-life	Digoxin total body CL significantly reduced by 29% (from 2.05 ± 0.76 to 1.46 ± 0.64 mL/min/kg). Digoxin half-life nonsignificant increase by 31% (from 49.5 ± 8.8 to 65.0 ± 28.8 hours).	36
Dronedarone	Crossover, dronedarone 400 mg BID with/without digoxin 0.25 mg daily for 10 days	Healthy adults	10	Digoxin CL • SDC maximum • Digoxin area under the curve • Digoxin steady state • Dronedarone steady state	Decreased digoxin CL by 1.7 fold. SDC maximal concentration increased by 1.75 (CI 1.58–1.93) fold. Digoxin area under the curve increased by 2.57 (CI 2.21–2.98) fold. Digoxin steady state reached by day 2. Dronedarone steady state reached by day 4.	37
Diltiazem	Double blind crossover 10 days of digoxin with/without diltiazem 180 mg/day	Patients with heart failure	8	SDC • Digoxin area under the curve • Digoxin half-life	Steady state SDC increased 50% (from 1.34 ± 0.14 to 2.01 ± 0.29 ng/mL). Digoxin area under the curve increase 51% (from 18.24 ± 1.34 to 26.18 ± 3.62 ng/h/mL). Digoxin half-life increased by 29% (from 18.05 ± 6.92 to 23.3 ± 7.8 hours).	38
	Diltiazem 60 mg 3 times daily added to patients on digoxin >2 weeks	Patients with heart failure	11	SDC at 3 days coadministration • SDC at 7 days coadministration	SDC after 3 days (from 1.11 ± 0.18 ng/mL to 1.54 ± 0.22 ng/mL) coadministration. SDC at 7 days (from 1.11 ± 0.18 ng/mL to 1.54 ± 0.23 ng/mL) coadministration.	39
	Diltiazem 60 mg 3 or 4 times daily added to patients on digoxin >2 weeks	Patients with atrial fibrillation	19 (3 times daily) 9 (4 times daily)	SDC	SDC after 1 week (from 1.05 ± 0.61 ng/mL to 1.06 ± 0.43 ng/mL) coadministration (not significant).	40
	Single oral digoxin dose of 0.75mg given before and after 1 week diltiazem 30 mg 3 times daily	Healthy adults	6	Digoxin renal CL • Digoxin absorption half-life • Digoxin peak concentration • Digoxin peak concentration time • Digoxin distribution half-life • Digoxin elimination half-life • Digoxin VD	Digoxin renal CL after 1 week decreased (from 3.05 ± 0.126 to 2.31 ± 0.234 mL/min/kg) coadministration. No significant difference in other measures.	41
	Single intravenous digoxin dose of 1 mg given before and after 1 week diltiazem 30 mg 4 times daily	Healthy adults	5	Digoxin total body CL • Digoxin distribution half-life • Digoxin elimination half-life • Digoxin VD	No significant change with any measure after 1 week coadministration.	42
Verapamil	Randomized crossover digoxin with/without diltiazem 90 mg 2 times daily	Healthy adults	24	SDC • Digoxin half-life	SDC increase 22.4% within 48 hours. Digoxin half-life increased (from 36.2 ± 11.2 to 44.5 ± 11.5 hours) within 48 hours.	43
	Digoxin dose given before and after 10 days of verapamil 80 mg 3 times daily	Healthy Adults	8	Digoxin total body CL • Digoxin half-life • Digoxin VD	Digoxin CL decreased 35% (from 3.28 ± 0.58 to 2.15 ± 0.66 mL/min) after 10 days coadministration. Digoxin half-life increased 20% (from 38.6 ± 8.5 to 50.5 ± 8.3 hours) after 10 days coadministration. Digoxin VD decreased 23% (from 0.83 ± 0.25 to 0.64 ± 0.171/kg) after 10 days coadministration.	44
	Verapamil 320–480 mg/day added to patients on digoxin $(0.46 \pm 0.18$ mg/day)	Patients with atrial fibrillation	10	SDC after 1 week • SDC after 4 weeks	SDC increased from 1.6 ± 0.35ng/mL to 2.2 ± 0.6ng/mL after 1 week coadministration. SDC increased from 1.6 ± 0.35ng/mL to 2.7 ± 0.9ng/mL after 4 weeks coadministration.	45
St. John's Wort	Digoxin single oral dose of 0.5 mg given before and after 14 days of St. John's wort (300 mg 3 times daily)	Healthy adults	8	Digoxin bioavailability area under the curve	Digoxin bioavailability AUC decreased by 18% after 14 days coadministration.	46
	Digoxin 0.25 mg and St. John's wort (900 mg/day) or placebo coadministration	Healthy adults	25 (13-St. John's wort, 12-placebo)	SDC difference between group • SDC with St. John's wort	SDC 25% net decrease between placebo and St. John's wort groups after 10 days. SDC 37% decrease after 10 days coadministration with St. John's wort.	46

Note: All data shown in results column represents a statistically significant change unless otherwise noted.

TABLE 6-2 Clinical Manifestations of Acute and Chronic Digoxin Toxicity[50-53]

Acute		Chronic	
Gastrointestinal	*Neurologic*	*Gastrointestinal*	*Neurologic*
Usually occur early	*Usually preceded by gastrointestinal complaints*	Anorexia	Delirium
Nausea	Lethargy	Abdominal pain	Confusion
Vomiting	Confusion	Nausea	Drowsiness
Abdominal pain	Weakness	Vomiting	Headaches
			Visual disturbances
			Blurred vision
			Discoloration
Electrolyte		*Electrolyte*[a]	
Hyperkalemia		Hyperkalemia	
		Hypokalemia	
		Hypomagnesemia	
		Hypercalcemia	
		Cardiotoxicity[b]	
		Premature ventricular contractions	
		Junctional tachycardia	
		Junctional rhythm	
		AV dissociation	
		First-, second-, or third-degree heart block	
		Paroxysmal atrial tachycardia	
		Atrial fibrillation	
		Atrial flutter	
		Premature atrial contractions	
		Premature junctional concentrations	
		Sinus arrest	
		Sinus bradycardia	
		Sinus tachycardia	
		Ventricular tachycardia	
		Ventricular fibrillation	

[a]These electrolyte abnormalities can be seen with chronic exposures. They are not due to digoxin effect but due to concurrent medications such as diuretics or disease states such as renal failure. These abnormalities can exacerbate digoxin toxicity.
[b]Cardiotoxicity can occur with both acute and chronic toxicity. Cardiac manifestations can be seen at presentation with chronic exposures. Conversely, with acute exposures these effects can be absent at presentation and they can progress as the clinical course evolves.

nodal blocks with toxicity.[51] Thus, with the exception of a supraventricular tachycardia with rapid ventricular response, digoxin toxicity can precipitate almost any arrhythmia, with premature ventricular contractions being the most common.[50-51] Bidirectional ventricular tachycardia is considered a pathognomonic finding, as it is uncommon for almost all other toxins.[51] Finally, digoxin achieves its therapeutic effect by inhibiting myocardial sodium-potassium ATPase, increasing extracellular potassium concentrations.[50] Hyperkalemia can occur, typically with acute overdoses, and is considered a prognostic factor. Prior to the advent of digoxin-specific Fab, death occurred in 50 percent and 100 percent of acutely poisoned digoxin patients with serum potassium levels of 5.0–5.5 mEq/L and >5.5 mEq/L, respectively.[54] Additionally, patients chronically on digoxin are frequently on medications such as loop diuretics, which can exacerbate digoxin toxicity and cause other electrolyte abnormalities, such as hypokalemia and hypomagnesemia.[55] Hypokalemia, like digoxin inhibits myocardial sodium-potassium ATPase and can independently precipitate arrhythmias. Therefore, hypokalemia could precipitate toxicity at lower and sometimes therapeutic digoxin concentrations.[53]

Digoxin follows a two-compartment model with compartments displaying rapid and slow distribution.[5] SDCs are sampled from the rapidly distributing compartment. Conversely, the myocardium is found within the slowly distributing portion. The rapid and slowly distributing compartments do not reach distribution equilibrium until approximately 4 hours and 6 hours after the last administered intravenous or oral dose, respectively.[55-56] Predistribution values can be falsely elevated, making interpretation difficult. One review of toxic levels (SDC >2 ng/mL) noted that 16 percent of toxic

specimens were drawn during the predistribution period.[49] When assessing a toxic SDC it is important to assess this value in the context of a patient's symptoms and the timing of the level in relation to the last administered digoxin dose.

Digoxin-specific Fab (DSFab) is the definitive therapy for digoxin toxicity and is indicated with life-threatening or potentially life-threatening toxicity (see Table 6-3).[57-58] Digibind® and DigiFab® are the commercially available preparations of DSFab, and the pharmacokinetic properties of these products are detailed in Table 6-4.[57-58]

TABLE 6-3 Indications for Digoxin-Specific Fab (DSFab)[57,58]

Progressive bradydysrhythmias or second/third-degree heart block not responsive to atropine
Severe ventricular dysrhythmias or tachydysrhythmias
Serum potassium >5 mEq/L in acute digoxin intoxication
Postdistribution SDC ≥10 ng/mL or a SDC ≥15 ng/mL at any time-point
Acute digoxin ingestion ≥10 mg (adult) or ≥4 mg (child)
Rapidly progressing clinical signs/symptoms in combination with an increasing serum potassium level

TABLE 6-4 Pharmacokinetic Parameters of DSFab Formulations[57,58]

	Digibind®	DigiFab®
Onset of action (hr)	≤0.5	≤0.5
VD (L/kg)	0.4	0.3
Elimination half-life (hr)	23	15
Route of elimination	Urine	Urine

Each vial of DSFab binds 0.5 mg of digoxin. Considering its VD, which is 0.4 L/kg, DSFab will bind with free digoxin within the circulatory system, creating a concentration gradient moving free drug from the tissue into the systemic circulation and effectively reducing digoxin concentrations within the myocardium. The elimination half-life of the DSFab-digoxin complex (15–23 hours) is significantly shorter than free digoxin (36 hours), indicating enhanced elimination. It must be noted that SDCs are no longer useful after DSFab administration unless free digoxin concentrations can be measured. The standard digoxin assay measures both free and bound digoxin and will measure the DSFab-digoxin complex in addition to both bound and unbound digoxin, which will lead to a falsely elevated value that will not likely correspond with clinical status.[57-58]

The dose of DSFab is dependent on the total body load (TBL) of digoxin. Empiric dosing of DSFab can be performed if the ingested quantity is unclear or if a SDC is not available. In acute exposures, 10–20 DSFab vials are recommended empirically for adult and pediatric patients.[57-58] An adequate clinical effect with 10 vials will be achieved in most patients. An additional 10 vials can be administered if a sufficient response is not achieved. In acute exposures the following equation can be used to calculate the DSFab dose if ingested amount is known[57]:

$$\text{Equation 1: } Number\ of\ vials = \frac{Amount\ ingested\ (mg)}{0.5\left(\frac{mg}{vial}\right)} \times 0.80$$

Additionally the following equation can be used in acute or chronic exposures to calculate the DSFab dose if a postdistribution SDC is known[57]:

$$\text{Equation 2: } Number\ of\ vials = \frac{SDC\left(\frac{ng}{mL}\right) \times Patient\ weight\ (kg)}{100}$$

Regardless of the method, the number of vials should be rounded up to the next whole vial and should be administered as an IV infusion over 30 minutes as a diluted solution. In critically ill patients both Digibind and DigiFab can be administered as an IV bolus.[57-58] The manufacturer warns about use in patients with an allergy to papaya extracts.[57] Patients with a history of atrial fibrillation or heart failure should be monitored for disease emergence as DSFab not only reverses toxic effects but therapeutic effects as well. Hypokalemia can develop due to reactivation of myocardial sodium-potassium ATPase. Serum potassium concentrations should be closely monitored for the first few hours after administration and cautious supplementation should be performed when necessary.[57-58] Finally, DSFab is renally eliminated and its clearance probably decreases with renal insufficiency.[57] One series noted no recrudescence of toxicity in patients with renal failure.[59] However, in one case, an anephric patient developed an atrioventricular block 10 days after DSFab administration and symptom resolution.[59] Therefore, it may be prudent to monitor for reemergence of digoxin toxicity in anephric patients after DSFab administration.

Digoxin has a large VD and is extensively tissue bound.[5] Because the majority of digoxin is not within the circulation, extracorporeal elimination is not effective.

DIGOXIN-LIKE IMMUNOREACTIVE SUBSTANCES

Some patients have detectable serum digoxin concentrations despite never taking the medication. This phenomenon is related to the presence of chemicals that interfere with digoxin immunoassays due to similarities in chemical structure. It should be noted that some of these chemicals are functionally similar to digoxin and are typically classified as endogenous or exogenous in nature.[60]

Endogenous digoxin-like immunoreactive substances (EDLISs) are thought to be natriuretic hormones, with some having the ability to inhibit sodium-potassium ATPase.[60-61] These compounds are typically undetectable in healthy individuals and are found in a variety of patient populations and disease states. Examples include uremic syndrome, liver disease and liver failure, renal insufficiency, pregnancy, preeclampsia, congestive heart failure, and neonates or premature infants.[61] It has been postulated that an endogenous synthesis pathway produces these compounds, which are absent in healthy adults and are not commonly found in edible plants. Clinical observations indicate that the contributions of EDLISs are generally less than 2.0 ng/mL but can be higher.[61] However, the magnitude of these contributions is dependent on the immunoassay. Positive interference has been noted with the digoxin fluorescence polarization immunoassay, making the SDC appear falsely elevated. Conversely, negative interference has been noted with the microparticle enzyme immunoassay, making the SDC appear falsely low.[62]

A variety of exogenous digoxin-like immunoreactive substances (ExDLISs) have been noted. Like EDLISs, they are structurally similar to digoxin. However, these compounds are foreign and synthesis is not endogenous in nature. Examples include spironolactone, canrenone (spironolactone's active metabolite), potassium canrenoate, and an array of Chinese medications, including chan su, oleander-containing herbs, Siberian ginseng, Asian ginseng, Ashwagandha, and danshen.[61,63] Like EDLISs, reports of both positive and negative interference have been noted with ExDLISs.[61] The nature of these differences varies with the type of immunoassay.[61]

EDLISs and ExDLISs can complicate digoxin therapeutic drug monitoring. Positive interference can make a SDC appear falsely elevated. This value could be potentially misinterpreted as a supratherapeutic or toxic level. More dangerously, negative interference can make a SDC appear falsely low and toxicity could occur secondary to dosage increases in response to an artificially low value. Thus, it is important to assess any given SDC in the context of a patient's individual clinical status. Medication histories, including herbal supplements, should be obtained. Dosage adjustments should likely be driven by the combined assessment of the SDC and signs or symptoms of inadequate therapeutic response or toxicity. Additionally, interference is assay-dependent and the degree of interference is continually changing as assays evolve. Clinicians need to assess which assays are used at their institution and the effect that EDLISs and ExDLISs have on a given assay. Contacting the laboratory performing the SDC could provide insight. Interestingly, EDLISs and ExDLISs are highly protein bound and assessment of free digoxin concentrations could reduce EDLIS and ExDLIS interference. Clinical evidence suggests that assessment of free digoxin concentrations eliminates the interference seen with some immunoassays.[64-65] Assessment of free digoxin concentrations could be considered if a patient has an abnormal SDC and if EDLIS and ExDLIS interfere with the immunoassay used in the assessment. However, this approach is not universally effective; interference still occurred with some assays when only free digoxin concentrations were estimated.[66]

CASES

CASE 1: DIGOXIN LOADING DOSE CASE

A 47-year-old female is to be initiated on digoxin for atrial fibrillation. Calculate an appropriate digoxin loading dose and maintenance dose if the patient is to be started on an intravenous loading and oral maintenance dose using digoxin tablets. Assume her CrCl is 80 mL/min and her target Css is 1 ng/mL.

Answer:

$$\text{Loading dose} = (VD)(C)/(F)$$

First calculate Volume of distribution.

$$VD = 226 + [298(CrCl)/(29.1 + CrCl)]$$
$$= 226 + [298(80 \text{ mL/min})/(29.1 + 80 \text{ mL/min})]$$
$$= 444.5 \sim 445 \text{ L}$$

$$\text{Loading dose} = (VD)(C)/(F)$$
$$= (444.5 \text{ L})(1 \text{ ng/mL})/(1)$$
$$= 444.5 \text{ mcg} \sim 0.5 \text{ mg}$$

$$\text{Maintenance dose} = (CL)(Css)(T)/(F)$$

First calculate CL.

$$CL = 1.303 \text{ CrCl (mL/min)} + CL_m, (CL_m = 40 \text{ mL/min})$$
$$= 1.303 \times 80 \text{ mL/min} + 40 \text{ mL/min}$$
$$= 144.2 \text{ mL/min}$$

$$\text{Converting to L/day} = [(144.2 \text{ mL/min})(1,440 \text{ min/day})]/ \\ 1,000 \text{ mL/L} = 207.7 \text{ L/day}$$

$$\text{Maintenance Dose} = (CL)(Css)(T)/(F)$$
$$= [(207.7 \text{ L/day})(1 \text{ ng/mL})(1 \text{ day})]/(0.7)$$
$$= 296.7 \text{ mcg} \sim 250 \text{ mcg, or } 0.25 \text{ mg}$$

CASE 2: DIGOXIN MAINTENANCE DOSE CASE (EMPIRIC)

A 73-year-old male with moderate CHF is to be initiated on digoxin. Calculate an appropriate oral regimen to target a goal of 0.8 ng/mL using digoxin tablets via his orogastric (OG) tube. Assume his CrCl is 35 mL/min.

Answer:

$$\text{Maintenance dose} = (CL)(Css)(T)/(F)$$

First calculate CL.

$$CL = 1.303 \text{ CrCl (mL/min)} + CL_m, (CL_m = 20 \text{ mL/min})$$
$$= 1.303 \times 35 \text{ mL/min} + 20 \text{ mL/min}$$
$$= 65.6 \text{ mL/min}$$

$$\text{Converting to L/day} = [(65.6 \text{ mL/min})(1,440 \text{ min/day})]/ \\ 1,000 \text{ mL/L} = 94.5 \text{ L/day}$$

$$\text{Maintenance dose} = (CL)(Css)(T)/(F)$$
$$= [(94.5 \text{ L/day})(0.8 \text{ ng/mL})(1 \text{ day})]/(0.7)$$
$$= 108 \text{ mcg} \sim 125 \text{ mcg tablets}$$

His final regimen is 125 mcg tablet daily. A loading dose is not needed because the indication is CHF and not atrial fibrillation.

CASE 3: DIGOXIN MAINTENANCE DOSE CASE (BASED ON LEVEL)

A 45-year-old male admitted for right hip surgery develops atrial fibrillation postoperatively. His past medical history includes moderate-severe HF, chronic kidney disease, and hypertension. He was loaded with 750 mcg intravenously (IV) and started on a maintenance dose of 0.125 mg PO daily. In 16 days the digoxin level is obtained at steady state. Calculate a new oral regimen to target a level of 1.0 ng/mL for adequate ventricular control.

Assume his CrCl is 60 mL/min and digoxin level is 0.4 ng/mL on a digoxin maintenance dose of 0.125 mg IV daily.

Answer:

First calculate his true CL.

$$Css = (MD)(F)/(CL)(T), \text{ rearranging}$$
$$CL = (MD)(F)/(Css)(T)$$
$$= (125 \text{ mcg})(0.7)/0.4 \text{ ng/mL}(1)$$
$$= 218.8 \text{ L/day}$$

Next, estimate his new oral tablet regimen.

$$\text{Maintenance dose} = (CL)(Css)(T)/(F)$$
$$= [(218.8 \text{ L/day})(1.0 \text{ ng/mL})(1 \text{ day})]/(0.7)$$
$$= 312.6 \text{ mcg} \sim 250\text{-}375 \text{ mcg, or } 0.25 \text{ mg to} \\ 0.375 \text{ mg}$$

His dose can be increased to 0.25 mg or 0.375 mg orally daily.

CASE 4: DIGOXIN DOSING IN PATIENTS WITH EXCESSIVE BODY MASS

PL is a 56-year-old male who is admitted under the cardiology service with newly diagnosed atrial fibrillation. The team decides to administer an oral loading dose of digoxin for rate control. You, as the pharmacist on the team, are asked to recommend an appropriate loading dose that will yield a level of 0.8 ng/mL.

Height: 5′7″

Weight: 250 lbs

SCr = 1

IBW = 50 kg + (2.3)(7) = 66.1 kg

ABW = 250 lb/2.2 = 113.6 kg

When the ABW is greater than 30 percent above IBW, patient is obese.

Answer:

$$\text{Loading dose} = \frac{(VD)(C)}{(F)}$$

$$\text{Volume of distribution} = \left(7\frac{L}{kg}\right) \times 66.1 \ kg = 463 \ L$$

$$\text{Loading dose} = \frac{(463.5 \ L)(0.8 \ mcg/L)}{(0.7)} = 529 \approx 500 \ mcg$$

Because this patient's ABW is more than 30 percent above IBW, he is classified as obese. The volume of distribution of digoxin is not affected by increased adipose tissue and, therefore, it is appropriate to utilize IBW when calculating doses in obese patients. In this example, we use PL's IBW to calculate the volume of distribution (utilizing the average population value). We then in-putted the rest of the information into the loading dose equation, with F (bioavailability) = 0.7. Because commercially available tablets come in multiples of 125 mcg, a dose of 529 mcg can be rounded down to 500 mcg.

CASE 5: DIGOXIN DOSING IN PATIENTS WITH LOW BODY MASS

What would be the loading dose if PL was underweight?

Height: 5′7″

Weight: 100 lbs

SCr = 1

IBW = 66.1 kg

ABW = 45.5 kg

Answer:

$$Volume\ of\ distribution = 7\frac{L}{kg} \times 45.5\ kg = 318.5\ L$$

$$Loading\ dose = \frac{(318.5\ L)(0.8\ mcg/L)}{(1)(0.7)} = 364 \approx 375\ mcg$$

As you can see in this example, PL's ABW is below his IBW, therefore, he is underweight. Underweight patients have a reduced amount of total body water and, therefore, would have a reduced volume of distribution. Here we used the patient's ABW to calculate the volume of distribution and, ultimately, the loading dose.

CASE 6: DIGOXIN DOSING IN PATIENTS WITH KIDNEY DISEASE

RM is a 75-year-old female with a history positive for CKD, CAD, and type 2 DM presenting to the ED with dizziness and fatigue for several days. Electrocardiogram reveals atrial fibrillation. Her cardiologist is ordering IV digoxin loading dose and oral maintenance dose with a target serum level of 1.2 ng/mL.

Height = 66 inches

Weight = 62 kg

SCr = 1.7 mg/dL

IBW = 45 + 6(2.3) = 58.8 kg

$$CrCl = \frac{(140 - 75)(58.8)}{72(1.7)}\ [0.85] = 26\ mL/min$$

QUESTIONS

1. *What is an appropriate IV loading dose?*

Answer:

VD = 226 + [298(CrCl)/(29.1 + CrCl)]

VD = 226 + [298(26) / 29.1 + 26] = 366 L

LD = (VD)(C)/(F) = (366)(1.2)/(1) = 439 mcg ~ 500 mcg

2. *What would you recommend as an oral maintenance dose?*

Answer:

CL = 1.303 CrCl (mL/min) + CL$_m$

CL = (1.303)(26) + 40 = 73.8 mL/min

MD = (CL)(C$_{ss}$)(T)/(F)

= (73.8)(1.2)(1)/(0.7) = 87.6/0.7 = 126 mcg ~125 mcg

3. *What is the calculated half-life of digoxin in this patient?*

Answer:

Change CL from mL/min to L/day.

CL L/day = (CL mL/min)(1,440 min/day)/1,000 mL/L

CL L/day = (73.8)(1,440)/1,000 = 105 L/day

T1/2 = (0.693)(VD)/CL = (0.693)(366)/105 = 2.4 days

CASE 7: DIGOXIN INTERACTION WITH AMIODARONE

DW is a 78-year-old female with estimated creatinine clearance of 45 mL/min and has been on the following medications for more than three months.

-Metoprolol 25 mg by mouth twice daily

-Digoxin 0.125 mg by mouth daily

-Levothyroxine 25 mcg by mouth daily

Her most recent digoxin level was 1.1 ng/mL, 2 weeks ago. Since that time, she has had no appreciable change in renal function and her medication compliance is good. She has had some symptomatic atrial fibrillation episodes, and her cardiologist begins her on amiodarone 200 mg by mouth 3 times daily with a taper to 200 mg daily.

QUESTIONS

1. *When would DW's digoxin be at new steady state, and what is the expected serum concentration?*

Answer:

To determine true steady state of digoxin, we would need to determine when amiodarone steady state would be achieved. Based on half-life of amiodarone of 15 to 65 days, at a fixed dose of amiodarone, the new steady state would be 1.5 months to 1 year. However, in this patient we are starting with a higher dose (200 mg 3× daily) for the purpose of obtaining a therapeutic concentration more quickly. Based on Pollack and colleague's[67] pharmacokinetic modeling study, if a high-dose amiodarone "loading" regimen is utilized, a "therapeutic" amiodarone concentration is obtained within a few days and maintained thereafter. However, the regimen described in the Pollack study (1,600 mg/day for 2 days, 1,200 mg/day for 5 days, 1,000 mg/day for 7 days, 800 mg/day for 7 days, 600 mg/day for 7 days, then 400 mg/day) is substantially different from the regimen mentioned in this case. In Nademanee and colleagues,[36] a fixed dose of amiodarone was used for the first 16 days and resulted in increasing amiodarone concentrations and increasing digoxin concentrations over that time. The authors of that study felt that due to the long and variable half-life of amiodarone and the kinetic analysis of amiodarone concentrations, the steady state of amiodarone had not been reached by 16 days. Also in Nademanee, an amiodarone-digoxin dose-related interaction was demonstrated when amiodarone increased from 200 mg per day to 600 mg per day; digoxin concentration increased from 0.4 to 0.7 ng/mL (see Table 6-1).

As far as impact of amiodarone on the patient's serum digoxin concentration, the expected increase could be minimal with a low dose (e.g., 200 mg daily) to substantial with larger doses (e.g., >400 mg per day) with potential expected doubling of concentration. To summarize expected effect upon digoxin steady state, we would expect new steady state within variable time period based upon dosing regimen of 1 week to 1 year and potential doubling of new steady-state serum digoxin concentration. For practical purposes, monitoring of digoxin serum concentrations should be established for several months after an addition of amiodarone to a patient taking digoxin. The frequency of levels should take into consideration the current digoxin level, which may potentially double.

In the case of DW, her most recent serum concentration is 1.1 ng/mL. We can expect to see doubling of this concentration within a few weeks, and therefore, a dose decrease of digoxin to every other day or routine serum digoxin concentration measurements weekly to avoid toxicity would be prudent.

2. *Should we take a level before expected new steady state?*

Answer:

If the current regimen is maintained, based on details in answer to question 1, it would be prudent to obtain digoxin serum concentrations routinely for the next few months.

3. *Should we reduce digoxin dose empirically prior to any serum concentration measurement?*

Answer:

Because DW's current digoxin concentration is 1.1 ng/mL, it would be prudent to decrease digoxin dosing by 50 percent when we expect the digoxin concentration to potentially double. On the other hand, if DW's baseline serum concentration was lower, perhaps 0.4 ng/mL, then concentration doubling would not put her at risk of toxicity and may increase therapeutic benefit, meaning no empiric dose adjustment would be necessary.

4. *How would DW's case differ if amiodarone was started at 200 mg per day rather than 200 mg 3 times daily?*

Answer:

The expected effect on serum digoxin concentration would be less than doubling. However the exact effect is not known based on current pharmacokinetic trials. Additionally, a full effect will take several months to determine. In this case, routine digoxin monitoring may be applied.

CASE 8: DIGOXIN INTERACTION WITH DRONEDARONE

QUESTION

How would DW's case differ if dronedarone was used instead of amiodarone?

Answer:

Based on pharmacokinetic studies in healthy adults, we would expect to see a significant increase in serum digoxin concentration within days and new steady state within a week (see Table 6-1). It is suggested that digoxin discontinuation be considered as coadministration has been associated with increased risk of arrhythmia or sudden death in dronedarone-treated patients compared to placebo. If treatment is continued, decrease the dose of digoxin by 50% and monitor serum concentrations closely.[68]

Digoxin toxicity occurred in an 82-year-old female after she received a loading dose of 0.25 mg for three doses. The patient experienced bradycardia with an elevated digoxin level (>5 ng/mL).[69]

CASE 9: DIGOXIN INTERACTION WITH VERAPAMIL

After 2 days on amiodarone 200 mg three times daily and digoxin 0.125 mg daily, DW reports intolerable abdominal pain.

A stat digoxin level prior to this morning's dose was 1.4 ng/mL. Digoxin toxicity was ruled out. The cardiologist decides to discontinue amiodarone and metoprolol and begins verapamil at 80 mg twice daily.

QUESTION

When would DW be at new steady state, and what is the expected serum concentration?

Answer:

Based on verapamil's usual half-life of 3–12 hours, expected verapamil steady state would be within a few days, and full impact on

digoxin serum concentration should be seen within a week. Based on pharmacokinetic studies (Table 6-1), a significant decrease in digoxin clearance and volume of distribution occurs, as well as an increase in digoxin half-life. These changes result in potential doubling of digoxin serum concentration.

CASE 10: DIGOXIN INTERACTION WITH DILTIAZEM

Instead of choosing verapamil, the clinician changes DW to diltiazem 60 mg three times daily.

QUESTION

When would DW be at new steady state, and what is her expected serum concentration?

Answer:

Although diltiazem is included in the FDA summary of those drugs that interact with digoxin through inhibition of p-glycoprotein transport system, the results of pharmacokinetic studies have shown variable impact of coadministration of diltiazem and digoxin (Table 6-1). A rough summary of the studies reviewed seems to indicate that studies performed in healthy adults and patients with atrial fibrillation tend to show little change in digoxin pharmacokinetics with the addition of diltiazem. On the other hand, those pharmacokinetic studies completed in patients with heart failure have shown increased digoxin area under the curve and half-life, resulting in increased serum digoxin concentration of approximately 40–50 percent within a week of coadministration.

Based on this information, with the addition of diltiazem to a patient already receiving digoxin, monitoring digoxin serum concentration in approximately a week would be prudent. Determination of levels would be particularly applicable to those patients with heart failure as well as those with higher baseline digoxin concentrations who may be at risk for toxicity.

CASE 11: DIGOXIN DOSING WITH P-GLYCOPROTEIN INDUCERS (E.G., ST. JOHN'S WORT)

JN is a 65-year-old male with estimated creatinine clearance of 20 mL/min and has been on digoxin 0.125 mg every other day for 1 year along with other medications for his heart failure. Since beginning therapy, he has had several serum concentrations that have been between 0.6 ng/mL and 1 ng/mL. Three weeks ago his routine serum digoxin concentration was 1 ng/mL. JN notifies you that his friend suggested St John's Wort and will be starting it as soon as he picks up a bottle from the pharmacy.

QUESTION

What is the expected impact of St John's Wort on digoxin serum concentration, and should you obtain a level?

Answer:

The coadministration of St. John's Wort and digoxin has been well studied in Europe (Table 6-1). In general, a decrease in digoxin bioavailability results in a 25–40 percent decrease in serum digoxin concentrations after 10 days.

However, the preparation of St. John's Wort greatly influences the impact on digoxin pharmacokinetics. A pharmacokinetic study of various St. John's Wort preparations was performed in 96 healthy volunteers.[70] These volunteers were given a 7-day loading phase of digoxin and then 14 days of comedication with placebo or one of 10 St. John's Wort preparations. Preparations that contained lower amounts of hyperforin had no apparent effect on digoxin trough concentration and nonsignificant changes in digoxin maximal concentration and AUC of -14 percent and 9 percent, respectively. On the other hand, St. John's Wort preparations with increased hyperforin and hypericin content showed significant decreases in digoxin trough, maximal concentration, and AUC of 19 percent, 38 percent, and 27 percent, respectively, after 14 days of comedication. When exposed to a half-dose of this St. John's Wort preparation, the impact on digoxin pharmacokinetic parameters was roughly half of the full dose.

To summarize, if JN's last serum concentration was 1 ng/mL, a 25–40 percent reduction in serum concentration would be acceptable for management of heart failure. However, because JN's serum concentration is lower, it would be prudent to obtain a serum digoxin concentration in about 1 week to ensure therapeutic concentration.

CASE 12: DIGOXIN TOXICITY (ACUTE)

A 31-year-old male (weight 82 kg) with no PMH history presents after ingesting four of his grandmother's digoxin 0.125 mg tablets in an attempt to get high. He stated that the ingestion occurred approximately an hour ago, and he denied any coingestants or use of any chronic medications. Currently he has no complaints. He denies any headaches, nausea, vomiting, abdominal pain, or visual disturbances. He is currently awake, alert, and oriented and is answering questions appropriately.

VS: T 36.7°C; BP 132/88 mm Hg; HR 84 bpm; RR 16 rpm; O2sat 99% RA

Physical examination is nonremarkable.

BMP: Na^+ 140 mEq/L; K^+ 4.0 mEq/L; Cl^- 104 mEq/L; HCO_3^- 24 mmol/L; BUN 14 mg/dL; SCr 1.0 mg/dL; glucose 120 mg/dL

Digoxin level (drawn two hours after ingestion): 3.94 ng/mL

ECG: Normal sinus rhythm; ventricular rate 84 bpm; QRS 90 msec; QTc 425 msec

QUESTIONS

1. *Does this patient have signs or symptoms consistent with digoxin toxicity? If so what signs or symptoms of digoxin toxicity does this patient exhibit, and what is the likely cause?*

Answer:

This patient has no signs or symptoms consistent with digoxin toxicity. He has no gastrointestinal or neurological complaints at this time. His ECG does not show any dysrhythmias or conduction abnormalities, and he is hemodynamically stable. His serum potassium is within normal limits.

Additionally based on the size of this patient's dose, toxicity would not be expected. DSFab is indicated with acute exposures ≥10 mg and ≥4 mg in adults and children, respectively. This patient was exposed to 0.5 mg, which is <10 mg.

2. *Is the patient's digoxin level a pre- or postdistribution level? Why would knowing this information impact the interpretation of this digoxin level?*

Answer:

Digoxin's therapeutic range is 0.8–2.0 ng/mL. It is important to note that this range refers to a postdistribution, steady-state concentration.

Digoxin obeys a two-compartment model, with a rapidly distributing compartment and a slowly distributing compartment. The vasculature and the myocardium are respective parts of the rapidly distributing and slowly distributing compartments. Once a distribution equilibrium is reached between the compartments, the concentrations in the rapidly distributing compartment are proportional to the concentrations in the slowly distributing compartment. This equilibrium occurs approximately 4 hours and 6 hours after the administration of IV and oral doses, respectively. Concentrations assessed prior to distribution equilibrium will appear falsely elevated because digoxin has not yet fully distributed throughout the body.

This patient's digoxin level was 3.94 ng/mL, which, if drawn appropriately, could be potentially toxic. However, this level was drawn approximately 2 hours postingestion and is a predistribution level. Our reference range is based on postdistribution levels and cannot be used for comparison. Additionally, this patient has no signs or symptoms of toxicity at this time. A digoxin level should be repeated at least 6 hours postingestion and should be interpreted in the context of the clinical picture at that time.

3. *Should this patient receive digoxin-specific Fab (DSFab)? If so, what dose should the patient receive?*

Answer:

DSFab is indicated with the following:

- Progressive bradydysrhythmias or second-/third-degree heart block not responsive to atropine.
- Severe ventricular dysrhythmias or tachydysrhythmias.
- Serum potassium >5 mEq/L in an acute digoxin intoxication.
- Postdistribution serum digoxin concentration (SDC) ≥10 ng/mL, or a SDC ≥15 ng/mL at any time.
- Acute digoxin ingestion ≥10 mg (adult) or ≥4 mg (child).
- Rapidly progressing signs or symptoms of digoxin toxicity in combination with an increasing potassium level.

This patient does not meet any of these criteria and DSFab is not indicated at this time.

CASE 13: DIGOXIN TOXICITY (CHRONIC)

An 89-year-old female (weight 52 kg) presents with complaints of confusion, nausea, and vomiting over the past week. Four weeks prior to presentation, the patient had been admitted for palpations and atrial fibrillation poorly controlled on metoprolol. The patient was started on digoxin 0.25 mg once daily and discharged home. Her last digoxin dose was the evening prior to presentation (>12 hours). An initial ECG demonstrated atrial fibrillation with frequent premature ventricular contractions (PVCs).

Past medical history includes atrial fibrillation, congestive heart failure, hypothyroidism, hypertension, and diabetes mellitus.

She is currently taking metoprolol 100 mg twice daily, verapamil XR 240 mg once daily; digoxin 0.25 mg once daily, fosinopril 20 mg once daily; furosemide 40 mg twice daily, spironolactone 100 mg once daily, levothyroxine 100 mcg once daily, insulin glargine 35 units subcutaneously every bedtime, and insulin aspart 8 units subcutaneously before every meal.

VS: T 37.5°C; BP 78/54; HR 60 bpm; RR 26 rpm; O2sat 100% 6L NC

BMP: Na^+ 135 mEq/L; K^+ 5.2 mEq/L; Cl^- 104 mEq/L; HCO_3^- 22 mmol/L; BUN 60 mg/dL; SCr 2.1 mg/dL; Glucose 145 mg/dL

Serum digoxin concentration: 4.5 ng/mL

ECG: atrial fibrillation with frequent premature ventricular contractions

QUESTIONS

1. *Does this patient have signs or symptoms consistent with digoxin toxicity? If so what signs or symptoms of digoxin toxicity does this patient exhibit, and what is the likely cause?*

Answer:

A number of the patient's signs and symptoms are consistent with digoxin toxicity. She has gastrointestinal (nausea), neurologic (confusion, altered mental status), and cardiac (hypotension, atrial fibrillation with frequent PVCs) manifestations. The patient's hyperkalemia is likely multifactorial and could be the result of renal insufficiency or concurrent medications. Hyperkalemia due to digoxin effect is more commonly associated with acute exposures.

The patient has a number of factors that could have attributed to the signs and symptoms of digoxin toxicity. First, this patient appears to have some degree of renal insufficiency. Digoxin is eliminated 60–80 percent unchanged in the urine, and renal insufficiency could lead to accumulation and increased serum digoxin concentrations. Secondly, the patient was started on an inappropriate digoxin dose for an 89-year-old female. Elderly patients frequently have reduced lean body mass, decreased renal function, and are on an assortment of medications that could interact with digoxin. All these factors can increase SDCs and could have played a role in the development of digoxin toxicity.

2. *Is the patient's digoxin level a pre- or postdistribution level? Why would knowing this information impact the interpretation of this digoxin level?*

Answer:

The patient's serum digoxin concentration was drawn greater than 6 hours after her last dose. Therefore, this level is a postdistribution level and can be compared to the conventional reference range. The patient's serum digoxin concentration and her clinical effects are consistent with digoxin toxicity.

3. *Should this patient receive digoxin-specific Fab? If so, what dose should the patient receive?*

Answer:

This patient has demonstrated arrhythmias, hemodynamic changes, and mental status changes. The hyperkalemia is multifactorial.

Arrhythmias and hemodynamic instability are consistent with significant, potentially life-threatening toxicity and digoxin-specific Fab is clearly indicated. The patient's dose would be calculated as follows:

$$Number\ of\ vials = \frac{SDC(ng/mL) \times weight(kg)}{100}$$

$$Numbers\ of\ vials = \frac{4.5\ ng/ml \times 52\ kg}{100}$$

$$Number\ of\ vials = 2.34 \sim 3\ vials$$

CASE 14: ENDOGENOUS AND EXOGENOUS DIGOXIN-LIKE IMMUNOREACTIVE SUBSTANCES

A 78-year-old male (weight = 98 kg) presents to his cardiologist's office for a routine follow-up appointment. The patient has been maintained on digoxin 0.25 mg every other day for 2 years with serum digoxin concentrations (SDCs) between 0.8 and 1.2 ng/mL. He is on the medication for congestive heart failure; he has noted symptomatic improvement since digoxin started. He has no complaints today. He denies any nausea, vomiting, visual changes, mental status changes, or palpations. He denies any increasing shortness of breath or swelling in his lower extremities. He has had no changes in his prescribed medications since his last SDC assessment. However, the patient stated he has started taking danshen, a Chinese herbal medication he heard about on the news, about 2 weeks ago. The patient stated he took his last digoxin dose last evening, which was 12 hours prior to the appointment, and that he has been taking the medication as prescribed.

A SDC is obtained and analyzed at the office's laboratory during the appointment. The office's laboratory uses the fluorescence polarization immunoassay for digoxin.

Past medical history includes congestive heart failure, hypertension, coronary artery disease, and diabetes mellitus. Current medications include digoxin 0.25 mg every other day, lisinopril 40 mg every day, furosemide 40 mg twice daily, aspirin 81 mg every day, metoprolol 100 mg twice daily, metformin 1,000 mg twice daily, and glipizide XL 2.5 mg once daily.

VS: T 37.5°C; BP 124/82; HR 84 bpm; RR 16 rpm; breathing comfortably on room air

Physical examination is unremarkable.

BMP: Na^+ 141 mEq/L; K^+ 4.2 mEq/L; Cl^- 104 mEq/L; HCO_3^- 23 mmol/L; BUN 10 mg/dL; SCr 0.9 mg/dL; glucose 147 mg/dL (Values are stable when compared to his last appointment.)

Digoxin level: 2.9 ng/mL

ECG: Normal sinus arrhythmia; QRS 90 msec; QTc 425 msec

QUESTIONS

1. *Does this patient have any signs or symptoms consistent with digoxin toxicity? If so, what are they, and should this patient receive digoxin-specific Fab?*

Answer:

This patient has no signs or symptoms consistent with digoxin toxicity. He does not have any gastrointestinal or neurologic complaints. His ECG is not abnormal. He is hemodynamically stable. Digoxin-specific Fab is not indicated in this patient.

2. *What are some potential causes for the patient's elevated digoxin level?*

Answer:

Elevations in SDCs can be explained by a variety of factors including renal insufficiency, drug interactions, improper sampling, and improper digoxin administration. The patient's SCr is stable compared to previous values. The patient's prescribed medications are unchanged from previous visits. The digoxin level was sampled greater than 6 hours after the patient's last dose and is a postdistribution level. Additionally, the patient stated that he has been taking his digoxin as prescribed. The only thing that has changed with the patient's medications is that he started taking the Chinese herb danshen.

Danshen is an exogenous digoxin-like immunoreactive substance (ExDLIS) that is structurally similar to digoxin, which also possesses some activity at sodium-potassium ATPase. It can cause interference with some digoxin immunoassays and leads to both falsely low and falsely elevated values depending on which immunoassay is used. Therefore, the elevated SDC is most likely related to danshen.

3. *What interventions could potentially be attempted to more thoroughly assess this serum digoxin concentration?*

Answer:

You could contact the laboratory to see if danshen interferes with the digoxin immunoassay used in the assessment. Danshen has been shown to have positive interference with the fluorescence polarization immunoassay for digoxin, leading to falsely elevated values. Clinical evidence suggests that assessing free digoxin concentrations with this assay eliminates danshen interference.

It should be noted that interference is assay-dependent and varies with different ExDLISs. Additional follow-up would be required for different herbal supplements and different immunoassays. For some herbal preparations and some immunoassays, assessment of free digoxin concentrations does eliminate DLIS interference.

REFERENCES

1. Gheorghiade M, Veldhuisen DJ, Colucci W. Contemporary use of digoxin in the management of cardiovascular disorders. *Circulation.* 2006;113:2556–2564.

2. Maron BA, Rocco TP. Chapter 28. Pharmacotherapy of congestive heart failure. In Brunton LL, Chabner BA, Knollmann BC, (Eds.). *Goodman & Gilman's The Pharmacological Basis of Therapeutics,* 12th ed. New York: McGraw-Hill, 2011. Available at: http://www.accessmedicine.com/content.aspx?aID=16668047 (accessed January 11, 2013).

3. Gheorghiade M, Adams K, Colucci W. Digoxin in the management of cardiovascular disorders. *Circulation.* 2004;109:2959–2964.

4. Aronson JK. Clinical pharmacokinetics of digoxin 1980. *Clin Pharmacokinet.* 1980;5(2):137–149.

5. Lisalo E. Clinical pharmacokinetics of digoxin. *Clin Pharmacokinet.* 1977;2(1):1–16

6. Reuning RH, et al. Role of pharmacokinetics in drug dosage adjustment: I. Pharmacologic effect kinetics and apparent volume of distribution of digoxin. *J Clin Pharmacol.* 1973;13:127.

7. Abernethy DR, et al. Digoxin disposition in obesity: Clinical pharmacokinetic investigation. *Am Heart J.* 1981;102:740–744.

8. Perrier D, Mayersohn M, Marcus FJ. Clinical Pharmacokinetics of digitoxin. *Clin Pharmacokinet.* 1977;2:292–311.

9. Graves PE, Fenster PE, MacFarland RT, et al. Kinetics of digitoxin and the bis- and mono-digitoxosides of digitoxigenin in renal insufficiency. *Clin Pharmacol Ther.* 1984;36(5):607–612.

10. Gault MH, Longerich LL, Loo JC, et al. Digoxin biotransformation. *Clin Pharmacol Ther.* 1984;35(51):74–82.

11. Maron BA, Rocco TP. Chapter 28. Pharmacotherapy of congestive heart failure. In Brunton LL, Chabner BA, Knollmann BC, (Eds.). *Goodman & Gilman's The Pharmacological Basis of Therapeutics,* 12th ed. New York: McGraw-Hill, 2011. Available at: http://www.accessmedicine.com/content.aspx?aID=16668047 (accessed January 11, 2013).

12. Chan KE, Lazarus JM, Hakim RM. Digoxin associates with mortality in ESRD. *J Am Soc Nephrol.* 2010;21(9):1550–1559.

13. Jusko W, Szefler S, Goldfarb A. Pharmacokinetic design of digoxin dosage regimens in relation to renal function. *J Clin Pharmacol.* 1974;14(10):525–535.

14. Ahmed A, Rich MW, Love TE, et al. Digoxin and reduction in mortality and hospitalization in heart failure: A comprehensive post hoc analysis of the DIG trial. *Eur Heart J.* 2006;27:178–186.

15. Gheorghiade M, Hall VB, Jacobsen G, et al. Effects of increasing maintenance dose of digoxin on left ventricular function and neurohormones in patients with chronic heart failure treated with diuretics and angiotensin-converting enzyme inhibitors. *Circulation.* 1995;92:1801–1807.

16. Heart Failure Society of America. Executive summary: HFSA 2006 comprehensive heart failure practice guidelines. *J Card Fail.* 2006;12:10–38.

17. Fuster V, Rydén LE, Cannom DS, Crijns HJ, Curtis AB, Ellenbogen KA, et al. ACC/AHA/ESC 2006 guidelines for the management of patients with atrial fibrillation: A report of the American College of Cardiology/American Heart Association Task Force on Practice Guidelines and the European Society of Cardiology Committee for Practice Guidelines (writing committee to revise the 2001 guidelines for the management of patients with atrial fibrillation). Developed in collaboration with the European Heart Rhythm Association and the Heart Rhythm Society. *Circulation.* 2006;114(7):e257–e354.

18. Bauman LJ, DiDomenico JR, Viana M, et al. A method of determining the dose of digoxin for heart failure in the modern era. *Arch Intern Med.* 2006;166:2539–2545.

19. Koup JR, Jusko WJ, Elwood CM, Kohli RK. Digoxin pharmacokinetics: Role of renal failure in dosage regimen design. *Clin Pharmacol Ther.* 1975;18:9–21.

20. Lisalo E. Clinical pharmacokinetics of digoxin. *Clin Pharmacokinet.* 1991;2:1–16.

21. Cheng JW, Charland SL, Shaw LM, Kobrin S, Goldfarb S, Stanek E, Spinler SA. Is the volume of distribution of digoxin reduced in patients with renal dysfunction? *Pharmacother.* 1997;17(3):584–590.

22. Reuning RH, Sams RA, Notari RE. Role of pharmacokinetics in drug dosage adjustment, I. Pharmacologic effect kinetics and apparent volume of distribution of digoxin. *J Clin Pharmacol.* 1973;13:127.

23. Ackerman GL, Dougherty JE, Flanagan WI. Peritoneal dialysis and hemodialysis of tritiated digoxin. *Ann Intern Med.* 1967;67:718–723.

24. Cusack B. Pharmacokinetics in older persons. *American Journal of Geriatric Pharmacotherapy.* 2004;2(4):274–302.

25. Currie GM, Wheat JM, Kiat K, Pharmacokinetic considerations for digoxin in older people. *Open Cardiovasc Med J.* 2011;5:130–135.

26. Sheiner LB, et al. Estimation of population characteristics of pharmacokinetic parameters from routine clinical data. *J Pharmacokinet Biopharm.* 1977;5:445.

27. Doherty JE, Perkins WH. Digoxin metabolism in hypo- and hyperthyroidism: Studies with tritiated digoxin in thyroid disease. *Ann Intern Med.* 1966;64(3):489–507.

28. Croxson MS, Ibbertson HK. Serum digoxin in patients with thyroid disease. *Br Med J (Clin Res Ed).* 1975;3:555–556.

29. Zilley W, Richter E, Rietbrock N. Pharmacokinetics of digoxin and methyldigoxin in patients with acute hepatitis. *Med Klin.* 1978;73(13):463–469.

30. Verschraagen M, Koks CHW, Schellens JHM, Beijnen JH. P-glycoprotein system as a determinant of drug interactions: The case of digoxin-verapamil. *Pharmaco Res.* 1999;40:301–306.

31. Koren G, Woodland C, Ito S. Toxic digoxin-drug interactions: The major role of renal p-glycoprotein. *Vet Human Toxicol.* 1998;40:45–46.

32. U.S. Food and Drug Administration. Drug interaction studies: Study design, data analysis, implications for dosing, and labeling recommendations. 2012. Available at: http://www.fda.gov/Drugs/GuidanceComplianceRegulatoryInformation/Guidances/default.htm.

33. Bigger JT, Leahey EB. Quinidine and digoxin. *An important reaction. Drugs.* 1982;24(3):229–239

34. Moysey JO, Jaggarao NSV, Grundy EN, Chamberlain DA. Amiodarone increases plasma digoxin concentrations. *Br Med J.* 1981;282:272.

35. Fenster PE, White NW, Hanson CD. Pharmacokinetic evaluation of the digoxin-amiodarone interaction. *J Am Coll Cardiol.* 1985;5:108–112.

36. Nademanee K, Kanna R, Hendrickson J, Ookhtens M, Kay I, Singh B. Amiodarone-digoxin interaction: Clinical significance, time course of development, potential pharmacokinetic mechanisms and therapeutic implications. *J Am Coll Cardiol.* 1984;4:111–116.

37. Gaud C, Hurbin F, Brunet A, Sultan E, Galleyrand J, Guenole E. Effects of dronedarone on the pharmacokinetics of digoxin in healthy subjects [abstract]. *Basic Clin Pharmacol Toxicol.* 2010;107(suppl 1):298; Abstract 1262.

38. Mahgoub AA, El-Medany AH, Abdulatif AS. A comparison between the effects of diltiazem and isosorbide dinitrate on digoxin pharmacodynamics and kinetics in the treatment of patients with chronic ischemic heart failure. *Saudi Med J.* 2002;23:725–731.

39. Andrejak M, Hary L, Andrejak MTH, Lesbre J. Diltiazem increases steady-state digoxin serum levels in patients with cardiac disease. *J Clin Pharmacol.* 1987;27:967–970.

40. Maragno I, Santostasi G, Gaion RM, Trento M, Grion AM, Miraglia G, Volta SD. Low- and medium-dose diltiazem in chronic atrial fibrillation: Comparison with digoxin and correlation with drug plasma levels. *Am Heart J.* 1988;116:385–392.

41. Yoshida A, Fujita M, Kurosawa N, Nioka M, Shichinohe T, Arakawa M, Fukuda R, Owada E, Ito K. Effects of digoxin on plasma level and urinary excretion of digoxin in healthy subjects. *Clin Pharmacol Ther.* 1984;35:681–685.

42. Beltrami TR, May JJ, Bertino JS. Lack of effect of diltiazem on digoxin pharmacokinetics. *J Clin Pharmacol.* 1985;25:390–392.

43. Rameis H, Magometschnigg D, Ganzinger U. The diltiazem-digoxin interaction. *Clin Pharmacol Ther.* 1984;36:183–189.

44. Pedersen KE, Dorph-Pedersen A, Hvidt S, Klitgaard NA, Nielsen-Kudsk F. Digoxin-verapamil interaction. *Clin Pharmacol Ther.* 1981;30: 311–316.

45. Schwartz JB, Keefe D, Kates RE, Kirsten E, Harrison DC. Acute and chronic pharmacodynamic interaction of verapamil and digoxin in atrial fibrillation. *Circulation.* 1982;65:1163–1170.

46. Durr D, Stieger B, Kullak-Ublick GA, Rentsch KM, Steinert HC, Meier PJ, Fattinger K. St. John's wort induces intestinal P-glycoprotein/MDRI and intestinal and hepatic CYP3A4. *Clin Pharmacol Ther.* 2000;68: 598–604.

47. Johne A, Brockmoller J, Bauer S, Maurer A, Langheinrich M, Roots I. Pharmacokinetic interaction of digoxin with an herbal extract from St. John's wort (hypericum perforatum). *Clin Pharmacol Ther.* 1999;66:338–345.

48. Beller GA, Smith TW, Abelmann WH, et al. Digitalis intoxication: A prospective clinical study with serum level correlations. *N Engl J Med.* 1971;284:989–997.

49. Williamson KM, Thrasher JA, Fulton KB, et al. Digoxin toxicity: An evaluation in current clinical practice. *Arch Intern Med.* 1998;158(22):2444–2449.

50. Bauman JL, DiDomenico RJ, Galanter WL. Mechanisms, manifestations and management of digoxin toxicity in the modern era. *Am J Cardiovasc Drugs.* 2006;6(2):77–86.

51. Ma G, Brady WJ, Pollack M, et al. Electrocardiographic manifestations: Digitalis toxicity. *J Emerg Med.* 2001;20(2):145–152.

52. Cooke D. The use of central nervous system manifestations in the early detection of digitalis toxicity. *Heart Lung.* 1993;22:477–481.

53. Sundar S, Burma DP, Vaish SK. Digoxin toxicity and electrolytes: A correlative study. *Acta Cardiol.* 1983;38(2):115–123.

54. Bismuth C, Gaultier M, Conso F, et al. Hyperkalemia in acute digitalis poisoning: Prognostic significance and therapeutic implications. *Clin Toxicol.* 1973;6:153–162.

55. Shapiro W, Narahara K, Taubert K. Relationship of plasma digitoxin and digoxin to cardiac response following intravenous digitalization in man. *Circulation.* 1970;42:1065–1072.

56. Walsh FM, Sode J. Significance of non-steady-state serum digoxin concentrations. *Am J Clin Pathol.* 1975;63(3):446–450.

57. DigiFab [package insert]. West Conshohocken, PA: BTG International Inc., 2012.

58. Digibind [package insert]. Research Triangle Park, NC: GlaxoSmithKline, 2003.

59. Wenger TL. Experience with digoxin immune Fab (ovine) in patients with renal impairment. *Am J Emerg Med.* 1991;9(2 Suppl 1):21–23; discussion 33–34.

60. Stone JA, Soldin SJ. An update on digoxin. *Clin Chem.* 1989;35(7): 1326–1331.

61. Dasgupta A. Therapeutic drug monitoring of digoxin: Impact of endogenous and exogenous digoxin-like immunoreactive substances. *Toxicol Rev.* 2006;25(4):273–281.

62. Dasgupta A, Trejo O. Suppression of total digoxin concentrations by digoxin-like immunoreactive substances in the MEIA digoxin assay. Elimination of negative interference by monitoring free digoxin concentrations. *Am J Clin Pathol.* 1999;111(3):406–410.

63. Dasgupta A. Endogenous and exogenous digoxin-like immunoreactive substances: Impact on therapeutic drug monitoring of digoxin. *Clin Chem.* 2002;118:132–140.

64. Dasgupta A, Saldana S, Heimann P. Monitoring free digoxin instead of total digoxin in patients with congestive heart failure and high concentrations of digoxin-like immunoreactive steroids. *Clin Chem.* 1990;36(12):2121–2123.

65. Datta P, Dasgupta A. Effect of Chinese medicine Chan Su and Danshen on EMIT2000 and Randox digoxin immunoassays: Wide variation in digoxin-like immunoreactivity and magnitude of interference in digoxin measure by different brands of the same product. *Ther Drug Monit.* 2002;24(5):637–644.

66. Reyes MA, Actor JK, Risin SA, et al. Effect of Chinese medicines Chan Su and Lu-Shen-Wan on serum digoxin measurement by Digoxin III, a new digoxin immunoassay. *Ther Drug Monit.* 2008;30(1):95–99.

67. Pollak PT, Bouillon T, Shafer SL. Population pharmacokinetics of long-term oral amiodarone therapy. *Clin Pharmacol Ther.* 2000;67: 642–652.

68. Multaq [package insert]. Bridgewater, NJ: Sanofi Aventis U.S. LLC, 2012.

69. Vallakati A, Chandra P, Pednekar M, Frankel R, Shani J. Dronedarone-induced digoxin toxicity: New drug, new interactions. *Amer J of Ther.* 2013;20(6):e717–e719.

70. Mueller SC, Uehleke B, Woehling H, Petzsch M, Majcher-Peszynska J, Hehl E, Sievers H, Frank B, Riethling A, Drewelow B. Effect of St. John's wort dose and preparations on the pharmacokinetics of digoxin. *Clin Pharmacol Ther.* 2004;75:546–557.

CHAPTER

7

Unfractionated Heparin and Low-Molecular Heparins

LIZ G. RAMOS, BS, PharmD, BCPS
AMY L. DZIERBA, PharmD, FCCM, BCPS

UNFRACTIONATED HEPARIN

OVERVIEW

Unfractionated heparin (UFH) is considered an indirect parenteral anticoagulant, as it has little or no intrinsic anticoagulant activity and works by potentiating the effect of antithrombin (AT), by UFH binding to it, and thereby inhibiting various activated clotting factors.[1]

UFH is a glycosaminoglycan found in the secretory granules of mast cells.[2] UFH is a heterogeneous mixture of various lengths and properties. Each heparin molecule is made up of alternating D-glucuronic acid and N-acetyl-D-glucosamine residues with varying molecular size from 5,000 to 30,000 daltons (mean 15,000 daltons).[3-5] The anticoagulant effect of UFH is mediated through a specific pentasaccharide sequence on the heparin molecule that binds to AT, which causes a conformational change to antithrombin.[3] This UFH-AT complex inhibits the activity of factors IXa, Xa, XIIa, and thrombin (IIa). Only one-third of the heparin molecule possesses this unique pentasaccharide sequence with affinity to antithrombin. This complex is 100 to 1,000 times more potent as an anticoagulant compared to antithrombin alone.[6] Through its action on thrombin, this UFH-AT complex also inhibits factors V and VIII. Not only does UFH prevent the growth of formed thrombus, it may also have effects on the patient's own thrombolytic system.[7] The factors that are most sensitive to this complex are IIa and Xa. Only molecules that contain >18 pentasaccharides can bind to both antithrombin and thrombin simultaneous. Conversely, molecules with as few as 5 pentasaccharides can inhibit factor Xa.[8] In addition, heparin binds to platelets, thereby inhibiting platelet function by either inducing or inhibiting platelet aggregation, which may contribute to the bleeding effects of heparin by a mechanism independent of its anticoagulation effect.

Commercially available UFH preparations are derived from porcine intestinal mucosa.[9]

PHARMACOKINETICS

Due to its large molecular size and anionic structure, UFH is not absorbed reliably from the gastrointestinal tract when taken orally.[2] Intramuscular (IM) injection is discouraged, given its erratic absorption. In addition, IM administration may result in hematomas. Therefore, the preferred route of UFH administration is either by a continuous intravenous (IV) infusion or by subcutaneous injection. It is recommended to give UFH as an IV bolus if an immediate anticoagulant effect is required rather than via a subcutaneous route, because its anticoagulant effect is seen in one to two hours.[10]

The bioavailability of UFH is dose dependant, which ranges from 30 percent at lower doses to as high as 70 percent at the higher doses.

Therefore, if the subcutaneous route is chosen to deliver a dose, this dose should be higher than the usual intravenous dose.[11,12] The bioavailability and anticoagulant activity of UFH is limited by the binding of UFH to a number of circulating plasma proteins such as platelet factor-4, macrophages, fibrinogen, lipoprotein, and endothelial cells, which may account for the inter- and intrapatient variability.[13] The circulating plasma proteins levels can rapidly change in acutely ill patients or patients with active thrombosis. The volume of distribution of UFH is similar to blood volume (60 mL/kg) and binds extensively to low-density molecules. UFH does not cross the placenta and does not distribute in breast milk.[10]

The half-life of UFH is also dose-dependent and can range from 30 to 90 minutes or more in patients receiving high doses. Heparin clearance consists of a rapid saturable phase and slower first-order process. In the saturable phase, heparin binds to endothelial cells and macrophages, and once bound it is internalized and eliminated from the circulation. The slower nonsaturable phase is the renal elimination of heparin.[14,15] Therefore, a disproportionate anticoagulant response may occur at therapeutic doses with the duration and intensity of anticoagulation rising nonlinearly with increasing dose. At therapeutic doses, a large proportion of heparin is cleared through the rapid saturable, dose-dependent mechanism. In addition, the apparent half-life of heparin increases from approximately 30 minutes after an IV bolus of 25 units/kg, to 60 minutes with an IV bolus of 100 units/kg, to 150 minutes with a bolus of 400 units/kg.[8]

UFH is used to treat various cardiovascular disorders including the prevention and treatment of arterial and venous thromboembolism, treatment of unstable angina, acute myocardial infarction, cardiac and vascular surgery, coronary angioplasty, stent placement and is also used as an adjunctive medication during thrombolysis.[16] UFH still remains the anticoagulant of choice for any interventional or surgical procedures, despite the availability of newer agents on the market. It also remains the anticoagulant of choice for patients during pregnancy, given its favorable pharmacokinetics.

DOSING

The dose and route of UFH is dependent on the indication, the therapeutic goals and the patient's response. For the prevention of venous thromboemolism, the recommended UFH dose is 5,000 units subcutaneous every 8 to 12 hours[17] and a weight-based intravenous continuous infusion is preferred when immediate and full anticoagulation is required.[8] The efficacy of heparin in the initial treatment of VTE is critically dependent on dose.

In a randomized trial by Raschke and colleagues,[18] patients received heparin at fixed doses (5,000-unit bolus followed by 1,000 units/h by infusion) or adjusted doses using a weight-based nomogram (starting dose, 80 units/kg bolus followed by 18 units/kg/h by infusion). This trial showed that while patients receiving UFH via a weight-based nomogram received higher doses within the first 24 hours than those given fixed doses of heparin, the rate of recurrent thromboembolism was significantly lower with the weight-based UFH regimen. The 2012 guidelines from the American College of Chest Physicians[8] recommend that the initial parenteral heparin dosing for VTE be administered as weight-based (80 units/kg IV bolus and 18 units/kg/h IV infusion). If continuous intravenous heparin administration is not possible, then it is recommended to administer UFH subcutaneously SC via two options: (1) an initial IV bolus of 5,000 units followed by 250 units/kg SC twice daily[19]; or (2) an initial SC dose of 333 units/kg followed by 250 units/kg SC twice daily thereafter.[20] For the treatment of acute coronary syndromes, the recommended doses are much lower than that used for VTE. The American College of Cardiology[21] recommends a heparin bolus of 60 to 70 units/kg (maximum 5,000 units) followed by an infusion of 12 to 15 units/kg/h (maximum 1,000 units/h) for unstable angina and non-ST-segment elevation myocardial infarction. If UFH is used in combination with a fibrinolytic agent for the treatment of ST-segment elevation myocardial infarction, the recommended dose is 60 units/kg (maximum 4,000 units) as a bolus and the infusion is 12 units/kg/h (maximum of 1,000 units/kg/h).[22]

MONITORING

The risk of heparin-associated bleeding increases as the UFH dose increases[23,24] and if used in conjunction with other antithrombotic agents such as fibrinolytic agents[25] or glycoprotein IIb/IIIa inhibitors.[26] This risk also increases when patients have had recent surgery or other invasive procedures or have other comorbidities that can worsen hepatic function. The dose of UFH is adjusted based on the activated partial thromboplastin (aPTT), while the evidence is weak to maintain a "therapeutic range" (which is hospital-specific and only based on a subgroup analysis). A strong correlation is found, however, between subtherapeutic aPTT value and recurrent VTE, but a relationship between a supratherapeutic aPTT value and bleeding is not as clear.[27] The activated clotting time can be used to monitor the higher heparin doses given to patients undergoing percutaneous coronary interventions or cardiopulmonary bypass surgery. The recommended aPTT ratio that has been associated with a reduced risk of recurrent VTE is between 1.5 and 2.5 times control.[28]

As stated before, this range has not been confirmed by any randomized trials, but has been accepted as the standard. The therapeutic aPTT ranges vary from hospital to hospital as it is dependent on the various reagents and instruments used to measure the aPTT. Therefore, no weight-based heparin nomogram is the same from hospital to hospital, nor can they be applied to all reagents; each hospital must determine there own anti-Xa assay dependent on the reagent being used. One study established a therapeutic range for an aPTT ratio of 1.5 to 2.5 that corresponded to a heparin level of 0.2 to 0.4 units by protamine titration and a heparin level of 0.3 to 0.7 units measured by an anti-Xa assay.[28] Again, given the variability between aPTT and anti-Xa assays between each laboratory, more research is needed to identify which is the best monitoring tool for UFH. Therefore, in 2012, the American College of Chest Physicians[8] recommended that each lab calibrate specifically for each reagent/coagulometer in determining aPTT values and correlating these values with therapeutic UFH levels. Prior to initiating therapeutic UFH, it is recommended to obtain a baseline PT, aPTT, CBC with platelet count, and subsequent aPTT levels every six hours after initiation and for any dosing changes, until therapeutic aPTT values have been achieved.

ADVERSE EFFECTS

A well-known adverse effect of UFH is thrombocytopenia in addition to hemorrhagic complications. The relationship between supratherapeutic aPTT and bleeding has not been clearly delineated.[27] The

occurrence of bleeding complications in patients receiving UFH ranges from 1.5 to 20 percent with an increased risk in patients with preexisting risk, which includes renal or liver disease, malignancy, and age greater than 65 years, to name a few. Thrombocytopenia is defined as platelet count of <150,000/mm^3. Of the two types of heparin-induced thrombocytopenia (HIT), the first type of HIT presents within the first 2 days after exposure to heparin, and the platelet count normalizes with continued heparin therapy. It is well known that this type of HIT is a nonimmune disorder, and occurs with the direct effect of heparin on platelet activation. The second type of HIT is an immune-mediated disorder that typically occurs 4–10 days after exposure to heparin, and it has life-threatening prothrombotic complications if not quickly identified.[29]

Immune-mediated HIT should be suspected when a patient has a fall in platelet count while receiving heparin—particularly if the fall is more than 50 percent of the baseline count, even if the platelet count >150,000/mm^3—and is evidenced by skin lesions at heparin injection sites. To help clinicians with determining the probability that a patient has this type of HIT, the 4Ts score has been developed and the most studied.[30-32] This pretest clinical scoring system, helps clinicians in the diagnosis of HIT, but should never be used alone. Other nonhemorrhagic side effects are uncommon and include skin reactions that can progress to necrosis, alopecia, and hypersensitivity reactions manifested by chills, fever, pruritus, or anaphylactoid reactions. Other adverse effects that are seen with UFH therapy include elevations of serum transaminases, but are usually transient, and osteoporosis. Osteoporosis is caused by binding of heparin to osteoblasts, which has been reported in patients receiving long-term (>6 months) large daily doses of UFH.

REVERSAL OF ANTICOAGULANT EFFECT OF UFH

Given all the new anticoagulants coming to market, UFH has one advantage over these new agents in that protamine can rapidly reverse its anticoagulant effect. Protamine sulfate is a basic protein derived from fish sperm that binds to heparin to form a stable salt. The recommended dose is 1 mg of protamine sulfate to neutralize approximately 100 units of heparin.[8] For example, if a patient bleeds immediately after receiving an IV bolus of 4,000 units of heparin then this patient should receive about 40 mg of protamine sulfate. Protamine sulfate is quickly cleared from circulation with a half-life of about 7 minutes.

As stated previously, the half-life of IV heparin is about 60–90 minutes when heparin is given as an IV infusion. The calculated dose of protamine that needs to be administered should take into account the amount of heparin only given in the previous few hours. If a patient is receiving UFH as a continuous IV infusion at 2,000 units/h, then you require approximately 50 mg of protamine sulfate to neutralize the heparin that was given in the past 2–2.5 hours. It is important that the correct dose of protamine be used to reverse UFH, because protamine can exert its own anticoagulant effect if used in doses larger than required. Additional protamine adverse effects include hypotension or bradycardia, which can be minimized by administering protamine no faster than 5 mg/min.[9]

LOW-MOLECULAR-WEIGHT HEPARIN

OVERVIEW

The development of low-molecular-weight heparin (LMWH) from either chemical or depolymerization of UFH has increased clinical options for the management of thromboembolic disorders.

LMWHs primarily exert their anticoagulant effect by inactivating active factor X with less affinity for thrombin.[8] Each LMWH has a different amount of antifactor Xa activity; therefore, each preparation should be considered an individual drug that cannot be used interchangeably.

It is well-established that LMWHs are approximately one-third the molecular weight and exhibit decreased binding to macrophages, endothelial cells, platelets, and platelet factor 4.[8] These differences offer several advantages of LMWHs when compared to UFH. These advantages include a more predictable pharmacokinetic response, improved subcutaneous bioavailability, longer half-life, and lower incidence of HIT. As a result, LMWHs have largely replaced UFH for the prevention and treatment of venous thromboembolism (VTE) and in the management of unstable angina and non-ST elevation myocardial infarction (NSTE-MI).

PHARMACOKINETICS

After SC administration, the bioavailability of LMWH approaches 100 percent.[33] Low-molecular-weight heparins predominately concentrate in the plasma and highly vascular tissues with little distribution in fat tissue.[34] The half-life of LMWHs is approximately 3–6 hours after SC administration, significantly longer as compared to UFH. Antifactor Xa activity persists longer than antifactor IIa activity, reflecting the more rapid clearance of longer heparin chains.[35] The peak anticoagulant effect is observed with LMWHs 3–5 hours after administration.[8] Even though UFH is mainly cleared by a cellular mechanism, LMWHs are strongly dependent on the renal route for elimination. Renal impairment will lead to a reduction in clearance with a subsequent increase in elimination half-life and augmented anticoagulant activity leading to an increased risk of bleeding.

MONITORING

Routine monitoring of traditional measures of coagulation is not necessary for the vast majority of patients receiving LMWHs as a result of the predictable anticoagulant response. Baseline coagulation factors along with a complete blood count and serum creatinine should be obtained at the initiation of a LMWH and periodically throughout therapy.[8] Monitoring of plasma anti-Xa activity is the recommended test if monitoring is desired; however, it is not essential in patients with stable and uncomplicated conditions.[36,37] Peak anti-Xa level, drawn four hours after SC administration, is dependent on the drug and dosing interval. Target anti-Xa levels for twice daily treatment of VTE with enoxaparin are 0.6–1.0 units/mL.[37,38] Target anti-Xa levels for once daily administration of enoxaparin, dalteparin, or tinzaparin are >1.0 units/mL, 1.05 units/mL, and 0.85 units/mL, respectively.[37,39]

GENERAL DOSING

Fixed or weight-based dosing for LMWH is based on product and indication (see Table 7-1). For each product, doses should be based on actual body weight. It is important to note that enoxaparin dosing is expressed in milligrams, whereas dalteparin and tinzaparin are expressed in units of antifactor Xa activity.[40-42]

Dosing Considerations in the Obese Patient

Obese patients, defined as individuals with a body mass index (BMI) of greater than 30 kg/m^2, have a lower proportion of lean body mass as compared to their total body weight.[43] Controversy surrounds the appropriate dosing in this patient population because of a paucity of data on the optimal dosing strategy of LMWHs.

Two retrospective subgroup analyses of obese patients receiving a fixed prophylactic dose of enoxaparin or dalteparin did not demonstrate a significant difference in VTE occurrence compared with placebo in nonobese patients.[44,45] However, unadjusted prophylactic doses of LMWHs may be insufficient to prevent VTE in this patient population because of an inverse correlation between total body weight and antifactor Xa activity.[46] A prospective study of bariatric surgical patients demonstrated a lower incidence of DVT in patients receiving a higher dose of enoxaparin without an increase in bleeding rate.[47] A small nonrandomized trial demonstrated effectiveness without increased bleeding when enoxaparin was dosed per weight for the prevention of thromboembolism in medically ill, morbidly obese patients.[48] Based on these and other clinical studies, increasing VTE prophylactic doses of enoxaparin or dalteparin may be appropriate in obese patients, especially the morbidly obese bariatric surgical patient.[46,47,49,50]

Small studies including obese patients treated for VTE using enoxaparin or dalteparin have demonstrated that dosing regimens based on actual body weight were effective without an increase in bleeding events.[51,52] In a prospective registry of patients with acute VTE, thrombotic and bleeding outcomes did not differ between obese and nonobese patients, despite the low doses of LMWH in the patients weighing more than 100 kg.[53] In a retrospective analysis of the TIMI IIb and ESSENCE trials, about half of the patients who received enoxaparin or UFH for NSTE-MI were obese with a mean BMI of 31.4 kg/m^2.[54] In this analysis the composite endpoint of death, MI, and urgent revascularization were lower in patients receiving enoxaparin in both obese and nonobese patients. Rates of major bleeding were similar between obese and nonobese patients. A prospective study enrolling patients with NSTE-MI compared dalteparin to placebo on the rate of death and new MI during the first 6 days.[55] Dalteparin doses were capped at 10,000 IU twice daily. Patients weighing less than 76 kg demonstrated a 1.3 percent incidence of death or MI, compared to 2.2 percent in patients weighing more than 76 kg at study day 6. Based on these results, obese patients with VTE or ACS should have their LMWH dosed based on total body weight. Until further elucidated, obese patients with VTE receiving enoxaparin should be treated with twice daily dosing.[56]

Dosing Considerations in Patients with Kidney Injury

Low-molecular-weight heparin is primarily eliminated through the kidneys. As such, the use of LMWHs in patients with renal impairment leads to accumulation and a higher risk of bleeding.[8] The risk of LMWH accumulation and bleeding is dependent on the severity of renal injury along with the dose and the LMWH administered.

At prophylactic doses, LMWHs have not demonstrated a significant increase in bleeding risk in patients with mild-to-moderate renal impairment. The available evidence suggests that dose adjustments of dalteparin and tinzaparin are not necessary in patients with renal impairment. In a prospective study, prophylactic subcutaneous dalteparin was administered to consecutive critically ill patients with an estimated CrCl of less than 30 mL/min.[57] No evidence indicated accumulation or an increased risk of bleeding. A small study enrolling elderly patients with an estimated CrCl between 20 and 50 mL/min showed no evidence of accumulation of tinzaparin over an eight-day period when administered at prophylactic doses.[58] However, accumulation of enoxaparin occurs with repeated prophylactic doses in patients with renal impairment.[58,59] As a result, the manufacture recommends a dose reduction of enoxaparin to 30 mg SC daily in patients with a CrCl of 30 mL/min or less.[40] No specific recommendations are given for other LMWHs. Bleeding rates from LMWH when used as prophylactic treatment of VTE appear to be low with little accumulation; however, the risk of bleeding in patients with moderately impaired renal function over an extended time period remains elusive.

TABLE 7-1 Dosing and Indications of LMWH

Generic Name (brand name)	Prophylaxis in Hip-Replacement Surgery	Prophylaxis in Knee-Replacement Surgery	Prophylaxis Abdominal Surgery	Prophylaxis in Acute Medical Illness	Treatment of Deep Vein Thrombosis with or without Pulmonary Embolism	Unstable Angina or Non-Q Wave Myocardial Infarction
Enoxaparin (Lovenox)	30 mg SC q12h administered 12–24 hrs after surgery[a] OR 40 mg SC q24h administered 12 hrs prior to surgery[a]	30 mg SC q12h administered 12–24 hrs prior to surgery[a]	40 mg SC q24h administered 2 hrs prior to surgery[a]	40 mg SC q24h[a]	1 mg/kg SC q12h[a] OR 1.5 mg/kg SC q24h[a]	1 mg/kg SC q12h[a]
Dalteparin (Fragmin)	2,5000 IU SC administered 2 hrs prior to surgery, followed by 2,500 IU SC the evening after surgery and at least 6 hrs after the first dose, then 5,000 IU SC q24h[a] OR 5000 IU SC q24h administered the evening prior to surgery[a]		2,500 IU SC q24h administered 1–2 hrs prior to surgery (without malingancy)[a]	5,000 IU SC q24h[a]	200 IU/kg SC q24h OR 100 IU/kg SC q12h	120 IU/kg SC q12h (max dose: 10,000 IU)[a]
Tinzaparin (Innohep)	75 units/kg SC q24h administered the evening prior to surgery or 12 hrs after surgery OR 4,500 IU SC q24h administered 12 hrs prior to surgery	75 units/kg SC q24h administered the evening prior to surgery or 12 hrs after surgery	3,500 units SC q24h administered 1–2 hrs prior to surgery		175 units/kg SC q24h[a]	

[a]FDA approved dose

At therapeutic doses, a reduction is noted in LMWH elimination in patients with renal insufficiency, which is associated with an increased risk of bleeding.[60,61] A meta-analysis including 4,971 patients demonstrated an increased risk of major bleeding in patients receiving enoxaparin with a CrCl of 30 mL/min or less when compared to patients with a CrCl greater than 30 mL/min.[62] The rate of bleeding for daltaparin or tinzaparin could not be determined because of insufficient data. Empiric dose reductions of enoxaparin decreased bleeding rates; however, did not reach statistical significance. Several large registries have also demonstrated an increase in major bleeding when LMWHs were used in patients with a CrCl of 30 mL/min or less in the treatment of VTE or ACS.[54,63-66] Enoxaparin is the only LMWH that has dosing recommendations for use in patients with severe renal impairment.[40] A 50 percent dose reduction is recommended compared to the standard dose for patients with VTE yielding peak antifactor Xa levels within target range.[67,68]

Although limited, available data suggests that therapeutic dose tinzaparin has little accumulation when administered to patients with age-related renal impairment over a 10- to 30-day period.[69,70] This difference in clearance may be related to the higher molecular weight as compared to other LMWHs.[8]

In patients with severe kidney injury requiring therapeutic anticoagulation, alternative agents such as UFH may be a safer choice. If a LMWH is initiated in a patient with renal impairment, along with dose reductions, antifactor Xa measurements may be prudent with extended use.

Dosing Considerations in the Elderly

Older populations are frequently underrepresented or not included in clinical trials making the assessment of LMWH safety and efficacy limited in this patient population. Many elderly patients have pharmacokinetic alterations based on age-related renal impairment and a reduction in lean body mass. In addition, the elderly are at twofold increase risk for a major bleeding event when anticoagulated for the treatment of VTE.[71] Among the three LMWHs, only enoxaparin has a recommended dose reduction in patients aged 75 or greater for the treatment of ACS.[40]

The use of tinzaparin is not recommended in elderly patients with renal insufficiency based on the interim findings of a clinical trial that compared tinzaparin to UFH in the initial treatment of DVT and/or PE in elderly patients aged 70 years or older with estimated creatinine clearance below 30 mL/min or patients aged 75 years or older with estimated creatinine clearance below 60 mL/min.[42] Overall mortality rates were 6.3 percent in patients treated with UFH and 11.5 percent in patients treated with tinzaparin.[72]

Dosing Considerations in the Critically Ill Patient

In the absence of any contraindications, all critically ill patients should receive pharmacologic thromboprophylaxis. In patients with active bleeding or an acquired coagulopathy, intermittent pneumatic compression devices may serve as an alternative. In critically ill patients, the bioavailability of subcutaneously administered drugs has been shown to be reduced in ICU patients because of the concomitant use of vasoactive drugs or the presence of edema; therefore, potentially providing a reduced effect.[73,74]

REVERSAL

Neutralization of LMWH by protamine sulfate is incomplete neutralization of antifactor Xa. In scenarios when the reversal of LMWH is clinically indicated, protamine sulfate should be administered in a dose of 1 mg for every 100 antifactor Xa units of LMWH (1 mg of enoxaparin is approximately equal to 100 antifactor Xa units) if the dose of LMWH was given within the previous 8 hours.[8] The maximum single dose of protamine sulfate is 50 mg. Smaller doses of protamine sulfate may be considered if more than 8 hours have elapsed from the last dose of LMWH.

ADVERSE EFFECTS

The most common adverse effect associated with LMWHs is bleeding. Major bleeding from LMWH has been reported to be less than 3 percent and varies among the different preparations.[8] Minor bleeding, particularly at the site of injection, may occur frequently. Epidural or spinal hematomas may occur in patients who are receiving LMWH and neuraxial anesthesia or undergoing spinal puncture, potentially resulting in long-term or permanent paralysis.[40-42]

CASE STUDIES

CASE 1

JT is an 85-year-old man (80 kg, 5′11″) admitted to Hospital X with right calf swelling and pain of one day in duration. He denies any trauma but reports he was a passenger on a lengthy trip where he was sitting for long hours. He denies any shortness of breath, cough, or chest pain. JT has a history of MI and hypercholesterolemia. Initial relevant labs include SCr = 1.5, INR = 1, PT = 10.8 s, aPTT = 23.6 s, and platelet count is 200,000/mm³. JT is diagnosed with a DVT of his right calf.

QUESTION

Which anticoagulant is recommended for JT and at what dose and route?

Answer:

Given JT's elevated SCr of 1.5, UFH is recommended via the intravenous route. The 2012 guidelines for the American College of Chest Physicians[8] recommends the initial IV heparin dosing for VTE to be administered as weight-based (80 units/kg bolus and 18 units/kg/h infusion). Therefore, JT should receive an initial bolus of 6,400 units (80 units/kg × 80 kg) of UFH, followed by an initial infusion of 1,400 units/hr (18 units/kg/h × 80 kg), round to the nearest 100 units. In addition, you recommend that an aPTT level be drawn 6 hours after heparin infusion has begun.

QUESTION

Seven hours later the results for JT's aPTT level comes back at 50 s and the attending on call wants JT's goal aPTT level to be 90 s, which was the therapeutic aPTT goal at the previous institution where he worked at. What do you want to tell the attending? What is your recommendation? (See Table 7-2.)

Answer:

The therapeutic aPTT ranges vary from hospital to hospital and are dependent on the various reagents and instruments used to measure the aPTT. At Hospital X, the therapeutic aPTT corresponds to 56–80 s. Therefore, based on Hospital X's weight-based nomogram and JT's current aPTT level of 50 s, it recommends to bolus with

3,200 units (40 units/kg × 80 kg) and to increase the infusion rate by 200 units/hr (i.e., 1,600 units/hour, keeping in mind to round to the nearest 100 units). Additionally, the serum aPTT level should be ordered and monitored in 6 hours.

QUESTION

This time, JT's aPTT serum level is drawn 2 hours later and comes back at 100 s with no signs of any bleeding. The resident wants to hold the UFH infusion and decrease the rate. What do you recommend?

Answer:

It is recommend to continue the same rate and drawing an appropriate serum aPTT level in 4 hours and adjusting infusion based on that level.

QUESTION

JT has been therapeutic on his heparin infusion (1,600 units/hr) for the last 24 hours and a morning aPTT is drawn and comes back >100 s, hemoglobin and hematocrit drops from 8.9 g/dL to 6.9 g/dL and 36.5% to 20.8 % respectively, and blood is present in JT's urine and stool. The resident wants to reverse the heparin. What do you recommend?

Answer:

Bleeding is the most common adverse effect associated with UFH administration. Protamine is used to neutralize UFH by forming an inactive protamine-heparin complex. The recommended dose is 1 mg of protamine sulfate to neutralize approximately 100 units of heparin. Because JT was receiving a continuous infusion of 1,600 units/hr, you want to give enough protamine sulfate to neutralize the heparin that was being administered in the past 2.5 hours. It is important that the correct dose of protamine be used to reverse UFH, because protamine can exert its own anticoagulant effect if used in doses larger than required. Therefore, administer 40 mg (1,600 units/hr × 2.5 hr = 4,000 units; 4,000 units/100 units = mg of protamine to administer) of protamine intravenous, no faster than 5 mg/min, to help minimize hypotension or bradycardia.[9]

CASE 2

KL is a 55-year-old man (80 kg, 5′10″) admitted to Hospital Z with a swollen left calf, which has gradually increased and is affecting the entire left leg to the groin. Now admitted, he is complaining of new onset right-sided pleuritic chest pain with SOB and no hemoptysis. His chest X-ray and VQ scan are highly suggestive of a PE. A pulmonary angiography is performed and a PE is diagnosed. Initial relevant labs include SCr = 2.5, INR = 1, PT = 12.8 s, aPTT = 27 s, and platelet count is 250,000/mm³. It was difficult to obtain baseline labs, and

TABLE 7-2	Hospital X's Weight-Based Nomogram			
	Heparin Bolus	Infusion Hold Time	Infusion Rate Adjustment	When to Draw Next aPTT
aPTT <45 s	80 units/kg	0	↑ 4 units/kg/h	In 6 hours
aPTT 45–55 s	40 units/kg	0	↑ 2 units/kg/h	In 6 hours
aPTT, 56–80 s	**(Corresponds to therapeutic heparin serum level at this institution)**			Every 6 hours until 2 consecutive therapeutic levels
aPTT 81–100 s	0	0	↓ 2 units/kg/h	In 6 hours
aPTT >100 s	0	1 hour	↓ 3 units/kg/h	In 6 hours

IV access is difficult to maintain in this patient. Which anticoagulant is recommended for KL and at what dose and route?

Answer:

Based on KL's SCr of 2.5, UFH is the best anticoagulant. Because intravenous access is difficult to obtain, it is recommended to administer UFH subcutaneously via one of two options: (1) an initial IV bolus of 5,000 units followed by 250 units/kg SC twice daily[19]; or (2) an initial SC dose of 333 units/kg followed by 250 units/kg SC twice daily thereafter.[20]

If you choose option 1, then administer initial bolus of 5,000 units, followed by 20,000 units (250 units/kg × 80 kg) twice daily; or using option 2, then administer initial bolus of 26,500 units (333 units/kg × 80 kg, round to nearest 500 units), followed by 20,000 units (250 units/kg × 80 kg) twice daily, with serum aPTT levels drawn every 6 hours.

QUESTION

After being on therapeutic subcutaneous UFH for the last 4 days, KL's CBC reveals a platelet count of 100,000/mm³ (baseline of 250,000/mm³). What do you think is the cause of KL's platelet count drop, and what do you recommend?

Answer:

Immune-mediated HIT is a disorder that typically occurs 4–10 days after exposure to heparin, and it has life-threatening prothrombotic complications if not quickly identified.[29] HIT should be suspected when a patient has a fall in platelet count while receiving heparin—particularly if the fall is more than 50 percent of the baseline count. To help clinicians with determining the probability that a patient has HIT, the 4Ts score has been developed and the most studied.[30-32] If the 4Ts score results in intermediate or high probability for HIT, all UFH should be immediately discontinued, a Heparin PF4 AB/HIT assay sent, and anticoagulation with a direct thrombin inhibitor (e.g., Argatroban) considered.

CASE 3: DOSING AND ADMINISTRATION OF LMWH FOR DVT PROPHYLAXIS

MH is a 66-year-old woman admitted to the intensive care unit after her hip replacement surgery. She is 5′4″ and weighs 59 kg. Her latest laboratory values indicate that she is not anemic and has normal kidney function. It is decided to initiate DVT prophylaxis with enoxaparin. What dose should be initiated in MH? How should enoxaparin be administered to MH?

Answer:

Two dose regimens of enoxaparin are approved for DVT prophylaxis in patients having hip-replacement surgery. One regimen would be to initiate enoxaparin 30 mg subcutaneously every 12 hours beginning 12–24 hours after surgery, providing that hemostasis has been established.[40] Alternatively, 40 mg subcutaneously every 24 hours beginning 12 hours prior to surgery may be considered.[40] Because this patient in not underweight/overweight and does not have renal impairment, no dose adjustments need to be made at this time. Of note, dalteparin and tinzaparin also have approved dosing regimens for DVT prophylaxis in patients undergoing hip replacement surgery.

Each dose of enoxaparin would be administered as a subcutaneous injection while in the supine position in the abdominal area or the upper, outer part of the thigh. It is recommended to alternate injection sites.

CASE 4: DOSING AND ADJUSTMENT OF LMWH FOR ACUTE DVT

AH is a 35-year-old woman who presents to the emergency room with new onset left calf swelling. She is 5′3″ and weighs 158 kg. Venous dopplers are performed, and a blood clot is confirmed in the left leg. It is decided to initiate therapeutic anticoagulation with enoxaparin. Her latest laboratory values indicate that she is not anemic and has normal kidney function. What dose should be initiated in AH?

Answer:

The enoxaparin dose for the treatment of DVT with or without PE is 1 mg/kg administered subcutaneously twice daily or 1.5 mg/kg once daily. Despite the patient having a BMI >30 kg/m², total body weight should be used to calculate the patients dose. Therefore, the patient should receive enoxaparin 160 mg subcutaneously every 12 hours if using the twice daily dosing regimen.

QUESTION

In general for patients <190 kg, anti-Xa monitoring is not necessary; however, after 1 week of therapy of enoxaparin, it was decided to obtain an anti-Xa level. The level comes back at 0.3 IU/mL. Would you make any adjustments to AH's dose at this time?

Answer:

First it is important to determine when the anti-Xa level was drawn in relation to the last administered dose. Peak anti-Xa levels should be drawn 4 hours following subcutaneous injection.[8] Target peak anti-Xa of 0.6–1.0 IU/mL (4 hours after subcutaneous injection) have been suggested for twice-daily administration of enoxaparin.[8] No well-established guidelines indicate how to adjust the dose of enoxaparin to achieve the desired concentration; however, a suggestion of a 25 percent increase in dose may be considered with repeat anti-Xa monitoring.[75]

CASE 5: DOSING OF LMWH FOR PE IN RENAL DYSFUNCTION WITHOUT DIALYSIS

JJ is a 66-year-old man presenting to the emergency department with pleuritic chest pain and shortness of breath. A pulmonary angiography is performed and a PE is diagnosed. It is decided to initiate JJ on enoxaparin. He is 5′9″ and weighs 115 kg. His latest laboratory values indicate that he is not anemic, but has a serum creatinine of 2.5 mg/dL. JJ has chronic kidney disease with a baseline serum creatinine of 2.1–2.5 mg/dL. What dose should be initiated in MH? How would enoxaparin be monitored in this patient?

Answer:

Because this patient has an elevated serum creatinine with known chronic kidney disease, it is imperative to calculate the patient's creatinine clearance. His creatinine clearance is estimated to be <30 mL/min, but greater than 20 mL/min, then JJ's calculated enoxaparin dose would be adjusted to 120 mg subcutaneously daily (or 1 mg/kg subcutaneously daily).[40] Limited data are available for treatment doses of dalteparin or tinzaparin in patients with a creatinine clearance less than 30 mL/min.[41,42]

Patients with renal impairment given a LMWH require careful assessment for potential bleeding risks and observation for signs and symptoms of bleeding. If a LMWH is initiated in a patient with renal impairment, along with dose reductions, antifactor Xa measurements may be prudent with extended use.

REFERENCES

1. Brinkhous KM, Smith HP, Warner ED, et al. The inhibition of blood clotting: An unidentified substance which acts in conjunction with heparin to prevent the conversion of prothrombin into thrombin. *Am J Physiol.* 1939;125:683–687.

2. Majerus PW, Tollefsen DM. Anticoagulant, thrombolytic, and anti-platelet drugs. In *Goodman & Gilman's The Pharmacological Basis of Therapeutics*, 10th ed. New York: McGraw-Hill, 2001.

3. Johnson EA, Mulloy B. The molecular weight range of commercial heparin preparations. *Carbohydr Res.* 1976;51:119–127.

4. Andersson L-O, Barrowcliffe TW, Holmer E, et al. Molecular weight dependency of the heparin potentiated inhibition of thrombin and activated factor X: Effect of heparin neutralization in plasma. *Thromb Res.* 1979;5:531–541.

5. Harenberg J. Pharmacology of low-molecular-weight heparins. *Semin Thromb Hemost.* 1990;16:12–18.

6. Lam LH, Silbert JE, Rosenberg JD. The separation of active and inactive forms of heparin. *Biochem Biophys Res Commun.* 1976;89:570–577.

7. Danielsson A, Raub E, Lindahl U, Bjork I. Role of ternary complexes, in which heparin binds both antithrombin and proteinase, in the acceleration of the reactions between antithrombin and thrombin or factor Xa. *J Biol Chem.* 1986;261:15467–15473.

8. Garcia DA, Baglin TP, Weitz JI, et al. Parenteral anticoagulants: Antithrombotic therapy and prevention of thrombosis, 9th ed: American College of Chest Physicians evidence-based clinical practice guidelines. *Chest.* 2012;141(2 suppl):e24S–e43S.

9. Lexicomp. Available at: http://www.crlonline.com/lco/action/doc/retrieve/docid/patch_f/7022 (accessed April 2012).

10. Bara L, Billaud E, Garamond G, et al. Comparative pharmacokinetics of low molecular weight heparin (PK 10169) and unfractionated heparin after intravenous subcutaneous administration. *Thromb Res.* 1985;39:631–636.

11. Pini M, Pattachini C, Quintavalla R, et al. Subcutaneous vs intravenous heparin in the treatment of deep venous thrombosis—a randomized clinical trial. *Thromb Haemost.* 1990;64(2):222–226.

12. Berkowitz SD. Treatment of established deep vein thrombosis: a review of the therapeutic armamentarium. *Orthopedics.* 1995;18(suppl):18–20.

13. Bick RL, Frenkel EP, Walenga J, et al. Unfractionated heparin, low molecular weight heparins, and pentasaccharide: Basic mechanism of actions, pharmacology, and clinical use. *Hematol Oncol Clin N Am.* 2005;19:1–51.

14. Bjornsson TD, Wolfram KM, Kitchell BB. Heparin kinetics determined by three assay methods. *Clin Pharmacol Ther.* 1982;31(1):104–113.

15. de Swart CA, Nijmeyer B, Roelofs JM, Sixma JJ. Kinetics of intravenously administered heparin in normal humans. *Blood.* 1982;60(6):1251–1258.

16. Bick RL. Heparin and low-molecular-weight heparins. In Bick RL (Ed.). *Disorders of Thrombosis and Hemostasis: Clinical and Laboratory Practice.* Philadelphia: Lippincott Williams & Wilkins, 2002: 359–377.

17. Kahn SR, Lim W, Dunn AS, et al. Prevention of VTE in nonsurgical patients. Antithrombotic therapy and prevention of thrombosis, 9th ed: American College of Chest Physicians evidence-based clinical practice guidelines. *Chest.* 2012;141(2)(suppl):e195S–e226S.

18. Raschke RA, Reilly BM, Guidry JR, Fontana JR, Srinivas S. The weight-based heparin dosing nomogram compared with a "standard care" nomogram. A randomized controlled trial. *Ann Intern Med.* 1993;119(9):874–881.

19. Prandoni P, Carnovali M, Marchiori A; Galilei Investigators. Subcutaneous adjusted-dose unfractionated heparin vs fixed-dose low-molecular-weight heparin in the initial treatment of venous thromboembolism. *Arch Intern Med.* 2004;164(10):1077–1083.

20. Kearon C, Ginsberg JS, Julian JA, et al; Fixed-Dose Heparin (FIDO) Investigators. Comparison of fixed-dose weight adjusted unfractionated heparin and low-molecular-weight heparin for acute treatment of venous thromboembolism. *JAMA.* 2006;296(8):935–942.

21. Braunwald E, Antman E, Beasley J, et al. ACC/AHA Guidelines for the management of patients with unstable angina and non-ST-segment elevation myocardial infarction. A report of the American College of Cardiology/American Heart Association Task Force on Practice Guidelines. *J Am Coll Cardio.* 2000;36(3):970–1062.

22. Ryan T, Antman E, Brooks N, et al. 1999 update: ACC/AHA guidelines for the management of patients with acute myocardial infarction. A report of the American College of Cardiology/American Heart Association Task Force on Practice Guidelines. *J Am Coll Cardiol.* 1999;34(3):890–911.

23. Levine M, Hirsh J, Kelton J. Heparin-induced bleeding. In Land DA, Lindahl U (Eds.). *Heparin: Chemical and Biological Properties, Clinical Applications.* London: Edward Arnold, 1989:517–532.

24. Morabia A. Heparin doses and major bleedings. *Lancet.* 1986;1(849):1278–1279.

25. Antman EM. Hirudin in acute myocardial infarction. Thrombolysis and Thrombin Inhibition in Myocardial Infarction (TIMI) 9B trial. *Circulation.* 1996;94(5):911–921.

26. EPILOG Investigators. Platelet glycoprotein IIb/IIIa receptor blockade and low-dose heparin during percutaneous coronary revascularization. *N Engl J Med.* 1997;336(24):1689–1696.

27. Hull RD, Raskob GE, Rosenbloom D, et al. Heparin for 5 days as compared with 10 days in the initial treatment of proximal venous thrombosis. *N Engl J Med.* 1990;322:1260–1264.

28. Basu D, Gallus A, Hirsh J, Cade J. A prospective study of the value of monitoring heparin treatment with the activated partial thromboplastin time. *N Engl J Med.* 1972;287(7):324–327.

29. Linkins L-A, Dans AL, Moores LK, et al. Treatment and prevention of heparin-induced thrombocytopenia: Antithrombotic therapy and prevention of thrombosis, 9th ed: American College of Chest Physicians evidence-based clinical practice guidelines. *Chest.* 2012;141(2)(suppl):e495S–e530S.

30. Pouplard C, Gueret P, Fouassier M, et al. Prospective evaluation of the '4Ts' score and particle gel immunoassay specific to heparin/PF4 for the diagnosis of heparin-induced thrombocytopenia. *J Thromb Haemos.* 2007;5(7):1373–1379.

31. Bryant A, Low J, Austin S, Joseph JE. Timely diagnosis and management of heparin-induced thrombocytopenia in a frequent request, low incidence single centre using clinical 4Ts score and particle gel immunoassay. *Br J Haematol.* 2008;143(5):721–726.

32. Warkentin TE, Linkins LA. Non-necrotizing heparin-induced skin lesions and the 4Ts score. *J Thromb Haemost.* 2010;8(7):1483–1485.

33. Handeland GF, Abildgaard U, Holm HA, Arnesen KE. Dose adjusted heparin treatment of deep venous thrombosis: A comparison of unfractionated and low molecular weight heparin. *Eur J Clin Pharmacol.* 1990;39:107–112.

34. Frydman A. Low-molecular-weight heparins: An overview of their pharmacodynamics, pharmacokinetics and metabolism in humans. *Haemostasis.* 1996;26(suppl 2):24–38.

35. Boneu B, Caranobe C, Cadroy Y, et al. Pharmacokinetic studies of standard unfractionated heparin, and low molecular weight heparins in the rabbit. *Semin Thromb Hemost.* 1988;14:18–27.

36. Alhenc-Gelas M, Jestin-Le Guernic C, Vitoux JF, Kher A, Aiach M, Fiessinger JN. Adjusted versus fixed doses of the low-molecular-weight heparin fragmin in the treatment of deep vein thrombosis. Fragmin-Study Group. *Thromb Haemost.* 1994;71:698–702.

37. Laposata M, Green D, Van Cott EM, Barrowcliffe TW, Goodnight SH, Sosolik RC. College of American Pathologists Conference XXXI on laboratory monitoring of anticoagulant therapy: The clinical use and laboratory monitoring of low-molecular-weight heparin, danaparoid, hirudin and related compounds, and argatroban. *Arch Pathol Lab Med.* 1998;122:799–807.

38. Boneu B. Low molecular weight heparin therapy: Is monitoring needed? *Thromb Haemost.* 1994;72:330–334.

39. Boneu B, de Moerloose P. How and when to monitor a patient treated with low molecular weight heparin. *Semin Thromb Hemost.* 2001;27:519–522.

40. Lovenox (enoxaparin sodium injection) [package insert]. Bridgewater, NJ, April 2011.

41. Fragmin (dalteparin sodium injection) [package insert]. New York, April 2007.

42. Innohep (tinzaparin sodium injection) [package insert]. Parsippany, NY, December 2002.

43. Kuczmarski RJ, Flegal KM. Criteria for definition of overweight in transition: Background and recommendations for the United States. *Am J Clin Nutr.* 2000;72:1074–1081.

86

CHAPTER 7

Unfractionated Heparin and Low-Molecular Heparins

44. Alikhan R, Cohen AT, Combe S, et al. Prevention of venous thromboembolism in medical patients with enoxaparin: A subgroup analysis of the MEDENOX study. *Blood Coagul Fibrinolysis.* 2003;14:341–346.

45. Kucher N, Leizorovicz A, Vaitkus PT, et al. Efficacy and safety of fixed low-dose dalteparin in preventing venous thromboembolism among obese or elderly hospitalized patients: A subgroup analysis of the PREVENT trial. *Arch Intern Med.* 2005;165:341–345.

46. Frederiksen SG, Hedenbro JL, Norgren L. Enoxaparin effect depends on body weight and current doses may be inadequate in obese patients. *Br J Surg.* 2003;90:547–548.

47. Scholten DJ, Hoedema RM, Scholten SE. A comparison of two different prophylactic dose regimens of low molecular weight heparin in bariatric surgery. *Obes Surg.* 2002;12:19–24.

48. Rondina MT, Wheeler M, Rodgers GM, Draper L, Pendleton RC. Weight-based dosing of enoxaparin for VTE prophylaxis in morbidly obese, medically ill patients. *Thromb Res.* 2010;125:220–223.

49. Hamad GG, Choban PS. Enoxaparin for thromboprophylaxis in morbidly obese patients undergoing bariatric surgery: Findings of the prophylaxis against VTE outcomes in bariatric surgery patients receiving enoxaparin (PROBE) study. *Obes Surg.* 2005;15:1368–1374.

50. Borkgren-Okonek MJ, Hart RW, Pantano JE, et al. Enoxaparin thromboprophylaxis in gastric bypass patients: Extended duration, dose stratification, and antifactor Xa activity. *Surg Obes Relat Dis.* 2008;4:625–631.

51. Al-Yaseen E, Wells PS, Anderson J, Martin J, Kovacs MJ. The safety of dosing dalteparin based on actual body weight for the treatment of acute venous thromboembolism in obese patients. *J Thromb Haemost.* 2005;3:100–102.

52. Bazinet A, Almanric K, Brunet C, et al. Dosage of enoxaparin among obese and renal impairment patients. *Thromb Res.* 2005;116:41–50.

53. Barba R, Marco J, Martin-Alvarez H, et al. The influence of extreme body weight on clinical outcome of patients with venous thromboembolism: findings from a prospective registry (RIETE). *J Thromb Haemost.* 2005;3:856–862.

54. Spinler SA, Inverso SM, Cohen M, Goodman SG, Stringer KA, Antman EM. Safety and efficacy of unfractionated heparin versus enoxaparin in patients who are obese and patients with severe renal impairment: Analysis from the ESSENCE and TIMI 11B studies. *Am Heart J.* 2003;146:33–41.

55. Low-molecular-weight heparin during instability in coronary artery disease, Fragmin during Instability in Coronary Artery Disease (FRISC) study group. *Lancet.* 1996;347:561–568.

56. Merli G, Spiro TE, Olsson CG, et al. Subcutaneous enoxaparin once or twice daily compared with intravenous unfractionated heparin for treatment of venous thromboembolic disease. *Ann Intern Med.* 2001;134:191–202.

57. Douketis J, Cook D, Meade M, et al. Prophylaxis against deep vein thrombosis in critically ill patients with severe renal insufficiency with the low-molecular-weight heparin dalteparin: An assessment of safety and pharmacodynamics: The DIRECT study. *Arch Intern Med.* 2008;168:1805–1812.

58. Mahe I, Aghassarian M, Drouet L, et al. Tinzaparin and enoxaparin given at prophylactic dose for eight days in medical elderly patients with impaired renal function: A comparative pharmacokinetic study. *Thromb Haemost.* 2007;97:581–586.

59. Sanderink GJ, Guimart CG, Ozoux ML, Jariwala NU, Shukla UA, Boutouyrie BX. Pharmacokinetics and pharmacodynamics of the prophylactic dose of enoxaparin once daily over 4 days in patients with renal impairment. *Thromb Res.* 2002;105:225–231.

60. Chow SL, Zammit K, West K, Dannenhoffer M, Lopez-Candales A. Correlation of antifactor Xa concentrations with renal function in patients on enoxaparin. *J Clin Pharmacol.* 2003;43:586–590.

61. Schmid P, Brodmann D, Odermatt Y, Fischer AG, Wuillemin WA. Study of bioaccumulation of dalteparin at a therapeutic dose in patients with renal insufficiency. *J Thromb Haemost.* 2009;7:1629–1632.

62. Lim W, Dentali F, Eikelboom JW, Crowther MA. Meta-analysis: Low-molecular-weight heparin and bleeding in patients with severe renal insufficiency. *Ann Intern Med.* 2006;144:673–684.

63. Falga C, Capdevila JA, Soler S, et al. Clinical outcome of patients with venous thromboembolism and renal insufficiency. Findings from the RIETE registry. *Thromb Haemost.* 2007;98:771–776.

64. Spinler SA, Mahaffey KW, Gallup D, et al. Relationship between renal function and outcomes in high-risk patients with non-ST-segment elevation acute coronary syndromes: Results from SYNERGY. *Int J Cardiol.* 2009;144:36–41.

65. Santopinto JJ, Fox KA, Goldberg RJ, et al. Creatinine clearance and adverse hospital outcomes in patients with acute coronary syndromes: Findings from the global registry of acute coronary events (GRACE). *Heart.* 2003;89:1003–1008.

66. Collet JP, Montalescot G, Agnelli G, et al. Non-ST-segment elevation acute coronary syndrome in patients with renal dysfunction: Benefit of low-molecular-weight heparin alone or with glycoprotein IIb/IIIa inhibitors on outcomes. The Global Registry of Acute Coronary Events. *Eur Heart J.* 2005;26:2285–2293.

67. Fox KA, Antman EM, Montalescot G, et al. The impact of renal dysfunction on outcomes in the ExTRACT-TIMI 25 trial. *J Am Coll Cardiol.* 2007;49:2249–2255.

68. Lachish T, Rudensky B, Slotki I, Zevin S. Enoxaparin dosage adjustment in patients with severe renal failure: Antifactor Xa concentrations and safety. *Pharmacotherapy.* 2007;27:1347–1352.

69. Siguret V, Pautas E, Fevrier M, et al. Elderly patients treated with tinzaparin (Innohep) administered once daily (175 anti-Xa IU/kg): Anti-Xa and anti-IIa activities over 10 days. *Thromb Haemost.* 2000;84:800–804.

70. Pautas E, Gouin I, Bellot O, Andreux JP, Siguret V. Safety profile of tinzaparin administered once daily at a standard curative dose in two hundred very elderly patients. *Drug Saf.* 2002;25:725–733.

71. Spencer FA, Gore JM, Lessard D, et al. Venous thromboembolism in the elderly. A community-based perspective. *Thromb Haemost.* 2008;100:780–788.

72. http://www.fda.gov/Drugs/DrugSafety/PostmarketDrugSafety InformationforPatientsandProviders/DrugSafetyInformationfor HeathcareProfessionals/ucm136254.htm (accessed April 2012).

73. Dorffler-Melly J, de Jonge E, Pont AC, et al. Bioavailability of subcutaneous low-molecular-weight heparin to patients on vasopressors. *Lancet.* 2002;359:849–850.

74. Rommers MK, Van der Lely N, Egberts TC, van den Bemt PM. Anti-Xa activity after subcutaneous administration of dalteparin in ICU patients with and without subcutaneous edema: A pilot study. *Crit Care.* 2006;10:R93.

75. Monagle P, Michelson AD, Bovill E, Andrew M. Antithrombotic therapy in children. *Chest.* 2001;119:344S–370S.

8

Colistin and Polymyxin B

LISA M. VOIGT, PharmD, BCPS
KIMBERLY T. ZAMMIT, PharmD, BCPS, FASHP

Antimicrobial resistance has become a worldwide health care crisis with many pathogens showing limited or no susceptibility to currently available antimicrobial treatments. Gram-negative infections are of even more concern because of the lack of currently effective treatments, as well as the lack of new antibiotics in development to treat these potentially lethal pathogens. It is currently estimated that no new antibiotics with activity against multiresistant gram-negative bacteria will be released within the next five years, emphasizing the need for last-line options, such as colistin, in cases where pathogens are resistant to all other antibiotics. In the last two decades, the paucity of novel antibiotics with which to treat drug-resistant infections, especially those caused by gram-negative pathogens, has led to their reconsideration as a therapeutic option.[1]

Polymyxins are a group of polypeptide antibiotics that consists of five chemically different compounds (polymyxins A–E) discovered in 1947. Only polymyxin B and polymyxin E (colistin) have been used in clinical practice. They differ by a single amino acid change (D-phenylalanine in polymixin B replaces D-leucine in colistin). Polymyxins have been used extensively worldwide in topical otic and ophthalmic solutions for decades.[2] The mechanism behind colistin's bactericidal ability is considered to be identical to that of polymyxin.[1]

Colistin was discovered in 1949 and was nonribosomally synthesized by *Bacillus polymyxa* subspecies *colistinus* Koyama.[3-4] Colistin was initially used therapeutically in Japan and in Europe during the 1950s and in the United States in the form of colistimethate sodium in 1959.[5] However, the intravenous formulations of colistin and polymyxin B were gradually abandoned in most parts of the world in the early 1980s because of the reported high incidence of nephrotoxicity.[6-8]

This chapter review focuses on colistin, rather than polymyxin B, because of its wider use in current clinical practice.

MECHANISM OF ACTION

The initial target of the antimicrobial activity of polymyxins is the lipopolysaccharide (LPS) component of the outer membrane. The polymyxins have a strong positive charge and a hydrophobic acyl chain that give them a high binding affinity for LPS molecules. They interact electrostatically with these molecules and competitively displace divalent cations (Mg^{2++} and Ca^{2++}) from them, causing disruption of the membrane. The result of this process is an increase in the permeability of the cell envelope, leakage of cell contents, and, subsequently, cell death. The exact mechanism by which the polymyxins induce bacterial killing is still unknown, and multiple bacterial cell targets may be involved. Polymyxins also bind to the lipid A portion of LPS and, in animal studies, block many of the biological effects of endotoxin.[9]

FORMULATIONS, DOSAGE, AND ROUTE OF ADMINISTRATION

Colistin is composed of at least 30 different polymyxin compounds, mainly colistin A and B. Two forms of colistin are available: colistin sulfate and the commercially available parenteral formulation colistimethate sodium (CMS, also called sodium colistin methanesulphonate, colistin methanesulphonate, colistin sulfomethate, or colistimethate). It is extremely important to note that the two forms are not interchangeable. CMS is an inactive prodrug and in aqueous solution, CMS undergoes spontaneous hydrolysis to the active form colistin.[10]

As a prodrug, CMS is readily hydrolyzed to form partially sulfomethylated derivatives, as well as colistin sulfate, the active form of the drug. This hydrolysis of CMS to colistin is an important step in providing the drug's antimicrobial activity. Up until colistin is formed, CMS by itself has been shown to display little to no antibacterial activity, and is therefore considered an inactive prodrug of colistin.[11] CMS is eliminated mainly by the renal route, with a fraction of the dose being converted to active colistin in vivo. Colistin undergoes extensive renal tubular reabsorption and therefore is mainly cleared by nonrenal mechanisms. CMS is administered intravenously or intramuscularly, because it is less toxic than colistin sulfate. The intramuscular injection, which is rarely used in clinical practice, may cause severe local pain, and absorption is variable.[9] Solutions of colistimethate sodium for IM injection, IV injection, or continuous IV infusion should be freshly prepared and used within 24 hours.[9]

Colistin sulfate is administered either orally (for bowel decontamination, without absorption) or topically (for the treatment of bacterial skin infections). Both colistimethate sodium and colistin can be given via inhalation, but colistin may result in a higher frequency of bronchoconstriction than colistimethate sodium. Colistimethate sodium can also be administered by the intrathecal or intraventricular routes.[9]

LACK OF A UNIVERSAL DOSAGE UNIT FOR COLISTIN

Coly-Mycin M Parenteral, which is manufactured and used in the United States, contains 150 mg of colistin base activity (CBA) per vial, equivalent to 400 mg of colistimethate sodium per vial and to 5 × 10⁶ international units (IU) of colistimethate sodium. Colomycin injection, which is manufactured and used in Europe, is provided in vials containing 5 × 10⁶ or 2 × 10⁶ IU of colistimethate sodium. An IU is defined as the minimal concentration that inhibits the growth of *Escherichia coli* 95 I.S.M in 1 mL broth at pH 7.2 and 10⁶ IU is considered to be equivalent to 80 mg of colistimethate sodium.[9]

The complexity of the nomenclature used to define colistin dosing has resulted in much confusion, increasing the potential for drug errors. The need for utilization of a uniform dosing unit to avoid such confusion is obvious.[12,13] In June 2011, a National Alert for Serious Medication Errors was issued by the American Society of Health-System Pharmacists (ASHP) and the Institute for Safe Medication Practices (ISMP), warning that potentially fatal errors may occur with dosing for colistimethate for injection.[13] Particular attention must be paid to the dosing units used in various drug information sources and scientific literature to avoid utilization of incorrect doses.

ASHP/ISMP Recommendations for Safe CMS Use[13]

- In the United States, colistimethate for injection must ONLY be prescribed as colistin in terms of base activity with dose range of 2.5–5 mg/kg/day in patients with normal renal function. As per package insert, use ideal body weight for obese patients. This total daily dose should be given in 2 to 4 divided doses.

- Dosage reduction in the setting of renal insufficiency is recommended (see product labeling for suggested modification of dosage schedules).

- If the drug is ordered as "colistimethate" or "colistimethate sodium," the prescriber should be contacted to verify the dose in terms of colistin base.

- Consider restricting ordering to infectious disease specialists or intensivists.

- To prevent errors, preapproved printed guidelines or computer order sets should be made available with dosing only as colistin base. Include adjustments for renal dysfunction.

- Dose limits should be established with immediate investigation required for doses outside hospital guidelines. Guidelines should define any circumstances where dosing outside the 2.5–5 mg/kg/day range may be appropriate. Testing of CPOE and pharmacy computer systems should be accomplished to assure proper function of alerts.

- Monitoring of renal function while receiving colistin is important to detect signs of renal toxicity associated with colistin, and the appropriateness of dosage should be reevaluated periodically while on treatment.

The ASHP/ISMP recommendation for dosing unit convention will be followed in this chapter (see Table 8-1). Unless otherwise specified all dose recommendations are made in milligrams of colistin base activity (CBA).

NEPHROTOXICITY

One of the commonly observed adverse effects following intravenous administration of colistimethate sodium is nephrotoxicity, with incidences reported to be as high as 55 percent in the following studies.

TABLE 8-1	Comparison of Colistimethate Sodium Products	
	Colomycin®	**Coly-Mycin M®**
Availability	Europe	USA, Australia
Dosing units	IU (international units)	milligram colistin base (CBA)
Dosing conversion	5 million IU = 400 mg colistimethate	150 mg CBA = 400 mg colistimethate

30 mg colistin base = 80 mg CMS = 1 MIU (European international units)
1 mg colistin base = 2.67 mg CMS = 33,333 IU; 1 mg CMS = 12,500 IU
Source: Adapted from van Duin D, Kaye KS, Neuner EA. Carbapenem-resistant Enterobacteriaceae: A review of treatment and outcomes. *Diagn Microbiol Infect Dis.* 2013;75(2):115–120.

In studies comparing treatment with colistimethate sodium with or without other antibiotics versus other antibiotic regimens, nephrotoxicity was significantly higher with colistimethate sodium (or polymyxin B) in six studies, similar to that with comparators in five (two of which claimed no events), and lower in two that may actually be less nephrotoxic than aminoglycosides. Rates of nephrotoxicity in recent studies designed to assess this outcome have ranged from 6 percent to 14 percent in some[20-24] and from 32 percent to 55 percent in others.[25-30]

The wide range of nephrotoxicity rates can be at least partly explained by different definitions of renal failure. Some studies used any of the RIFLE criteria (risk, injury, failure, loss, and end-stage kidney disease).[31] Some used the threshold of failure or above, and others defined renal failure as creatinine >2 mg/dL. Risk factors for nephrotoxicity found in different studies included older age,[26,29] preexisting renal insufficiency,[32] hypoalbuminaemia,[27] and concomitant use of nonsteroidal anti-inflammatory drugs[27] or vancomycin.[29] Higher dosing is associated with renal failure, with some studies identifying the total cumulative dose as predictive of renal failure,[3,24,25] and others the daily dose.[26,29-30] The time to nephrotoxicity was not reported in most studies. Four studies reported that most cases occurred within the first week of treatment.[26,28-30] Studies monitoring patients for 1–3 months after treatment demonstrated reversibility of renal failure in at least 88 percent of patients.[21,25,27] Overall, rates of nephrotoxicity are probably lower today than those observed in old studies.[3] Explanations for the lower toxicity include fewer chemical impurities in colistimethate sodium, better intensive care unit (ICU) monitoring, and avoidance of coadministration of other nephrotoxic drugs.[33,34] Recent observations have suggested that, at least in CF patients, colistimethate sodium may actually be less nephrotoxic than aminoglycosides.[35]

NEUROTOXICITY

Neurotoxicity is less common than nephrotoxicity. Clinical manifestations include dizziness, muscle weakness, paresthesias, partial deafness, visual disturbances, vertigo, confusion, hallucinations, seizures, ataxia, and neuromuscular blockade. Paresthesias constitute the most common clinical manifestation, being reported in approximately 27 percent of cases with the use of intravenous colistimethate sodium. Neurotoxic effects are usually mild and resolve after prompt discontinuation of the antibiotic.[34] Apnea and respiratory failure, which are feared complications of neuromuscular blockade, have not been reported with intravenous colistimethate sodium in the recent literature.[34]

RESPIRATORY EFFECTS

Bronchoconstriction[15-19] and hypersensitivity pneumonitis[36] have been reported in adult and pediatric cystic fibrosis patients who received oral nebulized CMS. Bronchoconstriction occurs almost immediately after initiation of nebulization and may persist for more than 30 minutes.[16] Administration of bronchodilators prior to colistin nebulization may reduce the potential for development of bronchoconstriction.[15-19] Pre- and posttreatment pulmonary function tests may have clinical utility to identify individuals at risk for bronchoconstriction.[16] In those individuals who are unable to perform pulmonary function tests (especially young children), bronchodilator premedication is recommended.[19] It should also be noted that in critically ill patients without CF, these adverse events have not yet been demonstrated.[37-45]

Both CMS and colistin can be given via inhalation, but colistin may result in a higher frequency of pulmonary adverse effects than colistimethate sodium. A component of colistin (polymyxin E1) has been shown to cause pulmonary inflammatory reactions in animals and may contribute to such local toxicity in humans. Given the fact that colistmethate sodium is hydrolyzed to colistin in aqueous solutions and potentially serious pulmonary toxicity, including fatal respiratory failure, has been associated with the administration of premixed product, inhalation solutions should be prepared immediately prior to administration.[15] The Food and Drug Administration and the Cystic Fibrosis Foundation underscored the importance of this practice by issuing an alert recommending that patients not use colistmethate for inhalation premixed by pharmacies and that patients should prepare their colistmethate nebulizer inhalation solutions immediately prior to use.[15]

SPECTRUM OF ACTIVITY AND RESISTANCE

Colistin is bactericidal against most strains of gram-negative bacilli, including *Enterobacter aerogenes*, *Escherichia coli*, *Haemophilus influenza*, *Bordetella pertussis*, *Legionella pneumophilia*, *Salmonella* species, *Shigella* species, *Pasteurella* species, *Klebsiella pneumonia*, *Pseudomonas aeruginosa*, and *Stenotrophomonas maltophilia*. However, some bacteria are resistant to colistin, including the gram-negative organisms of *Proteus* species, *Burkholderia cepacia*, *Providencia* species, *Serratia marcescens*, *Moraxella catarrhalis*, and *Morganella morganii*. Gram-positive bacteria, fungi, and gram-negative cocci (*Neisseria gonorrhoeae* and *Neisseria meningitides*) are inherently resistant to colistin.[46-48]

P. aeruginosa and *A. baumannii* susceptibility are defined as MICs of ≤4 and ≤2 mg/L colistin sulfate, respectively, according to the European Committee on Antimicrobial Susceptibility Testing,[49] and as an MIC of ≤2 mg/L for both bacteria according to the Clinical and Laboratory Standards Institute (CLSI).[50]

Isolates with intrinsic resistance to polymixins have alterations in lipid A that account for reduced binding.[47] But acquired resistance to colistin has been historically deemed to be infrequent, although this may simply be a function of the drug's relatively limited use. Emergence of resistance has been increasingly reported and it is likely mediated by alteration in the negatively charged bacterial cell membrane, although additional mechanisms may also be involved. Inadequate dosing may also be a factor in the development of resistance due to preferential growth within heteroresistant subpopulations. As such, optimization of dosing is necessary to achieve desired therapeutic outcomes.[51,52]

DRUG INTERACTIONS[53]

Colistmethate may increase the levels/effects of neuromuscular-blocking agents. Case reports have described potentiation of neuromuscular blockade of pancuronium when concomitantly given polymyxin B. Antagonizing the block was not successful with pyridostigmine or calcium chloride.[54] Neuromuscular blockade from Polymyxin B alone has been reported in both medical and surgical patients not receiving anesthetic or other neuromuscular blocking drugs. It also potentiates d-tubocurarine- and succinylcholine-induced blockades.[55] The levels/effects of colistmethate may be increased by aminoglycosides, amphotericin B, and vancomycin. Concomitant use with BCG (*M. tuberculosis* vaccine) should be avoided.

PHARMACOKINETICS

The pharmacokinetics of colistmethate sodium and colistin are complex and incompletely characterized. The antimicrobial activity of colistmethate requires conversion to colistin, and thus its rate of conversion impacts peak concentrations.[11] The overall disposition of colistin is rate limited by the elimination of the parent compound, because the colistin has a substantially longer terminal half-life than CMS.[51] Complete understanding of the pharmacokinetics of colistmethate sodium and colistin continues to evolve, as studies using HPLC and not immunoassays allow better characterization of the disposition of each drug. It is important to note that the pharmacokinetic and prescribing information supplied with currently available parenteral products was obtained using microbiological assays.[51]

Palchouras and colleagues[60] conducted a pharmacokinetic study of 18 critically ill patients administered CMS 3 million units (240 mg CMS) every 8 hours, with a reduction to 160 mg q8h for those whose creatinine clearance was less than 50 mL/min. Plasma samples for drug concentration analysis were obtained with the first and fourth dose. A nonlinear mixed-effects model analysis was performed in which all concentration-time data were modeled simultaneously. The predicted maximum concentrations of drug in plasma were 0.60 mg/liter and 2.3 mg/liter for the first dose and at steady state, respectively. Colistin displayed a half-life that was significantly long in relation to the dosing interval (14.6 hours). This study suggests that administration of a loading dose may be more beneficial in critically ill patients as plasma colistin concentrations are insufficient before steady state.

A subsequent study[57] evaluated the disposition of the prodrug, CMS, and formed colistin in 105 critically ill patients, including 12 on intermittent hemodialysis and 4 on continuous renal replacement therapy. Of the 105 patients, 69 had creatinine clearances of less than 40 mL/min/1.73 m2. This study demonstrated important information concerning the disposition of CMS and colistin. First, it revealed the significant role of renal function as a determinant of the plasma concentrations of the active antibacterial, formed colistin. Second, it is apparent that in patients with moderate-to-good renal function, utilization of a daily dose of CBA at the high end of manufacturer recommended doses (300 mg CBA per day)[53] was not able to generate plasma colistin concentrations that would be expected to be reliably efficacious.

It is also important to note that the disposition of the active component colistin is remarkably flat for >14 hours, which may limit the optimization of the dose without unacceptable toxicity. Therefore, based on our current understanding of colistin PK and pharmacodynamic relationships, colistin may best be used as part of a highly active combination, especially for patients with moderate-to-good renal function and/or for organisms with MICs of ≥1.0 mg/L.[57]

DISTRIBUTION

Following IM or IV administration of colistmethate sodium, it is widely distributed into body tissues, but only negligible concentrations of antimicrobial activity are attained in synovial, pleural, or pericardial fluids. Animal studies indicate that colistin reversibly binds to and persists in body tissues such as the liver, kidneys, lung, heart, and muscle.[61]

In cystic fibrosis, patients 14–53 years of age receiving IV colistmethate sodium in a dosage of 5–7 mg/kg of colistin daily given in 3 equally divided doses, the volume of distribution at steady state was 0.09 L/kg.[5]

Colistin is approximately 50 percent bound to serum proteins, especially alpha 1 acid glycoprotein. This binding may be higher in critically ill patients due to a greater production of this protein during acute illness.

Only minimal concentrations of antimicrobial activity are attained in CSF following IM or IV administration of colistmethate sodium in patients with normal or inflamed meninges.[61]

Colistin crosses the placenta and is distributed into milk.[61]

ELIMINATION

Approximately 60 percent of CMS is cleared renally with a component of tubular secretion,[63] whereas for colistin less than 1 percent of the dose is excreted in urine, likely due to extensive renal tubular reabsorption.[64] The low in vivo conversion of CMS to colistin occurs because CMS is cleared more quickly than colistin can be formed.[63] As a result, the overall disposition of CMS and formed colistin is complex.

In adults with normal renal function, the plasma half-life of antimicrobial activity following IM or IV administration of colistimethate sodium is 1.5–8 hours, while in children the decline in serum concentrations of antimicrobial activity occurs more rapidly.

Patients with renal dysfunction demonstrate higher serum concentrations and prolonged half-lives. In patients with creatinine clearances less than 20 mL/min, the half-life of colistin ranges from 10–20 hours. Following administration of colistimethate sodium in a few anuric patients, half-life of antimicrobial activity reportedly ranged up to 2–3 days.

The mean plasma half-life in cystic fibrosis patients 14–53 years of age who received IV colistimethate sodium in a dosage of 5–7 mg/kg of colistin daily given in 3 equally divided doses was 3.4 hours after the first dose and 3.5 hours at steady state.[5]

With a dosage of 66.66 mg of colistin (2 million international units) the plasma half-life following oral inhalation via nebulization of colistimethate sodium in cystic fibrosis patients 12–48 years of age was 4.1–4.5 hours.[62]

Urine antimicrobial activity is generally higher than seen in the serum. Following IM or IV administration of a single 150 mg dose of colistin as colistimethate sodium in patients with normal renal function, antimicrobial concentrations in urine are 200–270 mcg/mL at 2 hours after the dose and 15–25 mcg/mL at 8 hours after the dose.[61]

PHARMACODYNAMICS

Colistin is rapidly bactericidal in a concentration-dependent manner against susceptible strains of *P. aeruginosa, A. baumannii,* and *K. pneumoniae,* including multi-drug resistant (MDR) strains.[58,65,67]

Colistin concentrations near or above the bacteria's MIC result in extremely rapid killing.[58,65,67] The pharmacodynamic parameter most closely associated with efficacy is the fAUC/MIC (area under the plasma-concentration time curve/ minimum inhibitory concentration)[67,68] and degree of bactericidal activity is greater with low versus high inoculums.[69] Frequency of dosing is also an important factor, because bacterial growth recovery occurs early.[58] Indeed, a dosing regimen with 8-hour frequency demonstrated a lower likelihood of the emergence of resistance.[66] Aggressive colistin regimens have been suggested in vitro to overcome the potential for resistance. Regrowth[58] has been reported in static time-kill studies utilizing colistin concentrations up to 64× MIC. The role of colistin may ultimately be a part of a highly active combination regimen.[51] Studies have demonstrated synergy with the combination of colistin and cefepime, carbapenems, or rifampicin and have also noted suppression of resistance.[51]

DOSING

PACKAGE INSERT

The doses of CMS used for systemic infections in adults range widely, from 240 to 720 mg daily (i.e., 3–9×10^6 IU/day), in two to four divided doses,[9] yet the optimal dose of colistin is currently unknown.[51] This issue is due in part to the differences in dosing units as well as a lack of systematic investigation. Table 8-2 describes dosing as recommended in the current package insert.[53] As more of the true disposition of colistimethate sodium and colistin continues to unfold, optimal colistin dosing may be better ascertained from the primary literature rather than the manufacturer recommendations.

CRITICALLY ILL

The dose required to provide therapeutic concentrations of colistin may be significantly different than package insert labeling. Table 8-3 outlines dosing recommendations based on the pharmacokinetics in critically ill patients.[57] It has been reported that CMS and its active metabolite colistin in critically ill patients are removed

TABLE 8-2[53] Package Insert Dosage Recommendations in Terms of Colistin Base Activity (CBA)[a]

Renal Function	Degree of Impairment			
	Normal	Mild	Moderate	Considerable
Plasma creatinine, mg/100 mL	0.7–1.2	1.3–1.5	1.6–2.5	2.6–4
Urea clearance, % of normal	80–100	40–70	25–40	10–25
Dosage				
Unit dose of colistimethate for injection, mg	100–150	75–115	66–150	100–150
Frequency, times/day	4 to 2	2	2 or 1	Every 36 hours
Total daily dose, mg CBA	300	150–230	133–150	100
Approximate daily dose, mg/kg/day CBA	5	2.5–3.8	2.5	1.5
Summary	2.5–5 mg/kg/day in 2 to 4 divided doses	2.5–3.8 mg/kg/day in 2 divided doses	1.6–2.5 mg/kg/day in 1 to 2 divided doses	~1.5 mg/kg q36h

- **Intermittent Hemodialysis**
  For patients who have complete hemodialysis sessions three times per week, administer CMS after hemodialysis on dialysis days: 1.5 mg/kg every 24–48 hours.
- **Continuous Renal Replacement Therapy (CRRT)**
  General recommendations based on dialysate flow rate of 1–2 L/hour and minimal residual renal function: CVVH/CVVHD/CVVHDF: 2.5 mg/kg every 24–48 hours (frequency dependent on site or severity of infection or susceptibility of pathogen).
- **Direct Intermittent Administration**
  Slowly inject one-half of the total daily dose over a period of 3–5 minutes every 12 hours.
- **Continuous Infusion**
  Slowly inject one-half of the total daily dose over 3–5 minutes. Add the remaining half of the total daily dose of colistimethate for injection, USP, to one of the following: Administer the second half of the total daily dose by slow intravenous infusion, starting 1–2 hours after the initial dose, over the next 22–23 hours. In the presence of impaired renal function, reduce the infusion rate depending on the degree of renal impairment.

[a]**In obese individuals, dosage should be based on ideal body weight.**

TABLE 8-3 Estimating colistin loading and maintenance doses.[57] All doses expressed as colistin base activity (CBA).

Dose Type	Category	Dosing Strategy (CBA)
Loading	All patients	Loading dose = Colistin $C_{ss,avg}$ target $\times$ 2.0 $\times$ body wt (kg) • $C_{ss,avg}$ in mg/liter and dependent on MIC, infection site, and severity • Use either ideal or actual body weight whichever is LOWER. Loading doses greater than 300 mg /day should be used with extreme caution, as risk of toxicity is unknown(see reference 57 for additional details) Administer first maintenance dose within 24 hours
Maintenance	No renal replacement	Total daily dose = Colistin $C_{ss,avg}$ target $\times$ (1.50 $\times$ CrCL + 30) • $C_{ss,avg}$ in mg/liter and dependent on MIC, infection site, and severity Recommended dosage intervals: (CrCL determined by Jeliffe equation) Below 10 ml/min/1.73 m², every 12 h 10–70 ml/min/1.73 m² every 8–12 h Above 70 ml/min/1.73 m² every 8–12 h • In patients with CrCL values above 70 ml/min/1.73 m² or when targeting a "high" colistin $C_{ss,avg}$, predicted daily doses may be substantially greater than the current upper limit in the product label (300 mg). Utilization of this equation is recommended only when targeting lower $C_{ss,avg}$ targets to avoid exceeding 300 mg (see reference 57 for additional details)
	Intermittent hemodialysis (HD)	Total daily dose = 30 mg non-HD day to achieve each 1.0-mg/liter colistin $C_{ss,avg}$ target Supplemental dose on HD day add: (assuming dialysis is toward the end of dose interval) 50% to the daily dose if administered during the last hour of the HD session OR 30% to the daily dose if administered after the HD session Twice-daily dosing is suggested
	Continuous renal replacement	Total daily dose = 192 mg to achieve each 1.0-mg/liter colistin $C_{ss,avg}$ target Doses may be given every 8–12 h. • Dosing estimate based on pharmacokinetic analysis of 4 critically ill patients

by CVVHDF. Unfortunately, colistin is notorious for its ability to be adsorbed to many different materials including hemodialysis filters. Based on PK studies, colistin has been shown to be eliminated by CRRT and doses may need to be adjusted upward.[59]

CENTRAL NERVOUS SYSTEM

Multidrug-resistant CNS infections with *A. baumannii* is increasingly more common due to few if any therapeutic choices.[70,71] CNS penetration of colistin is poor[70-72] and literature supporting its direct CNS administration involves single case reports and case series.[70,71] Although no comparative efficacy data are available, in a comprehensive review of the published literature (which included both colistin and polymyxin B),[71] overall clinical cure rates with or without systemic therapy ranged between 80–91 percent. In addition, therapy was generally well tolerated, with a dose-dependent, reversible meningeal irritation occurring in 20 percent of patients.

A recently published pharmacokinetic study evaluated nine patients (aged 18 to 73 years) treated with intraventricular CMS (daily doses of 2.61–10.44 mg).[72] Colistin concentrations were measured using a selective high-performance liquid chromatography (HPLC) assay. When CMS was administered at doses of >5.22 mg/day, measured CSF concentrations of colistin were continuously above the MIC of 2 mcg/mL, and measured values of trough concentration ranged from 2.0 to 9.7 mcg/mL. Microbiological cure was observed in eight of nine patients. The authors concluded that daily doses of CMS >5.22 mg were appropriate but given the variability in external CSF efflux the daily dose of 10 mg suggested by the Infectious Diseases Society of America[73] may be more prudent.

CYSTIC FIBROSIS

The Cystic Fibrosis Foundation (CFF) guidelines for treatment of acute pulmonary exacerbations (APE) recommend utilization of two intravenous (IV) antipseudomonal antibiotics, with different mechanisms of action to improve antibacterial activity and reduce resistance.[74] Despite the emergence of multidrug-resistant pseudomonas complicating the treatment of APE the guideline does not address optimal dosing of antibiotics or the utilization of CMS.[74]

Three CMS efficacy studies have been published in CF patients,[75-77] which demonstrated good clinical outcomes with minimal toxicity utilizing a dose of 8 mg/kg/day (CBA dose = 3 mg/kg/day) divided every 8 hours (maximum daily CMS dose of 480 mg) for 12–14 days. Combination therapy was utilized for the majority of patients. In the one trial that did compare colistin alone to combination therapy,[75] both treatment groups experienced significant improvements in FEV1 and clinical score (P <0.05) but only those patients who received combination therapy had significant improvements in FVC, WBC, and weight (P <0.01). An additional study,[78] using the aforementioned dose, evaluated the development of renal impairment in combination with aminoglycosides or a beta-lactam. Results showed a strong correlation between aminoglycoside use and poor renal function, which was potentiated by concurrent utilization of colistin. When colistin was coadministered with other antibiotics, however, it did not show significant nephrotoxicity. Taken together, recent literature supports the use of a lower dose of CMS: 8 mg/kg/day divided every 8 hours (maximum daily CMS dose of 480 mg = 3 mg/kg/day, or 180 mg colistin base activity).

It should be noted this dose is lower than that recommended by the 1994 CFF Microbiology and Infectious Disease in CF Consensus Conference: 2.5–5 mg/ kg/day (CMS 6.67–13.3 mg/kg/day) divided every 8 hours,[79] and the UK CF Trust Antibiotic Working Group: 1–2 million units (MU) (CMS 80–160 mg) every 8 hours of IV colomycin.[80]

Clinical Pearls

• Until such time that its role is fully delineated (i.e., combination therapy), use should be reserved for patients with MDR pathogens such as *P. aeruginosa* and *A. baumannii.* As such, particular attention should be paid to appropriate dosing to prevent the emergence of resistant organism during treatment.

- Currently no convention exists with regard to a standard dosage unit for colistin/CMS. Drug references and literature provide dosing based on either colistin base activity (package insert recommendations) **or** CMS **or** international units. Close attention MUST be paid to which unit is used to prevent serious medication errors.

- Proper dosing for renal function and close monitoring should minimize the development of adverse effects. If nephrotoxicity does develop, it is generally reversible. Strategies to minimize risk of nephrotoxcity include avoidance of concomitant nephrotoxins and close monitoring of renal function. In CF patients, colistin may have a lower risk of nephrotoxicity than aminoglycosides.

- Neurotoxicity is less common but may be more difficult to detect in ICU patients. Close monitoring is recommended here as well.

- Older literature used methods of drug detection that did not distinguish between CMS and colistin. Only studies that determine plasma concentrations with non immune assays (i.e., HPLC) can appropriately characterize the time course of CMS and colistin.

- Colistin exhibits limited postantibiotic effect and rapid regrowth. Concentrations above MIC should be maintained for the entirety of the dosing interval to prevent resistance. As such for patients with normal renal function, an 8-hour interval is recommended.

- Initiation of therapy without a loading dose will result in a significant delay to attaining therapeutic colistin concentrations, as the half-life in critically ill patients is 14 hours. Although outside the standard dosing recommendations, a loading dose should be used to ensure the patient is promptly receiving a therapeutic dose and maintaining serum concentrations above the organism's MIC.

- Optimal dosing for CRRT has not been established, but its removal/binding to dialysis circuits may warrant higher doses.

- The true characterization of the PK/PD of CMS and colistin has yet to be elucidated and information about its optimal utilization will continue to evolve. The reader is encouraged to review the primary literature for the most recent studies that will complement the information contained herein.

CASES

CASE 1: COLISTIN LOADING DOSE

JC is a 68-year-old male admitted to the intensive care unit with SOB and is intubated for acute hypoxic respiratory failure. His PMH includes HTN, COPD, and Type II DM. He is an active drinker with family reporting about six beers per day. He quit smoking 10 years ago. He has multiple admissions to the hospital for pneumonia. He is empirically started on broad spectrum antibiotics to cover for gram-negative and gram-positive organisms. The ICU team obtains blood, sputum, and urine cultures.

Height: 165 cm

Weight: 60 kg

Creatinine 0.98 mg/dl

On day 2, his sputum grows many *Acinetobacter baumanii* susceptible to colistin and amikacin. Based on recent PK data to target a concentration of 2.5 mg/L, calculate JC's loading dose of CMS.

Answer:

Using the equations from Table 8-3:

Loading dose of CBA (mg) = colistin $C_{ss,avg}$ target × 2 × body weight (kg)

= 2.5 mg/L × 2 × 60 kg

= 300 mg IV of colistin base activity

Calculate JC's maintenance dose:

Daily dose of CBA (mg) = colistin $C_{ss,avg}$ target × (1.5 × CrCl + 30)

= 2.5 mg/L × (1.5 × 61 mL/min + 30)

= 304 mg, or 300 mg per day

Recommended dose would be 100 mg IV q8h.

QUESTION

JC requires a contrasted CT of his chest, abdomen, and pelvis and 48 hours later develops acute kidney injury. The decision is made to place him CRRT due to his hemodynamics.
    Recommend a new CMS dose while he is on CVVHDF.

Answer:

Based on the equation in Table 3, which included 4 patients receiving CRRT:

Daily dose of CBA to achieve each 1 mg/liter colistin $C_{ss,avg}$ target = 192 mg. May divide dose every 8–12 hours. Suggest a dose of 100 mg IV q12h.

QUESTION

JC becomes more hemodynamically stable and now is being changed over to intermittent hemodialysis. What is his new CMS dose?

Answer:

Using Table 8-3:

Daily dose of CBA on a non-HD day to achieve each 1 mg/liter colistin $C_{ss,avg}$ target = 30 mg. Because CrCl is zero, Dose = colistin $C_{ss,avg}$ target × (1.5 × CrCl + 30).

On HD days, a supplemental dose is needed. Add 50 percent to the daily maintenance dose if the supplemental dose is administered during the last hour of HD. Add 30 percent to the daily maintenance dose if the supplemental dose is administered after the HD session. Twice daily dosing is suggested.

Therefore, daily maintenance dose is 30 mg per day and 45 mg on HD day if being administered during the last hour of HD, or 30 mg of CBA per day and 39 mg on HD days if being administered after the HD session.

QUESTION

Drug Interaction with NMBAs.

JC's respiratory status deteriorates and is placed on high-frequency ventilation and requires a neuromuscular blocking agent to assist with his oxygenation. What is your recommendation to the team regarding the drug interaction between colistin and the neuromuscular blocking agent?

Answer:

Because the effects of the NMBA are increased with colistin, he may require a lower dose of the NMBA than what is recommended. Monitoring parameters for NMBAs include the train of four with a goal of 2–3 twitches. It is important to monitor the effect of the NMBA frequently and adjust the dose downward as needed.

CASE 2: UTI

RH is a 75-year-old female who resides in a nursing home after suffering a stroke two years ago. She has a chronic urinary catheter and is repeatedly treated for urinary tract infections. She is admitted to the ED with a fever and dysuria. Her urine culture grows a MDR A. baumanii. The decision is made to initiate colistin therapy. Using traditional dosing, what would be your recommendation? RH's serum creatinine is 1.4 mg/dL, and she weighs 65 kg.

Answer:

Traditional dosing is used due to the fact RH is not critically ill or showing signs of sepsis. A serum creatinine of 1.4 puts her degree of renal dysfunction as mild impairment.

A dose of 2.5–3.8 mg/kg in 2 divided doses equals 162.5 mg–247 mg/day. A suggested dose would be 100 mg IV q12h of colistin base activity (or anywhere in this range). Remember to monitor for signs of nephrotoxicity or neurotoxicity.

CASE 3: CNS

BD, a 52-year-old male, presents with SAH and obstructive hydrocephalus. An EVD was inserted and was replaced once (day 7). The patient is intubated, sedated in the ICU with persistent fevers. Multiple cultures were obtained. CSF and the EVD tip from day 7 grew MDR Acinetobacter baumanii. In addition, blood cultures were positive for the same organism. Patient is now exhibiting signs and symptoms of sepsis and requiring vasopressors to maintain blood pressure.

Height: 172 cm

Weight: 125 kg

Creatinine: 1.2 mg/dL

What is an appropriate IV and intraventricular dose for this patient?

Answer:

IV Dose

Calculate IBW (use calculations for obese patient).

Males: IBW = 50 kg + 2.3 kg for each inch over 5 feet
IBW = 50 + 2.3(7.7) = 67.7 kg

Using the equations from Table 8-3:

$$\text{Loading dose of CBA (mg)} = \text{colistin } C_{ss,avg} \text{ target} \times 2 \times \text{body weight (kg)}$$
$$= 2.5 \text{ mg/L} \times 2 \times 67.7 \text{ kg}$$
$$= \text{Calculated dose} = 338 \text{ or } 340 \text{ mg IV of colistin base activity}$$

Recommend a maximum of 300 mg IV daily based on the author's recommendations.[57]

Calculate BD's maintenance dose.

$$\text{Daily dose of CBA (mg)} = \text{colistin } C_{ss,avg} \text{ target} \times (1.5 \times \text{CrCl} + 30)$$
$$= 2.5 \text{ mg/L} \times (1.5 \times 99 \text{ mL/min} + 30)$$
$$= 483 \text{ or } 480 \text{ mg IV per day divided q8h}$$

Recommended dose would be 160 mg IV q8h.

This dose is significantly greater than the current maximum labeled dose, and some clinicians may not accept exceeding 150 mg IV q12h or 5 mg/kg/d to a maximum of 300 mg.

Intraventricular Dose

10 mg CMS intraventricularly daily (= 3.75 mg CBA)

Close monitoring for renal and neurotoxicity is recommended. Neurotoxicity from intraventricular administration is dose-related, may respond to a dose reduction, and is typically reversible upon discontinuation.

CASE 4: CYSTIC FIBROSIS

AR is a 27-year-old female with progressively worsening pulmonary symptoms and presumed acute exacerbation. She has had several previous exacerbations and received multiple courses of IV antibiotics. She does not receive inhaled colistin as she did not tolerate the nebulizer administrations.

Height: 155 cm

Weight: 42 kg

Creatinine 0.3 mg/dL

Her sputum grows many *Pseudomonas aeruginosa* susceptible to colistin and amikacin. Therapy will be initiated with both agents. What is the best colistin dosing regimen for this patient?

Answer:

8 mg/kg/day CMS (3 mg/kg/day CBA) in 3 divided doses
= 112 mg IV q8h CMS
OR = 42 mg IV q8h CBA

REFERENCES

1. Lim LM, Ly N, Anderson D, et al. Resurgence of colistin: A review of resistance, toxicity, pharmacodynamics, and dosing. *Pharmacotherapy*. 2010;30(12):1279–1291.
2. Falagas ME, Kasiakou SK. Colistin: The revival of polymyxins for the management of multidrug-resistant gram-negative bacterial infections. *Clin Infect Dis*. 2005;40(9):1333–1341.
3. Komura S, Kurahashi K. Partial purification and properties of L-2,4-diaminobutyric acid activating enzyme from a polymyxin E producing organism. *J Biochem*. 1979;86(4):1013–1021.
4. Koyama Y, Kurosasa A, Tsuchiya A, et al. A new antibiotic "colistin" produced by spore-forming soil bacteria. *J Antibiot* (Tokyo). 1950;3: 457–458.
5. Reed MD, Stern RC, O'Riordan MA, et al. The pharmacokinetics of colistin in patients with cystic fibrosis. *J Clin Pharmacol*. 2001;41: 645–654.
6. Brown JM, Dorman DC, Roy LP. Acute renal failure due to overdosage of colistin. *Med J Aust*. 1970;2(20):923–924.
7. Koch-Weser J, Sidel VW, Federman EB, et al. Adverse effects of sodium colistimethate. Manifestations and specific reaction rates during 317 courses of therapy. *Ann Intern Med*. 1970;72:857–868.
8. Ryan KJ, Schainuck LI, Hickman RO, et al. Colistimethate toxicity. Report of a fatal case in a previously healthy child. *JAMA*. 1969;207(11):2099–2101.

9. Yahav D, Farbman L, Leibovici L et al. Colistin: New lessons on an old antibiotic. *Clin Microbiol Infect*. 2012;18(1):18–29.

10. Couet W, Grégoire N, Marchand S, et al. Colistin pharmacokinetics: The fog is lifting. *Clin Microbiol Infect*. 2012;18(1):30–39.

11. Bergen PJ, Li J, Rayner CR, Nation RL. Colistin methanesulfonate is an inactive prodrug of colistin against Pseudomonas aeruginosa. *Antimicrob Agents Chemother*. 2006;50(6):1953–1958.

12. Li J, Nation RL, Turnidge JD. Defining the dosage units for colistin methanesulfonate: Urgent need for international harmonization. *Antimicrob Agents Chemother*. 2006;50:4231.

13. American Society of Health-System Pharmacists (ASHP) and Institute for Safe Medication Practices (ISMP) press release: *National Alert Issued: Dosing Confusion with Colistimethate for Injection* (released June 30, 2011). Available at: http://www.ashp.org/menu/AboutUs/ForPress/PressReleases/PressRelease.aspx?id=645.

14. van Duin D, Kaye KS, Neuner EA. Carbapenem-resistant Enterobacteriaceae: A review of treatment and outcomes. *Diagn Microbiol Infect Dis*. 2013;75(2):115–120.

15. US Food and Drug Administration: Information for Healthcare Professionals: Colistimethate (marketed as COLY-MYCIN M(R) and generic products). US Food and Drug Administration. Rockville, MD. 2007. Available from URL: http://www.fda.gov/cder/drug/InfoSheets/HCP/colistimethateHCP.htm.

16. Beringer P. The clinical use of colistin in patients with cystic fibrosis. *Curr Opin Pulm Med*. 2001;7:434–440.

17. Shirk M, Donahue K, Shirvani J. Unlabeled uses of nebulized medications. *Am J Health Syst Pharm*. 2006;63:1704–1716.

18. Alothman G, Ho B, Alsaadi MM, et al. Bronchial constriction and inhaled colistin in cystic fibrosis. *Chest*. 2005;127:522–529.

19. Cunningham S, Prasad A, Collyer L, et al. Bronchoconstriction following nebulised colistin in cystic fibrosis. *Arch Dis Child*. 2001;84:432–433.

20. Falagas ME, Rizos M, Bliziotis IA, et al. Toxicity after prolonged (more than four weeks) administration of intravenous colistin. *BMC Infect Dis*. 2005;5:1.

21. Falagas ME, Kasiakou SK, Kofteridis DP, et al. Effectiveness and nephrotoxicity of intravenous colistin for treatment of patients with infections due to polymyxin-only-susceptible (POS) gram-negative bacteria. *Eur J Clin Microbiol Infect Dis*. 2006;25(9):596–599.

22. Pintado V, San Miguel LG, Grill F, et al. Intravenous colistin sulphomethate sodium for therapy of infections due to multidrug-resistant gram-negative bacteria. *J Infect*. 2008;56(3):185–190.

23. Cheng CY, Sheng WH, Wang JT, et al. Safety and efficacy of intravenous colistin (colistin methanesulphonate) for severe multidrug-resistant gram-negative bacterial infections. *Int J Antimicrob Agents*. 2010;35(3):297–300.

24. Falagas ME, Fragoulis KN, Kasiakou SK, et al. Nephrotoxicity of intravenous colistin: A prospective evaluation. *Int J Antimicrob Agents*. 2005;26.504–507.

25. Hartzell JD, Neff R, Ake J, et al. Nephrotoxicity associated with intravenous colistin (colistimethate sodium) treatment at a tertiary care medical center. *Clin Infect Dis*. 2009;48:1724–1728.

26. Deryke CA, Crawford AJ, Uddin N, et al. Colistin dosing and nephrotoxicity in a large community teaching hospital. *Antimicrob Agents Chemother*. 2010;54:4503–4505.

27. Kim J, Lee KH, Yoo S, et al. Clinical characteristics and risk factors of colistin-induced nephrotoxicity. *Int J Antimicrob Agents*. 2009;34:434–438.

28. Ko H, Jeon M, Choo E, et al. Early acute kidney injury is a risk factor that predicts mortality in patients treated with colistin. *Nephron Clin Pract*. 2011;117:c284–c288.

29. Rattanaumpawan P, Ungprasert P, Thamlikitkul V. Risk factors for colistin-associated nephrotoxicity. *J Infect*. 2011;62:187–190.

30. Pogue JM, Lee J, Marchaim D, et al. Incidence of and risk factors for colistin-associated nephrotoxicity in a large academic health system. *Clin Infect Dis*. 2011;53:879–884.

31. Bellomo R, Ronco C, Kellum JA, et al. Acute renal failure—definition, outcome measures, animal models, fluid therapy and information technology needs: The Second International Consensus Conference of the Acute Dialysis Quality Initiative (ADQI) Group. *Crit Care*. 2004;8:R204–R212.

32. Levin AS, Barone AA, Penco J, et al. Intravenous colistin as therapy for nosocomial infections caused by multidrug-resistant Pseudomonas aeruginosa and Acinetobacter baumannii. *Clin Infect Dis*. 1999;28:1008–1011.

33. Falagas ME, Rafailidis PI. Nephrotoxicity of colistin: New insight into an old antibiotic. *Clin Infect Dis*. 2009;48:1729–1731.

34. Falagas ME, Kasiakou SK. Toxicity of polymyxins: A systematic review of the evidence from old and recent studies. *Crit Care*. 2006;10(1):1–13.

35. Nation RL, Li J. Optimizing use of colistin and polymyxin B in the critically ill. *Semin Respir Crit Care Med*. 2007;28:604–614.

36. Leong KW, Ong S, Chee HL, et al. Hypersensitivity pneumonitis due to high-dose colistin aerosol therapy. *Int J Infect Dis*. 2010;14:e1018–e1019.

37. Falagas ME, Siempos II, Rafailidis PI, et al. A. Inhaled colistin as monotherapy for multidrug-resistant gram (-) nosocomial pneumonia: A case series. *Respir Med*. 2009;103:707–713.

38. Ghannam DE, Rodriguez GH, Raad II, et al. Inhaled aminoglycosides in cancer patients with ventilator-associated gram-negative bacterial pneumonia: Safety and feasibility in the era of escalating drug resistance. *Eur J Clin Microbiol Infect Dis*. 2009;28:253–259.

39. Kofteridis DP, Alexopoulou C, Valachis A, et al. Aerosolized plus intravenous colistin versus intravenous colistin alone for the treatment of ventilator-associated pneumonia: A matched case-control study. *Clin Infect Dis*. 2010;51:1238–1244.

40. Korbila IP, Michalopoulos A, Rafailidis PI, et al. Inhaled colistin as adjunctive therapy to intravenous colistin for the treatment of microbiologically documented ventilator-associated pneumonia: A comparative cohort study. *Clin Microbiol Infect*. 2010;16:1230–1236.

41. Kwa AL, Loh C, Low JG, et al. Nebulized colistin in the treatment of pneumonia due to multidrug-resistant Acinetobacter baumannii and Pseudomonas aeruginosa. *Clin Infect Dis*. 2005;41:754–757.

42. Lin CC, Liu TC, Kuo CF, et al. Aerosolized colistin for the treatment of multidrug-resistant Acinetobacter baumannii pneumonia: Experience in a tertiary care hospital in northern Taiwan. *J Microbiol Immunol Infect*. 2010;43:323–331.

43. Michalopoulos A, Fotakis D, Virtzili S, et al. Aerosolized colistin as adjunctive treatment of ventilator-associated pneumonia due to multidrug-resistant gram-negative bacteria: A prospective study. *Respir Med*. 2008;102:407–412.

44. Michalopoulos A, Kasiakou SK, Mastora Z, et al. Aerosolized colistin for the treatment of nosocomial pneumonia due to multidrug-resistant gram-negative bacteria in patients without cystic fibrosis. *Crit Care*. 2005;9:R53–R59.

45. Rattanaumpawan P, Lorsutthitham J, Ungprasert P, et al. Randomized controlled trial of nebulized colistimethate sodium as adjunctive therapy of ventilator-associated pneumonia caused by gram-negative bacteria. *J Antimicrob Chemother*. 2010;65:2645–2649.

46. Sarkar S, DeSantis ER, Kuper J. Resurgence of colistin use. *Am J Health Syst Pharm*. 2007;64(23):2462–2466.

47. Landman D, Georgescu C, Martin DA, et al. Polymyxins revisited. *Clin Microbiol Rev*. 2008;21(3):449–465.

48. Walkty A, DeCorby M, Nichol K, et al. In vitro activity of colistin (polymyxin E) against 3,480 isolates of gram-negative bacilli obtained from patients in Canadian hospitals in the CANWARD study, 2007–2008. *Antimicrob Agents Chemother*. 2009;53:4924–4926.

49. European Committee on Antimicrobial Susceptibility Testing (EUCAST). Breakpoint tables for interpretation of MICs and zone diameters. Version 13, 5 January 2011. Available at: http://www.eucast.org/clinical_breakpoints (accessed March 1, 2013).

50. Clinical and Laboratory Standards Institute. Performance standards for antimicrobial susceptibility testing. Twenty-First Informational Supplement [serial on the Internet]. Wayne, PA: CLSI, 2011. Available at: http://www.clsi.org (accessed December 1, 2011).

51. Bergen PJ, Li J, Nation RL. Dosing of colistin-back to basic PK/PD. *Curr Opin Pharmacol*. 2011;11:464–469.

52. Bergen PJ, Bulitta JB, Forrest A, et al. Pharmacokinetic/pharmacodynamic investigation of colistin against Pseudomonas aeruginosa using an in vitro model. *Antimicrob Agents Chemother*. 2010;54:3783–3789.

53. Colistimethate for injection [package insert]. Big Flats, NY: X-Gen pharmaceuticals, 2010.

54. Pittinger C, Adamson R. Antibiotic blockade of neuromuscular function. *Ann Rev Pharmacol.* 1972;12:169–184.

55. Fogdall RP, Miller RD. Prolongation of a pancuronium-induced neuromuscular blockade by polymyxin B. *Anesthesiology.* 1974;40(1):84–87.

56. Dudhani RV, Turnidge JD, Coulthard K, Milne RW, Rayner CR, Li J, Nation RL. Elucidation of the pharmacokinetic/pharmacodynamic determinant of colistin activity against Pseudomonas aeruginosa in murine thigh and lung infection models. *Antimicrob Agents Chemother.* 2010;54:1117–1124.

57. Garonzik SM, Li J, Thamlikitkul V, Paterson DL, Shoham S, Jacob J, Silveira FP, Forrest A, Nation RL. Population pharmacokinetics of colistin methanesulfonate and formed colistin in critically ill patients from a multicenter study provide dosing suggestions for various categories of patients. *Antimicrob Agents Chemother.* 2011;55:3284–3294.

58. Owen RJ, Li J, Nation RL. In vitro pharmacodynamics of colistin against *Actinetobacter baumanni* clinical isolates. *J Antimicrob Chemother.* 2007;59:473–477.

59. Karvanen M, Plachouras D, Friberg LE, et al. Colistin methanesulfonate and colistin pharmacokinetics in critically ill patients receiving continuous venovenous hemodiafiltration. *Antimicrob Agents Chemother.* 2013;57(1):668–671.

60. Plachouras D, Karvanen M, Friberg LE. Population pharmacokinetic analysis of colistin methanesulfonate and colistin after intravenous administration in critically ill patients with infections caused by gram-negative bacteria. *Antimicrob Agents Chemother.* 2009;53(8):3430–3436.

61. AHFS Drug Information. © Copyright, 1959–2012. Selected Revisions June 30, 2011, American Society of Health-System Pharmacists, Inc., 7272 Wisconsin Avenue, Bethesda, MD 20814.

62. Ratjen F, Rietschel E, Kasel D, et al. Pharmacokinetics of inhaled colistin in patients with cystic fibrosis. *J Antimicrob Chemother.* 2006;57:306–11.

63. Li J, Milne RW, Nation RL, Turnidge JD, Smeaton TC, Coulthard K. Pharmacokinetics of colistin methanesulphonate and colistin in rats following an intravenous dose of colistin methanesulphonate. *J Antimicrob Chemother.* 2004;53:837–840.

64. Li J, Milne RW, Nation RL, Turnidge JD, Smeaton TC, Coulthard K. Use of high-performance liquid chromatography to study the pharmacokinetics of colistin sulfate in rats following intravenous administration. *Antimicrob Agents Chemother.* 2003;47:1766–1770.

65. Li J, Turnidge J, Milne R, Nation RL, Coulthard K. In vitro pharmacodynamic properties of colistin and colistin methanesulfonate against Pseudomonas aeruginosa isolates from patients with cystic fibrosis. *Antimicrob Agents Chemother.* 2001;45:781–785.

66. Bergen PJ, Li J, Nation RL, et al. Comparison of once-, twice- and thrice-daily dosing of colistin on antibacterial effect and emergence of resistance: Studies with Pseudomonas aeruginosa in an in vitro pharmacodynamic model. *J Antimicrob Chemother.* 2008;61:636–642.

67. Bergen PJ, Bulitta JB, Forrest A, Tsuji BT, Li J, Nation RL. Pharmacokinetic/pharmacodynamic investigation of colistin against Pseudomonas aeruginosa using an in vitro model. *Antimicrob Agents Chemother.* 2010;54:3783–3789.

68. Dudhani RV, Turnidge JD, Nation RL, Li J. fAUC/MIC is the most predictive pharmacokinetic/pharmacodynamic index of colistin against Acinetobacter baumannii in murine thigh and lung infection models. *J Antimicrob Chemother.* 2010;65:1984–1990.

69. Bulitta JB, Yang JC, Yohonn L, Ly NS, Brown SV, D'Hondt RE, Jusko WJ, Forrest A, Tsuji BT. Attenuation of colistin bactericidal activity by high inoculum of Pseudomonas aeruginosa characterized by a new mechanism-based population pharmacodynamic model. *Antimicrob Agents Chemother.* 2010;54:2051–2062.

70. Ng J, Gosbell IB, Kelly J, et al. Cure of multiresistant Acinetobacter baumannii central nervous system infections with intraventricular or intrathecal colistin: Case series and literature review. *J Antimicrob Chemother.* 2006;58(5):1078–1081.

71. Falagas ME, Bliziotis JA, Tam VH. Intraventricular or intrathecal use of polymyxins in patients with Gram-negative meningitis: A systematic review of the available evidence. *Int J Antimicrob Agents.* 2007;29:9–25.

72. Imberti R, Cusato M, Accetta G, et al. Pharmacokinetics of colistin in cerebrospinal fluid after intraventricular administration of colistin methanesulfonate. *Antimicrob Agents Chemother.* 2012;56:4416–4421.

73. Tunkel AR, et al. Practice guidelines for the management of bacterial meningitis. *Clin Infect Dis.* 2004;39:1267–1284.

74. Flume PA, Flume PA, Mogayzel PJ Jr, Robinson KA, Goss CH, Rosenblatt RL, Kuhn RJ, Marshall BC. Clinical Practice Guidelines for Pulmonary Therapies Committee. Cystic fibrosis pulmonary guidelines: Treatment of pulmonary exacerbations. *Am J Respir Crit Care Med.* 2009;180:802–808.

75. Conway SP, Pond MN, Watson A, Etherington C, Robey HL, Goldman MH. Intravenous colistin sulphomethate in acute respiratory exacerbations in adult patients with cystic fibrosis. *Thorax.* 1997;52:987–993.

76. Conway SP, Etherington C, Munday J, Goldman MH, Strong JJ, Wootton M. Safety and tolerability of bolus intravenous colistin in acute respiratory exacerbations in adults with cystic fibrosis. *Ann Pharmacother.* 2000;34:1238–1242.

77. Ledson MJ, Gallagher MJ, Cowperthwaite C, Convery RP, Walshaw MJ. Four years' experience of intravenous colomycin in an adult cystic fibrosis unit. *Eur Respir J.* 1998;12(3):592–594.

78. Al-Aloul M, Miller H, Alapati S, Stockton P, Ledson MJ, Walshaw MJ. Renal impairment in cystic fibrosis patients due to repeated intravenous aminoglycoside use. *Pediatr Pulmonol.* 2005;39:15–20.

79. Foundation CF. Microbiology and infectious disease in cystic fibrosis. In Cystic Fibrosis Foundation Consensus Conference. 1994

80. Trust UCF. Antibiotic treatment for cystic fibrosis. In UK Cystic Fibrosis Trust Antibiotic Working Group, 2009.

Lidocaine

TUDY HODGMAN, PharmD, FCCM, BCPS

Lidocaine is a local anesthetic that also has Vaughan Williams classification type IB antiarrhythmic properties. It is indicated for ventricular fibrillation in patients who cannot undergo synchronized cardioversion and are hemodynamically stable who do not require electrical cardioversion. It can also be used for both monomorphic and polymorphic ventricular tachycardias. Lidocaine is considered an alternative to amiodarone as a second-line agent in patients with ventricular tachycardia or pulseless electrical activity who are resistant to electric cardioversion and intravenous epinephrine or vasopressin.[1] The use of intravenous lidocaine has decreased with the elimination of lidocaine as the standard of practice for prophylaxis of asymptomatic premature ventricular contractions or nonsustained ventricular tachycardia after acute myocardial infarction.

PHARMACOKINETIC PARAMETERS

Lidocaine serum concentrations decrease biexponentially, and intravenous lidocaine follows a two-compartment pharmacokinetic model (see Figure 9-1).[2] After an intravenous loading dose, lidocaine distributes into cardiac tissue rapidly, with an alpha t½ of approximately 8 minutes (range 7–30 minutes), achieving maximum serum concentrations within an hour. The cardiac tissue is considered to be part of the central compartment for lidocaine with onset of effects quickly after a loading dose. The beta elimination phase is due to transfer of drug from the larger volume of distribution (Vdss) back into the central compartment (Vdc) with t½ of 87–108 minutes. Therefore, even if a maintenance infusion is started simultaneously to the loading dose, rapid redistribution can lead to subtherapeutic concentrations that may place the patient at risk for life-threatening arrhythmia.[3] This rapid distribution phase justifies the repetition of a "loading dose," generally 50 percent of the initial load, given at 5- to 20-minute intervals to maintain a therapeutic concentration.[1,4,5,6]

THERAPEUTIC CONCENTRATION

Most sources suggest therapeutic concentrations fall in the range of 1.5–5 mcg/mL.[1,5 6,7] Unfortunately, lidocaine has a narrow therapeutic index and adverse effects are both dose- and concentration-related. As you approach the upper end of this range, adverse events such as paresthesias, dizziness, drowsiness, and euphoria may appear. If lidocaine concentrations rise above the therapeutic range into toxic concentrations, a host of adverse consequences may be seen, including general adverse events like confusion, dysarthria, muscular twitching or seizures, agitation, psychosis, and even coma.[6,7] Cardiovascular adverse events include hypotension, atrioventricular blockade with concurrent hyperkalemia, and circulatory collapse.[2,8,9,10,11] However, lidocaine-induced adverse drug events are often missed and attributed to the underlying disease pathology. Routine serum concentration monitoring is not recommended unless the clinician suspects an adverse drug event, the patient experiences recurrent ventricular arrhythmias, or the patient has

disease states or conditions known to change the pharmacokinetics of lidocaine.[12,13]

METABOLISM AND ELIMINATION

Lidocaine is almost exclusively (>95%) eliminated by cytochrome P450 hepatic metabolism. The CYP1A2 and 3A enzyme groups, which are abundant in both the intestinal wall and liver, metabolize efficiently, leading to a large first-pass effect with low oral bioavailability (30%).[14] The primary active metabolite is mono-ethylglycinexylidide (MEGX), which is both renally excreted and further hepatically broken down to glycinexylidide (GX) and other inactive metabolites. Both GX and a portion of MEGX are renally eliminated and have been associated with some of the adverse effects seen with lidocaine.[15] Because these metabolites are renally eliminated, patients with significant renal dysfunction can exhibit signs of toxicity despite a concentration within the therapeutic range.[4,6] When lidocaine is administered as a prolonged infusion, the metabolites MEGX and GX can compete for hepatic metabolism and lead to accumulation.[1,3,4,16–20] Because lidocaine has a low sieving coefficient, it is not removed by hemodialysis or by hemofiltration[21]; however, no specific dosing guidelines are provided for patients with renal dysfunction either with or without dialysis.

With normal circulatory function, lidocaine has 100 percent bioavailability after intravenous injection. Intramuscular administration is generally avoided because it may interfere with assessment of creatine kinase enzyme concentrations used in the evaluation of acute myocardial infarction and also the need for rapid onset. Lidocaine is a drug with an extraction ratio of about 70 percent, placing it in the category of high extraction ratio where clearance is approximated by liver blood flow, approximately 10 ml/kg/min.[9] Therefore, diseases that affect liver blood flow are likely to significantly affect lidocaine clearance. In either CHF or cirrhosis, clearance decreases by about 40 percent to 6 ml/kg/min, whereas in major trauma or critical illness clearance is approximately 6.8 ml/kg/min.[6,17,22,23]

Unlike the general usefulness of using a serum creatinine to estimate the degree of renal insufficiency, no serum hepatic marker correlates to significant changes in hepatic dysfunction. Therefore, since hepatic disease leads to variable protein binding and elimination, some have used an objective measurement of hepatic function, the Child-Pugh classification (see Table 9-1).[24]

A Child-Pugh score of ≥8 would suggest poor hepatic function that would necessitate decreased dose.[14] Although lidocaine has a high extraction ratio, in decompensated cirrhotic patients, the clearance is not related to blood flow, but likely decreases relative to the amount of circulating hepatic enzymes that are produced. Additionally many of the patients with hepatic dysfunction will also be treated with a nonselective beta blocker that is known to decrease hepatic enzyme activity as well.[14] Patients with known hepatic dysfunction would best have serum lidocaine concentrations utilized to prevent toxicity in this high-risk population.

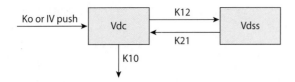

FIGURE 9-1. Two-compartment model.[2]

Changes in plasma protein binding are also likely to affect high-extraction-ratio drugs like lidocaine.[6] Normally, plasma protein binding is about 70 percent, with a small portion (30%) to albumin and the rest bound to alpha 1-acid glycoprotein (AAG).[20] AAG is an acute phase reactant secreted in high quantities during stress situations (e.g., acute MI, CHF, or trauma that leads to even lower free concentrations of lidocaine as the bound fraction increases). The pharmacokinetics of AAG are also known to be effected by other disease processes such as rheumatoid arthritis, cancer, morbid obesity, nephritic syndrome, or drugs (estrogen).[20,25,26] After a myocardial infarction, AAG concentrations may increase for the first 72 hours leading to a decrease in the unbound percentage of lidocaine from 30 percent to 20 percent. This process may be exhibited by decreased lidocaine clearance, placing these patients at risk for adverse effects. It has been suggested that monitoring of unbound drug may be necessary for the most accurate assessment of drug effect.[27]

The terminal half-life of lidocaine with normal hepatic function is 1–2 hours and increases to more than 5 hours in patients with hepatic dysfunction.[1,4,9] In order to estimate steady state, three to five half-lives should pass (8–24 hours) before assessing steady-state serum concentrations. To avoid the delay in achieving a therapeutic serum concentration and allowing the potential for breakthrough arrhythmias, it is suggested a loading dose be given prior to instituting the maintenance dose. The maintenance dose should then be started immediately to avoid subtherapeutic serum concentrations until steady state is reached. One to two repeat bolus doses can be given after 5- to 20-minute intervals to accommodate the initial distribution phase, because the maintenance dose causes only a slow rise in serum concentrations.[1,15] The half-life of lidocaine can increase to approximately 5 hours with liver disease (cirrhosis, hepatitis) due to the lack of hepatic enzyme activity. With prolonged infusions, greater than 24 hours, the terminal t½ increases.[3,18,19,28] Obesity—defined as total body weight (TBW) >130 percent of lean body weight (LBW)—is not known to specifically affect terminal t½.

The volume of central compartment (Vdc) is not easily measurable, therefore, most clinicians use a population average of 0.5 L/kg for this parameter with a total body volume of distribution (Vdss) of 1.5–2 L/kg.[4] The volume of distribution increases minimally with hepatic dysfunction to approximately 0.6 L/kg with Vdss of 2.3 L/kg due to decreased protein stores (albumin and AAG).[9] Vdc decreases with acute heart failure to approximately 0.3 L/kg due to increases in AAG, with a Vdss of 0.88 L/kg.[4,9] Trauma patients or the critically ill have a Vdc of 0.25 and Vdss of 0.75 L/kg.[22,23] Renal failure does not change the volume of distribution. Obesity (TBW >130% LBW) is not associated with a larger Vdc; therefore, doses should be based

upon LBW. However, because Vdss does increase with weight, controversy exists as to which weight is best to utilize for computing the total bolus (i.e., the number of bolus doses given).[29] Of note, the volume of distribution changes should not lead to changes in individual loading doses administered, but rather changes the total "loading dose" administered as several intermittent boluses (e.g., decreasing or increasing the number of repeat boluses at a dose of 0.5–0.75 mg/kg).

MONITORING

Because lidocaine is an antiarrhythmic agent, the electrocardiogram should be monitored for its effect on the presenting dysrhythmia. The standard goal of therapy is suppression of dysrhythmia with concurrent avoidance of adverse effects. Commonly lidocaine is only employed for a short duration while other therapeutic interventions are done, as there is not a therapeutic class oral agent to transition to. Rarely lidocaine is continued for recalcitrant ventricular dysrhythmias while assessing other long-term antiarrhythmic options. Monitoring of serum lidocaine concentrations is often not necessary as it used short term. However, in the case when a prolonged course is necessary for recalcitrant dysrhythmia or evaluation of drug-related adverse events, serum concentrations should be assessed to avoid lidocaine toxicity or increase morbidity.[30,31] Some clinicians suggest stopping lidocaine infusions after 6–24 hours to assess the need for continued therapy.

DRUG INTERACTIONS

Lidocaine is a substrate for the cytochrome P450 (CYP) enzymes, specifically 1A2, 2B6, and 3A4, but can also inhibit the CPY1A2 enzymes. Drug interactions can occur due to changes in metabolic enzyme activity or due to changes in hepatic blood flow. Beta-adrenergic blockers reduce clearance due to decreased cardiac output and hepatic blood flow. Cimetidine is thought to inhibit enzyme activity leading to decreased clearance. Medications such as phenobarbital isoniazid, chloramphenicol, or phenytoin can induce hepatic enzymes leading to increased clearance of lidocaine.[1,6]

PHARMACOKINETIC MODIFICATIONS FOR DISEASE STATES

Hepatic dysfunction as seen with cirrhosis or hepatitis may lead to wide variation in lidocaine clearance.[32] The protein binding of lidocaine is reduced, so the Vd is larger than normal. Concurrently metabolic processes may be depressed due to decreased CYP3A activity, leading to decreased clearance. These opposing parameters make prediction of lidocaine clearance in this population difficult to predict, and lidocaine serum concentrations are useful in guiding therapy.[1,9] The effect of age is unclear as many of these patients also have some degree of cardiac dysfunction that indirectly effects hepatic blood flow and therefore clearance.[1,7]

Myocardial infarction precipitates a surge in AAG release leading to decreased percentage of unbound lidocaine and therefore a decrease in clearance. Because the rise in AAG can continue for up to 72 hours after a myocardial infarction and persist up to several weeks, widely variable changes in clearance are reported.[17]

Heart failure and cardiogenic shock can significantly impair clearance due to decreased cardiac output and altered hepatic blood flow. Elevated AAG concentrations lead to increased plasma protein binding with lower unbound fraction of lidocaine (a smaller Vd = 0.3 L/kg). Half-life is quite variable depending on acute changes in cardiac function and is difficult to predict, again

Test or symptom	1 point	2 points	3 points
Total bilirubin (mg/dL)	<2.0	2.0–3.0	>3.0
Serum albumin (g/dL)	>3.5	2.8–3.5	<2.8
Prothrombin time (sec. prolonged over control)	<4	4–6	>6
Ascites	Absent	Slight	Moderate
Hepatic encephalopathy	None	Moderate	Severe

TABLE 9-1 Child-Pugh Classification[24]

Disease State	Estimated t½ (hr)	Vdc (L/kg)	V area (L/kg)
None	1–1.5	0.5	1.5
AMI	4	0.5	1.5
CHF	2	0.3	1
Liver dysfunction Child-Pugh >8	5	0.6	2.6

TABLE 9-2 Estimated Pharmacokinetic Parameters Based on Concurrent Disease State

necessitating serum lidocaine concentrations if lidocaine infusion is continued.[6,9,18] Some have suggested that clearance be estimated as 2.1–14.5 ml/kg/min based upon the degree of heart failure present (class IV to class I, respectively).[33]

It is difficult to obtain specific pharmacokinetic parameters for individual patients, so most lidocaine dosing is based on population parameters (shown in Table 9-2). The patient should be assessed for disease states known to change kinetic variables, specifically t½. The Kel can then be estimated and clearance calculated utilizing estimated Vd.[6,9]

DOSING

Traditional literature-based recommendations for loading dose 1–1.5 mg/kg, with repeat loading doses of 0.5–1 mg/kg every 5–20 minutes (up to total 3 mg/kg) administered at maximum rate of 50 mg/min. For patients with heart failure, half the normal loading doses are recommended.[6] Unfortunately, unpredictable results have been noted with this approach to dosing.

Maintenance doses ranges are 1–4 mg/min, or 10–30 mcg/kg/min.[1,6] Patients with decreased clearance secondary to liver dysfunction should start at half the normal maintenance dosage.[6]

An alternative dosing schedule that has been advocated is a loading dose of 8 mg/min for up to 25 minutes followed by maintenance dose 2 mg/min.[34] Another scheme suggested is 75 or 100 mg IV push bolus followed by 8 mg/min (120 mcg/kg/min) × 25 minutes, then 2 mg/minute (30 mcg/kg/min) thereafter, which resulted in only 52 percent of patients achieving a serum lidocaine concentration greater than 2.5 mcg/ml.[3] Wheeler[35] employed two dosing regimens: 100 mg IV push followed by 6.5 mg/min for 15 minutes, then 2 mg/min thereafter; or 100 mg IV push followed by 4.5 mg/min over 30 minutes, 3.1 mg/min over 30 minutes, then 2 mg/min. Computer-assisted dosing using nonlinear least squares regression analysis to adjust clearance and volume of distribution has been proposed as a method for attaining desired therapeutic concentrations during both the distributive and elimination phases of therapy.[36]

These complex dosing schemes may mathematically improve the time within a desired therapeutic range; however, their use is discounted by the inherent disadvantages of increases in dosing errors or calculations, and close monitoring by nursing staff due to the need for multiple pump setting changes.[37]

Theoretically, Bayesian forecasting techniques that incorporate expected population parameters and two or three serum measurements could be utilized to overcome the errors in dosing when applying one-compartment kinetic equations for a two-compartment drug like lidocaine.[38] Again, the need for multiple serum samples and computer programs combined with the short duration of infusions in current practice preclude use of Bayesian dosing.

Two-compartment model kinetics are complicated by trying to calculate the amount of drug lost from the central compartment and adjust the infusion rate to maintain a steady concentration of lidocaine. It leads most clinicians to estimate the concentration

when the two compartments are at a steady-state equilibrium using one-compartment model kinetics.[2]

Bolus loading dose:

$$LD = \frac{Css \times Vdc}{S \times F}$$

Css = desired lidocaine concentration at steady state (mcg/ml = mg/L)

Vdc = volume of the central compartment

S = active fraction of drug (0.87)

F = bioavailability (1 for intravenous)

Repeat loading doses after infusion has begun:

$$LD = \frac{(Cdes - Css) \times Vdc}{S \times F}$$

Cdes = desired serum concentration

Kel = 0.693/ t½   t½ = half-life

Steady-state clearance CL = Kel × Vd area (see Table 9-2)

$$\text{Infusion (maintenance) dose (mg) Ko} = \frac{Css \text{ (mg/L)} \times CL \text{ (L/hr)}}{S \times F}$$

Individual patient pharmacokinetic parameters can be utilized if steady-state serum lidocaine concentrations are obtained.

$$Cl \text{ (L/min)} = Dose \text{ (mg/min)}/Css \text{ (mcg/ml)}$$

ASSAYS

Lidocaine can be measured in either whole blood or plasma, with plasma concentrations of 120 percent of what is found in blood.[6] The most desirable assay would provide good reliability and also a quick turnaround time. Gas liquid chromatography (GLC) is one modality used to evaluate serum lidocaine concentrations. The sensitivity is from 0.1–10 mcg/mL with a coefficient of variation of 7.5 percent. Unfortunately with GLC, some of the metabolites are detected along with the parent compound. GLC requires trained technicians and requires a time-consuming separation extraction prior to testing. High-pressure liquid chromatography (HPLC) has a sensitivity of 0.1 mcg/mL with a coefficient of variation of 5–10 percent. The use of lidocaine, as well as the duration of lidocaine infusions, has decreased. This decrease, along with the lack of rapid turnaround, limits the use of some of these more traditional methods of assay for lidocaine.

Enzyme immunoassay (EIA) or enzyme immunoassay technique (EMIT) using the competitive binding principle correlates well with standard chromatographic methods. EMIT uses an inexpensive spectrophotometer and is completed in about 1 minute. EMIT measures lidocaine concentrations of 1–2 mcg/ml with a coefficient of variation of <10 percent.[3] EIA allows rapid turnaround with little cross-reactivity or interference with some plasma proteins, and it does not assay lidocaine metabolites. EMIT also has the advantage of decreased technician time for performing the assay, and decreased expertise needed for operating the equipment.

CASES

CASE 1

WM, a 44-year-old man, is admitted to the ED with probable AMI and associated ventricular tachycardia. After successive shocks, he is to be administered lidocaine as an intravenous infusion. He has no known prior medical history and does not smoke or drink.

Height = 73 inches

Weight = 80 kg

QUESTION

What are the loading and maintenance doses for this patient for a serum level of 2.5 mcg/mL utilizing pharmacokinetic dosing methods?

Answer:

$$T\frac{1}{2} = 4 \text{ hr}$$
$$Kel = 0.693/t\frac{1}{2} = 0.693/4 = 0.173/\text{hr}$$
$$Vdc = 0.5 \text{ L/kg} \times 80 \text{ kg} = 40 \text{ L}$$
$$V \text{ area} = 1.5 \text{ L/kg} \times 80 \text{ kg} = 120 \text{ L}$$
$$Cl = 0.173/\text{hr} \times 120 \text{ L} = 20.76\text{L/hr}$$

$$LD = Css \times Vdc = 2.5 \times 40 = 100 \text{ mg}$$
$$MD = Css \times Cl = \frac{2.5 \times 20.76/\text{hr}}{60 \text{ min/hr}} = 0.9 \text{ mg/min}$$

Utilizing the literature-based dose for a patient without disease states known to affect lidocaine clearance:

$$\text{Loading dose} = 1\text{--}1.5 \text{ mg/kg} \times 80 \text{ kg} = 80\text{--}120 \text{ mg}$$

Maintenance dose = 2–3 mg/min to achieve midtherapeutic range.

When would you obtain a steady-state serum concentration?

$$T\frac{1}{2} \times 5 = 4 \times 5 = 20 \text{ hr}$$

You would get a serum lidocaine level to ensure efficacy of the infusion or to rule out toxicity.

CASE 2

A 43-year-old female is found in a parking lot unresponsive. Paramedics evaluate the patient and find her in ventricular fibrillation. She is treated according the ACLS standard protocol, including defibrillation and epinephrine. Amiodarone is initiated, but leads to significant hypotension. Lidocaine is to be initiated as an alternative.

The patient has a long history of ETOH abuse, with known cirrhosis, and substance abuse.

Height = 66 inches

Weight = 47.9 kg

QUESTION

What would your recommended target steady-state concentration be for this patient?

Because the patient is at high risk for accumulation, should you aim for the lower end of the therapeutic range (1–2 mcg/mL) provided this concentration controls the patient's ventricular dysrhythmia. What would be your suggested loading and maintenance doses to achieve a serum concentration of 2 mcg/ml for this patient?

Answer:

$$T\frac{1}{2} = 5 \text{ hr}$$
$$Kel = 0.693/t\frac{1}{2} = 0.693/5 = 0.139/\text{hr}$$
$$Vdc = 0.6 \text{ L/kg} \times 47.9 \text{ kg} = 28.7 \text{ L}$$
$$V \text{ area} = 2.6 \text{ L/kg} \times 47.9 \text{ kg} = 124.5 \text{ L}$$
$$Cl = 0.139/\text{hr} \times 124.5 \text{ L} = 17.31 \text{ L/hr}$$

$$LD = Css \times Vdc = 2 \times 28.7 = 57.4 \text{ mg, rounded to 50 mg}$$
$$MD = Css \times Cl = \frac{2 \times 17.31/\text{hr}}{60 \text{ min/hr}} = 0. 58 \text{ mg/hr, rounded to 0.5 mg/min}$$

The patient should be assessed for suppression of dysrhythmia during the first 24 hours. If the infusion is to continue past 24 hours, she should be assessed for adverse effects secondary to accumulation of lidocaine. Remember this level will be difficult to assess in a patient with hepatic cirrhosis, so serum lidocaine concentration may be necessary to guide further therapy.

CASE 3

A 63-year-old male with a history of cardiomopathy and NYHA class IV heart failure presents with SOB and fatigue. Over the next 24 hours, he is aggressively diuresed leading to severe hyponatremia, hypokalemia, and hypomagnesemia. His electrolyte disturbances are thought to have led to the occurrence of ventricular fibrillation. ACLS procedure is followed, but based on the patient's past history of lack of response to amiodarone, the cardiologist wants to treat him with lidocaine. Please suggest an initial dosing regimen to achieve a lidocaine concentration of 3 mcg/mL.

Height = 69 inches

Weight = 104.6 kg

$$T\frac{1}{2} = 2 \text{ hr}$$
$$Kel = 0.693/t\frac{1}{2} = 0.693/2 = 0.347/\text{hr}$$
$$Vdc = 0.3 \text{ L/kg} \times 70.7 \text{ kg} = 21.2 \text{ L, use LBW secondary to obesity} = 70.7 \text{ kg}$$
$$V \text{ area} = 1 \text{ L/kg} \times 70.7 \text{ kg} = 70.7 \text{ L}$$
$$Cl = 0.347/\text{hr} \times 21.2 \text{ L} = 7.36 \text{ L/hr}$$

Answer:

$$LD = Css \times Vdc = 3 \times 21.2 = 63.6 \text{ mg, rounded to 75 mg}$$
$$MD = Css \times Cl = \frac{3 \times 7.36 \text{ L/hr}}{60 \text{ min/hr}} = 0.37 \text{ mg/min rounded to 0.5 mg/min}$$

CASE 4

A 49-year-old male is admitted s/p cardiopulmonary arrest. His current rhythm is ventricular tachycardia, and he is to be started on a lidocaine infusion. He has a long history of diabetes poorly controlled, renal insufficiency (CKD stage 4), hyperlipidemia, morbid obesity, and severe CAD with several stents placed.

Height = 70 inches

Weight = 158.8 kg

QUESTION

What is a typical loading and maintenance dose for this patient?

Answer:

Without liver dysfunction or heart dysfunction, the typical loading dose is 1–1.5 mg/kg based on LBW.

$$LBW = 73 \text{ kg}$$
$$73 \times 1\text{--}1.5 \text{ mg/kg} = 73\text{--}110 \text{ mg}$$

Rounding doses of 75 or 100 mg would be appropriate.

Due to long diabetes history and known renal insufficiency, the patients' serum target for lidocaine should be on the low end of the therapeutic range, therefore, maintenance dose should start at the lower end, 1–2 mg/min.

CASE 5

An elderly female with a history of CHF presents with an acute 6-pound weight gain and complaints of increasing pedal edema leading to an inability to ambulate. She is placed on a furosemide continuous infusion for acute pulmonary edema that necessitates intubation. Concurrent medications include heparin 5,000 units subcutaneous q8h, cimetidine 300 mg via tube q12h, metoprolol 12.5 mg via tube q12h, ramipril 5 mg via tube daily, aspirin 81mg via tube daily, propofol at 25 mcg/kg/min, and fentanyl 25 mcg/hr.

Height = 59 inches

Weight = 49.9 kg

QUESTION

Based upon her disease state and current medications, what would your initial loading and maintenance dosing be?

Answer:

With CHF, the typical loading dose is 0.5–0.75 mg/kg. The patient is not obese, so dosing is based on TBW.

$$0.5–0.75 \text{ mg/kg} \times 49.9 \text{ kg} = 25 \text{ mg to } 37.4 \text{ mg,}$$
round to 25–37.5 mg IV push over at least 2 min

Considering her heart failure and significant drug interaction with cimetidine, would aim for lower end of the therapeutic range (1–2 mcg/mL) for maintenance dosing with lower dose 0.5–2 mg/min.

On day 2 of therapy, the patient is observed to have facial twitching and appears oriented x 0. Her current sedation has been stopped. A serum lidocaine level was reported to be 6 mcg/mL with the lidocaine infusing at 2 mg/min. The physician asks for your assistance in decreasing the serum lidocaine to 2 mcg/mL.

Because lidocaine kinetics are linear, a simple dose proportion can be set up:

Dose new/Css new = Dose old/Css old

$$\text{New dose} = \frac{2 \text{ mg/min} \times 2 \text{ mcg/mL}}{6 \text{ mcg/mL}} = 0.67 \text{ mg/min, rounded to } 0.75 \text{ mg/min}$$

CASE 6

A 49-year-old female with a history of Down syndrome, hypothyroidism, morbid obesity, and epilepsy is initiated on a lidocaine infusion for recurrent ventricular tachycardia. Her current meds are famotidine 20 mg oral q12h, furosemide 20 mg oral daily, levothyroxine 88 mcg daily, phenytoin 150 mg po qam, and 300 mg po qHS, lidocaine 2 mg/min. She has a steady-state lidocaine level of 4 mcg/mL. Her cardiologist would like to maintain the serum lidocaine at 2 mcg/mL. Calculate and suggest a new dose based upon her current serum concentration.

$$Cl = \text{dose/Css} = \frac{2 \text{ mg/min}}{4 \text{ mcg/mL (mg/L)}} = 0.5 \text{ L/min}$$

Dose = Cl × desired Css = 0.5 L/min × 2 mcg/mL (mg/L) = 1 mg/min

This dose would be appropriate since lidocaine and phenytoin may have additive antiarrhythmic effects, so it should be started immediately.

CASE 7

An 88-year-old male presents with a syncopal episode which if found to be slow monomorphic ventricular tachycardia. He has no previous cardiac history. Hepatic and renal function are normal. He is 74 inches and 64.8kg. He is given lidocaine 100mg IV push, and placed on lidocaine 2 mg/min infusion. After 24 hours, he reverts back into his previous monomophic ventricular tachycardia and a lidocaine concentration is drawn. His Css is 1.3 mcg/mL. While awaiting transfer to the cath lab, the physician requests a dose to rapidly achieve 2.5 mcg/mL.

Answer:

Loading dose = (2.5 – 1.3) × 64.8 kg
= 77.8 mg, rounded to 75 mg

Dose new/Css new = Dose old/Css old

$$\text{New dose} = \frac{2 \text{ mg/min} \times 2.5 \text{ mcg/mL}}{1.3 \text{ mcg/mL}} = 3.85 \text{ mg/min, rounded to } 3.75 \text{ mg/min}$$

REFERENCES

1. AHFS Drug Information 2011;(section 24:04.04.08):1672–1675.
2. Pieper JA, Rodman JH. Lidocaine. In Evans WE, Schenteg JJ, Jusko WJ (Eds.). Applied pharmacokinetics: principles of therapeutic drug monitoring, 2nd ed. Spokane, WA. *Applied Therapeutics.* 1986;639–681.
3. Salzer LB, Weinrib AB, Marina RJ, Lima JJ. A comparison of methods of lidocaine administration in patients. *Clin Pharmacol Ther.* 1981;29:617–624.
4. Boyes RN, Scott DV, Jepson PJ, Goodman MJ, Julian DJ. Pharmacokinetics of lidocaine in man. *Clin Pharmacol Therap.* 1971;12:105–116.
5. Benowitz NL, Meister W. Clinical pharmacokinetics of lignocaine. *Clin Pharmacokin.* 1978;3:177–201.
6. Collinsworth KA, Kalman SM, Harrison DC. The clinical pharmacology of lidocaine as an antiarrhythmic drug. *Circ.* 1974;50:1217–1230.
7. Buckman K, Claiborne K, deGuzman M, Walberg CB, Haywood LJ. Lidocaine efficacy and toxicity assessed by a new rapid method. *Clin Pharmacol Ther.* 1980;177–181.
8. Selden R, Sasahara AA. Central nervous system toxicity induced by lidocaine. *J Am Med Assn.* 1967;202(9):908–909.
9. Thomson PD, Melmon KL, Richardson JA, Cohn K, Steinbrunn W, Cudihee R, Rowland M. Lidocaine pharmacokinetics in advanced heart failure, liver disease and renal failure in humans. *Ann Intern Med.* 1973;78:499–508.
10. Cheng TO, Wadhwa K. Sinus standstill following intravenous lidocaine administration. *J Am Med Assn.* 1973;223:790–792.
11. McLean SA, Paul ID, Spector PS. Lidocaine –Induced conduction disturbance in patients with systemic hyperkalemia. *Ann Emerg Med.* 2000;36:615–618.
12. Deglin SM, Deglin JM, Wurtzbacker J, et al. Rapid serum lidocaine determination in the critical care units. *J Am Med Assn.* 1980;44(6):571–573.
13. Vaisrub S. Laboratory testing: Routine or on demand? *J Am Med Assn.* 1980;244(6):592.
14. Orlando R, Piccoli P, De Martin S, Padrini R, Floreani M, Palatini P. Cytochrome P450 1A2 is a major determinant of lidocaine metabolism in vivo: Effects of liver function. *Clin Pharmacol Ther.* 2004;75:80–88.
15. Collinsworth KA, Strong JM, Atkinson AJ Jr, Winkle RA, Perlroth F, Harrison AC. Pharmacokinetics and metabolism of lidocaine in patients with renal failure. *Clin Pharmacol Ther.* 1975;18:59–64.
16. Strong JM, Mayfield DE, Atkinson AJ, et al. Pharmacological activity, metabolism and pharmacokinetics of glycine xylide. *Clin Pharmacol Ther.* 1975;17:184–194.
17. Prescott LF, Adjepom-Yamoah KK, Talbot RG. Impaired lignocaine metabolism in patients with myocardial infarction and cardiac failure. *Brit Med J.* 1976;1:939–941.

18. LeLorier J, Grenon D, Latour Y, Caille G, Dumont G, Brosseau A, Solignac A. Pharmacokinetics of lidocaine after prolonged intravenous infusions in uncomplicated myocardial infarction. *Ann Intern Med.* 1977;87:700–706.

19. Ochs HR, Carstens G, Greenblatt DJ. Reduction in lidocaine clearance during continuous infusion and by coadministration of propranolol. *N Engl J Med.* 1980;303:373–377.

20. Routledge PA, Shand DG, Barchowsky A, Wagner G, Stargel WW. Relationship between α1-acid glycoprotein and lidocaine disposition in myocardial infarction. *Clin Pharmacol Ther.* 1981;30:154–157.

21. Jacobi J, McGory RS, McCoy H, Matzke, GR. Hemodialysis clearance of total and unbound lidocaine. *Clin Pharm.* 1983;2:54–57.

22. Berkenstadt H, Segal E, Mayan H, Almog S, Rotenberg M, Perel A, Ezra D. The pharmacokinetics of morphine and lidocaine in critically ill patients. *Intensive Care Med.* 1999;25:110–112.

23. Berkenstadt H, Mayan H, Segal E, Rotenberg M, Almog S, Perel A, Ezra D. The pharmacokinetics of morphine and lidocaine in nine severe trauma patients. *J Clin Anesth.* 1999;11(8):630–634.

24. Pugh RNH, Murray-Lyon IM, Dawson JL, Pietroni MC, Williams R. Transection of the esophagus in bleeding oesophageal varices. *Br J Surg.* 1973;60:648–652.

25. Piafsky KM, Knoppert D. Binding of local anesthetics to α-1-acid glycoprotein. *Clin Res.* 1979;26:836a.

26. Slaughter RL, Hassett JM. Hepatic drug clearance following traumatic injury. *Drug Intell Clin Pharm.* 1985;19(11):799–806.

27. Valdes R Jr, Jortani SA, Gheorghiade M. Standards of laboratory practice: Cardiac drug monitoring. *Clin Chem.* 1998;44(5):1096–1109.

28. Bauer LA, Brown T, Gibaldi M. Influence of long-term infusions on lidocaine kinetics. *Clin Pharmacol Ther.* 1982;31:433–437.

29. Abernethy DR, Greenblatt DJ. Lidocaine disposition in obesity. *Am J Cardiol.* 1984;53:1183–1186.

30. Zeisler JA Jr, Skovseth JR, Anderson JR, Meister FL. Lidocaine therapy: Time for reevaluation. *Clin Pharm.* 1993;12:527–528.

31. Sadowski ZP, Alexander JH, Skrabucha B, et al. Multicenter randomized trial and a systematic overview of lidocaine in acute myocardial infarction. *Am Heart J.* 1999;137:792–798.

32. Testa R, Campo N, Caglieris S, et al. Lidocaine elimination and mono-ethylglycinexylidide formation in patients with chronic hepatitis or cirrhosis. *Hepatogastroenterology.* 1998;45:154–159.

33. Zito RA, Reid P. Lidocaine kinetics predicted by indocyanine green clearance. *N Engl J Med.* 1978;298:1160–1163.

34. Greenblatt DJ, Bolognini F, Koch-Weser J, Hormatz JS. Pharmacokinetic approach to the clinical use of lidocaine intravenously. *J Am Med Assn.* 1976;236:273–277.

35. Wheeler LA, Sheiner LB, Melmon KL. Pharmacokinetics of lidocaine. *J Am Med Assn.* 1977;237(14):1433–1434.

36. Rodman JH, Jelliffe RW, Kolb E, et al. Clinical studies with computer-assisted initial lidocaine therapy. *Arch Intern Med.* 1984;144:703–709.

37. Greenblatt DJ. Reply. Pharmacokinetics of lidocaine. *J Am Med Assn.* 1977;237(14):1434.

38. Vozeh S, Berger M, Wenk M, et al. Rapid prediction of individualized dosage requirements for lignocaine. *Clin Pharmacokinet.* 1984;9(4):354–363.

CHAPTER

10

Lithium

HENRY COHEN, MS, PharmD, FCCM, BCPP, CGP

Lithium was discovered in 1818, and its psychiatric benefits were discovered in the 1940s. Until 1950, the popular beverage 7-Up contained lithium citrate and was positioned for people with hangovers. The number "7" in 7-Up is in reference to the atomic mass of lithium and the word "Up" is in reference to the uplifting effects of the lithium citrate.

Lithium is indicated for the management of bipolar disorders, the acute treatment of manic episodes or mixed episodes in patients with bipolar 1 or bipolar 2 disorder, and maintenance therapy in bipolar disorders to prevent or decrease the intensity of subsequent manic episodes.[1-5] Lithium is also indicated for refractory unipolar depression (60–80% efficacy).[3] Lithium has also been used for the management of bulimia, tardive dyskinesia, alcoholism, cluster headaches, postpartum psychosis, corticosteroid psychosis, posttraumatic stress disorder, aggression, as an augmentation agent for patients with depression, disorders of impulse control, schizoaffective and schizophrenic disorders, neutropenia or anemia, and hyperthyroidism.[3-6] Lithium has been used for the syndrome of inappropriate antidiuretic hormone, however, due to the perils of using lithium in patients with water imbalances and the availability of demeclocycline and the newer vaptans such as conivaptan, lithium should only be used as a refractory agent.

Lithium has several mechanisms of action that influence its clinical effects in psychiatry. Lithium reduces cation transport such as calcium, magnesium, sodium, and potassium into cell membranes in the nerves and muscles.[2,3] These univalent and divalent cations are involved in the synthesis, storage, release, and reuptake of catecholamines. Lithium also reduces the reuptake of catecholamines and attenuates supersensitive receptors, resensitizing the receptor and reestablishing the effects of norepinephrine, epinephrine, serotonin, and dopamine.[3] Both norepinephrine and dopamine may be involved in the pathogenesis of mania, and serotonin may be involved with depression. The effects of lithium may be noted within 7–14 days, and 14–21 days for a full effect.

THERAPEUTIC AND TOXIC PLASMA CONCENTRATIONS

Lithium has a narrow therapeutic index but a well-defined plasma concentration range. The usual lithium target serum level for acute manic or mixed episodes in patients with bipolar 1 or bipolar 2 disorder is 0.8–1.2 mEq/L; rarely levels of 1.2–1.5 mEq/L are needed.[6] Once the patient's manic episode is stabilized, maintenance lithium serum levels are 0.6–1.0 mEq/L and rarely 1.0–1.2 mEq/L. In order to minimize lithium-adverse effects, the target ranges of lithium for the elderly are usually 0.2 mEq/L or less.[7] The available target serum levels for lithium assume a multiple daily dose model; no target level has been established for once-daily dosing.

ADVERSE EFFECTS

Two of the most common adverse effects associated with lithium are gastrointestinal and central nervous system (CNS) related, and generally resolve with continued treatment.[2] Gastrointestinal side effects may occur in up to 30 percent of patients and include nausea, vomiting, diarrhea, and bloating and are more problematic with the extended release lithium dosage forms.[8] Central nervous system adverse effects occur in 40–50 percent of patients, and include confusion, lethargy, fatigue, headache, mild memory impairment, muscle weakness, and tremor.[8] The hand tremor occurs in up to 50 percent of patients and manifests as a fine, rapid intention tremor.[9,10] The CNS adverse effects of lithium may be associated with high peak levels, and may be minimized by administering the immediate-release lithium products with food or by using the extended-release lithium products.[11]

Lithium may reversibly increase the WBC count by 10–30 percent and has been used to treat neutropenia secondary to a variety of causes, with well-controlled studies completed in patients with antineoplastic drug-induced neutropenia.[3,12-13] Lithium-induced leukocytosis, with leukocyte counts of 10,000–15,000/mm^3 have been observed.[3] Lithium should not be used in patients with leukemia.

Lithium decreases the response to antidiuretic hormone (arginine vasopressin) and may cause nephrogenic diabetes insipidus (DI). The incidence of lithium-induced DI is 30–50 percent and occurs shortly after treatment is started and persists in 10–25 percent with chronic treatment.[14] Polyuria followed by polydipsia and xerostomia occur with increased urine volumes to greater than 5 L/day. Polyuria has been successfully ameliorated with the potassium-sparing diuretics amiloride or triamterene.[15]

Lithium may cause hypothyroidism—the incidence is 1–4 percent. Lithium inhibits organification of iodine and inhibits conversion of tetraiodothyronine (T_4) to triiodothyronine (T_3). Elevated thyroid-stimulating hormone (TSH) occurs in 6–25 percent of patients.[16,17] Patients may present with goiters, with or without hypothyroidism. All patients receiving lithium should be monitored for signs and symptoms of hypothyroidism such as fatigue, depression, brittle hair, coarse skin, cold intolerance, and hypotension. The TSH levels should be completed at baseline and monitored every 6–12 months. Other endocrine effects of lithium include mild asymptomatic hyperparathyroidism, and manifests with increased calcium and decreased phosphate serum levels.[3]

Lithium-induced dermatologic adverse effects occur in 1 percent of patients—acneform eruptions, folliculitis, and psoriasis exacerbation are most common.[18,19] A Raynaud's disease-like effect occurs rarely and after one day of use, presenting with painful discolored fingers and toes and coldness of extremities.[19] Lithium may cause benign electrocardiogram changes, specifically T-wave inversion with an incidence of 30 percent.[3] Lithium causes nonspecific renal morphologic

TABLE 10-1 Concentration-Related Lithium Toxicity

Mild Toxicity <1.5 mEq/L	Moderate Toxicity 1.5–2.5 mEq/L	Severe Toxicity >2.5 mEq/L
Fine tremor of limbs	Coarse tremors of limbs	Coarse tremors of limbs
Cog-wheel rigidity	Muscle weakness	Delirium
Gastrointestinal disturbances	Muscle twitching	Stupor
Polyuria	Hyperreflexia	Clonus
Polydipsia	Slurred speech	Seizures
Agitation	Blurred vision and nystagmus	QTc interval prolongation
Confusion	Ataxia	Renal failure
Delirium	Sedation	Respiratory-complications
	Lethargy	Coma
	Hyperthermia	Death

changes such as glomerular fibrosis and interstitial fibrosis, nephron and tubular atrophy.[20] Sclerosis of up to 10–20 percent of glomeruli have been observed in some patients. The relationship between these changes and renal function are unknown and generally have not been associated with decreased renal function.[21] Nevertheless, it is prudent to monitor renal function with chronic lithium use.

Lithium is a teratogen and is classified as pregnancy category D.[3] Lithium readily crosses the placenta and fetal lithium levels are equal to that of the mother. Lithium has caused an increased risk of Ebstein's anomaly of the tricuspid valve to 1:1,000 from 1:20,000 in the normal population. Other lithium-induced cardiac anomalies such as ventricular conduction delay have been reported.[22] Teratogenic effects seen with lithium include Down syndrome and club foot. Lithium should not be used in the first trimester because of the highest risk of teratogenic effects.[23] If lithium is used during pregnancy, the lithium daily dose will have to be increased due to increased lithium clearance. Immediately, postpartum renal clearance of lithium decreases to prepregnancy levels, and the lithium daily dose will have to be reduced.

Lithium is a neurotoxin and toxicity can be life-threatening, presenting with coarse tremors, stupor, seizures, dysrhythmias, renal failure, coma, and death.[24] Poor clinical outcomes with lithium toxicity can be predicted by the duration of lithium toxic exposure and can lead to permanent basal ganglia damage.[25] The syndrome of irreversible lithium-effectuated neurotoxicity (SILENT) describes irreversible neurologic and neuropsychiatric sequelae from chronic lithium toxicity that persists for at least two months after lithium has been discontinued.[26] See Table 10-1 for concentration-related toxicities of lithium. In order to avoid lithium toxicity patients should avoid scenarios that cause dehydration, such as excessive sun exposure, diarrhea, vomiting, fever, and diaphoresis. The loss of sodium and water will lead to reabsorption of lithium and lithium toxicity. Patients should be instructed to maintain a regular diet with special attention to sodium intake, drink 8–12 eight-ounce glasses of liquid daily, and maintain a daily fluid input at 2,500–3,000 mL.

BIOAVAILABILITY

Lithium is not available intravenously, so the syrup liquid dosage form is used to determine bioavailability and is considered to be 100 percent bioavailable. Lithium is absorbed rapidly and achieves peak plasma concentrations with the liquid syrup dosage form within 30–60 minutes, with immediate-release tablets and capsules in 1–3 hours, and with sustained-release dosage forms in 3–12 hours.[3] The gastrointestinal absorption from immediate-release dosage forms

of lithium in tablets, capsules, or syrup is 95–100 percent, hence the bioavailability of lithium is 1 (F = 1).[27] The absorption of the sustained release dosage forms is 60–90 percent, in clinical practice 80 percent (F = 0.8) may be used.[3] Food decreases the peak plasma concentrations of lithium but does not decrease the bioavailability of lithium.

VOLUME OF DISTRIBUTION

Lithium is not protein bound and is widely distributed and approximately equal to that of body water. Lithium has a molecular weight of 74 daltons and is a monovalent cation. Lithium distribution follows a two-compartment open pharmacokinetic model. Lithium distributes rapidly to the central compartment, organs with a good blood supply (blood, heart, lungs, liver, and kidneys) and less rapidly to the peripheral compartments (fat, skin, muscle, bone, thyroid, and brain).[28] The initial volume of distribution of lithium is 0.2–0.3 L/kg, and after distribution is complete the final volume of distribution is 0.7 L/kg. The range of the lithium volume of distribution is 0.6–1.2 L/kg. The lithium volume of distribution in the elderly is 20–40 percent less due to less total body water and lean body weight.[29] The alpha (distribution) half-life is 6 hours and is complete in 10 hours.[28] Due to lithium following a two-compartment model, serum levels of lithium should be taken only after distribution is complete.

CLEARANCE

Lithium is not metabolized and is almost exclusively eliminated renally via proximal tubule.[2] Negligible amounts of lithium are eliminated in the saliva, sweat, and feces. Lithium is filtered via the glomerular membrane and 80 percent of lithium is reabsorbed through the proximal tubule.[3] Tubular reabsorption of lithium is closely linked to sodium. Lithium clearance is proportional to the GFR and renal blood flow, and in patients with a normal sodium balance is 25 percent of the creatinine clearance.[30] The adult lithium clearance is 0.024 L/hr/kg and is reduced in the elderly to 0.015 L/hr/kg.[31]

HALF-LIFE

The alpha half-life of lithium is 6 hours, and the beta half-life is 20–24 hours.[3,29] The plasma half-life of lithium increases to 48 hours in patients with renal failure. The time to achieve steady state with lithium is 3–5 days. Although lithium concentrations plateau at steady state within 3–5 days allowing for precise dosing adjustments in order to achieve target lithium serum levels, clinicians should be cognizant that the clinical effects of lithium may take up to 14–21 days.

LITHIUM BLOOD SAMPLING

Because lithium distribution follows a two-compartment model, lithium plasma levels need to be sampled after equilibrium between the first and second compartments is complete. This process generally takes 8–12 hours after the last dose.[28,29,32] Lithium levels may be drawn just before the first morning dose of lithium and at least 8–12 hours after the last evening dose, which is a postabsorption and postdistribution level. If necessary, clinicians may hold the morning lithium dose for several hours in order to obtain a true trough lithium level. During acute management with lithium, serum lithium levels should be monitored once or twice weekly and then monthly. When patients are stable on chronic lithium therapy, serum lithium levels may be taken every 1–6 months.

TABLE 10-2 Lithium Dosage Forms and Strengths

Dosage Form	Carbonate	Citrate	Lithium Salt
Immediate-release tablets	300 mg		8.12 mEq
Immediate-release capsules	150 mg		4.06 mEq
	300 mg		8.12 mEq
	600 mg		16.24 mEq
Extended-release tablet	300 mg		8.12 mEq
	450 mg		12.18 mEq
Syrup		560 mg	8 mEq

DOSAGE FORMS

Lithium is available in immediate-release and extended-release tablets and capsules as the lithium carbonate salt. Lithium carbonate 300 mg equals 8.12 mEq of the lithium salt. Table 10-2 depicts the lithium dosage forms and available strengths. Lithium capsules are preferred over the tablets because the tablets cause stomatitis.[33] The extended-release lithium dosage forms have several advantages: they can be dosed twice or three times daily, they improve compliance, and they minimize toxic peaks and subtherapeutic trough lithium levels.[2] The extended-release dosage forms should not be crushed, chewed, or halved.

Lithium oral solution is available as the citrate salt in a syrup dosage form. Lithium citrate is prepared with citric acid and has a pH of 4–5. It is raspberry flavored in sorbitol and available in a concentration of 300 mg/5 mL.[3] In order to minimize gastrointestinal distress, lithium citrate should be diluted with water or flavored juices. Lithium citrate should never be mixed with antidepressant or antipsychotic liquids, especially chlorpromazine because it forms an insoluble, unabsorbable citrate salt.[3] Lithium citrate is available as citrate 560 mg/5 mL, which is equivalent to 300 mg or 8 mEq of lithium carbonate.[2] In order to prevent medication errors, lithium liquid should only be ordered in milligrams and *not* milliequivalents.

DOSING

The product labeling for immediate-release lithium carbonate lists a start dose of 600 mg (16 mEq) three or four times a day or lithium extended-release 900 mg (24 mEq) twice daily. At these doses, 50 percent of adult patients would develop lithium toxicity. Empiric dosing for lithium in acute mania is 15 mg/kg or 300 mg (8 mEq) three times a day and 300 mg (8 mEq) four times a day for larger patients. Generally, for every lithium 8 mEq increase or decrease in daily dose, the lithium level will increase or decrease by 0.3 mEq/L.[28] Generally, immediate- or extended-release lithium can be administered twice daily; however, to decrease gastrointestinal and CNS adverse effects immediate-release lithium is administered three to four times a day. Although lithium may be dosed once daily, daily dosing achieves high peak plasma levels and is associated with higher risk of CNS adverse effects.

DRUG INTERACTIONS

Thiazide diuretics may decrease lithium renal clearance by 30–70 percent.[34] Despite thiazides exerting their diuretic effect on the distal convoluted tubule and lithium excretion occurring at a different site of the kidney in the proximal convoluted tubule, the interaction occurs with a rapid onset, usually within days, and the increase in lithium level is significant. Thiazides cause sodium and water loss on the distal convoluted tubule of the kidney, and because the kidney cannot distinguish between sodium and lithium, the sodium loss is compensated by lithium reabsorption in the proximal convoluted tubule. Adjustment factors are the fraction of the usual dose or clearance that would be suggested when both lithium and the interacting agent are used concomitantly. The adjustment factor for lithium with thiazide diuretics is 0.3–0.75 depending on the thiazide's potency, dose, and duration of effect. Loop diuretics are more potent in their diureses effect than thiazides; however, they are short acting and hence less likely to interact with lithium.[35] When loop diuretics are administered via continuous infusion or with multiple daily doses (three or four times a day), significant water and sodium depletion and subsequent lithium toxicity may occur—these combinations should be avoided. Osmotic diuretics such as mannitol, urea, and glycerin increase lithium excretion and may lower lithium serum levels; however, due to their propensity to cause dehydration, lithium reabsorption may occur and lead to lithium toxicity.

Angiotensin-converting enzyme inhibitors (ACEIs) and angiotensin II receptor blockers (ARBs) induce sodium repletion resulting in lithium reabsorption from the proximal tubule.[36] The ACEIs increase lithium serum levels by 15–30 percent.[37] The interaction can occur within days or weeks and can intensify after dosage increases. Several manufactures do not recommend the concomitant use of ACEs and lithium. The adjustment factor for lithium with ACEs or ARBs is 0.87 for patients less than 50 years old and 0.7 for patients over 50 years.[34]

Nonsteroidal anti-inflammatory drugs (NSAID) may decrease lithium excretion and increase lithium serum levels by 20–80 percent.[34] The magnitude of the interaction is based on the potency, dose, and duration of effect of the NSAID; however, significant magnitude variability with each NSAID exists among different patients. The mechanism of this interaction is due to the NSAID-induced renal inhibition of vasodilatory prostaglandins E_2 and I_2, decreasing hydrostatic pressure, causing sodium and water reabsorption, and subsequent lithium reabsorption. The NSAIDs that cause minimal renal prostaglandin effects such as sulindac, nabumetone, and etodolac are not likely to interact with lithium; however, it is prudent to monitor for lithium toxicity and serum levels.[38] Additionally, acetaminophen and low-dose aspirin do not interact with lithium.[39] The adjustment factor for lithium with NSAIDs is 0.2–0.8 depending on the NSAID's potency, dose, and duration of effect. The usual lithium adjustment factor when usual doses of NSAIDs are used is 0.7 to 0.8.

Theophylline and aminophylline increase the glomerular filtration rate and subsequently increases lithium clearance by 20–60 percent.[34] Similar increases on lithium clearance are seen with caffeine, sodium-containing intravenous fluids, and the administration of sodium bicarbonate intravenously or orally.[40] Cases of depressive and manic relapse have occurred when theophylline products have been started and doses of lithium have not been increased. The adjustment factor for lithium with theophylline, its derivatives, and sodium-containing intravenous fluids is 1.2 to 1.3.

A pharmacodynamic interaction exists between lithium and the nondihydropyridine calcium channel blockers (CCB) verapamil and diltiazem.[41-42] Lithium can decrease the calcium transport into cells and alter CNS neurotransmitter secretion; it is plausible that CCBs have a similar effect as lithium in the CNS. Patients will present with signs and symptoms of lithium toxicity, especially neurotoxicity and movement disorders with generally no increases in lithium serum levels. The interaction with lithium and CCBs does not generally occur with dihydropyridine CCBs.[43] Because of this pharmacodynamic interaction, adjustment factors cannot be used in this setting. It is prudent to avoid lithium with nondihydropyridine CCBs, and when administered concomitantly clinicians and patients should carefully monitor for signs and symptoms of lithium toxicity.

CASES

CASE 1: DETERMINING THE LITHIUM MAINTENANCE DOSE

MS is a 43-year-old white female to be placed on lithium carbonate for refractory acute mania. Her serum creatinine = 1.1 mg%. Calculate a maintenance dose to achieve a steady-state lithium serum level of 1.5 mEq/L.

Height: 5'6"

Weight: 70 kg

Answer:

Step 1. Calculate the patient's creatinine clearance and convert to L/hr by multiplying by 0.06.

The patient's creatinine clearance is 61.7 mL/minute.

$$Creatinine\ clearance = 61.7\ mL/min\ (0.06)$$
$$Creatinine\ clearance = 3.7\ L/hr$$

Step 2. Calculate the patient's lithium clearance using population data.

$$Lithium\ clearance = 0.25(Creatinine\ clearance)$$
$$Lithium\ clearance = 0.25(3.7\ L/hr)$$
$$Lithium\ clearance = 0.92\ L/hr$$

The lithium clearance in this patient is 0.92 L/hr.

Step 3. Calculate the maintenance dose (MD) using the following equation:

$$MD = \frac{(Cl\ in\ L/hr)(C_{pss\ AVG})(\tau[hr/day])}{(S)(F)}$$

$$MD = \frac{(0.92\ L/hour)(1.5\ mEq/L)(24\ hr)}{(1)}$$

$$MD = 33.1\ mEq$$

Step 4. Convert lithium carbonate milliequivalents into the equivalent lithium carbonate dose in milligrams using the following formula:

$$Lithium\ carbonate\ (mg) = \frac{[lithium\ dose\ in\ mEq] \times 300\ mg}{8.12\ mEq}$$

$$Lithium\ carbonate\ (mg) = \frac{[33.1\ mEq] \times 300\ mg}{8.12\ mEq}$$

$$Lithium\ carbonate\ (mg) = 1,222.9\ mg$$

The total daily dose of lithium carbonate may be rounded down from 1,222.9 mg daily to 1,200 mg daily. This patient will need four capsules of 300 mg (8.12 mEq) lithium carbonate daily.

This patient may be placed on any of the following regimens:

1. Lithium carbonate 300 mg: 1 capsule qid
2. Lithium carbonate 300 mg: 2 capsules bid
3. Lithium carbonate 600 mg: 1 capsule bid

CASE 1A: DETERMINING THE LITHIUM MAINTENANCE DOSE USING THE PATIENT'S ACTUAL LITHIUM CLEARANCE

MS is on lithium carbonate capsules 600 mg twice daily for the past two weeks, and her steady state lithium serum level is 1.9 mEq/L. She

has developed mild muscle twitching, hand tremor, and occasional confusion. Calculate a new maintenance dose to achieve a steady state lithium serum level of 1.5 mEq/L.

Answer:

Step 1. Calculate the patient's actual lithium clearance, and compare it to the patient's lithium clearance that was determined using population lithium clearance data.

$$Cl = \frac{\dfrac{(S)(F) \times Dose}{\tau[hr/day]}}{C_{pss\ AVG}}$$

$$Cl = \frac{\dfrac{(1)(1) \times 32.48\ mEq}{24\ hr}}{1.9\ mEq/L}$$

$$Cl = 0.71\ L/hr$$

The patient's actual lithium clearance is 0.71 L/hr versus the patient's lithium clearance of 0.92 L/hr that was determined using population lithium clearance data. The slower lithium clearance explains why the original maintenance dose yielded a high and toxic lithium level of 1.9 mEq/L rather than the 1.5 mEq/L target lithium level.

Step 2. Calculate the new maintenance dose using the patient's actual lithium clearance using the following maintenance dose equation:

$$MD = \frac{(Cl\ in\ L/hr)(C_{pss\ AVG})(\tau[hr/day])}{(S)(F)}$$

$$MD = \frac{(0.71\ L/hr)(1.5\ mEq/L)(24\ hr)}{(1)(1)}$$

$$MD = 25.6\ mEq$$

Step 3. Convert lithium carbonate milliequivalents into the equivalent lithium carbonate dose in milligrams using the following formula:

$$Lithium\ carbonate\ (mg) = \frac{[Lithium\ dose\ in\ mEq]}{8.12\ mEq} \times 300\ mg$$

$$Lithium\ carbonate\ (mg) = \frac{[25.6\ mEq] \times 300\ mg}{8.12\ mEq}$$

$$Lithium\ carbonate\ (mg) = 945.8\ mg$$

The total daily dose of lithium carbonate may be rounded down from 945.8 mg daily to 900 mg daily. This patient will need three capsules of 300 mg (8.12 mEq) lithium carbonate daily.

This patient may be placed on any of the following regimens:

1. Lithium carbonate 300 mg: 1 capsule tid
2. Lithium carbonate 150 mg : 3 capsules bid

CASE 2: LITHIUM DRUG-DRUG INTERACTION WITH THIAZIDE DIURETICS

AA is a 52-year-old Hispanic male, who is stable on lithium carbonate 300 mg tid for acute bipolar disorder. His steady-state lithium serum level is at target at 1.5 mEq/L. AA is diagnosed with hypertension and is to be placed on chlorthalidone 25 mg daily. Do you need to adjust the lithium maintenance dose?

Answer:

Chlorthalidone is a thiazide diuretic that decreases the renal clearance of lithium by 30 percent and may cause lithium toxicity. The adjustment factor for thiazide diuretics is 0.3–0.75, depending on the thiazide's potency, dose, and duration of effect. The average thiazide adjustment factor is 0.7. Chlorthalidone 25 mg daily is the recommended average daily dose and has a 24- to 72-hour duration of effect. The lithium dose should be adjusted using the adjustment factor of 0.7. The patient should also be counseled to monitor for the signs and symptoms of lithium toxicity.

The lithium maintenance dose should be adjusted by a factor of 0.7 using the following formula:

$$MD = (\text{Lithium daily dose in mEq})(\text{Adjustment factor})$$

Lithium daily dose = (24.36 mEq daily) or (900 mg daily) or (300 mg tid)

$$MD = (24.36 \text{ mEq/day})(0.7)$$

$$MD = 17.05 \text{ mEq/daily}$$

$$MD = \frac{17 \text{ mEq}}{8.12 \text{ mEq/Dose}}$$

$$MD = 2.09 \text{ capsules of 300 mg lithium carbonate}$$

The new lithium carbonate dose for this patient is 300 mg twice daily and takes into account the decreased renal clearance of lithium by chlorthalidone.

CASE 3: LITHIUM DRUG-DRUG INTERACTION WITH THIAZIDE DIURETICS PLUS NONSTEROIDAL ANTI-INFLAMMATORY DRUGS (NSAID)

BB 47-year-old white male, who is stable on lithium carbonate 300 mg tid for acute bipolar disorder. His steady state lithium serum level is 1.5 mEq/L. BB is to be placed on hydrochlorothiazide 12.5 mg twice daily and indomethacin 25 mg tid. Do you need to adjust the lithium maintenance dose?

Answer:

Hydrochlorothiazide is a thiazide diuretic that decreases the renal clearance of lithium by 30 percent (adjustment factor is 0.7). Indomethacin is a highly potent NSAID and decreases lithium clearance by 30 percent (adjustment factor is 0.7). However, indomethacin inhibits renal vasodilatory prostaglandins and blocks the diuretic effect of hydrochlorothiazide, thus negating the drug-drug interaction between hydrochlorothiazide and lithium.

$$MD = (\text{Lithium daily dose in mEq})(\text{Adjustment factor})$$

Lithium daily dose = (24.36 mEq daily) or (900 mg daily) or (300 mg tid)

$$MD = 24.36(0.7)$$

$$MD = 17.05 \text{ mEq/daily}$$

$$MD = \frac{17 \text{ mEq}}{8.12 \text{ mEq/Dose}}$$

$$MD = 2.09 \text{ capsules of 300 mg lithium carbonate}$$

The new lithium carbonate dose for this patient is 300 mg twice daily and takes into account the decreased renal clearance of lithium by indomethacin.

CASE 4: LITHIUM DRUG-DRUG INTERACTION WITH THIAZIDE DIURETICS PLUS NSAIDs

CC is a 39-year-old, 90 kg, male, who is stable on lithium carbonate 300 mg tid, with a steady-state lithium level of 1.5 mEq/L. CC is to be placed on chlorthalidone 25 mg, and sulindac 150 mg bid. Do you need to adjust the lithium maintenance dose?

Answer:

Chlorthalidone decreases renal clearance of lithium by 30 percent (adjustment factor is 0.7). Sulindac is an NSAID that may spare the kidneys and may not cause sodium and water retention, thus limiting the potential for a drug interaction with lithium (adjustment factor is 0) or with chlorthalidone. Heightened monitoring for lithium toxicity is recommended with sulindac therapy; however, no dosing adjustments need to be made.

$$MD = (\text{Lithium daily dose in mEq})(\text{Adjustment factor})$$

Lithium daily dose = (24.36 mEq daily) or (900 mg daily) or (300 mg tid)

$$MD = 24.36(0.7)$$

$$MD = 17.05 \text{ mEq/daily}$$

$$MD = \frac{17 \text{ mEq}}{8.12 \text{ mEq/Dose}}$$

$$MD = 2.09 \text{ capsules of 300 mg lithium carbonate}$$

The new lithium carbonate dose for this patient is 300 mg twice daily and takes into account the decreased renal clearance of lithium by chlorthalidone.

CASE 5: LITHIUM DRUG-DRUG INTERACTION WITH NSAIDS PLUS ASPIRIN

JJ is 42-year-old male and stable on lithium carbonate 300 mg tid, with a steady-state lithium level of 1.5 mEq/L. JJ is to be placed on ibuprofen 400 mg twice daily and aspirin 81 mg daily. Do you need to adjust the lithium maintenance dose?

Answer:

Ibuprofen is an NSAID and inhibits renal prostaglandins to cause sodium and water retention and decreases the renal clearance of lithium by 20–30 percent (ibuprofen adjustment factor is 0.8). Aspirin at high doses greater than 2 g daily may cause sodium and water retention; however, lower doses such as the doses used for acute coronary syndromes and stroke prevention (doses below 325 mg/daily) do not alter lithium clearance, and hence the low-dose aspirin adjustment factor is 0. In this case only the ibuprofen adjustment factor should be utilized to determine the new lithium dose.

$$MD = (\text{Lithium daily dose in mEq})(\text{Adjustment factor})$$

Lithium daily dose = (24.36 mEq daily) or (900 mg daily) or (300 mg tid)

$$MD = 24.36(0.8)$$

$$MD = 19.48 \text{ mEq/daily}$$

$$MD = \frac{19.48 \text{ mEq}}{8.12 \text{ mEq/Dose}}$$

$$MD = 2.4 \text{ capsules of 300 mg lithium carbonate}$$

The new lithium carbonate dose for this patient is 300 mg in the morning and 450 mg in the evening and takes into account the decreased renal clearance of lithium by ibuprofen.

REFERENCES

1. Price LH, Heninger GR. Lithium in the treatment of mood disorders. *New Engl J Med.* 1994;331:591–598. [IDIS 334509]
2. Lexi-Comp, Inc. Lithium drug information. In Rose, BD (Ed.). *UpToDate.* Wellesley, MA, 2014.
3. McEvoy GK, Snow ED (Eds.). *AHFS: Drug Information.* Bethesda, MD: American Society of Health-System Pharmacists, 2012: 2662–2671.
4. Suppes T, Dennehy EB, Swann AC, et al. Report of the Texas Consensus Conference Panel on medication treatment of bipolar disorder 2000. *J Clin Psychiat.* 2002;63:288–299.
5. Ereshefsky L, Gilderman AM, Jewett CM. Lithium therapy of manic depressive illness. Part I. Target symptoms, pharmacology, and kinetics. *Drug Intel Clin Pharm.* 1979;13:403–407.
6. American Psychiatric Association. Practice guideline for the treatment of patients with schizophrenia. 2nd ed. *Am J Psychiat.* 2004;161(Suppl):1–56.
7. Shulman KI, Herrmann N. The nature and management of mania in old age. *Psychiatric Clinics of North America.* 1999;22:649–665.
8. Reisberg B, Gershon S. Side effects associated with lithium therapy. *Arch Gen Psychiat.* 1979;36(8):879–887.
9. Gelenberg AJ, Jefferson JW. Lithium tremor. *J Clin Psychiat.* 1995; 56:283–287.
10. Miodownik C, Witztum E, Lerner V. Lithium-induced tremor treated with vitamin B6: A preliminary case series. *Intl J Psychiatry Med.* 2002;32:103–108.
11. Grof P. Some practical aspects of lithium treatment: blood levels, dosage prediction, and slow-release preparations. *Arch Gen Psychiat.* 1979;36(8):891–893.
12. Stein RS, Beaman C, Ali MY, Hansen R, Jenkins DD, Jumean HG. Lithium carbonate attenuation of chemotherapy-induced neutropenia. *N Engl J Med.* 1977;297:430–431.
13. Cohen MS, Zakhirch B, Metcalf JA, Root RK. Granulocyte function during lithium therapy. *Blood.* 1979;53:913–915.
14. MacNeil S, Jennings G, Eastwood PR, Paschalis C, Jenner FA. Lithium and the antidiuretic hormone. *Br J Clin Pharmacol.* 1976;3(2):305–313.
15. Boton R, Gaviria M, Battle DC. Prevalence, pathogenesis, and treatment of renal dysfunction associated with chronic lithium therapy. *Am J Kidney Dis.* 1987;10:329–324.
16. Lazarus JH. The effects of lithium therapy on thyroid and thyrotropin-releasing hormone. *Thyroid.* 1998;8:909–913.
17. Kleiner J, Altshuler l, Hendrick V, et al. Lithium-induced subclinical hypothyroidism: Review of the literature and guidelines for treatment. *J Clin Psychiat.* 1999;60:249–255.
18. Warnock JK, Morris DW. Adverse cutaneous reactions to mood stabilizers. *Am J Clin Dermatol.* 2003;4:21–30.
19. O'Brien M, Koo J. The mechanism of lithium and beta-blocking agents in inducing and exacerbating psoriasis. *J Drugs Dermatol.* 2006;5:426–432.
20. Walker RG. Lithium nephrotoxicity. *Kidney Intl.* 1993;42(Suppl.): S93–S98.
21. Jenner FA. Lithium and the question of kidney damage. *Arch Gen Psychiat.* 1979;36(8):888–890.
22. Weinstein MR, Goldfield M. Cardiovascular malformations with lithium use during pregnancy. *Am J Psychiat.* 1975;132:529–531.
23. Yonkers KA, Little BB, March D. 1998. Lithium during pregnancy: drug effects and their therapeutic implications. *CNS Drugs.* 9:261–269.
24. Amdisen A. Clinical features and management of lithium poisoning. *Med Toxicol Adverse Drug Exp.* 1988;3(1):18–32.
25. Adityanjee, Munshi KR, Thampy A. The syndrome of irreversible lithium-effectuated neurotoxicity. *Clin Neuropharmacol.* 2005;28: 38–49.
26. Apte SN, Langston JW. Permanent neurological deficits due to lithium toxicity. *Ann Neurol.* 1983;13:453–455.
27. Sugita ET, Stokes MD, Frazer A, Grof P, Mendels J, Goldstein FJ, Niebergal PJ. Lithium carbonate absorption in humans. *J Clin Pharmacol.* 1973;13:264–270.
28. Amdisen A. Serum level monitoring and clinical pharmacokinetics of lithium. *Clin Pharmacokin.* 1977;2:73–92.
29. Lehmann K, Merten K. Elimination of lithium in dependence on age in healthy subjects and patients with renal insufficiency. *Int J Clin Pharmacol.* 1974;10:292–298.
30. Thomsen K, Schou M. Renal lithium excretion in man. *Am J Physiol.* 1968;215:823–827.
31. Ward ME, Musa MN, Bailey L. Clinical pharmacokinetics of lithium. *J Clin Pharmacol.* 1994;34(4):280–285.
32. Dunner DL. Optimizing lithium treatment. *J Clin Psychiat.* 2000; 61(Suppl 9):76–81.
33. Hogan DJ, Murphy F, Burgess WR, Epstein JD, Lane PR. Lichenoid stomatitis associated with lithium carbonate. *J Am Acad Dermatol.* 1985;13(2,Pt 1):243–246.
34. Finley PR, Warner MD, Peabody CA. Clinical relevance of drug interactions with lithium. *Clin Pharmacokin.* 1995;29(3):172–191.
35. Colussi G, Rombolà G, Surian M, De Ferrari ME, Airaghi C, Benazzi E, Malberti F, Minetti L. Effects of acute administration of acetazolamide and furosemide on lithium clearance in humans. *Nephrol Dial Transplant.* 1989;4(8):707–712.
36. Navis GJ, de Jong PE, de Zeeuw D. Volume homeostasis, angiotensin-converting enzyme inhibition, and lithium therapy [letter]. *Am J Med.* 1989;86:621.
37. Correa FJ, Eiser AR. Angiotensin-converting enzyme inhibitors and lithium toxicity. *Am J Med.* 1992;93:108–109.
38. Ragheb MA, Powell RA. Failure of sulindac to increase serum lithium levels. *J Clin Psychiat.* 1986;47:33–34.
39. Reimann IW, Diener U, Frolich JC. Indomethacin but not aspirin increases plasma lithium ion levels. *Arch Gen Psychiat.* 1983;40: 283–286.
40. McSwiggan C. Interaction of lithium and bicarbonate. *Med J Aust.* 1978; 1:38–39.
41. Price WA, Shalley JE. Lithium-verapamil toxicity in the elderly. *J Am Geriatr Soc.* 1987;35:177–178.
42. Binder EF, Cayabyab L, Ritchie DJ, et al. Psychosis and a possible diltiazem-lithium interaction. *Arch Intern Med.* 1991;151:373–374.
43. Bruun NE, Ibsen H, Skott P. Lithium clearance and renal tubular sodium handling during acute and long-term nifedipine treatment in essential hypertension. *Clin Sci.* 1988;75:609–613.

MICHAEL BIGLOW, BS, PharmD, BCPS, BCPP
MEGAN FLINCHUM, PharmD, BCPS

CHAPTER 11

Long-Acting Injectable Antipsychotics

DRUG CLASS OVERVIEW

Antipsychotics are the mainstay of drug treatment for the management of schizophrenia and other psychotic disorders. The mechanism of action of the medication depends on the type of antipsychotic with the older "typical" antipsychotics focusing on the antagonism of postsynaptic dopamine type-2 (D_2) receptors. The newer "atypical" drugs antagonizing both D_2 and serotonin type-2A receptors elicit a comparable antipsychotic effect but with the potential for lessening iatrogenic movement disorders and improving negative symptoms (e.g., anhedonia, flattened affect, cognitive impairment).[1] The option of using depot formulations of these medications allows for a number of benefits including consistent drug delivery, assured patient compliance, predicable bioavailability, and avoidance of intentional or accidental overdose.[2] Available depot formulations exist for the typical antipsychotics haloperidol and fluphenazine and the atypical antipsychotics risperidone, paliperidone, and olanzapine. Dosing parameters vary due to different drug release mechanisms and intended time to response. (see Table 11-1) Their role in therapy has been established and they are recommended for patients who would prefer this method of treatment with the simplification of medication administration, who have a history of relapse due to noncompliance, and when avoiding noncompliance is a clinical priority.[2-4] Although patients on depot antipsychotics receive treatment on a more consistent and monitored basis, data are still limited on whether depot injections reduce relapse rates or long-term adverse drug events compared to oral antipsychotics.[5,6]

TYPICAL ANTIPSYCHOTICS

HALOPERIDOL AND FLUPHENAZINE

Haloperidol and fluphenazine are the two typical, or first-generation, antipsychotics available in a long-acting injectable form. Both are synthesized via esterification to a long chain fatty acid, decanoate. Previously, ethanate had been utilized as a lipid chain for fluphenazine but this formulation is no longer available in the United States. The esters are then dissolved in purified sesame oil for final preparation in the standard concentrations of 50 mg/mL and 100 mg/mL for haloperidol decanoate and 25 mg/mL for fluphenazine decanoate.[7,8,9] After intramuscular injection, the availability of the drug is presumed to be dependant on diffusion from the sesame oil because it has been observed that the hydrolysis of the ester is rapid and enzymatically mediated. The free drug is then allowed to pass through the blood brain barrier and elicit its antipsychotic effect (see Figure 11-1). Since the elimination rate constant remains the same after conversion to active drug, the absorption rate constant is the rate-limiting kinetic step, which has been described as a "flip-flop" kinetics model.[10]

Therefore, the time to steady-state concentration is dependent on the absorption and could take as long as 3 months to achieve.

Therapeutic Concentrations

Therapeutic plasma concentrations for both haloperidol and fluphenazine have been proposed, ranging from 5–14 ng/mL for haloperidol and <0.15–0.5 ng/mL for fluphenazine, but routine monitoring is not an established practice due to wide patient variability in response.[9,10,11] A linear correlation between haloperidol decanoate dose and steady-state plasma concentration has been established with a linear regression equation[9]:

$$Plasma\ concentration\ (ng/mL) = 0.0291 \times haloperidol\ decanoate\ dose\ (mg/month)$$

Effective doses generally require 60–80 percent of postsynaptic D_2 receptors to be antagonized, with lower percentages being less effective, except in the case of clozapine, and higher percentages being more associated with extrapyramidal symptoms (EPS).[12,13]

Bioequivalence to Oral Therapy

Due to the nature of the route of drug administration, depot administration bypasses oral absorption variability and first-pass or other predistribution metabolism. The conversion of stabilized patients to haloperidol decanoate can utilize a loading dose of 20 times the daily oral dose for the first injection and 10–15 times the oral dose for subsequent doses, or the prescriber can opt to give 10–15 times the oral dose but it is recommended to continue the oral dose of haloperidol for at least seven days. Fluphenazine decanoate is recommended to be dosed at 12.5–25 mg initially although a conversion ratio has been calculated at 1.6 times the daily oral dose being equivalent to the intramuscular fluphenazine decanoate requirement in mg/week but this conversion is rarely utilized.[10]

Clearance

Both medications undergo extensive hepatic metabolism with single-dose kinetic studies showing that after an initial peak within 24–48 hours, fluphenazine follows first-order elimination kinetics with an apparent half-life of 6.8–9.6 days, which increases to 14 days after multiple injections. Haloperidol decanoate has a peak after 7 days (range 3–9 days) and is noted to have a half-life of approximately 3 weeks.[9,10]

ATYPICAL ANTIPSYCHOTICS

RISPERIDONE

The first atypical or second-generation antipsychotic to be available in a long-acting injectable (LAI) formulation is risperidone. It differs significantly from the first depot injections in that it is

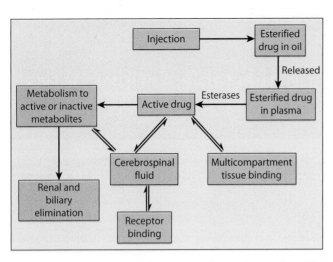

FIGURE 11-1. Disposition of depot antipsychotics. Source: Jann MW, Ereshefsky L, Saklad SR. Clinical pharmacokinetics of the depot antipsychotics. *Clin Pharmacokinet.* 1985;10(4):315–333. (With kind permission from Springer Science and Business Media.)

an aqueous formulation containing drug microencapsulated in a polylactide-co-glycolide (PLGA) polymer.[14] The polymer slowly hydrolyzes, releasing the drug in a slow but steady absorption pattern with clinically significant plasma levels of risperidone and its active metabolite, paliperidone (9-hydroxyrisperidone), developing in 3 weeks.

Therapeutic Concentration

After initial drug release, plasma concentration of risperidone continues to rise, reaching C_{MAX} in 4–5 weeks and lasting up to 7 weeks. This delay in drug absorption after the first injections necessitates the need for oral overlap for the first 3 weeks, although some practitioners would recommend covering for at least 6 weeks or after four injections to ensure the subject is at steady state. Kinetic studies (see Table 11-2) have shown that oral doses of 2 mg, 4 mg, and 6 mg daily are equivalent to 25 mg, 50 mg, and 75 mg of long-acting risperidone every 2 weeks, respectively, but current dosing conversion recommendations are 25 mg, 37.5 mg, and 50 mg every 2 weeks based on dose-repsonse studies.[15]

Bioequivalence to Oral Therapy

Bioequivalent conversion from oral to risperidone LAI as noted already has shown a slight decrease in AUC with an IM to oral ratio ranging from 88–94 percent as the dose increases from 25 mg to 75 mg.[15]

Clearance

As the drug is released from the polymer matrix the pharmacokinetics of oral and long-acting risperidone are similar. The metabolism of risperidone to 9-hydroxyrisperidone is mediated via cytochrome

P-450 (CYP) isoenzyme 2D6. Due to the difference in drug-release mechanism, the half-life of risperidone LAI is increased from 3 hours to 4–6 days.[19]

PALIPERIDONE

Paliperidone is another atypical antipsychotic developed into a long-acting injection formulation.[20] However, the formulation of paliperidone palmitate differs from the long-acting injection formulation of risperidone. Paliperidone palmitate is an extended-release aqueous-based nanosuspension, whereas risperidone has the unique microsphere formulation.[21,14]

Paliperidone palmitate has a low solubility and allows for an extended-release injectable product.[21] The isotonic aqueous buffer in which the drug is suspended penetrates muscle tissue and leaves a collection paliperidone palmitate particles locally at the injection site.[21,22] The drug particles dissolve slowly and are hydrolyzed into paliperidone and palmitic acid exhibiting biphasic absorption into systemic circulation.[21] The extended-release profile is a direct function of the paliperidone palmitate particle size, which is controlled by the wet grinding manufacturing process to increase surface area.[21]

Therapeutic Concentration

Paliperidone palmitate is initiated with a 234 mg injection on Day 1, and a 156 mg injection on Day 8 with monthly injections thereafter.[22] A paliperidone plasma concentration of 7.5 ng/mL, the threshold for antipsychotic efficacy, is generally reached within one week after the first injection.[23] However, plasma concentrations do not approach the C_{MAX} of 19 ng/mL until Day 13 after paliperidone palmitate initiation.[21] Due to its biphasic release pattern, supplemental oral antipsychotic doses are not recommended once the first dose of paliperidone palmitate is administered.[22,23] Previous kinetic studies have shown that monthly intramuscular paliperidone palmitate plus daily oral paliperdone doses of 6 mg or 12 mg daily results in a C_{MAX} range of 55–80 ng/mL.[22] Daily doses of 3 mg, 6 mg, and 12 mg are equivalent to monthly intramuscular paliperidone palmitate doses of 39 mg/78 mg, 117 mg, and 234 mg, respectively.[20]

Bioequivalence to Oral Therapy

Various kinetic trials have shown that median peak concentrations are 28 percent higher after the first injection into the deltoid muscle, compared to the gluteal muscle, which is most likely due to general anatomy of each site with more muscle and less adipose tissue within the deltoid.[20,22] For this reason, it is recommended to initiate paliperidone palmitate in the deltoid muscle to achieve therapeutic concentrations more rapidly.[22] However, the overall AUC resulting from both injection sites are within comparable ranges.[22] So when administering maintenance injections, it is acceptable to rotate injection sites.[22]

Bioequivalent doses of daily oral paliperidone to monthly intramuscular paliperidone palmitate are as mentioned previously. It is

TABLE 11-1	Dosing Parameters of Long-Acting Injectable Antipsychotics					
Drug	**Usual Starting Dose**	**Maximum Single Dose**	**Dosing Interval**	**T_{MAX} (days)**	**$T_{1/2}$ (days)**	**Injection Site**
Fluphenazine	12.5–25 mg	100 mg	q2–4weeks	0.3–1.5	14	gluteal, deltoid
Haloperidol	10–20x oral dose	450 mg	q4weeks	3–9	21	gluteal, deltoid
Risperidone	12.5–25 mg	50 mg	q2weeks	28 - 35	4 - 6	gluteal, deltoid
Paliperidone	234 mg & 156 mg loading doses, 117 mg maintenance dose	234 mg	q4weeks	13	25 - 49	gluteal after loading doses, deltoid
Olanzapine	210–405 mg	405 mg	q2 or q4weeks	7	30	gluteal only

TABLE 11-2	Steady-State Pharmacokinetics and Bioavailability of Long-Acting Risperidone Injection and Oral Risperidone[a]		
	Value at Indicate Dose		
Variable and Formulation	**2 mg Oral, 25 mg Long-Acting (n=21)**	**4 mg Oral, 50 mg Long-Acting (n=31)**	**6 mg Oral, 75 mg Long-Acting (n=26)**
Mean ± SD C_{MAX} (ng/mL)			
Oral	32.9 ± 9.2	74.1 ± 31.5	107.0 ± 49.0
Long-Acting	22.7 ± 9.2	57.3 ± 32.3	80.6 ± 40.0
Mean ± SD C_{MIN} (ng/mL)			
Oral	11.4 ± 3.6	22.3 ± 12.1	32.6 ± 15.7
Long-Acting	11.3 ± 4.5	24.3 ± 16.0	32.6 ± 16.5
Mean ± SD % fluctuation			
Oral	118 ± 33	137 ± 32	130 ± 45
Long-Acting	69 ± 44	83 ± 45	88 ± 54
AUC (ng*hr/mL)			
Oral[b]	5,996	12,027	18,056
Long-Acting[b]	5,303	11,571	16,886

[a]C_{MAX} = maximum plasma drug concentration, C_{MIN} = minimum plasma drug concentration, AUC = area under the concentration-versus-time curve.
[b]Least squares means (log transformed).
Source: Eerdekens M, Van Hove I, Remmerie B, Mannaert E. Pharmacokinetics and tolerability of long-acting risperidone in schizophrenia. *Schizophr Res.* 2004;70(1):91–100.

important to note that 156 mg of paliperidone palmitate is equivalent to 100 mg of active paliperidone. See Table 11-3 for equivalency conversions from long-acting intramuscular risperidone to paliperidone palmitate.[23]

Clearance

Paliperidone (active drug) undergoes hydroxylation, dehydrogenation, and benzisoxazole scission.[22] It has minimal involvement with CYP 2D6 and 3A4 isoenzymes, and is primarily eliminated renally.[20] Due to the drug release mechanism of the long-acting injection of paliperidone, the half-life is increased from 23 hours to 25–46 days.[20]

OLANZAPINE

Olanzapine pamoate monohydrate is a long-acting antipsychotic injection, specifically a salt-based depot combining olanzapine and pamoic acid.[24] This salt is poorly soluble, and its slow dissolution at the gluteal muscle injection site provides the mechanism for prolonged systemic absorption of olanzapine.[24,25]

Therapeutic Concentration

Upon intramuscular administration of olanzapine pamoate, the continuous dissolution of the salt begins immediately. A measurable serum concentration is reached within minutes to hours of

TABLE 11-3	Recommended Maintenance Equivalent Dose Conversions from Long-Acting IM Risperidone to IM Paliperidone Palmitate
Risperidone IM q2weeks	**Paliperidone palmitate IM q4weeks**
12.5 mg	39 mg
25 mg	78 mg
37.5 mg	117 mg
50 mg	156 mg
Unknown	234 mg

Source: National Drug Monograph. *Paliperidone palmitate [package inserts] (Invega Sustenna).* June 2010.

TABLE 11-4	Recommended Dose Conversion from Oral to LAI Olanzapine	
Oral Olanzapine Dose	**Olanzapine LAI Dose During First 8 Weeks**	**Olanzapine LAI Maintenance Dose After 8 Weeks**
10 mg/day	210 mg every 2 weeks OR 405 mg every 4 weeks	150 mg every 2 weeks OR 300 mg every 4 weeks
15 mg/day	300 mg every 2 weeks	210 mg every 2 weeks OR 405 mg every 4 weeks
20 mg/day	300 mg every 2 weeks	300 mg every 2 weeks

Source: National Drug Monograph. *Paliperidone palmitate [package inserts] (Invega Sustenna).* December 2010.

intramuscular injection.[24] Supplementation with concurrent oral antipsychotic medication is not necessary due to the salt's quick dissolution process. Therapeutic serum concentrations are generally reached within the first week of initiation and steadily decline over the next few weeks allowing for 2- or 4-week dosing.[24,25] Once olanzapine pamoate reaches steady state, plasma concentrations can range from 5 mg/mL to 73 mg/mL, which is equivalent to oral administration of olanzapine 5 mg to 20 mg once daily.[24,25]

Bioequivalence to Oral Therapy

Intramuscular injection of olanzapine pamoate 300 mg every 2 weeks delivers approximately 20 mg of olanzapine per day, and 150 mg of olanzapine pamoate every 2 weeks delivers approximately 10 mg per of olanzapine daily.[25] Refer to Table 11-4 for conversion dosing from oral to long-acting injection of olanzapine.[25]

Postinjection Delirium/Sedation Syndrome

Postinjection delirium and sedation syndrome (PDSS) is a serious adverse event that occurs following approximately 0.7 percent of all long-acting olanzapine injections.[24] The symptoms of this postinjection syndrome are consistent with an olanzapine overdose, and generally appear within 3 hours of administration.[24] Observed symptoms of PDSS include sedation (ranging from mild in severity to coma) and/or delirium (including confusion, disorientation, agitation, anxiety, and other cognitive impairment), extrapyramidal symptoms, dysarthria, ataxia, aggression, dizziness, weakness, hypertension, and convulsion.[25] Most olanzapine concentrations during a postinjection syndrome event have been found to exceed 100 ng/mL; some cases report concentrations reaching over 600 ng/mL.[24] Various factors have been investigated and excluded as possible mechanisms for this reaction, such as product quality issues, errors in reconstitution, and inappropriate dosing and administration.[24]

Evidence indicates that the mechanism of the overdose-like presentation of PDSS is a likely result of a more rapid than intended dissolution of olanzapine within hours of intramuscular administration. Simply stated, an amount of drug is inadvertently injected intravenously (refer to Figure 11-2).[24] Olanzapine pamoate solubility in plasma is substantially higher than in the extracellular fluid surrounding muscle tissue.[24] However, even in the plasma, the pamoate salt must still separate into active olanzapine and pamoic acid. Thus, the overdose-like symptoms do not occur immediately upon injection, but rather 1–3 hours after administration.[24]

The timing of the overdose-like symptoms and their resolution have appeared to correspond to the concentration-time profile, with symptoms resolving and olanzapine concentrations decreasing to therapeutic ranges within 24 to 72 hours.[24,25] The maximum plasma concentrations during PDSS have not been found to clearly correlate with the dose of olanzapine pamoate given.[24]

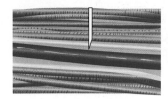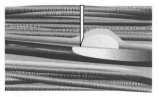

FIGURE 11-2. Illustration of proposed mechanism for olanzapine LAI distribution after vessel damage by nicking. The figure illustrates the proposed mechanism for distribution of the olanzapine LAI suspension during a PDSS event. The first panel depicts the tip of the syringe needle piercing the wall of the blood vessel situated within the muscle bed. In the second panel, the medication has been injected into the muscle tissue and is leaking into the blood vessel through the punctured vessel wall. Source: McDonnell DP, et al. Post-injection delirium/sedation syndrome in patients with schizophrenia treated with olanzapine long-acting injection, II: investigations of mechanism. *BMC Psychiatry.* 2010;10:45

Clearance

The major metabolic pathways for olanzapine include direct glucuronidation and CYP 450 mediated oxidation.[25] Studies have suggested that CYP 1A2 and 2D6 are the oxidation enzymes for olanzapine, 2D6 being the minor pathway.[25,25] This was determined because patients lacking this enzyme do not have issues adequately clearing olanzapine. The approximate half-life of olanzapine pamoate is 30 days, compared to the oral formulation, which is approximately 30 hours.[25]

CASES

CASE 1

LE is a 26-year-old male with a 4-year history of schizophrenia admitted to the acute psychiatric unit for recent decomposition with auditory hallucinations and paranoid delusions. LE's caregiver notes that he has not taken medications for the past 2 weeks and has a history of hospitalizations due to noncompliance. He is currently on haloperidol 3 mg po BID. After 3 days on the unit, LE begins to take medications and the psychiatrist places him on a new dose of 5 mg po BID with the option for converting to LAI. LE opts for haloperidol decanoate. The psychiatrist asks for options on the proper dosing practices of haloperidol decanoate.

Calculate a regimen utilizing a loading dose and maintenance dose based on LE new oral regimen as well as a regimen without a loading dose.

Answer:

Loading dose regimen:

Oral dose: 5 mg po BID = 10 mg/day
Conversion to LAI: 1 mg oral haloperidol per day = 20 mg IM haloperidol decanoate × 1 dose, then 10–15 mg IM haloperidol decanoate q4weeks
10 mg oral haloperidol × 20 = 200 mg haloperidol decanoate IM × 1
10 mg oral haloperidol × 10–15 = 100–150 mg haloperidol decanoate IM q4weeks

The conversion factor of 20 times the daily haloperidol dose closely approximates optimal plasma levels, taking into account the reported bioavailability of haloperidol (60–70%), but subsequent doses can increase plasma concentrations greater than twice that of oral therapy. So a dose reduction to 10 to 15 times that of the oral regimen is recommended.[9,16-18]

Nonloading dose regimen:

Conversion to LAI: 1 mg oral haloperidol per day
= 10–15 mg IM haloperidol decanoate q4 weeks plus oral haloperidol 5 mg po BID × 7 days
10 mg oral haloperidol × 10–15 = 100–150 mg haloperidol decanoate IM q4week + haloperidol 5 mg po BID × 7 days

Given that the time to peak for haloperidol decanoate is 7 days, it is generally recommended to continue oral medication for at least a week to ensure appropriate plasma concentrations in the interim.

QUESTION

Given that the psychiatrist chose to give LE the 100 mg dose, what is the expected plasma concentration after 4 months of therapy?

Answer:

Plasma concentration (ng/mL) = 0.0291 × 100 mg/month
= 29.1 ng/mL

This concentration is twice the proposed upper limit of normal for the proposed therapeutic range for haloperidol placing the patient at high risk for EPS but reflects the interpatient variability in treatment response. Efforts should be made to determine the lowest effective dose for all patients.

CASE 2

MJ is a 45-year-old female with a long history of schizoaffective disorder, controlled on risperidone 3 mg po bid. MJ notes that she heard about the long-acting injectable formulation of risperidone and would like to change her regimen.

QUESTION 1

What regimen would you recommend for converting MJ to risperidone LAI?

Answer:

Initiate risperidone LAI 50 mg IM q2 weeks. Continue oral therapy × 3 weeks.

As noted before, kinetic profiles do show that 6 mg/day of oral risperidone is equivalent to 75 mg of the LAI, but dose-response studies show a better correlation with the 50 mg dose. Also, due to the formulation of the injectable, oral therapy has to be continued for at least 3 weeks after the first injection in order to ensure adequate plasma concentration and prevent inadvertent relapse.

QUESTION 2

MJ returns for a routine checkup with no reports of psychotic features but does complain of worsening symptoms of depression. The psychiatrist initiates paroxetine 20 mg po daily. Three weeks later, MJ returns reporting no change in mood and noticeable tremors and complaints of restlessness. What could explain MJ's new onset adverse effects? What measures could be taken to resolve them?

Answer:

This situation is a case of CYP 2D6 drug-drug interaction between paroxetine and risperidone. Paroxetine is a potent 2D6 inhibitor and depending on the subject's 2D6 metabolic phenotype (e.g., ultra-rapid, extensive, intermediate, poor) can cause significant side effects. Clearance rates of risperidone can be reduced by as much as 36 percent if a subject's phenotype is changed from an extensive metabolizer to a poor metabolizer.[19] Also, the inhibition of 2D6 prevents the conversion to 9-hydroxirisperidone, which can impact patient response to the medication. In this case, MJ has developed two movement disorders, pseudoparkinsonism and akathisia, an extreme restlessness caused by antipsychotics.

In this case two options are available:

- Change the dose of risperidone LAI: Recommend reducing dose to 37.5 mg.
- Change paroxetine to a different antidepressant without 2D6 inhibition: Recommend switching to citalopram 20 mg po daily.

The preferred option depends on patient response to the antidepressant. Since 3 weeks have passed and MJ does not endorse any change in mood, possibly due to lack of efficacy of paroxetine or new onset adverse drug effects, a prudent approach would be to change the antidepressant.

CASE 3

JK is a 57-year-old male, with a history of chronic schizophrenia controlled on fluphenazine decanoate 25 mg IM q2weeks for the past three years, reporting to his new psychiatrist for increasing paranoia over the past 2 months. JK recently moved from another state and reports increased stress and is concerned that the fluphenazine doses that he is receiving from his new home care nurse is not working. JK has a history of hypertension for which he takes amlodipine 5 mg po daily and reports that he started smoking one pack per day due to the stress of the move.

Height = 67″

Weight = 75 kg

QUESTION

What pharmacokinetic changes could explain JK's worsening psychotic symptoms?

Answer:

JK has a couple of explanations for his worsening symptoms:

- Increased fluphenazine clearance secondary to smoking
- Improper administration technique by the "new" home care nurse, leading to impaired drug absorption

The first issue of increased clearance of fluphenazine decanoate is well established in smokers. Ereshefsky and colleagues noted that smoking increases oral fluphenazine clearance by a factor of 1.67 and fluphenazine decanoate by a factor of 2.33.[20] This significant increase in fluphenazine clearance could require a dose increase of up to 133 percent, or roughly 60 mg IM q2weeks.

The other concern is the potential of JK not receiving the full dose during administration. Experienced psychiatric care providers know to utilize the "z-track" method of administration in order to prevent leakage of the drug/lipid matrix as well as to use a needle of appropriate length. The former could be the case with JK in that he notes that the home care nurse is new; but without direct observation of the administration technique, it is only speculation.

The potential of incorrect needle length is mainly a concern with obese patients who may have a considerable amount of adipose tissue that prevents the needle tip from extending into the muscle, which would considerably delay absorption of the drug. Given JK is only 75 kg and has a BMI of 26, needle length is not likely an issue. Finally, repeated injections at the same site can potentially lead to reduced vascularization and thus lower absorption rate. Rotation of the site of injection is important for this reason.

CASE 4

CP is a 61-year-old African American male with a long history of schizoaffective disorder. He has recently become controlled on oral paliperidone 6 mg daily. Aside from his psychiatric illness, CP also has a complicated medical history including hypertension, hyperlipidemia, diabetes mellitus, and chronic kidney disease.

Height = 70″

Weight = 99 kg

IBW 73 kg, ABW 83.4 kg

SCr: 1.7 mg/dL

CP reports frustration with his medication regimen, and he would like reduce his pill burden. He remembers being on an injection a few years ago and expresses interest in trying a long-acting injection again.

QUESTION 1

This patient is currently on oral paliperidone. Does he still require a initial loading regimen? What if he was stabilized on a different long-acting antipsychotic injection?

Answer:

Yes, this patient still requires an initial loading regimen of paliperidone palmitate. However, if he was previously controlled on another LAI, no initial loading of paliperidone palmitate would be required. Once monthly administration, consistent with patients' previous injection schedules, is appropriate.

QUESTION 2

What would be the initial loading regimen of paliperidone palmitate when converting CP from oral paliperidone?

Answer:

Paliperidone has extensive renal elimination with 59 percent of unchanged drug removed via the kidneys. Drug accumulation and a prolonged half-life is a concern for patients with renal insufficiency with half-lives increasing from 23 hours to 51 hours in patients with severely impaired renal function. Dose adjustments are recommended in patients who have a creatinine clearance of 50–80 mL/min.

Day 1: 156 mg

Day 8: 117 mg, with maintenance doses of 78 mg every 4 weeks

$$[(140 - 61) \times 83.4]/(72 \times 1.7) = CrCl\ 53.8\ mL/min$$
(mild renal impairment)

QUESTION 3

In terms of renal function, when is the use of paliperidone palmitate not recommended?

Answer:

Use is not recommended in patients with CrCl <50 mL/min.

CASE 5

RM is a 32-year-old male with a nine-year history of schizophrenia, currently controlled on oral olanzapine 15 mg daily. The patient often has to keep his medication with him wherever he goes so that he can remember to take it at the same time every day. RM does not like to carry his medication with him because "it's annoying," and he does not want others to accidentally see what medication he does take. He has made some friends in various groups he attends and has heard about "shots" he can get every month.

QUESTION 1

What does this patient need to first be counseled on about olanzapine pamoate therapy?

Answer:

Because postdelirium/sedation syndrome (PDSS) or "postinjection syndrome" is a possibility, the patient needs to remain in a health care setting to be observed by a health care professional for at least 3 hours after *every* injection.

Symptoms of PDSS include sedation (ranging from mild in severity to coma) and/or delirium (including confusion, disorientation, agitation, anxiety, and other cognitive impairment), extrapyramidal symptoms, dysarthria, ataxia, aggression, dizziness, weakness, hypertension, and convulsion.

RM understands and agrees to the parameters surrounding injection administration.

QUESTION 2

What dosing regimen of olanzapine pamoate would you initiate in RM? And would this regimen need to be adjusted? If so, at what time point?

Answer:

Initial dosing would be olanzapine pamoate 300 mg IM every 2 weeks, but this regimen would need to be adjusted after the first 8 weeks.

At initiation, the patient is pleased with his new treatment. Despite adequate counseling before starting the long-acting injection, however, RM becomes frustrated that he's had to come in every 2 weeks.

QUESTION 3

It's Week 6 of therapy (3 injections given), what do you tell RM?

Answer:

The initiation period is 8 weeks, so he has one more 2-week injection remaining. After that, RM can be switched to monthly injections.

This situation isn't what RM prefers, but nonetheless he is understanding and agrees to continue with injection treatments.

QUESTION 4

What monthly maintenance dose of olanzapine pamoate do you recommend for RM?

Answer:

Maintenance dose: Olanzapine pamoate 405 mg IM every 4 weeks

REFERENCES

1. Haleem DJ. Serotonergic modulation of dopamine neurotransmission: A mechanism for enhancing therapeutics in schizophrenia. *J Coll Physicians Surg Pak.* 2006;16(8):556–562.
2. *Schizophrenia: Core Interventions in the Treatment and Management of Schizophrenia in Adults in Primary and Secondary Care.* NICE clinical guideline 82 (2009). Available at www.nice.org.uk/CG82 (accessed February 12, 2013).
3. American Psychiatric Association. *Practice Guideline for the Treatment of Patients with Schizophrenia,* 2nd ed. Arlington, VA: American Psychiatric Association, 2004. 114.
4. Kane JM, Aguglia E, Altamura AC, Ayuso Gutierrez JL, Brunello N, Fleischhacker WW, Gaebel W, Gerlach J, Guelfi JD, Kissling W, Lapierre YD, Lindström E, Mendlewicz J, Racagni G, Carulla LS, Schooler NR. Guidelines for depot antipsychotic treatment in schizophrenia. European Neuropsychopharmacology Consensus Conference in Siena, Italy. *Eur Neuropsychopharmacol.* 1998;8(1):55–66.
5. Quraishi S, David A. Depot haloperidol decanoate for schizophrenia (Cochrane Review). *The Cochrane Library.* 2003;3.
6. Adams CE, Fenton MK, Quraishi S, David AS. Systematic meta-review of depot antipsychotic drugs for people with schizophrenia. *BJP.* 2001;179:290–299.
7. Haloperidol decanoate [package insert]. APP Pharmaceuticals, LLC. Schaumberg, IL, November 2008.
8. Fluphenazine decanoate [package insert]. APP Pharmaceuticals, LLC. Schaumberg, IL, September 2010.
9. Ereshefsky L, Saklad SR, Jann MW, Davis CM, Richards A, Seidel DR. Future of depot neuroleptic therapy: Pharmacokinetic and pharmacodynamic approaches. *J Clin Psychiatry.* 1984;45(5 Pt 2):50–59.
10. Jann MW, Ereshefsky L, Saklad SR. Clinical pharmacokinetics of the depot antipsychotics. *Clin Pharmacokinet.* 1985;10(4):315–333.
11. Van Putten T, Marder SR, Mintz J, Poland RE. Haloperidol plasma levels and clinical response: A therapeutic window relationship. *Am J Psychiatry.* 1992;149(4):500–505.
12. Remington G, Kapur S. D2 and 5-HT receptor effects of antipsychotics: Bridging basic and clinical finding using PET. *J Clin Psychiatry.* 1999;60(suppl 10):15–19.
13. Kapur S, Zipursky RB, Remington G. Clinical and theoretical implications for 5-HT2 and D2 receptor occupancy of clozapine, risperidone, and olanzapine in schizophrenia. *Am J Psychiatry.* 1999;156:286–293.
14. Risperdal Consta® [package insert]. Janssen Pharmaceuticals, Inc. Titusville, NJ, 2011.
15. Eerdekens M, Van Hove I, Remmerie B, Mannaert E. Pharmacokinetics and tolerability of long-acting risperidone in schizophrenia. *Schizophr Res.* 2004;70(1):91–100.
16. Deberdt R, Elens P, Berghmans W, Heykants J, Woestenborghs R, Drelsens R, Reyntjens A, Wijngaarden I. Intramuscular haloperidol decanoate for neuroleptic maintenance therapy, efficacy, dosage schedule and plasma levels. *Acta Psychiatrica Scandinavia.* 1980;62:356–363.
17. Foresman A, Ohman R. Pharmacokinetic studies on haloperidol in man. *Current Therapeutic Research.* 1976;20:319–336.
18. Viukari M, Salo H, Hamminsevu U, Gordin A. Tolerance and serum levels of haloperidol during parenteral and oral haloperidol treatment in geriatric patients. *Acta Psychiatrica Scandinavia.* 1982;28:301–308.
19. Janssen Pharmaceutical Products, Inc. Risperidone long-acting injection (Risperdal Consta) U.S. prescribing information. Available at: www.risperdalconsta.com (accessed February 12, 2013).
20. Paliperidone palmitate [package insert]. Janssen Pharmaceuticals, Inc. Titusville, NJ, 2009.
21. Gopal S, Gassman-Mayer C, Palumbo J, Samtani MN, Shiwach R, Alphs L. Practical guidance for dosing and switching paliperidone palmitate treatment in patients with schizophrenia. *Curr Med Res Opin.* 2010;26(2):377–387.

22. Samtani MN, et al. Population pharmacokinetics of intramuscular paliperidone palmitate in patients with schizophrenia. *Clin Pharmacokinet.* 2009;48(9):585–600.

23. Coppola D, et al. A one-year prospective study of the safety, tolerability and pharmacokinetics of the highest available dose of paliperidone palmitate in patients with schizophrenia. *BMC Psychiatry.* 2012;12:26.

24. McDonnell DP, et al. Post-injection delirium/sedation syndrome in patients with schizophrenia treated with olanzapine long-acting injection, II: Investigations of mechanism. *BMC Psychiatry.* 2010;10:45.

25. Olanzapine pamoate [package insert]. Lilly USA, LLC. Indianapolis, IN, August 2012.

CHAPTER 12

Neuromuscular Blocking Agents

LESLY JURADO, PharmD, BCPS
TERESA A. ALLISON, PharmD, BCPS
BRIAN GULBIS, PharmD, BCPS
ELIZABETH FARRINGTON, PharmD, FCCP, FCCM, FPPAG, BCPS

DRUG OVERVIEW

Approximately 80 percent of critically ill intensive care patients require mechanical ventilation, thus administration of a one-time-only dose of a neuromuscular blocking agent (NMBA) is common. They are used to facilitate endotracheal intubation as they prevent laryngospasm and keep the patient from resisting the procedure. These agents should not be used, however, if the normalcy of the airway and the ability to successfully accomplish bag-mask ventilation and endotracheal intubation are questionable. Once intubated, only 1 percent to 15 percent of ICU patients are treated with continuous infusion or scheduled NMBAs (1%, surgical ICU; ≤10% medical ICU; ~15% trauma and pediatric ICU).[1] Aggressive use of analgesia and sedation is essential initially, and NMBAs are reserved for patients who fail to meet desired goals despite maximum sedative therapy. The clinical practice guideline for sustained neuromuscular blockade published by the Society of Critical Care Medicine states that "NMBAs should be used in an adult patient in an ICU to manage ventilation, manage increased ICP, treat muscle spasms, and decrease oxygen consumption ONLY when all other means have been tried without success."[2]

When used to manage ventilation, NMBAs allow improvement in pulmonary compliance. Neuromuscular blocking agents can assist ventilation therapy in at least three ways: (1) by reducing or eliminating spontaneous breathing; (2) preventing motor activity that might dislodge catheters, surgical dressings, or chest tubes; and (3) reducing oxygen consumption by patients with severely diminished cardiopulmonary function. However, the effect of neuromuscular blockade on ventilatory mechanics and chest wall compliance may be minimal in a patient who is maximally sedated. Although NMBAs are used in the mechanically ventilated patient, well-designed controlled trials do not exist that document improved patient outcomes when they are used to facilitate mechanical ventilation.[1,2] Most reports are limited to case studies, small prospective open-label trials, and small randomized open-label and double-blind trials. In addition, none of these reports compared NMBAs to placebos.

NMBAs may be used postoperatively for several reasons. First, neuromuscular blockade can prevent unacceptably high oxygen consumption due to the profound shivering that frequently accompanies rewarming from hypothermia. This condition is particularly deleterious for hypoxic patients or those with a history of cardiovascular disease. Further, postoperative neuromuscular blockade may be a useful adjunct to promote healing of specific surgical wounds (e.g., vascular anastomosis, supraglottoplasty) by immobilizing the patient for a defined period. Immobilization may prove of particular benefit after tracheal resection and anastomosis or when closure of the wound has been difficult or disruptive and its loss of integrity would place the patient at great risk. Improved patient outcomes have been documented in the surgical population when NMBAs are utilized postoperatively for complicated ENT procedures (cricoid split and supraglottoplasty) when compared to historical controls.[1]

Apart from mechanical ventilation and postoperative indications, situations in the ICU that may warrant administration of NMBAs are diverse. Therapeutic paralysis has been used appropriately in treating tetanus, status epilepticus, and uncontrolled intracranial hypertension or intracranial pressure (ICP). The use of NMBAs for prevention of rhabdomyolysis, myoglobinuria, and acute renal failure following status epilepticus and tetanus leads to improved patient outcomes. These benefits are intuitive and not extensively documented in the literature (mostly case reports). However, as paralytics do nothing to terminate seizures or protect the brain of seizing patients, concomitant antiepileptic therapy is mandatory and continuous or intermittent EEG monitoring is recommended. The routine use of NMBAs for patients post head injury has been discouraged, due to increased risk of pneumonia that may result in prolongation of ICU stay. Therapeutic paralysis may help control elevated intracranial pressure, so NMBAs may have a role after more conventional therapies post head injury.

The main use of NMBAs outside of the ED and ICU settings is to produce skeletal muscle relaxation during surgery after general anesthesia has been induced. When used in this setting, NMBAs allow a lighter level of anesthesia to be used.

PHYSIOLOGY

Although a detailed review of the physiology of the neuromuscular junction cannot be presented here, an understanding of the basic physiology is necessary for discussion of the pharmacodynamics of the neuromuscular blocking agent (NMBA). The neuromuscular junction consists of the prejunctional motor nerve ending, synaptic cleft, and postjunctional membrane, which contain nicotinic cholinergic receptors. The neurotransmitter acetylcholine (ACh) is synthesized in the motor nerve terminal and stored in vesicles. Normal neuromuscular transmission results from the release of ACh from the nerve terminal, its movement across the synaptic cleft, and subsequent binding to the postsynaptic nicotinic receptor on the sarcolemma of the skeletal muscle. The ACh molecules diffuse across the synaptic cleft and bind to the acetylcholine receptors, initiating a conformational change in the receptor that "opens" a potential channel formed by the receptor subunits. The opening of this channel allows the influx of sodium and calcium ions and the efflux of potassium ions, thereby facilitating the depolarization of the motor endplate and propagation of an action potential that spreads across the skeletal muscle fibers, leading to contraction. The enzyme acetylcholinesterase is responsible for rapid hydrolysis of ACh, which terminates the depolarization of the motor endplate.[3]

Neuromuscular blocking agents are designed to structurally resemble acetylcholine and all currently available NMBAs induce paralysis of skeletal muscle by occupying the ACh receptors on the muscle fiber, thereby preventing the binding of ACh to the receptors. They are classified as either depolarizing or nondepolarizing relaxants according to their effect on the motor end plate. The bulky nature of nondepolarizing NMBA, compared with that of ACh, causes drugs to interact with the receptors as antagonists, rather than agonists. Succinylcholine, the only depolarizing NMBA in clinical use, has a high affinity for ACh receptor sites. It binds with ACh receptors and depolarizes the motor end plate, but produces a more sustained depolarization than ACh, inactivating sodium channels and preventing impulse transmission. Transient twitching of skeletal muscle (fasciculation) is briefly produced, followed by paralysis. By contrast, nondepolarizing agents compete with ACh for access to receptors on the motor end plate, but once bound have no agonist activity. They have no effect on the resting electric potential of the motor end plate and do not cause muscle contraction. Evidence suggests that they also act to prevent ACh mobilization to some degree.[3]

SEQUENCE OF ONSET OF NEUROMUSCULAR BLOCKADE

Small, rapidly moving muscles such as those of the eyes and digits are affected by NMBA before those of the trunk and abdomen. Ultimately, intercostal muscles and finally the diaphragm are paralyzed. Recovery of skeletal muscles usually occurs in the reverse order to that of paralysis such that the diaphragm is the first to regain function.

Intravenous injection of an NMBA to a person who is awake initially produces difficulty in focusing and weakness in the mandibular muscles followed by ptosis, diplopia, and dysphagia. Relaxation of the small muscles of the ears improves acuity of hearing. Consciousness and sensorium remain undisturbed even in the presence of complete neuromuscular blockade. If time and patient condition permit, counseling the patient of what he or she will experience would most likely decrease any need for anxiolytics and sedation as the experience would be less terrifying.

BIOAVAILABILITY

All NMBA are poorly absorbed from the gastrointestinal tract. The onset of action varies between individual agents (Table 12-1), the route of administration, dosage, and concomitant drug therapy. In general, the first signs of neuromuscular blockade occur within 2 minutes following the IV administration of the nondepolarizing NMBA, and maximal effects occur in approximately 3–6 minutes. The maximal effects of succinylcholine occur within 1 minute. The onset of action following IM administration is slower and less predictable than following IV administration; therefore, the IM route is reserved for patients with no IV access.

TABLE 12-1 Summary of Available Neuromuscular Blocking Drugs

Drug	Adult Dose	Pediatric Dose	Onset of Action (min)	Duration of Action (min)	Elimination
Depolarizing Agents					
Succinylcholine	0.3–1.1 mg/kg (Max: 150 mg) MD: 0.04–0.07 mg/kg CI: 0.5–10 mg/min	1–2 mg/kg IM: 2.5–4 mg/kg MD: 0.3–0.6 mg/kg CI: not recommended	0.5–1	3–6	plasma cholinesterase
Nondepolarizing Agents					
Short-Acting					
Mivacurium*	0.15–0.2 mg/kg MD: 0.1–0.15 mg/kg CI: 1–15 mCg/min	0.2 mg/kg MD: 0.2 mg/kg CI: 10–14 mCg/kg/min (doses as high as 31 mcg/kg/min) have been used	1.5–3	15–20	plasma cholinesterase
Intermediate-Acting					
Atracurium	0.3–0.5 mg/kg MD: 0.08–0.2 mg/kg CI: 2–15 mCg/kg/min	0.3–0.4 mg/kg MD: 0.3–0.4 mg/kg CI: 0.6–1.2 mg/kg/hr OR 10–20 mCg/kg/min	3–5	20–35	Hoffman elimination, ester hydrolysis
Cisatracurium	0.15–0.2 mg/kg MD: 0.3 mg/kg CI: 1–3 mCg/kg/min	0.1 mg/kg MD: 0.03 mg/kg CI: 1–4 mCk/kg/min	1.5–3	40–60	Hoffman elimination, ester hydrolysis
Rocuronium	0.45–1.2 mg/kg MD: 0.1–0.2 mg/kg CI: 4–16 mCg/kg/min	0.6–1.2 mg/kg MD: 0.075–0.125 mg/kg CI: 10–12 mCg/kg/min	0.6–6	20–40	33% renal 54% biliary
Vecuronium	0.08–0.1 mg/kg MD: 0.05–0.1 mg/kg CI: 0.06–0.1 mg/kg/hr	0.1 mg/kg MD: 0.1 mg/kg CI: 0.09–0.15 mg/kg/hr	3–5	25–40	50% renal 40% biliary
Long-Acting					
Doxacurium[a]	0.05–0.08 mg/kg MD:0.005–0.1 mg/kg CI: 0.012 mg/kg/hr	0.03–0.05 mg/kg MD: 0.005–0.01 mg/kg CI: 0.012 mg/kghr	5	100–160	24–31% renal cholinesterase
Pancuronium	0.04–0.1 mg/kg MD: 0.01 mg/kg CI: 0.02–0.04 mg/kg/hr	0.1–0.15 mg/kg MD: 0.1–0.15 mg/kg CI: 0.05–0.1 mg/kg/hr	2–5	50–60	80% renal, 10–20% hepatic
Pipecuronium	0.07–0.085 mg/kg MD: 0.01–0.015 mg/kg	0.07 mg/kg MD: 0.01–0.015 mg/kg	2.5–5	60–120	>75% renal

MD, maintenance dose; CI, continuous infurion; [a]no longer manufactured in the United States.

TABLE 12-2	Pharmacokinetics of Neuromuscular Blocking Agents					
Drug	T½ (α)	T½ β	Volume of Distribution	Protein Binding	Clearance	Elimination
Succinylcholine	2					pseudocholinesterase 10% unchanged in the urine
Mivacurium[a]		2–3 min	0.15 L/kg		5.3 mL/kg/min	plasma cholinesterase
Atracurium	2–3.4 min	20 min	0.1 L/kg	82%	5.–1 6.1 mL/kg/min	Hoffman elimination, ester hydrolysis
Cisatracurium		22–31 min	0.16 L/kg		5.1 mL/kg/min	Hoffman elimination. ester hydrolysis
Rocuronium	1–2 min	1.4–2.4 hr	0.22–0.26 L/kg	30%	0.44 L/kg/hr	33% renal 54% biliary
Vecuronium	3.3–9 min	66–75 min	0.27 L/kg	60–80%	2.9–6.4 mL/min	30% renal 40% biliary
Doxacurium*		1.5 hr	0.22 L/kg	30%		24–31% renal cholinesterase
Pancuronium		2 hr	0.23 L/kg	87%	1.9 mL/min	80% renal 10–20% hepatic

t1/2, half life; [a]no longer available in the United States

Several blockers have been studied after intramuscular administration. The bioavailability of rapacuronium is 56 percent, and peak plasma concentrations occur 4–5 minutes after administration after 2.8 or 4.8 mg/kg during halothane anesthesia.[4] Rocuronium has better qualities than other nondepolarizers administered intramuscularly in that its bioavailability is greater than 80 percent, and less than 5 percent of the drug remains in muscle 30 minutes after administration.[5] Optimal intubating conditions exist 3 minutes after 1–1.8 mg/kg.[5] Succinylcholine may also be administered IM with intubating conditions in 2–3 minutes.[6]

VOLUME OF DISTRIBUTION (VD)/ DISTRIBUTION

A summary of individual Vd can be found in Table 12-2. Following IV administration, the drugs are distributed into the extracellular fluid and rapidly reach their site of action at the motor end plate. Conditions associated with an increase in extracellular fluid volume may require a higher dose of NMBA. These patients include those who have congestive heart failure, patients with peritonitis, and patients immediately postpartum.[7] In addition, newborn infants are known to have larger extracellular fluid volumes per unit of body weight. For all neuromuscular blockers that have been studied, the volume of distribution is greater in infants.[8] Most NMBA cross the blood-brain barrier to a small extent, if at all. Increased protein binding (possibly to alpha-1 acid glycoprotein) of nondepolarizing NMBA with a resulting decrease in free fraction of circulating drug has been reported in patients with burns.[6] Other conditions associated with an increase in alpha-1 acid glycoprotein are acute myocardial infarction, cancer, inflammatory diseases (Crohn's and inflammatory arthritis), surgery, trauma injury, and administration of phenytoin and carbamazepine.[9-11]

ELIMINATION

A summary of the method of elimination and clearance of individual NMBAs can be found in Table 12-2. Succinylcholine is metabolized rapidly by pseudocholinesterase and is excreted in the urine as active and inactive metabolites and small amounts of unchanged drug.[5] Pancuronium and pipecuronium are excreted primarily unchanged in the urine. Following IV administration, atracurium besylate and cisatracurium undergo rapid metabolism via Hoffman elimination and via nonspecific enzymatic ester

hydrolysis. Atracurium besylate and cisatracurium and their metabolites, including metabolic products of Hoffman elimination and ester hydrolysis are excreted primarily in the urine and also in feces via biliary elimination. Only a small fraction of the dose is excreted unchanged in the urine and bile. Vecuronium and rocuronium have both renal and biliary elimination; therefore, caution should be used when administering a continuous infusion to patients with either renal or hepatic dysfunction. Careful train-of-four monitoring is essential.

For NMBAs that are eliminated by renal elimination or hepatic metabolism, drug clearance is not proportional to the volume of distribution. A longer half-life, therefore, is observed in infants and children or any patient with renal or hepatic dysfunction. If the drug is metabolized in body fluids, however, as is the case for succinylcholine, mivacurium, atracurium, and cisatracurium; then, increasing the Vd results in increased clearance.[8]

PATIENT POPULATIONS WITH ALTERED PHARMACOKINETICS AND/OR PHARMACODYNAMICS

BURN PATIENTS

Patients with burn injury are resistant to the action of nondepolarizing NMBA. The magnitude of resistance depends on the extent of thermal injury and elapsed time since the burn, with patients having burns that extend over 25–30 percent or more of body surface area being most likely to exhibit resistance (increasing with increased injury) and the resistance only becoming apparent one week or longer after the burn.[12] NMBA resistance has been reported to peak two or more weeks after the burn, persists for several months or longer, and then decreases gradually with healing.[12] The mechanism of this resistance appears to be multifactorial and may involve pharmacokinetic, pharmacodynamic, and pathophysiologic factors. Increased production of alpha-1 acid glycoprotein will reduce the free (unbound) fraction of circulating NMBAs and may contribute to this resistance, however, the magnitude of the resistance cannot be solely explained by this mechanism. It also has been suggested that changes in the number of acetylcholine receptors and/or in anticholinesterase activity may contribute to this NMBA resistance. Other mechanisms (e.g., circulating substances in plasma that bind to or inactivate the drugs) also have been suggested. Higher and/or more frequent doses are required in patients with burn injury, especially when the injury is ≥30 percent.

OBESITY

For the majority of NMBAs, total body weight (TBW) dosing will result in a prolonged duration of effect in morbidly obese patients when compared with nonobese patients.

Succinylcholine

In morbidly obese patients, the concentration of pseudocholinesterase, the enzyme that metabolizes succinylcholine, is increased.[13] Because the level of plasma pseudocholinesterase activity and the volume of extracellular fluid determine the duration of action of succinylcholine, and both of these factors are increased in obesity, morbidly obese patients have larger absolute succinylcholine dose requirements than average-weight patients. When succinylcholine administration is based upon TBW, rather than upon lean body weight (LBW) or ideal body weight (IBW), a more profound neuromuscular block and better intubating conditions are achieved.[14]

Rocuronium

Nondepolarizing muscle relaxants such as rocuronium are only weakly or moderately lipophilic because the quaternary ammonium group they contain makes these molecules, as a whole, highly ionized at physiologic pH. The poor lipophilicity limits distribution outside the extracellular fluid space. However, the effect of the increased extracellular fluid volume is poorly understood. In one study,[15] after administration of 0.6 mg/kg of rocuronium, the pharmacokinetic parameters and spontaneous recovery to 75 percent of twitch height were similar in obese and lean patients. When administered to morbidly obese patients on the basis of both TBW and IBW, the duration of action was more than double when rocuronium was dosed on TBW.[16] Although higher doses of rocuronium result in a prolonged duration of action, no difference in onset time is observed when 0.6 mg/kg rocuronium is administered based on IBW, IBW and 20 percent of excess weight, or IBW and 40 percent of excess weight.[17] Therefore, the recommendation is to base rocuronium administration in morbidly obese patients on IBW. Similar results are reported for pancuronium.[17]

Vecuronium

Seven obese patients receiving TBW-based 0.1 mg/kg vecuronium took 60 percent longer to recover from neuromuscular blockade than did seven normal-weight controls.[18] However, pharmacokinetic parameters uncorrected for weight were similar between the two groups; therefore, basing administration on IBW is recommended.

Cisatracurium

Because cisatracurium is eliminated via Hoffman elimination, investigators have suggested it as the NMBA of choice for obese patients. However, when administered to both morbidly obese and normal-weight patients on the basis of both TBW and IBW, the duration of action was prolonged in morbidly obese patients.[19] When cisatracurium was administered to both obese patients and normal-weight patients according to IBW, its duration of action was shorter in the morbidly obese patient.[20]

In conclusion, succinylcholine should be dosed based on TBW. TBW dosing of nondepolarizing neuromuscular blockers will result in overdosing, therefore, IBW is recommended for these agents. If a nondepolarizing agent is needed, shorter-acting agents such as rocuronium or cisatracurium are recommended.

HYPOTHERMIA

During hypothermia, redistribution of blood away from the extremities, gastrointestinal tract, kidneys, and liver toward the coronary and cerebral circulation takes place. Vasodilation of skeletal muscles contributes to this redistribution. The intravascular distribution volume is reported to be decreased by 10–35 percent in animal models.[21] The Vd of pancuronium was reported to decrease by 40 percent in patients with moderate-to-severe hypothermia. The reduction in extracellular volume in addition to the reduced renal and hepatic blood flow and biliary clearance indicated that smaller doses may be required, along with less frequent dosing. Intermittent dosing as needed would be a more practical approach than continuous infusion with train-of-four monitoring.

Choice of Agents

NMBA may also be classified according to the duration of blockade they produce: short, intermediate, or long (Table 12-1). The selection of an NMBA must be based on the needs of the patient. Four variables that must be considered are time of onset, duration of action, side effects, and route of elimination for the agent chosen. Other equally important factors, often overlooked by physicians caring for the patient, are intravenous access, drug-drug compatibility, and volume of intravenous fluid required to administer a continuous infusion. One may choose a longer-acting agent dosed as needed over a continuous infusion in a severely fluid restricted patient. Lastly, one should not overlook cost when choosing an NMBA.

The medical condition of the patient also influences the NMBA decision. Patients with cardiovascular impairment are of special concern, because some NMBA produce cardiovascular effects such as hypotension and arrhythmias. Cardiovascular-stable NMBAs include vecuronium, pipecuronium, cisatracurium, and rocuronium. Pancuronium should be avoided in patients with preexisting tachycardia who cannot tolerate a further increase in the heart rate (angina, tachyarrhythmia). However, many young patients without preexisting cardiovascular disease can tolerate the increase in heart rate. Presence of hepatic and/or renal failure must be taken into consideration when choosing an NMBA, but is not a contraindication to agents metabolized and eliminated by these routes as long as appropriate monitoring is performed. In fact, use of these agents in concert with train-of-four (TOF) monitoring or dosing with movement may be used in an effort to reduce the overall costs of NMBA therapy. Atracurium and cisatracurium are often used in multisystem organ failure because their metabolism is via Hoffman elimination and ester hydrolysis, which is independent of the hepatic metabolism and renal elimination. Histamine release by some NMBAs (d-tubocurarine, atracurium) can place an asthmatic patient at increased risk. Pancuronium, vecuronium, pipecuronium, rocuronium, or cisatracurium is not associated with significant histamine release and may be preferred for asthmatics. Patients with extensive burns may also require dosage adjustments, because they may have increased synthesis of extrajunctional cholinergic receptors and thus react unpredictably to NMBAs. The accumulation of extrajunctional ACh receptors may be responsible for the risk of severe hyperkalemia that can occur following the use of succinylcholine in patients with burns, stroke, polio, spinal cord injury, severe muscle trauma, enforced immobilization, Guillain-Barré syndrome, or other conditions producing loss of nerve function. Succinylcholine should never be used in any of these situations.

The consensus statement of the Society for Critical Care Medicine (SCCM) states that the majority of patients in the ICU who are prescribed an NMBA can be managed effectively with pancuronium.[2] For patients for whom vagolysis is contraindicated (e.g., those with cardiovascular disease), NMBAs other than pancuronium may be used.[2] Many practitioners prefer vecuronium for those patients with cardiac disease or hemodynamic instability in whom tachycardia may be deleterious, based on the drug's cardiovascular stability, the low cost of the drug, and many years of experience in clinical practice. Lastly, because of their unique metabolism, cisatracurium or atracurium is recommended for patients with significant hepatic or renal disease.[2]

INTUBATION

Choice of appropriate NMBA for intubation is not always straightforward, especially when complicated by the need for tracheal intubation without bag and mask ventilation as in the case of a patient with a full stomach. Succinylcholine historically has been the gold standard for a rapid-sequence intubation because of the onset of 90 percent neuromuscular blockade within 60 seconds. However, large doses of some nondepolarizing agents such as mivacurium and rocuronium approach this onset: 2–2.5 minutes and 1–1.5 minutes, respectively. However, mivacurium is no longer commercially available in the United States. If practicing in an area where mivacurium is available, one should be aware that rapid bolus doses of mivacurium may cause some histamine release and hypotension in patients with preexisting cardiovascular instability.

The remainder of the nondepolarizing NMBAs generally take 3–4 minutes to reach intubating conditions. However, if succinylcholine is contraindicated and mivacurium or rocuronium are unavailable, two techniques can hasten the onset of neuromuscular blockade with nondepolarizing agents. One technique is *priming*. It involves the administration of one-tenth of an intubating dose of a nondepolarizing NMBA, followed 4 minutes later by an intubating dose. Then, after waiting an additional 90 seconds, intubation of the trachea may be performed.[3] The inherent risks of this method are related to the degree of weakness or respiratory distress in the patient before priming and to the fear and anxiety produced by the diplopia and dyspnea that often follow the priming dose. Informing the patient of what to expect can be extremely helpful in decreasing the anxiety and fear.

The second technique involves giving a relative overdose of the NMBA to flood the receptors, thereby shortening the time of onset. The usual practice is to administer two times the intubating dose of an NMBA as a rapid bolus. The complications of this technique are related to the cardiovascular effects of the relaxant, which can be avoided by the use of a drug with stable cardiovascular profile such as vecuronium, doxacurium (not available in the U.S.), cisatracurium, rapacuronium, or rocuronium.

MONITORING WITH CONTINUOUS INFUSION

It is now widely recommended that continuous NMBA be monitored using either a train-of-four (TOF) or a double-burst muscle twitch response to peripheral nerve stimulation (PNS). Monitoring by this method may prevent prolonged effect of the NMBA due to (1) changing organ function, (2) addition of medications that potentiate NMBA, or (3) accumulation of the drug or metabolite. In addition, investigators have documented that adjusting the dose of NMBA by PNS versus standard clinical dosing in critically ill patients reduces the drug requirements and results in cost savings.[1]

Nerve stimulators deliver an electrical current that is intended to activate a motor nerve, while the mechanical response of a muscle enervated by that nerve is measured. As the NMBA occupies an increasing number of the postsynaptic ACh receptors, the block becomes more profound and the muscle response to nerve stimulation diminishes. One must be careful to avoid direct muscle stimulation with the nerve stimulator as muscle will contract if stimulated electrically, regardless of the degree of block of the neuromuscular junction. This false positive result would cause the clinician to

increase the dose of NMBA that may lead to accumulation and prolonged paralysis after discontinuation of the NMBA.

Monitoring of neuromuscular function is uncomfortable and can be painful if tetanic stimulation is used. Therefore, monitoring should begin after sedation and analgesia, and optimally before any NMBA is given. The latter is not always possible. This sequence will assure that the nerve stimulator is functioning properly and the electrodes are placed correctly to assess the patient's baseline strength of response. The electrical current is delivered via surface electrodes (ECG electrodes are most commonly used), which should be placed over skin that is clean, dry, and hairless. Electrodes should be replaced every 24 hours as the conductive gel dries out. Substantial edema or obesity may result in insufficient current being delivered to the nerve by surface electrodes. Needle electrodes (23G) are available if ECG electrodes are ineffective.

Theoretically, any accessible nerve may be stimulated to assess neuromuscular blockade. However, stimulating the ulnar nerve while measuring the effect at the adductor pollicis has become the standard. If the ulnar nerve is not available or easily accessible, the facial nerve can be used, and the response at the orbicularis occuli can be observed. Lastly, the posterior tibial nerve can be stimulated behind the medial malleus and plantar flexion of the great toe can be observed, or the peroneal nerve can be stimulated around the fibular head, and dorsiflexion of the foot can be recorded. The evoked responses can be uncomfortable and, therefore, are not always practical in patients who are conscious, but most patients will be receiving analgesics and sedatives.

Train-of-Four

Train-of-four (TOF) is used most commonly in the ICU to monitor NMBA. This approach uses a train or series of four stimuli at a frequency of 2 Hz for 2 seconds. In the absence of NMBA, four twitches of equal amplitude should be observed. In the presence of a nondepolarizing NMBA, a progressive decrease in amplitude of each successive twitch is seen. Formally, the measured response is reported as the ratio of the amplitude of the fourth twitch to the first twitch, as measured with a force transducer, yielding the TOF ratio. However, it is not practical to measure the amplitude of twitches with a transducer in the clinical setting, therefore, the number of stimuli-induced palpable twitches is recorded. Because of the wide margin of safety of neuromuscular transmission, a single twitch is not abolished until 75 percent blockade is achieved (ratio 3/4; three twitches present out of four). Two palpable twitches correlate with approximately 80 percent suppression, one palpable twitch with approximately 90 percent suppression, and no twitches correlates with 100 percent or greater twitch suppression.

Although no prospective controlled trials have determined the degree of neuromuscular blockade required to achieve optimum mechanical ventilation in patients, it is recommended that the rate of infusion be titrated to a minimum presence of one or two twitches (80–90% blockade) at all times. Train-of-four stimulation should be monitored and recorded every 8 hours or more frequently when patient status dictates. Ablation of all four twitches during continuous infusion is considered a sign of relative overdose of NMBA. It is recommended that the NMBA infusion be discontinued until the return of one or two twitches, and then reinstated at a lower infusion rate. If intermittent boluses are used, TOF should be repeated every 15–30 minutes, and the next bolus not administered until at least a single twitch appears. Clinically as the muscles of the eyes and digits are the first to paralyze and the last to recover, they may be used with intermittent boluses as the indication to rebolus the NMBA in lieu of TOF monitoring. If TOF monitoring is not available, continuous infusion of NMBA should be stopped once a day and the time for return of some neuromuscular function noted. If this time is longer than 1 hour, the rate of infusion should be empirically decreased upon reinstatement of the continuous infusion. The amount of the decrease should be directly related to the duration of prolonged neuromuscular blockade. For example, if 1 hour was expected and 4 hours pass before movement, one might decrease the dose by 25 percent compared to 50 percent if 8–12 hours passes before movement. This approach should prevent accumulation of the NMBA. Regardless of whether TOF is used, all patients who receive continuous infusions of NMBA should have their infusions stopped once daily to assess blockade and to provide an opportunity for clinical evaluation to assess the adequacy of concomitant sedation and analgesia.[2]

PROBLEMS WITH TRAIN-OF-FOUR MONITORING

Substantial edema and obesity are the most often identified factors affecting TOF monitoring. Electrode placement too far from the nerve and pressure applied to the electrodes can also affect response. Pressure will decrease the electrode-skin resistance and distance from the skin to the nerve, thus increasing the amount of current delivered and possibly leading to overstimulation of response. Operator assessment of TOF is subjective and therefore, prone to misinterpretation. For example, two equal, strong thumb twitches with a faint third twitch may be interpreted by one operator as two twitches and by a second as three twitches. In fact, whether faint twitches should be included in the assessment is controversial and not addressed in the literature.

Equipment malfunction may produce a TOF error. Variability in current output has been documented at higher impedance with some peripheral nerve stimulator (PNS). Faulty connections of the stimulator to the electrodes, inadequate battery power, and improperly lubricated electrodes may contribute to erroneous TOF readings. Due to the numerous avenues to introduce error into TOF monitoring, the SCCM recommends that even with the use of peripheral nerve stimulation, neuromuscular blockade should be stopped at least once daily to produce an opportunity for clinical evaluation, to assess the adequacy of concomitant sedation and analgesia, and to determine if continued paralysis is needed.

Some patients will have no response to TOF testing, but still demonstrate movement or response to stimulation, such as a cough or gag when suctioned. Clinical assessment of patient response remains the standard when monitoring these patients. It is important to remember that TOF testing is performed to guide the maximal dose required by the patient. The minimum acceptable dose is determined by improvement in the parameter or condition being treated.

ADJUVANT THERAPY

The primary clinical effect of NMBA is to prevent movement. However, the need to provide adjuvant therapy should not be overlooked. The need for mechanical ventilation is obvious, but the need for other adjuvant therapy may not be as clear. Neuromuscular blocking agents provide no sedation or analgesia, therefore, it is imperative that patients are adequately sedated prior to being paralyzed and throughout the use of NMBA. Analgesics should be used when indicated but may not be necessary in every patient. The use of sedative or anxiolytic medications and narcotic analgesics prepare the patient to receive an NMBA by reducing awareness, relieving anxiety, and relieving pain. Without the adjuvant medications, the patient's experience of neuromuscular paralysis is likely to be terrifying. Choice of appropriate agents and dosing of sedatives and analgesics are patient-specific and will depend on the age of the patient, underlying condition, and other factors.

Even when sedated, all patients receiving NMBA should be treated as if they were fully awake. They should be given frequent verbal reassurance that their paralysis is purposely drug-induced and temporary. The use of sedatives causes anterograde amnesia, so patients must be frequently reoriented to their situation. They should be warned before anything is done to them (repositioning, needle sticks, dressing changes, suctioning of endotracheal tube, placement of bladder catheters, etc.). Too often, the patient is informed of a procedure only after the procedure has begun or not at all, which increases their fear and anxiety and the need for adjuvant medications

Patients receiving NMBA must be repositioned frequently to decrease the occurrence of pressure injury to nerves (most commonly knees or elbows) and the development of pressure injury to the skin or "bed sores." This task can be accomplished manually or with the aid of rotating beds or air mattresses. Lack of movement of the lower extremities also increases the risk of development of deep venous thrombosis (DVT) with subsequent pulmonary embolism (PE). Pharmacist should ensure that each patient receiving an NMBA receives heparin 5,000 units subcutaneously two to three times a day to prevent the development of a DVT. Low-molecular-weight heparins may also be used when clinically indicated. All ICU patients, not just those receiving NMBA are at an increased risk of DVT and PE and should receive prophylaxis. Patients who cannot receive an anticoagulant may benefit from the use of sequential compression devices or foot compression devices. Limited data are available to suggest a benefit of these devices, but the high-risk of DVT in patients receiving NMBA may justify their use. Lastly, as paralyzed patients cannot blink, their eyes must be protected with artificial tears or lubricant to prevent corneal abrasions.

Paralyzed patients cannot cough or swallow, so measures must be employed to ensure adequate clearing of pharyngeal and tracheal secretions. Lastly, disuse atrophy and contractions may develop during prolonged use of NMBA. Involvement of physical and occupational therapy to develop splints and perform range-of-motion exercises have been recommended to lessen potential for disuse atrophy and contractions in paralyzed patients.

Resistance to NMBA

Numerous authors have reported resistance or tachyphylaxis to the nondepolarizing NMBA in ICU patients. Resistance was demonstrated by an increasing dosage requirement over time to maintain adequate neuromuscular blockade. Seven of nine patients in one series received atracurium. Resistance was overcome by switching to low infusion rates of pancuronium in three and doxacurium in four. The remaining two patients developed resistance on vecuronium. The majority of the reports of NMBA resistance have been with vecuronium and atracurium. It is unclear whether these findings are due to increased use of these agents over other NMBA in the ICU, that one is more likely to identify an increased dose requirement with a continuous infusion than with PRN dosing as with pancuronium, or something unique to atracurium and vecuronium.

Adverse outcomes associated with NMBA resistance may include inadequate ventilatory management and an increased frequency of dose-dependent cardiovascular effects or adverse effects associated with frequent dosing with histamine release with some agents. Pharmacoeconomic issues must be considered as the cost of NMBA therapy in a resistant patient may be significant.

Proposed pharmacodynamic mechanisms of resistance include the up-regulation of the ACh receptors (AChR) caused by immobilization, sepsis, and polyneuropathy, alterations in AChR sensitivity, enhanced release of ACh at the neuromuscular junction, and inhibition of serum cholinesterase activity.[1] It is now clear that chronic administration of NMBA itself can lead to the development of extrajunctional receptors. An additional factor that may induce tolerance can be the qualitative change occurring in the AChR, which alters its affinity for NMBA. Pharmacokinetic alterations in NMBA, increased volume of distribution (hepatic disease and thermal injury), increased protein binding (inflammation, surgery, malignancy, myocardial infarction, or thermal injury), and an increase in clearance (thermal injury and acid base abnormalities) have been documented in ICU patients and are thought to contribute to NMBA resistance.

Factors Affecting Paralysis

Many factors can influence the degree of paralysis induced by NMBA. Effects can be antagonistic or may potentiate neuromuscular blockade. The resulting clinical manifestations depend on the degree of blockade induced, the agent used, and individual patient characteristics. Table 12-3 lists pathophysiologic variables and medications capable of altering the effects of nondepolarizing NMBA. Selected electrolyte and metabolic disturbances are known to contribute to enhanced blockade (e.g., hyponatremia, hypokalemia, hypermagnesemia, hypocalcemia, and acidosis) or decreased blockade (e.g., hypercalcemia, alkalosis). Alkalosis and acidosis are the most common impact on agents metabolized by Hoffman elimination. This pathway is increased by alkalosis and slowed by acidosis. Close monitoring of the patient after correction of any of these electrolyte or metabolic disturbances is critical. In addition, numerous drug interactions and underlying disease states can clinically affect the action of NMBA. These interactions are summarized in Table 12-3. Empiric dose adjustments combined with careful TOF monitoring is recommended. In addition the SCCM recommends stopping the NMBA once daily to assess the patient. These two monitoring parameters should allow for optimization of neuromuscular blockade while avoiding adverse effects.

Adverse Effects of Neuromuscular Blockade

The undesired effects of the NMBA can be divided into three categories (1) complications that result from the patient's inability to move and are therefore common to all NMBA, (2) side effects specific to individual NMBA, and (3) prolonged weakness after discontinuing the use of NMBA, a complication of unclear etiology. The complications of NMBA secondary to the patient's inability to move include pressure injury to nerves, pressure necrosis and ulceration, cough failure and retention of secretions, impaired ability to perform neurologic and abdominal examinations, and disuse atrophy.

Neuromuscular blocking agents are divided according to basic molecular structure into amino-steroid and benzylisoquinolinium compounds. Each class is associated with its own particular complications, and some complications are common to both. For example some benzylisoquinolinium agents are associated with histamine release, whereas steroidal NMBAs are not. Autonomic adverse effects, anaphylactic and anaphylactoid reactions are common to all classes of NMBA. Adverse effects may affect neuromuscular function or other organ systems. Molecular class and side effects specific to individual NMBAs are summarized in Table 12-4.

As the practice of intensive care medicine has become more sophisticated, reports of myopathies and neuropathies occurring in patients in the ICU have also been noted. Intravenous corticosteroids and NMBA, sepsis, and multiorgan failure have been strongly implicated in the development of these conditions, but the pathophysiology is poorly understood. Although the cause of prolonged weakness often maybe multifactorial, several distinct clinical syndromes have been identified. Critical illness polyneuropathy (CIP) can cause prolonged weakness in patients with sepsis or multisystem failure that generally is unrelated to the administration

TABLE 12-3 Clinical Variables Affecting Pharmacodynamics of Nondepolarizing NMBAs

Drug Interactions with NMBA

Effect	Drug	Mechanism

Enhanced blockade	Antibiotics
	  Aminoglycosides
	  Colistin
	  Tetracyclines
	  Clindamycin
	  Vancomycin
		Inhibition of neuromuscular transmission (Ag), decreased presynaptic Ach release, reduction of postsynaptic receptor sensitivity to Ach, blockade of Ach receptors, impairment of ion channels

	Cardiovascular Agents
	  Furosemide (high dose)
	  β-blockers
	  Calcium channel blockers
	  Procainamide
	  quinidine
		Decreased presynaptic Ach release, decreased muscle contractility

	Cyclophosphamide	Unsubstantiated mechanism
	Dantrolene	Unsubstantiated mechanism

	Immunosuppressive agents
	  Cyclosporine
	  Corticosteroids
		Inhibition of metabolism by cyclosporine suspected; corticosteroids may decrease sensitivity of end plate

	Inhaled anesthetics
	  Enflurane
	  Halothane
	  Isoflurane
	  Methoxyflurane
	  Nitrous oxide
		Reduction of postsynaptic receptor sensitivity to Ach, decreased muscle contractility

	Lithium	Unsubstantiated mechanism
	Local anesthetics	Decreased presynaptic Ach release, decreased muscle contractility
	Magnesium	Blocks repolarization
Decreased blockade	Carbamazepine	↑ CPP2C9, CYP3A4 ↑ production of α-1 acid glycoprotein
	Methylxanthines	Unsubstantiated mechanism, antagonist activity suspected
	Phenytoin	↑ CPP2C9, CYP3A4 ↑ production of α-1 acid glycoprotein Direct neuromuscular blocking effects, up-regulation of ACH receptors
	Ranitidine	Unsubstantiated mechanism

Clinical Variables

Variable	Potentiate blockade Decreased drug requirement	Antagonize blockade Increased drug requirement
Electrolyte disorders	Hypokalemia Hyponatremia Hypocalcemia Hyperemagnesemia Hypophosphatemia	Hypercalcemia Hyperkalemia
Metabolic disorders	Metabolic acidosis Respiratory acidosis Hypothermia	Alkalosis
Diseases	Myasthenia gravis Muscular dystrophy Neurofibromatosis Amyotrophic lateral Sclerosis Poliomyelitis Eaton-Lambert syndrome Multiple sclerosis Acute intermittent porphyria	Hemipareisis Demyelating lesions Peripheral neuropathies Diabetes mellitus Hepatic failure with ascites Endotoxin and sepsis

TABLE 12-4 Major adverse effects of NMBA

NMBA	Cardiovascular Effect	Vagal Stimulation	Histamine Release	Major Adverse Effects
Atracurium	+	None	+	
Cisatracurium	+	None	None	
D-tubocurarine (B)	++	None	+++	Hypotension doses of ≥0.25 mg/kg, repid IV. Decrease SVR and BP decondarily to ganglionic blockade
Doxacurium (B)	+	None	None	
Mivacurium (B)	+	None	+	CV effects >0.15 mg/kg
Pancuronium (S)	+++	Blocks ++	None	Increased HR, BP, CO due to vagolytic effects
Pipecuronium (S)	None	Blocks+	None	
Rocuronium (S)	+	None	None	
Succinylcholine	+++	Stimulates	Rare	Hyperkalemia, increased ICP and IOP
Vecuronium (S)	None	None	None	

S, steroidal structure; B, benzylisoquinolinium; IV, intravenous; SVR, systemic vascular resistance; BP, blood pressure; CV, cardiovascular; HR, heart rate; BP, blood pressure; CO, cardiac output; ICP, intracranial pressure; IOP, intraocular pressure; NMBA, neuromuscular blocking agent.

of NMBAs. Other neuromuscular diseases may emerge or become symptomatic in the ICU, including Guillain-Barré syndrome. The combination of corticosteroids and NMBA is associated with critical illness myopathy (CIM). Transient weakness may occur in the ICU patient as a result of metabolic derangements that include hypercalcemia, hypophosphatemia, and hypermagnesemia.[1]

SUMMARY

In addition to their use in the operating room and for intubation, specific situations may arise that require the use of NMBA in the ICU. When choosing an agent, the major issues include cardiovascular effects, metabolism, and cost. Because many patients in the ICU have some degree of hemodynamic instability, agents that cause excessive histamine release should be avoided. These agents should also be avoided in the asthmatic patient. In addition, the presence of hepatic or renal insufficiency may affect metabolism or elimination of some agents. Intermittent dosing may be preferable to continuous infusions in these cases. Atracurium or cisatracurium may be a more appropriate choice in patients with significant multiorgan dysfunction, because their metabolism is not altered by these conditions. Regardless of choice of agent, adjustment of the dose based on movement (with intermittent dosing) or with peripheral nerve stimulation is recommended. ICU patients' conditions are complex, and significant interpatient variability exists. Some of this variability may be explained by pharmacokinetic alterations, metabolic disorders, drug-drug interactions, or the patient's underlying disease state (Table 12-3). An additional problem that occurs in the ICU patient who received NMBAs for a prolonged period of time is the development of tachyphylaxis. The primary cause is thought to be an up-regulation of ACh receptors in patients who are chronically exposed to NMBAs. Given NMBAs' adverse effects profile, the SCCM recommends that they be administered only when aggressive attempts at sedation have failed to provide the desired level of patient immobilization, and that they should be discontinued as early as feasible.

CASE STUDIES

CASE 1: LOADING DOSE AND ADMINISTRATION

CJ is a 56-year-old male who has been in the medical intensive care unit with a diagnosis of respiratory failure. He weighs 70 kg. The ICU team decides to mechanically ventilate him and administer atracurium.

QUESTION

What loading dose of atracurium should be administered?

Answer:

To calculate the initial loading dose of atracurium, the pharmacokinetic dosing method is utilized. The initial dose can be administered as a range of 0.4 or 0.5 mg/kg.[22]

$$\text{Loading Dose} = 0.4 \text{ mg/kg} \times 70 \text{ kg} = 28 \text{ mg}$$

Bolus doses of neuromuscular blocker agents (NMBAs) are administered in order to achieve rapid neuromuscular blockade. Most NMBAs with a long t½, can be administered as bolus doses. Potential benefits of NMBA bolus administration include controlling tachyphylaxis, accumulation, and unwarranted paralysis.[2] Serum concentrations of NMBAs are not typically calculated.

Administration: NMBAs can be administered intravenously (IV) as an undiluted bolus. The continuous IV administration of atracurium, cisatracurium, doxacurium, mivacurium, pancuronium, pipecuronium, rocuronium, and vecuronium must be diluted appropriately and requires monitoring with a peripheral nerve stimulator and titration to ensure adequate paralysis with train-of-four (TOF) monitoring. Monitoring the depth neuromuscular blockade is imperative to reduce adverse events and minimize the amount of drug administered. The goal TOF as recommended by the Society of Critical Care Medicine is one to two twitches out of four, corresponding to 90 or 80 percent of receptors blocked. [2]

CASE 2: MAINTENANCE DOSE USING POPULATION PHARMACOKINETICS

MH is a 50-year-old female mechanically ventilated on adequate sedation and analgesia. She weighs 60 kg. Her O_2 saturation has decreased to 75 percent (>90%). The ICU team decides to start her on a pancuronium drip.

QUESTION

What loading dose of pancuronium should be administered and what continuous infusion should be started?

Answer:

The loading dose of pancuronium is 0.1 mg/kg. MH's loading dose is 6 mg. The continuous infusion of pancuronium ranges from

0.8 to 2 mcg/kg/min, or 1–5 mg/hr.[23] Maintenance of neuromuscular blockade with NMBAs can be sustained with a continuous infusion. Agents with short half-lives, such as atracurium and cisatracurium require administration as continuous infusions to maintain neuromuscular blockade.[2] To minimize the accumulation and potential adverse effects of NMBAs, monitoring TOFs frequently is recommended, along with clinically assessing the need for NMBA's continuous use at least daily. Patients receiving continuous infusions of NMBA could also develop tachyphylaxis. If tachyphylaxis occurs and neuromuscular blockade is still needed, a higher doses of NMBA can be used. Another alternative is to use a different neuromuscular blocking agent.[2]

CASE 3: DRUG INTERACTION THAT DECREASES LEVELS

CF is a 25-year-old male with history of seizure disorder and has been maintained and controlled on phenytoin therapy 400 mg daily. The patient is admitted for an elective excision of a posterior fossa brain tumor. A dose of 200 mg was given four hours prior to surgery. During surgery, pancuronium 0.8 mg/kg was administered. CF had an inadequate response to the first dose.

QUESTION

What can be done to overcome the resistance of neuromuscular blockade with pancuronium?

Answer:

Resistance to neuromuscular blockade can occur with concomitant administration of phenytoin and pancuronium.[25,26] Other NMBAs affected by this interaction include cisatracurium and vecuronium.[27,28] Concurrent administration of pancuronium and phenytoin has led to administration of incremental doses of pancuronium. In a case report by Hickey and colleagues, pancuronium was administered at doses up to 0.17 mg/kg over one hour and a decreased effect was observed with each additional dose.[29] Blood samples collected from a patient receiving phenytoin and pancuronium resulted in a short half-life of pancuronium, as well as a small volume of distribution.[26] The mechanism of pancuronium resistance may arise from induction of hepatic enzymes with phenytoin, alterations in plasma protein binding as well as tissue binding, or modifications in the myoneuronal junctional response to pancuronium.[24-26]

Chronic carbamazepine therapy can antagonize the action of NMBAs.[30] The nondepolarizing agents affected by this drug-drug interaction include vecuronium, pancuronium, rocuronium, and atracurium.[30,31,32,33] Case reports of patients on carbamazepine maintenance therapy by Whalley and colleagues and by Norman and colleagues showed that higher doses of vecuronium were required in order to achieve neuromuscular blocking effects comparable to patients with no carbamazepine therapy.[30,34] The mechanism of this drug-drug interaction can be due to increased metabolism and clearance of vecuronium.[34,35]

Theophylline and pancuronium therapy administered simultaneously has resulted in a reduced response in neuromuscular blockade.[36] The mechanism of this drug-drug interaction is unclear.

CASE 4: DRUG INTERACTION THAT INCREASES LEVELS

TR is a 23-year-old female who sustained injuries after a motor vehicle crash. She weighs 55 kg and is being treated with gentamicin 380 mg IV daily and cefazolin 1 g IV q8h for an open femur fracture. TR is taken to the operating room to fix the fracture and received rocuronium 20 mg to facilitate endotracheal intubation and muscle relaxation.

QUESTION

What drug-drug interaction exists between these agents?

Answer:

NMBAs' duration of action and time to recovery from paralysis are increased when administered concomitantly with aminoglycosides. This interaction could result in prolonged paralysis and acute myopathy. Potential patient risk factors for increased clinical duration of paralysis include continuous infusions, acid-base disorders, electrolyte disturbances, concurrent use of medications that may augment neuromuscular blockade (i.e., corticosteroids, calcium-channel blockers, aminoglycosides), and renal and hepatic insufficiency.[37] A study led by Dupuis assessed drug interactions between gentamicin and tobramycin and atracurium and vecuronium. The aminoglycosides increased the neuromuscular blockade of vecuronium, while atracurium was not affected.[38] The mechanism of this drug-drug interaction may result in increased binding of vecuronium to neuromuscular receptors.

Sustained concomitant administration of NMBAs and corticosteroids may also increase the risk of myopathy, resulting in prolonged paralysis. This interaction affects neuromuscular transmission. NMBAs should be discontinued if corticosteroids need to be administered.[39]

CASE 5: DISEASE STATE INTERACTIONS

YT is a 35-year-old male admitted with injuries sustained after a motorcycle crash 14 days ago. The patient is found to have a spinal cord injury (SCI) with cervical 4–5 fracture. YT will be paralyzed with pancuronium during a bedside tracheostomy, since he was unable to be weaned from the ventilator.

QUESTION

What risk factors does YT have for ICU myopathy?

Answer:

Critically ill patients are at risk of developing myopathy, as well as polyneuropathy, regardless of the primary injury.[40] Critical illness polyneuropathy (CIP) has been recognized in patients with sepsis or multiple organ dysfunction syndrome and the elderly.[41] Clinical manifestations of CIP are muscle atrophy and weaning failure. The mechanism or cause of CIP has not been elucidated.[42] Nerve and muscle disorders and syndromes that may exacerbate these conditions include myasthenia gravis, Lambert-Eaton syndrome, Guillain-Barré syndrome, central nervous system injury, spinal cord injury, mitochondrial myopathy, HIV-related myopathy, acute myopathy of intensive care, and disuse atrophy.[2,40,42] Recovery from CIP or ICU myopathy necessitates prolonged hospitalization, physical therapy, and rehabilitation. Critically ill patients who are paralyzed require venous thrombosis prophylaxis and prophylactic eye care to prevent keratitis and corneal abrasions.

YT's risk factors include his spinal cord injury, use of neuromuscular blockers, and being a critically ill patient.

CASE 6: DOSING IN RENAL DYSFUNCTION [NO HEMODIALYSIS]

ZG is an 86-year-old female who presents with pneumonia and requires intubation. ZG's past medical history is significant for chronic kidney disease stage III.

QUESTION

What paralytic agent would be ideal for ZG's intubation?

Answer:

The elimination of drugs in patients with impaired renal function is reduced. The kidney is not the only route for drug elimination, and alternate pathways for elimination such as biliary excretion, hepatic metabolism, ester hydrolysis, and Hofmann elimination exist.[43] The selection of NMBAs in patients with renal failure must be done with caution. The clearance of renally excreted drugs is reduced; therefore, NMBAs' active drug and metabolites can accumulate and prolong their duration of action. The metabolism of atracurium and cisatracurium is independent of renal function.[22,28,44] Rocuronium can be used in patients with renal dysfunction; however, neuromuscular blockade can be increased in patients with renal insufficiency.[45] Vecuronium is renally excreted, its duration of action is increased, and it can prolong neuromuscular blockade.[46,47] Renal insufficiency significantly increases the half-life and concentrations of pancuronium. Dosage adjustments are required in patients with mild-to-moderate renal insufficiency.[23]

Atracurium and cisatracurium could be used in ZG.

CASE 7: DOSING IN HEMODIALYSIS

ZG deteriorated overnight, became hypotensive (responded to fluid boluses), and her laboratory values today are as follows: Na 120 (135–145 mg/dL); K 4.6 (3.5–4.5 mg/dL); Cl 88 (98–107 mg/dL); CO2 20 (21–32 mmol/L); BUN 100 (7–18 mg/dL); SCr 8.4 (0.8–1.3 mg/dL); Gluc 111 (74–106 mg/dL); phosphorus 8.5 (2.5–4.9 mg/dL); arterial blood gas 7.27/21.2/14.4. The patient will start hemodialysis today secondary to metabolic acidosis and electrolyte imbalance.

QUESTION

If an NMBA is needed, which agent could be administered in this patient?

Answer:

Parameters that can affect patients requiring neuromuscular blockade and undergoing dialysis include a larger volume of distribution, reduced renal clearance, and increased duration of action.[48] Therefore, monitoring after NMBA administration in hemodialysis patients is critical. Administration of NMBAs in patients with renal dysfunction can lead to prolonged and profound neuromuscular blockade, which can continue despite hemodialysis.[49] The metabolism of atracurium and cisatracurium is independent of renal function.[22,28,50] A study conducted by Staals and others included patients with severe to end-stage renal failure who received rocuronium. The total plasma clearance of rocuronium was reduced in these patients compared to healthy controls.[51] A study compared vecuronium versus atracurium in patients with end-stage renal failure undergoing kidney transplantation.[52] The duration of action of initial and maintenance doses was prolonged with vecuronium. The study

suggested the use of atracurium in patients with end-stage renal failure. Pancuronium should be avoided in patients with severe renal dysfunction.[47] Cisatracurium can be administered in ZG.

CASE 8: DOSING IN CRITICALLY ILL WITH HIGH VOLUME OF DISTRIBUTION

AW is a 40-year-old, 80 kg male in the ICU for injuries sustained during a motor vehicle accident. He has a Tmax of 101.8° F, WBC 23,000 (3,700–10,400), mean arterial blood pressure >60 mm Hg, and heart rate >80 mm Hg on Norepinephrine 1 mcg/kg/min. In the operating room he received 10 liters of normal saline, two 6-pack of platelets, six units of fresh frozen plasma, and 4 units of whole blood. AW will be paralyzed with Vecuronium during a bedside bronchoscopy.

QUESTION

How do you expect a larger volume of distribution to affect the dose of Vecuronium?

Answer:

Acute increases in volume of distribution, which involves movement of fluid from the intravascular to the extracellular space, are often observed in critically ill patients due to disease states such as sepsis, congestive heart failure, burns, and renal failure. Additionally, hemodynamic instability or major surgical procedures may require patients to receive large volumes of fluid, which also contribute to an increase in volume of distribution. Because neuromuscular blockers are polar and hydrophilic, the volume of distribution in hemodilution is expected to increase. Xue and colleagues showed the effects of hemodilution on vecuronium pharmacokinetics in surgical patients.[53] The mean volume of the central compartment and volume of distribution at steady state were greater, and the elimination half-life was significantly longer (p <0.05) in the patients who received hemodilution compared to the control patients. No conclusive literature supports dosing adjustments of neuromuscular blockers in patients with altered volumes of distribution. It may be assumed based on the results of this study that patients with larger volumes of distribution will require an initial increase in dosage to achieve optimal neuromuscular blockage. Conversely, it may be assumed in conditions of hypovolemia or low volume of distribution that lower initial doses would be required and that the clinical duration of action would be shorter than in euvolemic patients. AW may need a larger initial dose of vecuronium. Monitoring with train-of-four should be initiated to ensure effective and safe dosing if repeated doses or a continuous infusion is administered.

CASE 9: DOSING IN OBESE PATIENTS

JR is a 30-year-old, 180 kg male who is in the intensive care unit with a subdural hematoma. Currently, he is hemodynamically stable and intubated. He has a ventriculostomy in place to monitor intracranial pressures. The cerebral perfusion pressure (CPP) was calculated to be 75–80 mm Hg. JR requires reintubation secondary to his endotracheal tube becoming dislodged and will be paralyzed with vecuronium.

QUESTION

What weight should be used to determine the dose?

Answer:

Because obesity affects all aspects of pharmacokinetics and pharmacodynamics, it is difficult to predict how an individual will respond to a particular agent. It is unclear whether weight-related dosage adjustments should be made and whether these agents should be based on actual weight, ideal weight, or an adjusted body weight. Lipophilicity of the agent can suggest the required dose. Lipophilic agents have an increased volume of distribution and an expected larger dose. However, lipophilicity is not always consistent due to other factors such as end-organ clearance and protein binding. Neuromuscular blockers are polar and hydrophilic.[54] The effect of obesity on the disposition and action of vecuronium 0.1 mg/kg was studied in seven obese and seven control surgical patients.[55] Pharmacokinetics, including volume of distribution, plasma clearance, and elimination half-life, were similar between groups. However, times to recovery were longer in the obese patients as compared to the control patients. The volume of distribution was calculated to be 50 percent smaller in the obese patients, consistent with the hydrophilicity of the drug. It was determined in order to reduce the risk of overdosing that obese patients should be administered on ideal body weight. JR should be administered vecuronium based on his ideal body weight. Monitoring with train-of-four should be initiated to ensure effective and safe dosing.

CASE 10: DOSING IN HYPOTHERMIA

MT is a 29-year-old, 85 kg male undergoing hypothermia secondary to a traumatic brain injury. He is being cooled to 33° C and requires paralysis to prevent shivering.

QUESTION

How does hypothermia affect the pharmacokinetics of neuromuscular blocking agents? Which neuromuscular blocking agent would be ideal to use in a hypothermic patient?

Answer:

The influence of hypothermia on the effect of drugs is becoming more clinically relevant as the use of therapeutic hypothermia expands to multiple patient populations. Human studies demonstrate a reduction in the adductor pollicis twitch response in the presence of hypothermia. A 2–10 percent reduction in the twitch response has been reported to occur for every degree Celsius decreased.[56] This response can complicate the study of hypothermia and its effects on neuromuscular blockers. However, *in vivo* animal and human studies consistently demonstrate that the duration of action of neuromuscular blocking agents is prolonged with hypothermia, even within the temperature range of 34–37° C. Hypothermia has been shown in pharmacokinetic studies to increase the duration of action by threefold for vecuronium and 1.5-fold for atracurium as compared to normothermic patients.[57,58,59] It has been shown to increase the duration of action of rocuronium by 5 minutes for every degree Celsius decrease in core body temperature.[60] Additionally, hypothermia has been shown to reduce the plasma clearance of vecuronium by 11 percent per degree Celsius and decrease the clearance of rocuronium by twofold.[60,61] Of note, moderate to deep hypothermia, 27–34° C, is frequently used during cardiopulmonary bypass. Despite significant changes in physiologic parameters secondary to changes in plasma volume and blood flow to the kidneys and liver, the actions of hypothermia appear to remain the same regarding its effects on neuromuscular blocking agents, which has been shown for *d*-tubocurarine, pancuronium, atracurium, and vecuronium.[56]

Currently, no ideal agent is available for use in hypothermia. Hypothermia appears to prolong the duration of action and recovery times with all agents. Lower doses and/or scheduled doses may be considered as opposed to continuous infusions. Continuous or frequent monitoring with train-of-four should be employed to reduce the risk of prolonged paralysis.

CASE 11: DOSING IN HEPATIC DYSFUNCTION

MM is a 62-year-old, 72 kg female, admitted to the cardiovascular surgery ICU following a three-vessel coronary artery bypass graft (CABG) surgery. MM had significant pulmonary edema during the surgery, and her chest had to be left open at the end of the surgery. When she arrives in the ICU, the surgeon would like to put the patient on NMBA to prevent any movement while her chest is open. Her vitals are: temperature 96.9 °F, blood pressure 109/72 mm Hg, heart rate 98 bpm, respiratory rate 14 breaths/minute. Her postoperative labs include: creatinine 0.9 mg/dL (0.8–1.2 mg/dL), AST 522 units/L (0–37 units/L), ALT 438 units/L (0–65 units/L).

QUESTION

Which neuromuscular blocking agents could be used in MM, and would they require a dosage adjustment due to her elevated liver enzymes?

Answer:

Pharmacokinetic properties of some NMBAs may be altered in the presence of hepatic impairment.[62] Patients with severe hepatic dysfunction receiving rocuronium have been shown to have approximately twice the volume of distribution (0.26 L/kg in normal hepatic function vs. 0.53 L/kg in severe hepatic dysfunction) and twice the plasma half-life (2.4 hours in normal hepatic function vs. 4.3 hours in severe hepatic dysfunction) compared with patients who have normal hepatic function.[63] As a result of these changes in volume of distribution and plasma half-life, the clinical duration of effect of rocuronium in hepatic dysfunction is prolonged 1.5 times the duration in a patient with normal hepatic function.[63] Doses for intubation up to 0.6 mg/kg have been used in patients with severe hepatic impairment; however, information on the use of a continuous infusion for extended neuromuscular blocking activity with rocuronium in hepatic dysfunction is limited.[63] Frequent monitoring of the TOF is recommended, and the minimum dose necessary to achieve the goal TOF should be used.

Vecuronium has also displayed an increased duration of effect and prolonged recovery time when used in patients with severe hepatic dysfunction. The dose of vecuronium may need to be reduced in patients with hepatic impairment, although the data recommending exactly how much to decrease the dose are limited.[46] If vecuronium is administered as a continuous infusion, the TOF should be frequently monitored and the infusion should be titrated to utilize the minimum dose necessary to achieve the goal TOF. Upon discontinuation of the infusion, the neuromuscular blocking effect may be prolonged.

Pancuronium is also dependent upon clearance through the liver (up to 20%), and prolonged neuromuscular blockage may occur in patients with severe hepatic dysfunction.[23] The volume of distribution of pancuronium increases by approximately 50 percent, and clearance from the plasma is decreased by 22 percent in the presence of severe hepatic impairment.[23] As a result, the elimination half-life is nearly double the half-life in a patient with normal hepatic function. Due to the greatly increased volume of distribution, patients with severe hepatic dysfunction may actually require an increased dose of pancuronium in order to achieve adequate neuromuscular blockade during intubation.[23] However, the duration of effect may then be significantly prolonged due to the significantly increased half-life.

Atracurium and cisatracurium may be used safely at normal doses in patients with hepatic dysfunction as they undergo Hofmann elimination, which is not dependent upon hepatic function.[61,22,27] Although a slight increase in volume of distribution and slight decrease in plasma clearance of cisatracurium were reported in patients with end-stage liver disease, the elimination half-life and clinical duration of effect were unaltered.[27] However, due to the greatly increased costs of atracurium and cisatracurium compared with other NMBAs, these agents are usually reserved for those patients with multiorgan dysfunction.

SPECIAL CONSIDERATIONS

DOSING IN THE ELDERLY

AG is an 86-year-old, 70 kg female, admitted to the ICU with septic shock. The ICU team is having difficulty ventilating her, and they decide to place her on an NMBA. Her most recent labs include: sodium 139 mEq/L (135–145 mEq/L), potassium 3.3 mEq/L (3.5–4.5 mEq/L), HCO_3^- 20 mEq/L, chloride 110 mEq/L, creatinine 0.9 mg/dL (0.8–1.2 mg/dL). AG is started on rocuronium.

QUESTION

What should be the initial bolus dose and initial infusion rate?

Answer:

Small studies have evaluated the effects of rocuronium in elderly patients. Advanced age has been associated with a prolonged time of onset and duration of action of rocuronium; however, time to recovery of neuromuscular function is unchanged compared to younger adults. No significant change in the clinical effectiveness of rocuronium in the elderly is apparent, and increasing the initial dose to overcome the delayed onset of action is not recommended. Therefore, recommended dosing in the elderly is the same as with younger adults. In this patient, an initial dose of 0.6 mg/kg followed by a continuous infusion starting at 10 mg/kg/minute would be appropriate.[62]

In general, the effects of NMBAs in the elderly may be altered slightly compared with younger adults.[63] A prolonged duration of action in the elderly is possible with the use of pancuronium or vecuronium, while other data suggest the effects are similar to younger adults.[45,23] However, no significant change in the elimination half-life of either agent in the elderly population is evident. The volume of distribution and elimination half-life are slightly increased in patients older than 65 years receiving cisatracurium.[63] However, these changes do not affect the time to clinical recovery of neuromuscular function, and no dosage adjustments are recommended. In general, when utilizing any NMBA in the elderly, it is recommended to start at the lower end of the recommended dosing range and monitor neuromuscular effects closely.[63]

DOSING IN PEDIATRICS

MR is a 2-year-old, 12 kg male, admitted to the pediatric ICU with severe asthma attack. He is unable to maintain his oxygenation and requires intubation.

QUESTION

What dose of vecuronium should be used for intubation of MR?

Answer:

Pediatric patients between 1 and 10 years old often require slightly higher initial doses of vecuronium than do adult patients.[45] This age group has a slightly faster onset of action and shorter duration of effect. Therefore, in this patient an appropriate initial dose would be 0.1–0.15 mg/kg (recommended adult dosing is 0.08–0.1 mg/kg). Children may also require more frequent supplementation of vecuronium than do adults. Patients older than 10 years of age may be dosed the same as an adult. Patients between 7 weeks and 1 year old appear to be more sensitive to vecuronium, and duration of effect may be prolonged approximately 1.5 times.

Dosing of many other NMBAs in the pediatric population is similar to the adult dosing. Rocuronium and pancuronium utilize the same dosing in pediatrics as with adults.[62,23] Dosing of atracurium in patients older than 2 years is the same as adults; however, in patients between 1 month and 2 years the dose should be decreased to 0.3–0.4 mg/kg.[22] The recommended dose of cisatracurium in children between 2 and 12 years old is 0.1–0.15 mg/kg, while the recommended dose in infants 1 month to 2 years old is 0.15 mg/kg.[26]

DOSING IN THE UNDERWEIGHT/CACHECTIC PATIENT

Limited data on the dosing of NMBAs in underweight patients are available. In one study, the duration of action and time to recovery following administration of rocuronium was compared in patients who were underweight, normal weight, and overweight.[64] No difference was noted in the onset of action, duration of effect, or time to recovery of neuromuscular function in patients who were underweight compared to those who were normal weight. In general, NMBAs in underweight adult patients should be dosed using standard adult doses based upon actual body weight. The neuromuscular blocking effect should be closely monitored in underweight patients.

CASES:

QUESTION 1

YG is a 57-year-old male mechanically ventilated, adequately sedated, and on analgesia. He weighs 70 kg. His O_2 saturation has decreased to 73 percent (>90%). The ICU team decides to start a pancuronium drip. What loading dose of pancuronium should be administered and what continuous infusion should be started?

Answer 1:

With a loading dose of pancuronium of 0.1 mg/kg, for YG 7 mg would be appropriate. The continuous infusion of pancuronium is usually 0.8–2 mcg/kg/min, or 56 mcg/min to 140 mcg/min. Patients receiving continuous infusion of NMBAs should have TOFs monitored frequently. It is necessary to clinically assess the need for NMBAs continuous use at least daily.

QUESTION 2

MA is a 26-year-old, 90 kg male undergoing hypothermia secondary to a traumatic brain injury. He is being cooled to 33⁰ C and requires paralysis to prevent shivering. Which neuromuscular blocking agent would be ideal to use in a hypothermic patient?

Answer 2:

No agent is ideal for use in hypothermia. Hypothermia may prolong the duration of action and recovery times with all agents. Lower doses or scheduled doses may be considered as opposed to continuous infusions. Continuous or frequent monitoring with train-of-four should be employed to reduce the risk of prolonged paralysis. Agents that have been utilized during hypothermia include pancuronium, atracurium, and vecuronium.

QUESTION 3

GB is a 55-year-old, 82 kg female, admitted to the medical intensive care unit after being found unresponsive at home. GB's past medical history is significant for end-stage liver disease. When she arrives in the ICU, the team would like to put the patient on a NMBA to improve her oxygenation. Her vitals are: temperature 96.9 °F, blood pressure 109/72 mm Hg, heart rate 98 bpm, respiratory rate 24 breaths/minute, O_2 sat 70%. Her labs include: creatinine 1.2 mg/dL (0.8–1.2 mg/dL), AST 522 units/L (0–37 units/L), ALT 438 units/L (0–65 units/L). Which neuromuscular blocking agents could be used in GB, and would they require a dosage adjustment due to her elevated liver enzymes?

Answer 3:

Atracurium and cisatracurium undergo Hofmann elimination, which is not dependent upon hepatic function, and these agents may be used safely at normal doses in patients with hepatic dysfunction. A slight increase in volume of distribution and slight decrease in plasma clearance of cisatracurium have been reported in patients with end-stage liver disease, but the elimination half-life and clinical duration of effect were unaltered.

REFERENCES

1. Jacobi J, Farrington E. Supportive care of the critically ill patient. *Critical Care Module of Pharmacotherapy Self-Assessment Program*, 3rd ed. American College of Clinical Pharmacy, 1998.
2. Murray MJ, Cowen J, DeBlock H, Erstad B, Gray AW, Tescher AN, McGee WT, et al. Clinical practice guidelines for sustained neuromuscular blockade in the adult critically ill patient. *Crit Care Med.* 2002;30(1):142–156.
3. Davis SL. Neuromuscular blocking agents. In Levin and Morriss (Eds.). *Essentials of Pediatric Intensive Care.* Quality Medical Publishing, 1997.
4. Reynolds RM, Infosino A, Brown R, et al. Pharmacokinetics of rapacuronium in infants and children with intravenous and intramuscular administration. *Anesthesiology.* 2000;92:376–386.
5. Reynolds LM, Lau M, Brown R. Intramuscular rocuronium in infants and children. Dose ranging and tracheal intubating conditions. *Anesthesiology.* 1996;85:231–239.
6. Lexicomp. Available at: http://online.lexi.com/crlsql/servlet/crlonline (accessed May 20, 2011).
7. Zaske DE. Aminoglycosides. In Evans WE, Schentag JJ and Jusko WJ (Eds.). *Applied Pharmacokinetics: Principles of Therapeutic Drug Monitoring*, 3rd ed. Vancouver, WA: Applied Therapeutics, Inc., 1992.
8. Brandom BW, Fine GF. Neuromuscular blocking drugs in pediatric anesthesia. *Anesthesiology Clinics of North America.* 2002;20(1):45–58.
9. Marathe PH, Dwersteg JF, Pavlin EG, et al. Effect of thermal injury on the pharmacokinetics and pharmacodynamics of atracurium in humans. *Anesthesiology.* 1989;70:752–755.
10. MacKichan JJ. Influence of protein binding and use of unbound (free) drug concentrations. In Evans WE, Schentag JJ and Jusko WJ (Eds.). *Applied Pharmacokinetics: Principles of Therapeutic Drug Monitoring*, 3rd ed. Vancouver, WA: Applied Therapeutics, Inc., 1992: 5–8.
11. Lexicomp. Available at: http://online.lexi.com/crlsql/servlet/crlonline (accessed May 20, 2011).
12. Blanchet B, Jullien V, Vinsonneau C, Tod M. Influence of burns on pharmacokinetics and pharmacodynamics of drugs used in the care of burn patients. *Clin Pharmacokinet.* 2008;47(10):635–654.
13. Bentley JB, Borel JD, Vaughan RW, Gandolfi AJ. Weight, pseudocholinesterase activity, and succinylcholine requirement. *Anesthesiology.* 1982;57:48–49.
14. Lemmens HJ, Brodsky JB. The dose of succinylcholine in morbid obesity. *Anesth Analg.* 2006;102:438–442.
15. Puhringer FK, Keller C, Kleinsasser A, et al. Pharmacokinetics of rocuronium bromide in obese female patients. *Eur J Anaesthesiol.* 1999;16:507–510.
16. Leykin Y, Pellis T, Lucca M, et al. The pharmacodynamic effects of rocuronium when dosed according to real body weight or ideal body weight in morbidly obese patients. *Anesth Analg.* 2004;99:1086–1089.
17. Meyhoff CS, Lund J, Jenstrup MT, et al. Should dosing of rocuronium in obese patients be based on ideal or corrected body weight? *Anesth Analg.* 2009;109:787–792.
18. Tsueda K, Warren JE, McCafferty LA, Nagle JP. Pancuronium bromide requirement during anesthesia for the morbidly obese. *Anesthesiology.* 1978;8:438–439.
19. Schwartz AE, Matteo RS, Ornstein E, et al. Pharmacokinetics and pharmacodynamics of vecuronium in the obese surgical patient. *Anesth Analg.* 1992;74:515–518.
20. Leykin Y, Pellis T, Lucca M, et al. The effects of cisatracurium on morbidly obese women. *Anesth Analg.* 2004;99:1090–1094.
21. Van den Broek, MPH, Groendaal F, Egberts ACG, Rademaker CMA. Effects of hypothermia on pharmacokinetics and pharmacodynamics. A systematic review of preclinical and clinical studies. *Clin Pharmacokinet.* 2010;49(5):277–294.
22. Atracurium [package insert]. Bedford, OH: Bedford Laboratories, 2010.
23. Pancuronium [package insert]. Irvine, CA: Sicor, 2005.
24. Ornstein E, Matteo R, Silverberg P, et al. Chronic phenytoin therapy and nondepolarizing muscular blockade. *Anesthesiology.* 1985;63:A331.
25. Liberman B, Norman P, Hardy B. Pancuronium-phenytoin interaction: A case of decreased duration of neuromuscular blockade. *Int J Clin Pharmacol Ther Toxicol.* 1988;26:371–374.
26. Gray H, Slater R, Pollard B. The effect of acutely administered phenytoin on vecuronium-induced neuromuscular blockade. *Anaesthesia.* 1989;44:379–381.
27. Cisatracurium [package insert]. Lake Forest, IL: Hospira, Inc., 2008.
28. Hickey D, Sangwan S, Bevan J. Phenytoin-induced resistance to pancuronium. *Anaesthesia.* 1988;43:757–759.
29. Whalley D, Ebrahim Z. Influence of carbamazepine on the dose-response relationship of vecuronium. *Br J Anaesth.* 1994;72:125–126.
30. Roth S, Ebrahim Z. Resistance to pancuronium in patients receiving carbamazepine. *Anesthesiology.* 1987;66:691–693.
31. Spacek A, Neiger F, Krenn C, et al. Rocuronium-induced neuromuscular block is affected by chronic carbamazepine therapy. *Aneshthesiol.* 1996;13:561–564.
32. Tempelhoff R, Modica P, Jellish W, et al. Resistance to atracurium-induced neuromuscular blockade in patients with intractable seizure disorders treated with anticonvulsants. *Anesth Analg.* 1990;71:665–669.
33. Alloul K, Whalley D, Shutway F, et al. Pharmacokinetic origin of carbamazepine-induced resistance to vecuronium neuromuscular blockade in anesthetized patients. *Anesthesiology.* 1996;84:330–339.
34. Soriano S, Sullivan L, Venkatakrishnan K, et al. Pharmacokinetics and pharmacodynamics of vecuronium in children receiving phenytoin or carbamazepine for chronic anticonvulsant therapy. *Br J Anaesth.* 2001;86(2):223–229.
35. Doll D, Rosenberg H. Antagonism of neuromuscular blockage by theophylline. *Anesth Analg.* 1979;58:139–140.
36. Watling S, Dasta J. Prolonged paralysis in intensive care unit patients after the use of neuromuscular blocking agents: A review of literature. *Crit Care Med.* 1994;22:884–893.

37. Dupuis J, Martin R, Tetrault J. Atracurium and vecuronium interaction with gentamicin and tobramycin. *Can J Anaesth.* 1989;36:407–411.

38. Marik P. Doxacurium-corticosteroid acute myopathy: another piece to the puzzle. *Crit Care Med.* 1996;24:1266–1267.

39. Bolton D, Laverty D, Brown J, et al. Critically ill polyneuropathy: Electrophysiological studies and differentiation from Guillain-Barré syndrome. *J Neurol Neurosurg Psychiatry.* 1986;49:563–573.

40. Nate J, Cooper D, Day B, et al. Acute weakness syndromes in critically ill patients: A reappraisal. *Anaesth Intensive Care.* 1997;25:502–513.

41. Hund E, Fogel W, Krieger D, et al. Critical illness polyneuropathy: Clinical findings and outcomes of a frequent cause of neuromuscular weaning failure. *Crit Care Med.* 1996;24:1328–1333.

42. Pollard B. Neuromuscular blocking drugs in renal failure. *Br J Anaesth.* 1992a;68:545–547.

43. Prielipp R, Jackson J, Coursin D. Comparison of the neuromuscular recovery after paralysis with atracurium versus vecuronium in an ICU patient with renal insufficiency. *Anesth Analg.* 1994;78:775–778.

44. Rocuronium (Zemuron®) [package insert]. Organon USA Inc., Rev Rec 10/98.

45. Vecuronium [package insert]. Bedford Laboratories, 2010.

46. Benett W, Aronoff G, Golper T, et al. Drug prescribing in renal failure. American College of Physicians, Philadelphia, 1987.

47. Head-Rapson A, Devlin J, Parker J, et al. Pharmacokinetics and pharmacodynamics of three isomers of mivacurium in health, in end-stage renal failure and in patients with impaired renal function. *Br J Anaesth.* 1995;75:31–36.

48. Smith C, Hunter J, Jones R. Prolonged paralysis following an infusion of atracurium in a patient with renal dysfunction. *Anaesthesia.* 1987;42:522–525.

49. Fahey M, Rupp S, Fisher D, et al. The pharmacokinetics and pharmacodynamics of atracurium in patient with and without renal failure. *Anesthesiology.* 1984;61:699–702.

50. Staals M, Snoeck M, Driessen J, et al. Reduced clearance of rocuronium and sugammadex in patients with severe to end-stage renal failure: a pharmacokinetic study. *Br J Anaesth.* 2010;104:31–39.

51. Lepage J, Malinge M, Cozian A. Vecuronium and atracurium in patients with end-stage renal failure. A comparative study. *Br J Anaesth.* 1987;59:1004–1010.

52. Xue FS, Liao X, Tong SY, et al. Pharmacokinetics of vecuronium during acute isovolaemic haemodilution. *Br J Anaesth.* 1997;79:612–616.

53. Cheymol G. Effects of obesity on pharmacokinetics: Implications for drug therapy. *Clin Pharmacokinet.* 2000;39:215–231.

54. Schwartz AE, Matteo RS, Ornstein E. Pharmacokinetics and pharmacodynamics of vecuronium in the obese surgical patient. *Anesth Analg.* 1992;74:515–518.

55. Heier T, Caldwell JE. Impact of hypothermia on the response to neuromuscular blocking drugs. *Anesthesiology.* 2006;104:1070–1080.

56. Heier T, Calwell JE, Sessler DI, et al. Mild intraoperative hypothermia increases duration of action and spontaneous recover of vecuronium blockade during nitrous oxide-isoflurane anesthesia in humans. *Anesthesiology.* 1991;74:815–819.

57. Heier T, Caldwell JE, Sharma ML, et al. Mild intraoperative hypothermia does not change the pharmacodynamics (concentration-effect relationship) of vecuronium in humans. *Anesth Analg.* 1994;78:973–977.

58. Leslie K, Sessler DI, Bjorksten AR, et al. Mild hypothermia alters propofol pharmacokinetics and increases the duration of action of atracurium. *Anesth Analg.* 1995;80:1007–1014.

59. Beaufort AM, Wierda JM, Belopalvlovic M, et al. The influence of hypothermia (surface cooling) on the time-course of action and on the pharmacokinetics of rocuronium in humans. *Eur J Anaesthesiol Suppl.* 1995;11:95–106.

60. Caldwell JE, Heier T, Wright PM, et al. Temperature-dependent pharmacokinetics and pharmacodynamics of vecuronium. *Anesthesiology.* 2000;92:84–93.

61. Craig RG, Hunter JM. Neuromuscular blocking drugs and their antagonists in patients with organ disease. *Anaesthesia.* 2009;64(Suppl. 1): 55–65.

62. Rocuronium (Zemuron®) [package insert]. Organon USA Inc., June 2002.

63. Vuyk J. Pharmacodynamics in the elderly. *Best Pract Res Clin Anaesth.* 2003;17:207–218.

64. Puhringer FK, Khuenl-Brady KS, Mitterschiffthaler G. Rocuronium bromide: Time-course of action in underweight, normal weight, overweight and obese patients. *Eur J Anaesthesiol Suppl.* 1995;11:107–110.

CHAPTER 3

Opioids

JEFFREY FUDIN, BS, PharmD, FCCP
RUTH J. PERKINS, BS, MA, PharmD, BCPS
ARTHUR G. LIPMAN, BS, PharmD, FASHP

OVERVIEW

Opioids are among the oldest documented medications used by humans. All opioids are derivatives of pharmacologically active alkaloids from the milky exudate of the opium poppy. These drugs act by binding at opioid receptors found in the CNS, the colon, and to a lesser extent, the periphery. Mu and kappa opioid receptors have clinical utility and delta opioid receptors offer promise, but no delta agonist has been found acceptable for human use to date. However, new work with biased legends offers promise of a possible future delta opioid agonist analgesic. Most clinically useful opioids are mu agonists that also have varying agonist activity at kappa receptors. The mu-1 aspect of the receptor is responsible primarily for analgesia and the mu-2 for other, largely adverse, opioid effects. Numerous subtypes of the mu-1 receptors have been isolated and cloned, clearly indicating genetic polymorphism. Recent work on opioid agonist G protein coupled receptors, and specifically beta arrestin, has elucidated our understanding of biased ligands that helps explain the mechanisms by which opioids cause some adverse effects. This offers promise of new agents which offer full analgesia with fewer adverse effects.[1-5]

The majority of opioid agents are indicated and FDA-approved for management of acute and chronic pain. However, some have indications other than pain (e.g., naloxone for opioid overdose reversal, naltrexone for abuse mitigation, naloxegol for opioid-induced constipation (OIC), buprenorphine for maintenance therapy in patients with a history of substance abuse, dextromethorphan and codeine for cough, diphenoxylate, codeine, and loperamide for diarrhea). In order to better understand and differentiate the therapeutic differences among natural, semisynthetic, and synthetic opioids, one must first appreciate the physiology and pharmacology associated with the class. This chapter will focus on those medications used specifically for analgesia but will include buprenorphine, as it too is indicated for pain.

These medications fall generally into four chemical classes: phenanthrenes, benzomorphans, phenylpiperidines, and diphenylheptanes. A fifth hybrid class of synthetics has some chemical similarities to several of these four groups. These dimethylamino compounds include tramadol and tapentadol and are seen in Figure 13-1. The chemical class of an opioid has little effect on its clinical utility. Note that Figure 13-1 lists cross-sensitivities as probable, possible, or low risk for each class from left to right. Although a true allergic reaction to any opioid is rare, pruritis is quite common. Pruritic reactions are a result of histamine release from mast cells. Such a reaction to one chemical class subjects a patient to histamine reactions to opioids within the same class. The fentanyl family has minimal histamine reactivity compared to all other opioids.[6]

Synthetic and semisynthetic opioids exhibit the same pharmacological properties as naturally occurring opium alkaloids and derivatives. Synthetic opioids do not contain the traditional phenanthrene nucleus found in the alkaloids isolated from opium. Available opioids all have similar activity, but vary considerably in potency, solubility, dosage form availability, and pharmacokinetics. Potency and solubility as outlined in Tables 13-1 through 13-4 do not generally impact therapeutic utility. However, when a small-volume opioid solution is desirable for parenteral administration due to volume restriction required because of comorbidity or for a continuous subcutaneous infusion, solubility becomes important.

For acute pain in an otherwise opioid-naive patient, it is generally best to initiate therapy with the lowest recommended dose proportionate to the intensity of the pain to assess tolerability and efficacy. The most common side effects are nausea and vomiting, constipation, sedation, urinary retention, and respiratory depression. For the chronic pain patient, sedation and respiratory depression are generally of less concern because some degree of tolerance develops to these relatively quickly. Conversely, constipation and urinary retention could remain an ongoing problem. For this reason, many acute and chronic pain patients often need stimulating laxatives during a course of opioid therapy. Depending on the dose, laxatives can sometimes be avoided if the patient is instructed to drink plenty of water and increase dietary fiber.

Nearly half of chronic nonmalignant pain patients do not have adequate bowel evacuation even with fiber, fluids, and stimulating laxatives.[7] For those patients, methylnaltrexone might be considered. It is currently approved for opioid-induced constipation as a subcutaneous injection in advanced disease patients and clinical trials are now ongoing with an oral form in CNMP patients.[8,9] Recent approval of naloxegol, a pegylated form of naloxone chemically similar to nor-oxymorphone was recently FDA approved for OIC in chronic non-cancer pain. It will be available at 12 mg and 25 mg tablets to be taken once daily. These drugs represent a new class known as peripherally active mu opioid receptor antagonists (PAMORAs).[10]

Opioids are available in a variety of dosage forms, including oral, transmucosal (buccal tablets, effervescent, lozenge), transdermal, intranasal, rectal, and parenteral (intravenous, subcutaneous, intramuscular, epidural, intrathecal). Moreover, because of genetic polymorphism and because some chronic pain patients (the minority) develop pharmacologic tolerance to opioid analgesia, clinical dosages vary widely.

THERAPEUTIC AND TOXIC CONCENTRATIONS

It is difficult to assign a "therapeutic concentration" or even range to most opioids because the dosage and corresponding blood levels required for adequate analgesia is variable and patient specific. Reported therapeutic and toxic serum levels for opioids overlap. For example, a starting morphine dose of 15 mg orally every 4 hours in an opioid-naive patient could cause significant lethargy. If the same dose were used to replace another patient's oxycodone sustained-release 160 mg PO every 12 hours, we would likely see withdrawal symptoms with little or no pain relief.

An important consideration in postmortem analysis is that decedents are often incorrectly assigned "narcotic overdose" as "cause of death" upon pathologist review. This conclusion could potentially be problematic for two reasons. The first is that postmortem blood

Phenanthrenes	Benzomorphans	Phenylpiperidines	Diphenylheptanes
Morphine	**Pentazocine**	**Meperidine**	**Methadone**

Rx examples >

Morphine	Pentazocine	Meperidine	Methadone
morphine	pentazocine	meperidine	methadone
codeine	diphenoxylate	fentanyl	propoxyphene
hydrocodone*	loperamide	sufentanil	
hydromorphone*		alfentanil	
levorphanol*		remifentanil	
oxycodone*			
oxymorphone*			
buprenorphine*			
nalbuphine			
butorphanol*			
naloxone*			
heroin (diacetyl-morphine)			

Cross-sensativity > risk

Probable	**Possible**	**Low Risk**	**Low Risk**

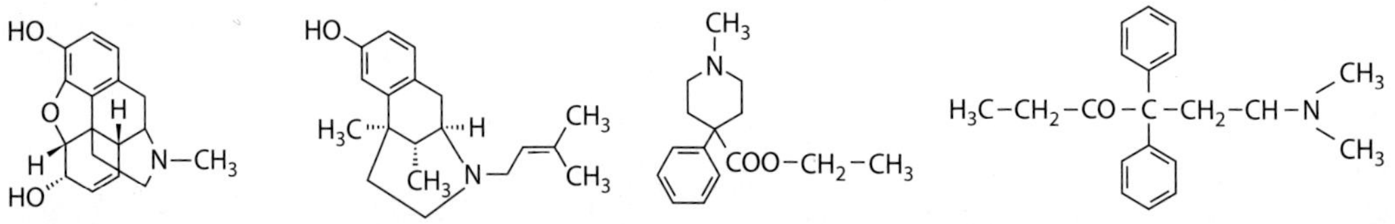

*These agents lack the 6-OH group of morphine, possibly decreasing cross-sensitivity within the phenanthrene group.

Tapentadol is a 3-[(1*R*,2*R*)-3-(dimethylamino)-1-ethyl-2-methylpropyl]phenol monohydrochloride.

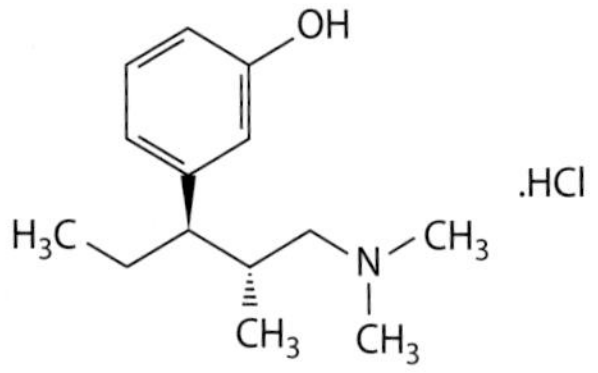

Tramadol is a (±)cis-2-[(dimethylamino)methyl]-1-(3-methoxyphenyl cyclohexanol hydrochloride.

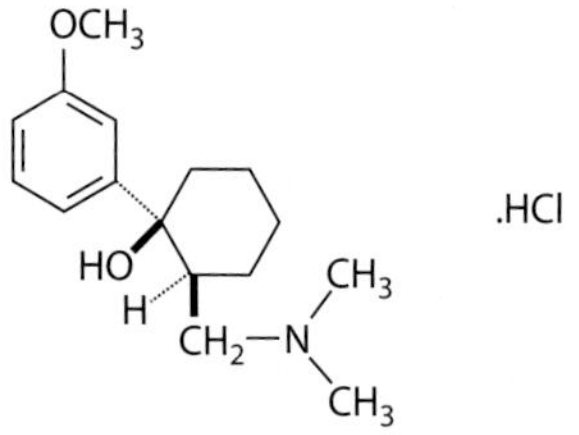

References:
1. Fudin J, Levasseur DJ, Passik SD, Kirsh KL, Coleman J. Chronic pain management with opioids in patients with past or current substance abuse problems. *Journal of Pharmacy Practice*. 2003;16;4:291–308.
2. Reisine T, Pasternak G. Opioid analgesics and antagonists. In Hardman JG, Limbird LE, Molinoff PB, Ruddon RW, Gilman AG (Eds.). *Goodman and Gilman's The Pharmacological Basis of Therapeutics*. 9th ed. New York: McGraw-Hill Companies; 1996:521–555.
3. Willette RE. Analgesic agents. In Delgado JN, Remers WA (Eds.). *Wilson and Grisvold's Textbook of Organic Medicinal Chemistry*. 9th ed. Philadelphia: JB Lippincott Company, 1991:629–654.

Used with permission from Jeffrey Fudin, B.S., Pharm.D., FCCP.

FIGURE 13-1. Chemical Classes of Opioids

analysis often yields higher numbers than antemortem samples due to redistribution of tissue.[11,12] For this reason, it is generally less accurate to obtain cavity blood from the heart or the pulmonary vessels to specifically match dose to concentration. More accurate specimens are achievable from the subclavian or femoral veins. Secondly, if the patient's opioid dose had been adjusted upward over time because of physical tolerance, what might otherwise appear as a lethal blood level in one patient will not necessarily correlate to death in another.

Nevertheless, important information can be gleaned from monitoring serum opioid levels clinically. These analyses have been used to monitor compliance, assess the possible effect of serum levels of one or more medications on the opioid, to compare pharmacokinetic parameters of single opioid formulation to alternative dosage forms, and to compare single opioid formulations to extemporaneously formulated products as single or combination formulations. The latter has become especially important with the newly instituted risk evaluation and mitigation strategies (REMS) imposed by the Food and Drug Administration (FDA).

A far less accurate, but popular strategy for monitoring opioid compliance is urine drug screen (UDS) analysis. These screens present an important fallacy in that they were initially developed to assess subjects for substances of abuse. Although it is important to ascertain whether a patient is abusing recreational drugs while concomitantly receiving prescribed opioids, UDSs are almost always enzyme-type screens where false positives and false negatives are ubiquitous. Because of potential for inaccurately assigning blame for noncompliance, the clinician needs to have a clear understanding of how to interpret these tests and the potential limitations. A suggested algorithm is outlined in Figure 13-2. Some authors, notably Gourlay and Heit,[13] advocate using the UDS as a "universal precaution," but the UDS is not always acceptable, may have legal implications, and may be inappropriate for some patients.[14]

AVAILABLE ASSAYS FOR DRUG-LEVEL MONITORING

Gas (or liquid) chromatography-mass spectrometry (GCMS, LCMS) are popular tests that may be employed to accurately measure specific opioids or substances of abuse. When using such tests, it is important to recognize the importance, practicality, and implications

TABLE 13-1 Pharmacodynamic and Pharmacokinetic Properties of Commonly Prescribed Opioids

Hydroxylated Phenanthrene	Receptor Binding	Mu Receptor Binding Affinity	Equivalent Doses	$T_{1/2}$	Duration of Action	Volume of Distribution (Vd)	Metabolism	Available Doses[a]
Morphine (Brand names: MSIR, Roxanol, MSContin, Avinza, Kadian)	Binds to both µ1 & µ2 ~equally Weak κ agonist M-6-G-6-receptor agonist	+	30 mg PO	2–4 hr	IR: 4 hr	3–4 L/kg	Phase II glucuronidation to morphine-3-glucuronide (not active for analgesia but will cause side effects) and morphine-6- glucuronide (active) Both major metabolites accumulate in renal failure Morphine (parent) accumulates in hepatic failure	IV: 2 mg/mL, 4 mg/mL, 5 mg/mL, 8 mg/mL, 10 mg/0.7 mL, 10 mg/mL, 15 mg/mL, 25 mg/mL, 50 mg/mL IR: 15 mg, 30 mg Solution: 2 mg/mL, 4 mg/mL, 20 mg/mL SA: MSContin 15 mg, 30 mg, 60 mg, 100 mg, 200 mg; Avinza 30 mg, 60 mg, 90 mg, 120 mg; Kadian 20 mg, 30 mg, 50 mg, 60 mg, 80 mg, 100 mg, 200 mg
Codeine	Prodrug, metabolized to morphine µ-receptor agonist with low binding affinity	+/– Metabolites responsible for analgesic properties	200 mg po	2.5–3.5 hr	4–6 hr	3.5 L/kg	2D6 mediated 0-demethylation to morphine (active) Phase II glucuronidation to codeine-6-glucuronide 3A4 mediated N-demethylation to norcodeine (inactive)	IV: 15 mg/mL, 30 mg/mL IR: phosphate 30 mg, 60 mg; sulfate 15 mg, 30 mg, 60 mg SA: (not available in U.S.) 50 mg, 100 mg, 150 mg, 200 mg
Diacetyl-morphine	not available	not available	not available	3–5 min	not available	60–100L	Peripheral Metabolism to 6-acetylmorphine, Morphine, Morphine-3-glucuronide, Normorphine, 6-acetylmorphine 3-glucuronide, Normorphine glucuronide	not available in the U.S.

Dehydroxylated phenanthrene	Receptor Binding	Mu Receptor Binding Affinity	Equivalent Doses	$T_{1/2}$	Duration of Action	Volume of Distribution (Vd)	Metabolism	Available Doses[a]
Levorphanol (Brand name: Levo-Dromoran)	µ-agonist κ1, κ3 >>κ2 Noncompetitive NMDA receptor antagonist SNRI activity	++	4 mg	~30 hr	6–15 hr	10–13 L/kg	Phase II glucuronidation to levorphanol-3-glucuronide	IV: 2 mg/mL IR: 1 mg, 2 mg, 3 mg
Hydromorphone (Brand name: Dilaudid)	µ receptor agonist	++	7.5 mg PO	1–3 hr	IR: 4–5 hr	4 L/kg	Phase II glucuronidation to hydromorphone-3-glucuronide and to some extent hydromorphone-6-glucuronide H3G accumulates in renal failure	IV: 1 mg/mL, 2 mg/mL, 4 mg/mL, 10 mg/mL IR: 2 mg, 4 mg, 8 mg
Hydrocodone (Brand names: Vicodin, Lortab, Lorcet, Vicoprofen)	µ receptor agonist with low binding affinity	+	30 mg PO	3.8 hr	4–6 hr	3.4–4.7 L/kg	0-demethylation, N-demethylation and 6-keto reduction to 6-α- and 6-β-hydroxymetabolites CYP3A4 mediated N-demethylation to norhydrocodone is the primary metabolic pathway." Nearly 60% of hydrocodone's metabolism is mediated through the combined CYP 2D6 and CYP 3A4 pathways resulting in the formation of hydromorphone and norhydrocodone[2]. Metabolism and excretion patterns of hydrocodone in urine found that norhydrocodone was the most abundant metabolite and frequently detected in combination with hydrocodone within 2 hours of drug administration.[b,c]	Combination with APAP: 2.5/500 mg, 5/325 mg, 7.5/325 mg, 10/325 mg, 5/500 mg, 7.5/500 mg, 10/500 mg, 7.5/750 mg 10/650 mg, 10/660 mg Combination with IBU: 5/200 mg, 7.5/200 mg

Source: Jeffrey Fudin, B.S., Pharm.D., FCCP. Ackowledgment: Jennifer L. Roy, Pharm.D. Candidate 2010.

Data from MSIR [package insert]. Perdue Pharma, Stamford, CT; March 2009. | MS Contin [package insert]. Perdue Pharma, Stamford, CT; Oct 2004. | MS Contin [package insert]. Richmond, VA: Reckitt Benckiser Pharmaceuticals 20Inc; April 2005. | Suboxone/Subutex [package insert]. Richmond, VA: Reckitt Benckiser Pharmaceuticals Inc; 2006. | Lacy CF, ed. *Drug Information Handbook*. 17th ed. Hudson, OH: Lexi-Comp; 2008. | Buprenex [package insert]. Richmond, VA: Reckitt Benckiser Pharmaceuticals Inc; 2009. | Methadose [package insert]. Hazelwood, Mo: Mallinckrodt Inc; 2009. | Duragesic [package insert]. Raritan, NJ: PriCara; July 2009. | OxyContin [package insert]. Stamford, CT: Purdue Pharma; April 2010. | Molina DK, Hargrove VM. What is the lethal dose of hydrocodone? *Am J Forensic Med Pathol*. 2010;31(3). | Koska AJ et al. Pharmacokinetics of high-dose meperidine in surgical patients. *Anesth Analg*. 1981;60(1). | Nucynta [package insert]. Raritan, NJ: Pricara; March 2010. | Rook E et al. Pharmacokinetics and pharmacokinetic variability of heroin and its metabolites: Review of the literature. *Curr Clin Pharmacol*. 2006;1:109–118. | Mayyas F et al. A systematic review of oxymorphone in the management of chronic pain. *J Pain Symptom Manage*. 2010;39(2);296–308.

TABLE 13-1 Adverse Effects Associated with Dronedarone and Amiodarone *(Continued)*

	Receptor Binding	Mu Receptor Binding Affinity	Equivalent Doses	T½	Duration of Action	Volume of Distribution (Vd)	Metabolism	Available Doses[a]
Dehydroxylated phenanthrene								
Oxycodone (Brand names: Oxy IR, OxyContin, Roxicodone, Percocet, Roxicet, Tylox)	μ receptor agonist with low binding affinity. Greater kappa agonist binding affinity than morphine suggesting it may be the opioid of choice for visceral pain because the viscera have relatively more kappa receptors than peripheral tissues	+	20 mg PO	IR: 2–3 hr; SA: ~5 hr	IR: 3–6 hr; SA: 12 hr	2.6 L/kg	*3A4 mediated N-demethylation to noroxycodone; *2D6 mediated 0-demethylation to oxymorphone (active)	IR: 5 mg, 15 mg, 30 mg; Solution: 1 mg/mL, 20 mg/mL; SA: 10 mg, 20 mg, 40 mg, 60 mg, 80 mg, 160 mg; Combination with APAP: 5/325 mg, 5/500 mg, 7.5/325 mg, 7.5/500 mg, 10/325 mg, 10/350 mg
Oxymorphone (Brand name: Opana, Opana ER)	μ receptor agonist with low binding affinity	*	10 mg PO	IV: 2 hr; IR: 7–9 hr; SA: 9–11 hr	IV: 3–6 hr; IR: 4–6 hr; SA: ~12 hr	1.9–4.2 L/kg	Phase II glucuronidation to oxymorphone-3-glucuronide	IV: 1 mg/mL; IR: 5 mg, 10 mg; SA: 5 mg, 10 mg, 20 mg, 40 mg
Buprenorphine (Brand names: Buprenex, Subutex, Suboxone)	Binds to μ1>>>>μ2 ~90% more doesn't block the alpha receptor as much as morphine means no withdrawal • not addicting • κ receptor antagonist	++++	0.3 mg IV	2.2 hr	6–8 hr	97–187 L/kg	3A4 mediated N-dealkylation to norbuprenorphine (weakly active); Phase II glucuronidation of both the parent compound and norbuprenorphine	IV/IM: 0.3 mg/mL; SL: 2 mg, 8 mg; SL combination with naltrexone: 2 mg/0.5 mg, 8 mg/2 mg
Phenylpiperidine	Receptor Binding	Mu Receptor Binding Affinity	Equivalent Doses	T½	Duration of Action	Volume of Distribution (Vd)	Metabolism	Available Doses[a]
Fentanyl (Brand names: Sublimaze, Actiq, Duragesic)	μ receptor agonist	+++	0.1 mg IV/IM	IV: 2–4 hr; Transdermal patch: 17–22 hr; Transmucosal lozenge: 7 hr	IV: 0.5–1 hr; IM: 1–2 hr; Transdermal: 48–72 hr	6 L/kg	3A4 mediated oxidative N-dealkylation to norfentanyl	IV: 0.05 mg/mL; Transdermal patch: 12 mcg/hr, 25 mcg/hr, 50 mcg/hr, 75 mcg/hr, 100 mcg/hr; Transmucosal lozenge: 200 mcg, 400 mcg, 600 mcg, 800 mcg, 1,200 mcg, 1,600 mcg
Meperidine (Brand name: Demerol)	μ receptor agonist; δ receptor agonist	**	300 mg PO	Parent: 2.5–4 hr; Liver Disease: 7–11 hr; Normeperidine: 15–30 hr	2–5 hr	3.7 L/kg	Phase II hydrolysis to meperidinic acid; N-demethylation to normeperidine (neurotoxic); normeperidine accumulates in hepatic failure	IM/SC: 25 mg/mL, 50 mg/mL, 100 mg/mL; Solution/Syrup: 10 mg/mL; IR: 50 mg, 100 mg
Diphenylheptanes	Receptor Binding	Mu Receptor Binding Affinity	Equivalent Doses	T½	Duration of Action	Volume of Distribution (Vd)	Metabolism	Available Doses[a]
Propoxyphene (Brand names: Darvon, Darvon-N, Darvon Compound 32, Darvon Compound 65, Darvocet A, Darvocet N)	μ receptor agonist	++	130 mg* or 200 mg** PO; *HCl salt; **napsylate salt	Parent: 6–12 hr; Norpropoxyphene: 30–36 hr	4–6 hr	16 L/kg	3A4 mediated N-demethylation to norpropoxyphene with is excreted by the kidneys; *metabolite accumulates in renal failure	IR: 65 mg, 100 mg; Combo with APAP: 50/325 mg, 65/650 mg, 100/325 mg, 100/650 mg
Methadone (Brand name: Dolophine, Methadose)	μ receptor agonist; Noncompetitive NMDA receptor antagonist; SNRI activity	++	7.5 mg PO	8–59 hr	15–60 hr	Vdss 1–8 L/kg	3A4, 2B6, 2C19 mediated N-demethylation to 2-ethylidene-1,5-dimethyl-3,3-diphenylpyrrolidene (EDDP)	IV/IM: 10 mg/mL; Solution: 1 mg/mL, 2 mg/mL, 10 mg/mL; Tablets: 5 mg, 10 mg
Analgesic-Miscellaneous								
Tapentadol (Brand name: Nucynta)	Strong mu receptor agonist with low binding affinity; NRI activity	– ; *18x less potent than morphine	75–100 mg	4 hr	4–6 hr	540 ± 98 L	Phase II glucuronidation to 0-glucuronide; 2C9/2C19 mediated methylation to N-desmethyl-tapentadol	50 mg, 75 mg, 100 mg

*Most common dosage forms listed; not all inclusive.

aCone E, et al. Prescription opioids. II. Metabolism and excretion patterns of hydrocodone in urine following controlled single-dose administration. *J Anal Toxicol.* 2013;37(8):486–494.

bVatier S and Bebarta VS (2012) Excretion profile of hydrocodone, hydromorphone and norhydrocodone in urine following single dose administration of hydrocodone to healthy volunteers. *J Anal Toxicol.* 36:507–514.

Gold MS, Redmond DE Jr, Kleber HD. Clonidine blocks acute opioid-withdrawal symptoms. *Lancet.* 1978;312(8090):599–602.

TABLE 13-2 Opioid Analgesic Comparison Table

Drug	Equianalgesic Doses Parenteral (IV, IM, SQ)	Equianalgesic Doses: Oral	Parenteral			Oral			Usual Dosing Interval (hr)
			Onset (min)	Peak (min)	Duration (hr)	Onset (min)	Peak (min)	Duration (hr)	
AGONISTS									
Morphine	10 mg	30 mg	<5	SQ: 30–60 IV: 20	3–6	15–60	30–60	3–6	3–4
Codeine	75–120 mg	130–200 mg	10–30	30–60	4–6	30–60	30–60	4–6	3–4
Fentanyl	0.1 mg	Transdermal 25 mcg/hr » 45 mg of oral sustained release morphine	IM: 7–15 IV: <1	ND	1–2 (TD: 48–72)				IV: 1 TD: 72
Hydrocodone		30 mg				ND	ND	4–8	3–4
Hydromorphone	1.5 mg	7.5 mg	ND	30–60	4–6	15–30	30–60	4–6	3–4
Levorphanol	2 mg	4 mg	ND	30–60	4–8	10–60	30–60	4–8	6–8
Meperidine	100 mg	300 mg	<5	30–60	2–4	10–15	30–60	2–4	2–3
Methadone	10 mg[a]	7.5 mg[a]	10–20	30–60	4–8	30–60	30–60	4–8	6–8
Oxycodone	ND	20 mg	<5	60	4	10–15	120–180	4–6	4
Oxymorphone	1 mg	10 mg	5–15	30–60	3–6	10–15	30	4–6	3–6
Tapentadol		100mg				ND	1.25 hr	4–6	4–6
PARTIAL AGONISTS									
Buprenorphine	0.4 mg	ND	15	60	4–8	~15 SL admin	40–210 SL admin		6–8
Butorphanol	2 mg	not available	IM: 30–60 IV: 4–5	30–60	3–5				3–4
Nalbuphine	10 mg	not available	IM: 30 IV: 1–3	60	3–6				3–4
Pentazocine	60 mg	150 mg	IV: 2–3	~15	2–3	15–30	~60	4–5	3–4

[a]The ratio of PO morphine: PO methadone is dependent on the dose of morphine prior to switching to methadone. With low doses of morphine (<90 mg/day), the ratio is approximately 4:1 (morphine: methadone). With higher doses of morphine (i.e., >300 mg/day), the ratio of PO morphine: PO methadone approaches 12:1. In between, a ratio of 8:1 has been studied. (Davis,2001).

The Fudin Factor equation eliminates significant peaks and troughs associated with previously accepted schematics and employs the most conservative dosing approach at morphine equivalents up to 300 mg per day.

Fudin J, Marcoux MD, Fudin JA. Mathematical model For methadone conversion examined. *Pract Pain Manag*. 2012;12(8):46–51.

ND – not determined.

The opioid analgesic comparison chart is meant to act as a guideline when switching patients from one opioid to another. It is important to recognize that response to opioids varies widely among individuals. Therefore, all doses should be titrated to effect for individual patients (Foley 1985; Pereira 2000).

Pereira J, Lawlor P, Vigano A, et al. Equianalgesic dose ratios for opioids: A critical review and proposals for long-term dosing. *J Pain Symptom Manage*. 2001;22:672–687.

Davis MP, Walsh D. Methadone for relief of cancer pain: a review of pharmacokinetics, pharmacodynamics, drug interactions and protocols of administration. *Support Care Cancer*. 2001;9:73–83.

Foley K. The treatment of cancer pain. *NEJM*. 1985;313:84–95.

TABLE 13-3 Dosage Recommendations for Opioids

Drug	Recommended Starting Dose for Adults >50 kg		Starting Dose for Children and Adults <50 kg	
	Oral	Parenteral	Oral	Parenteral
[a]Morphine	15–30 mg q3–4h	10 mg q3–4h	0.3 mg/kg q3–4h	0.1 mg/kg q3–4h
[β]Codeine	60 mg q3–4h	60 mg q2h (IM, Sq)	1 mg/kg q3–4h	not recommended
[a]Fentanyl	not available	0.5–1.0 mcg/kg/dose	not available	1–2 mcg/kg/dose
[a]Hydromorphone	2–6 mg q3–4h	0.5–2 mg q3–4h	0.06 mg/kg q3–4h	0.015 mg/kg q3–4h
[β]Hydrocodone	10 mg q3–4h	not available	0.2 mg/kg q3–4h	not available
[a]Levorphanol	4 mg q6–8h	2 mg q6–8h	0.04 mg/kg q6–8h	0.02 mg/kg q6–8h
[β]Meperidine	not recommended	100 mg q3h	not recommended	0.75 mg/kg q2–3h
[a]Methadone	10–20 mg q8h	10 mg q6–8h	0.2 mg/kg q6–8h	0.1 mg/kg q6–8h
[a]Oxycodone	10 mg q3–4h	not available	0.2 mg/kg q3–4h	not available
Oxymorphone	not available	1 mg q3–4h	not recommended	not recommended
[δ]Propoxyphene	65*or 100** mg q3–4h *hCl salt **napsylate salt	not available	not well established	not available
Buprenorphine	not available	0.4 q6–8h	not available	0.004 mg/kg q6–8h
Butorphanol	not available	2 mg q3–4h	not available	not recommended
Nalbuphine	not available	10 mg q3–4h	not available	0.1 mg/kg q3–4h
Pentazocine	50 mg q4–6h	not recommended	not recommended	not recommended

[a]For treatment of moderate to severe pain; [β]For treatment of mild-to-moderate pain; [δ]For treatment of mild pain, may be no more effective than ASA

Constipation

Because tolerance does not develop to narcotic-induced constipation, preventative measures should be initiated on day 1 of narcotic therapy. A stimulant laxative (e.g., Milk of Magnesia, senna) is necessary because opioids decrease propulsive contractions of the small intestine and increase tone of the large intestine, which slows transit time. Stool softeners as monotherapy for opioid-induced constipation are ineffective.

Meperidine should be reserved for brief courses in otherwise healthy patients who have demonstrated an unusual reaction or allergic response during treatment with other opioids (e.g., morphine, hydromorphone).

Converting patients from one opioid to another

Using conversion table, convert to morphine equivalents, then to opioid of choice. It is recommended to decrease the dose of the new opioid in half (after calculations) due to incomplete cross-reactivity between opioids in terms of analgesia and respiratory depression. Titrate up as necessary.

TABLE 13-4 Orally Administered Fentanyl Products

Trade Name	Generic Name	Administration	Available Strengths	Bioavailability	Cmax (ng/mL)	*Tmax (min)
Actiq	Fentanyl citrate	Lozenge that is placed between the lower gum and cheek and left in place for 15 min	200 mcg 400 mcg 600 mcg 800 mcg 1,200 mcg 1,600 mcg	Rapid ~25% from the mucosa, remaining swallowed with saliva and slowly absorbed from GI tract: **total 47%**	400 mcg – 0.63 800 mcg – 1.03	20–120
Fentora	Fentanyl citrate	Tablet for buccal administration: place in the buccal cavity above the rear molar, takes 14–25 min to dissolve, any remnants can be swallowed with water	100 mcg 200 mcg 300 mcg 400 mcg 600 mcg 800 mcg	Rapid ~50% absorbed from the mucosa, remaining swallowed with saliva and slowly absorbed from GI tract: **total 65%**	100 mcg – 0.25 200 mcg – 0.40 400 mcg – 1.02 800 mcg – 1.59	35–46.8
Onsolis	Fentanyl citrate	Two-layer film placed on the inside of the cheek, dissolves in 15–30 min	200 mcg 400 mcg 600 mcg 800 mcg 1,200 mcg	Rapid 51% absorbed from the mucosa, remaining swallowed with saliva and slowly absorbed from GI tract: **total 71%**	800 mcg – 1.67	60–150
Abstral	Fentanyl citrate	Sublingual tablet placed under the tongue	100 mcg 200 mcg 300 mcg 400 mcg 600 mcg 800 mcg	Rapid absorption occurs over about 30 minutes: **total 54%**	100 mcg – 0.187 200 mcg – 0.302 400 mcg – 0.765 800 mcg – 1.42	30–60

*Dose dependent; mucositis does not appear to affect peak plasma concentrations.

These products must not be used in opioid nontolerant patients due to the risk of life-threatening hypoventilation. They are not approved for the treatment of acute pain (e.g., postoperative, dental, migraine). In addition, switching between these fentanyl products must not occur at a 1:1 ratio due to differences in drug delivery and absorption profiles. Two of these products (Abstral and Onsolis) require REMS monitoring by the FDA and prescriber enrollment.
Prepared by: Ruth Perkins, B.S., M.A., Pharm.D., BCPS. Rev 04/2011

of the measurable metabolites as well. (See Table 13-5.) Assuming regular usage for example, if a patient is receiving codeine, we would expect to find measurable morphine metabolite; if a patient is receiving oxycodone we would expect to find measurable oxymorphone metabolite; if a patient is receiving fentanyl we would expect to find measurable norfentanyl metabolite; but if a patient is receiving morphine we should not expect the presence of, for example, meperidine, fentanyl, or methadone. (see Table 13-5, Figure 13-1)

Because of the enormous variability among opioids with regard to pharmacokinetics, therapeutics, and pharmacodynamics , this chapter provides a number of comprehensive tables. It is important to understand that any conversion tables within or outside the confines of this text reflect population averages, and—due to genetic polymorphism—individual patient conversions may vary considerably. Tables 13-2 and 13-3 can be used as a starting point, but titration to response is indicated.

Additionally, due to incomplete cross-tolerance among opioids (which is only an issue in the first 7–14 days of regularly scheduled dosing), clinicians should reduce the calculated equianalgesic conversion starting dose by 20 to 25 percent ; this practice will serve to reduce risk of inadvertent overdose, especially if the patient is more sensitive to the new opioid than the one it is replacing.

Table 13-5 illustrates various commonly prescribed opioids and their corresponding expected serum levels. Note that the half-life of most commonly prescribed immediate-release products is similar. Examples include morphine, codeine, hydrocodone, hydromorphone, oxycodone, oxymorphone, and others. Figure 13-1 provides a chemical categorization of these opioids. Those with high volumes of distribution and longer half-lives include methadone and levorphanol. Methadone has a unique pharmacokinetic profile, with broad patient metabolism variations and multiple metabolites. And unlike other opioids, the majority of methadone metabolism is mediated by CYP450 3A4 isoenzymes. Therefore, it presents an important therapeutic and potentially toxic conundrum, particularly if a potent 3A4 inducer or inhibitor is introduced or abruptly discontinued.

Moreover, methadone has two enantiomers (R– and S–). The "S" isomer depends on metabolism by CYP 2B6 isoenzymes and the accumulation of the "S" enantiomer is known to elevate risk of Torsade de pointes. Therefore, patients that are poor CYP 2B6 metabolizers are at higher risk of ventricular tachycardia due to accumulation of the "S" enantiomer.[15] When one considers that HIV pain is commonly caused by the AIDS virus itself and/or the antiretroviral agents used to treat it, methadone analgesia, maintenance, or both is relatively common. Because almost all of the antiretrovirals significantly affect several of the cytochrome P450 isoenzymes, use of methadone requires a clear understanding of these pharmacokinetic interactions.

SPECIAL CONSIDERATIONS FOR TRANSDERMAL FENTANYL

Pharmacokinetic interpatient and intrapatient variability can be significant. The elimination half-life after fentanyl transdermal patch removal is approximately 17 hours, ranging from 13 to 22 hours.[16] The extended half-life is due to slow release of drug from the skin depot, which is common with all transdermal delivery systems.

Another important consideration is that elimination half-life in the elderly may be prolonged.[16] This factor is especially noteworthy when switching a patient from fentanyl to an alternative opioid based solely on mathematical calculations because of the risk of overdosing the patient based on an incorrect presumption that the fentanyl is being absorbed. Homework case 2 illustrates this point when converting from fentanyl. The transition from fentanyl to the new opioid should be slow with use of immediate-release products for 2–4 days, until the lowest possible pain level is maintained. After the transition, a sustained-release formulation may be introduced. Following patch removal, the analgesic effects of fentanyl may continue for 12 to 24 hours.[17]

Absorbed transdermal fentanyl is proportional to the surface area of the patch. Fentanyl is released from the patch into the stratum corneum and epidermis as drug accumulates within these layers

Overall opioid drug classifications

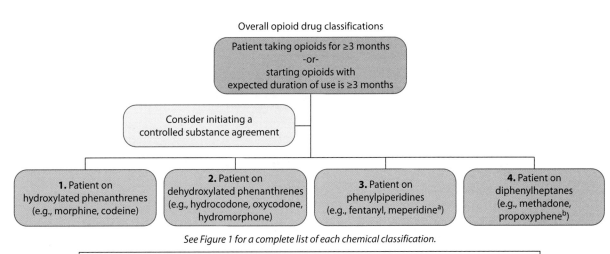

Patient taking opioids for ≥3 months
-or-
starting opioids with
expected duration of use is ≥3 months

Consider initiating a
controlled substance agreement

1. Patient on
hydroxylated phenanthrenes
(e.g., morphine, codeine)

2. Patient on
dehydroxylated phenanthrenes
(e.g., hydrocodone, oxycodone,
hydromorphone)

3. Patient on
phenylpiperidines
(e.g., fentanyl, meperidine[a])

4. Patient on
diphenylheptanes
(e.g., methadone,
propoxyphene[b])

See Figure 1 for a complete list of each chemical classification.

a. Meperidine should not be used chronically for pain based on toxicity profile.[1]
b. Propoxyphene is not available on the U.S. market.[2]

Urine drug screens are intended to **screen** for patients who may be diverting, supplementing, or abusing
prescribed drugs or other illicit substances.
They are not intended to predict or determine dose versus compliance.

1. Raymo LL, Camejo M, Fudin J. Eradicating analgesic use of meperidine in a hospital. *AJHP*. 2007;1150–1153.
2. Jonasson Ulf, Jonasson B, Saldeen T. Correlation between prescription of various dextropropoxyphene preparations and
    their involvement in fatal poisonings. *Forensic Science International*. 1999;103:125–132.

Is your patient a candidate for opioid medications?

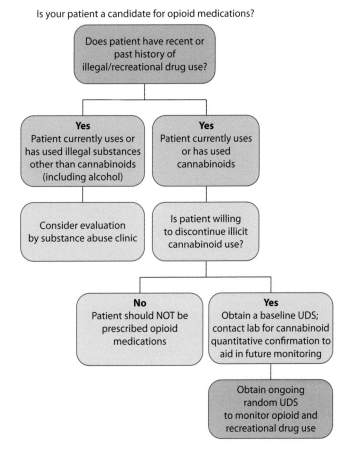

Does patient have recent or
past history of
illegal/recreational drug use?

Yes
Patient currently uses or
has used illegal substances
other than cannabinoids
(including alcohol)

Yes
Patient currently uses
or has used
cannabinoids

Consider evaluation
by substance abuse clinic

Is patient willing
to discontinue illicit
cannabinoid use?

No
Patient should NOT be
prescribed opioid
medications

Yes
Obtain a baseline UDS;
contact lab for cannabinoid
quantitative confirmation to
aid in future monitoring

Obtain ongoing
random UDS
to monitor opioid and
recreational drug use

FIGURE 13-2. Urine Drug Screen (UDS) Algorithm

Monitoring urine drug screens

Monitoring UDS for **Morphine/Codeine**

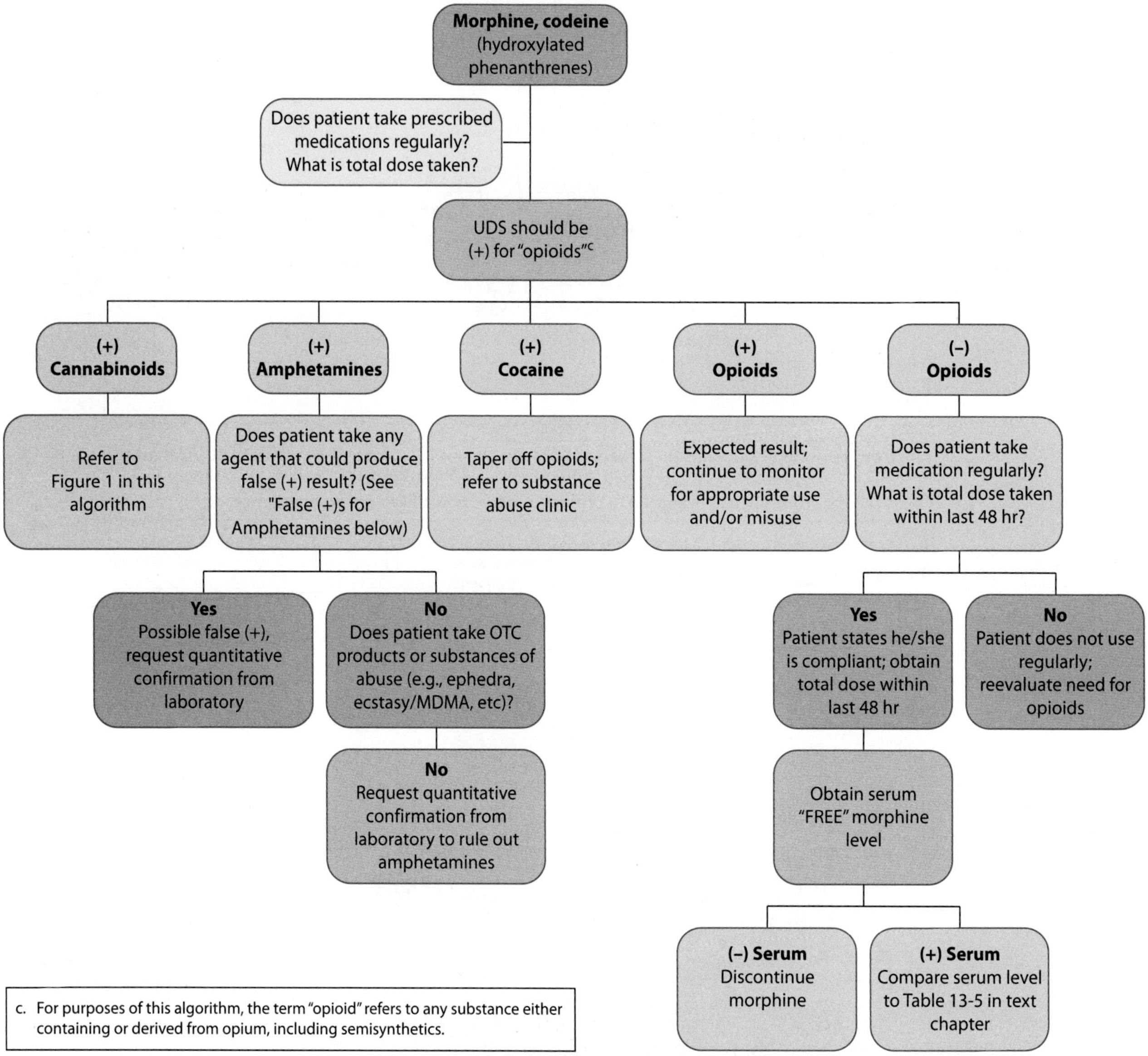

Morphine, codeine
(hydroxylated phenanthrenes)

Does patient take prescribed medications regularly? What is total dose taken?

UDS should be (+) for "opioids"ᶜ

(+) Cannabinoids

Refer to Figure 1 in this algorithm

(+) Amphetamines

Does patient take any agent that could produce false (+) result? (See "False (+)s for Amphetamines below)

(+) Cocaine

Taper off opioids; refer to substance abuse clinic

(+) Opioids

Expected result; continue to monitor for appropriate use and/or misuse

(–) Opioids

Does patient take medication regularly? What is total dose taken within last 48 hr?

Yes
Possible false (+), request quantitative confirmation from laboratory

No
Does patient take OTC products or substances of abuse (e.g., ephedra, ecstasy/MDMA, etc)?

No
Request quantitative confirmation from laboratory to rule out amphetamines

Yes
Patient states he/she is compliant; obtain total dose within last 48 hr

No
Patient does not use regularly; reevaluate need for opioids

Obtain serum "FREE" morphine level

(–) Serum
Discontinue morphine

(+) Serum
Compare serum level to Table 13-5 in text chapter

c. For purposes of this algorithm, the term "opioid" refers to any substance either containing or derived from opium, including semisynthetics.

Examples of drugs that may cause false positives for amphetamines (Note: This list is not all inclusive):

Any drug with a catecholamine nucleus:
- β-blockers (including propranolol, atenolol, timolol ophthalmic)
- β-agonists
- Dopamine congeners (e.g., levadopa, carbidopa, bupropion)
- α-agonist catecholamines [including chronic use of eye drops (Visine®), nasal decongestants (Afrin®)]
- Pseudoephedrine, phenylephrine, ephedra
- Adrenergic ophthalmic (e.g., dipivefrin, timolol, levobunolol)
NOTE: Methylphenidate will NOT show (+) for amphetamines.

FIGURE 13-2. (*Continued*)

Monitoring UDS for **Oxycodone/Hydrocodone/Hydromorphone**

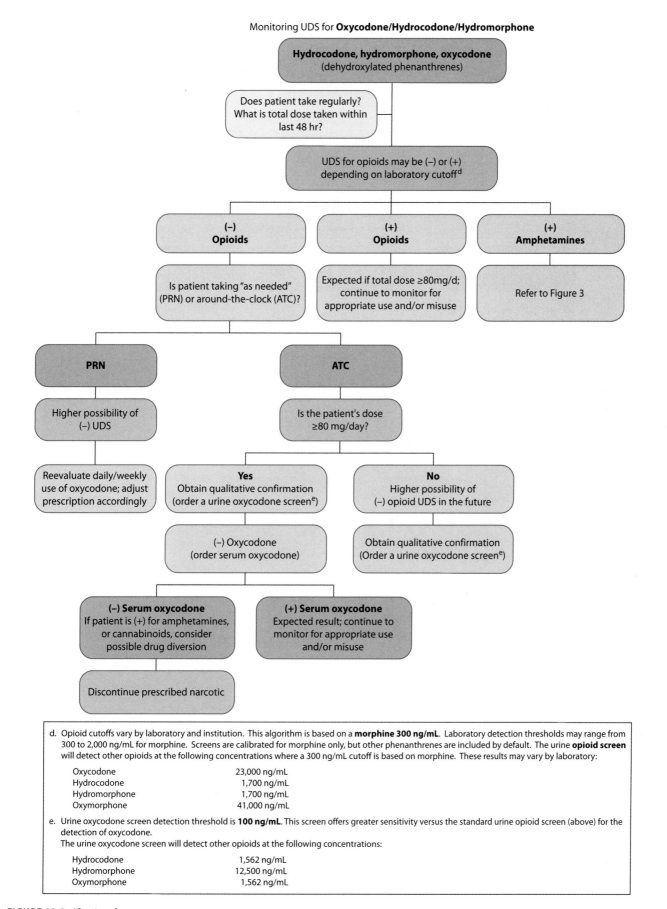

d. Opioid cutoffs vary by laboratory and institution. This algorithm is based on a **morphine 300 ng/mL**. Laboratory detection thresholds may range from 300 to 2,000 ng/mL for morphine. Screens are calibrated for morphine only, but other phenanthrenes are included by default. The urine **opioid screen** will detect other opioids at the following concentrations where a 300 ng/mL cutoff is based on morphine. These results may vary by laboratory:

Oxycodone	23,000 ng/mL
Hydrocodone	1,700 ng/mL
Hydromorphone	1,700 ng/mL
Oxymorphone	41,000 ng/mL

e. Urine oxycodone screen detection threshold is **100 ng/mL**. This screen offers greater sensitivity versus the standard urine opioid screen (above) for the detection of oxycodone.
The urine oxycodone screen will detect other opioids at the following concentrations:

Hydrocodone	1,562 ng/mL
Hydromorphone	12,500 ng/mL
Oxymorphone	1,562 ng/mL

FIGURE 13-2. *(Continued)*

Monitoring UDS for **Fentanyl**

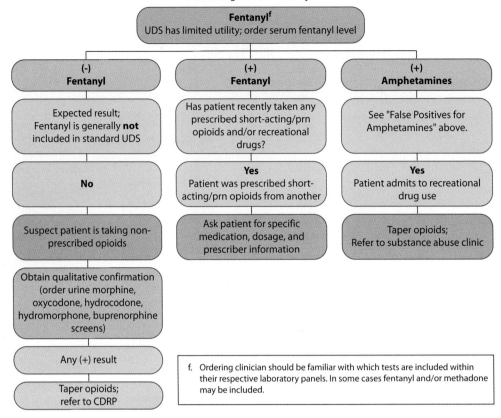

f. Ordering clinician should be familiar with which tests are included within their respective laboratory panels. In some cases fentanyl and/or methadone may be included.

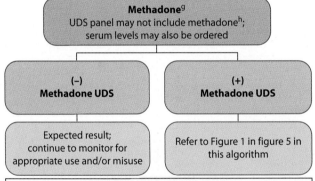

g. Methadone is CYP 3A4 substrate and is therefore prone to many drug interactions.
h. Some laboratory panels include methadone, but not fentanyl. Methadone UDS may be ordered as a separate test. In some cases fentanyl and/or methadone may be included in the UDS panel. If patient is on ≥ 20 mg/d of methadone, urine should remain (+) for 3 days.

Disclaimer: These flowcharts are not comprehensive, are not all inclusive, and may not include every possible permutation presented by the patient. These flow charts are intended as a simple guide; ordering clinician MUST know which drugs are included in the urine drug screen panel.

References:
1. Chronic Pain Treatment Guidelines. Available at: http://www.painmed.org/pdf/medical_treatment_utilization_schedule_guidelines.pdf (accessed August 2007): 35-41.
2. Florate OG. Urinary drug testing in pain management. *Practical Pain Management*. Glen Mills, PA: PPM Communications, Inc., April 2005: 38–42.
3. PainEDU.org. Screener and Opioid Assessment for Patients with Pain (SOAPP)*Version 1.0. ©2008 Inflexxion, Inc. Available at: http://painedu.org/soapp/SOAPP_24.pdf.
4. Probes LM. Opioid blood levels in chronic management. *Practical Pain Management*. Glen Mills, PA: PPM Communications, Inc., April 2005: 12–18.
5. Veterans Health Administration, Department of Defense. *VA/DoD Clinical Practice Guideline for the Management of Opioid Therapy for Chronic Pain*. Washington, DC: Veterans Health Administration, March 2003.
6. Virami A, Mailis A, Shapiro LE, Shear NH. Drug interactions in human neuropathic pain pharmacology. *Pain*. 1997;73:3–13.

Used with permission from Dr. Jeffrey Fudin http://paindr.com/resources/quick-references/

Prepared by: Jeffrey Fudin, B.S., Pharm.D., FCCP

FIGURE 13-2. *(Continued)*

TABLE 13-5 Opioid Pharmacokinetics and Expected Metabolites

Drug	Half-Life (hrs^a)	Time to Steady State (hrs^a)	Metabolites	Time to Peak Conc. (hrs^a)	Serum Predict-ability	Bioavailability	Serum Concentration (ng/mL)
buprenorphine/naloxone[44-46] (Suboxone)	24-42/2-12	120-294	norbuprenorphine	1.53-1.72/0.77-0.81	Y	15% / 3%	8 mg/2 mg Cmax = 3.37 +/- 1.8 ng/mL and 193 +/- 91.2 ng/mL
codeine[16,17,27]	2.5-3.5	12.5-17.5	morphine, norcodeine, normorphine, hydrocodone, codeine 6-glucuronide	1-2	Y	well absorbed	IR 180 mg = 222.9 +/- 48.9
transdermal fentanyl[8-11,27]	16-25	72	norfentanyl, 4-n-(n-propionylanilino) piperidine, 4-n-(n-hydroxypropionylanilino) piperidine, 1-(2-phenethyl)-4-n-(n-hydroxypropionylanilino) piperidine	24-72	Y	92%	25 mcg/hr = 0.6 +/- 0.3 50 mcg/hr = 1.4 +/- 0.5 75 mcg/hr = 1.7 +/- 0.7 100 mcg/hr = 2.5 +/- 1.2
transbuccal, transmucosal, sublingual fentanyl[8] **	14-19 (Onsolis) 2.6-11.7 (Fentora) 7 (Actiq) 5-13 (Abstral)	13-98	as above	0.75-4 (Onsolis) 0.58-0.78 (Fentora) 0.3-2 (Actiq) 0.25-1 (Abstral)	Y	Onsolis 71% Fentora 65% Actiq 47% Abstral 54%	800 mcg = 1.67^g (Onsolis) 800 mcg = 1.59^g (Fentora) 800 mcg = 1.03^g (Actiq) 800 mcg = 1.42^g (Abstral)
hydrocodone[18-20,27,321-41]	3.8	19-22.5	hydromorphone, norcodeine, 6-beta-hydrocodol, 6-alpha-hydrocodol, 6-beta-hydromorphol, 6-alpha-hydromorphol, norhydrocodone	1.3	Y	well absorbed	IR 10 mg = 23.6 +/- 5.2
heroin[24-27]	~3 min 1.7-5.3 min	~15 min	6-acetylmorphine, morphine, morphine-3-glucuronide, normorphine, 6-acetylmorphine 3-glucuronide, normorphine glucuronide	10 min for IM dose^b	Y	diacetylmorphine undergoes complete presystemic metabolism to morphine after oral administration	112 mcg/min for 5 min heroin level = 57 ng/mL^c 6-acetylmorphine level = 15ng/mL^c
hydromorphone[12-14,27]	2.5	12.5	hydromorphone-3-glucuronide, hydromorphone-3-glucoside, dihydroisomorphine-6-glucuronide, dihydroisomorphine-6-glucoside, dihydroisomorphine, dihydromorphine^e	48-60 min	Y	24%	IR 48 mg = 19.7 +/- 4.04
levorphanol	One dose 11-16 hr Chronic dosing up to 30hr	72 hr	3-glucuronide	approx. 1	?		
meperidine[21-23,27]	~3.6	3-6 days	normeperidine, meperidinic acid, normeperidinic acid	1-1.5	?	variable IM 57%	100 mg IM = 551 ng/mL
methadone[21-23,27]	15-60 (and up to 150)	~5 days	EDDP (2-ethyl-1,5-dimethyl-3,3-diphenylpyrrolinium), EMDP (2-ethyl-5-methyl-3,3-diphenylpyraline)	2-4	Y	85%	Linear drug levels increase 260 ng/mL for every 1 mg/kg consumed
morphine[4-7,27,28]	2-4	24	morphine-3-glucuronide, morphine-6-glucuronide, normorphine, codeine, 7,8-dihydromorphinone	IR = 1 CR = 2-3	Y	20-40%	IR 40 mg = 11.1 +/- 8.4 CR 100 mg = 36.9 +/- 15.5
morphine/naltrexone[43] (Embeda)	29	145-203	as above + 6-beta-naltrexol	7.5	Y	20-40%	lower Cmax and a higher Cmin than conventional immediate-release morphine at steady state
oxycodone[1-3,27]	IV, IR = 3.2 CR = 4.5-8	IR = 17.5 CR = 24-36	noroxycodone, oxymorphone, oxycodyl, oxymorphol, noroxycodyl	IR = 1.6 CR = 2.1-3.2	Y	60-87%	IV (0.14 mg/kg) = 34-38 IR 20 mg = 15.6 +/- 4.4 CR 20 mg = 15.1 +/- 4.7
oxymorphone[42]	IR = 7.2-9.4 hr ER 9.4-11.3	IR = 3-4 days ER = 3 days	oxyphorphone-3-glucuronide, 6-oh-oxymorphone,	IR = 30 min ER = 3 hr	Y	10%^F	IR 20 mg = 4.39 +/- 1.72 ER 20 mg = 2.54 +/- 1.35
tapentadol	4	20-28	tapentadol-o-glucuronide, desmethyl tapentadol, hydroxyl tapentadol	1.25-1.5	Y	32%	Cmax ~ 2.45 mcg/mL

IR, immediate release products; CR, continuous release products; SS, steady state

^aHours, unless otherwise indicated.

^bCan detect heroin and 6-acetyl morphine within 10-15 minutes of parenteral administration.

^cAdministered IV in a single patient over 180 minutes.

^dCumulative amount of fentanyl release from patch dose in 24 hours.

(Continued)

TABLE 13-5   Opioid Pharmacokinetics and Expected Metabolites (*Continued*)

*Hydromorphone is 7,8-dihydromorphinone: Please note that morphine metabolism to hydromorphone has been confirmed in 8 mammals other than humans. There is only data that correlates the conversion of morphine to hydromorphone in humans.[29]

*The bioavailability of oxymorphone increases significantly in hepatically (up to 12-fold) and renally impaired (65% with creatinine clearance less than 30 mL/min) patients.

*peak concentrations

*These products are not considered bioequivalent.

1. Reder RF, Oshlack B, Miotto JB, Benziger DD, Kaiko RF. Steady-state bioavailability of controlled-release oxycodone in normal subjects. *Clin Ther.* 1996;18(1):95–105.

2. Kaiko RF, Benziger DP, Fitzmartin RD, et al. Pharmacokinetic-pharmacodynamic relationships of controlled release oxycodone. *Clin Pharmacol Ther.* 1996;59(1):52–61.

3. Oxycodone - MICROMEDEX® Healthcare Series, Thomson MICROMEDEX, Greenwood Village, CO. Copyright © 1974–2008.

4. Christup LL, Sjogren P, Jensen NH, Banning AM, Elbaek K, Ersboll A. Steady-state kinetics and dynamics of morphine in cancer patients: Is sedation related to the absorption rate of morphine? *J Pain Symptom Manage.* 1999;18(3):164–173.

5. Gourlay GK, Cherry DA, Onley MM, et al. Pharmacokinetics and pharmacodynamics of twenty four hourly Kapanol compared to twelve-hourly Ms Contin in the treatment of severe cancer pain. *Pain.* 1997;69:295–302.

6. Morphine - MICROMEDEX® Healthcare Series, Thomson MICROMEDEX, Greenwood Village, CO. Copyright © 1974–2011.

7. Fentanyl - MICROMEDEX® Healthcare Series, Thomson MICROMEDEX, Greenwood Village, CO. Copyright © 1974–2011.

8. Portenoy RK, Southam MA, Gupta SK, et al. Transdermal fentanyl for cancer pain. *Anesthesiology.* 1993;78(1):36–43.

9. Ashburn MA, Ogdden LL, Ahang J, et al. The pharmacokinetics of transdermal fentanyl delivered with and without heat. *J Pain.* 2003;4(6):291–297.

10. Hagen N, Thirlwell MP Dhaliwal HS, et al. Steady-state pharmacokinetics of hydromorphone and hydromorphone-3-glucuronide in cancer patients after immediate and controlled release hydromorphone. *J Clin Pharmacol.* 1995;35:37–44.

11. Vallner JJ, Stewart JT, Kotzan JA, Kirsten EB, Honigberg IL. Pharmacokinetics and bioavailability of hydromorphone and hydromorphone following intravenous and oral administration to human subjects. *J Clin Pharmacology.* 1981;21:152–156.

12. Hydromorphone - MICROMEDEX® Healthcare Series, Thomson MICROMEDEX, Greenwood Village, CO. Copyright © 1974–2008.

13. Band CJ, Band PR, Deschamps M, et al. Human pharmacokinetic study of immediate-release (codeine phosphate) and sustained-release (codeine contin) codeine. *J Clin Pharmacol.* 1994;34:938–943.

14. Codeine - MICROMEDEX® Healthcare Series, Thomson MICROMEDEX, Greenwood Village, CO. Copyright © 1974–2008.

15. Cone EJ, Darwin WD, Gorodetzky CW, Tan T. Comparative metabolism of hydrocodone in man, rat, guinea pig, rabbit, and dog. *Drug Metab Dispos.* 1978 6(4):488–493.

16. Honigberg IL, Stewart JT. Radioimmunoassay of hydromorphone and hydrocodone in human plasma. *J Pharm Sci.* 1980;69(10):1171–1173.

17. Hydrocodone - MICROMEDEX® Healthcare Series, Thomson MICROMEDEX, Greenwood Village, CO. Copyright © 1974–2008.

18. Wolff K, Rostami-Hodjegan A, Hay AWM, et al. Population-based pharmacokinetic approach for methadone monitoring of opioid addicts: Potential clinical utility. *Addiction.* 2000;95(12):1771–1783.

19. Wolff K, Sanderson M, Hay AWM, Raistrick D. Methadone concentrations in plasma and their relationship to drug dosage. *Clin Chem.* 1991;37(2):205–209.

20. Methadone - MICROMEDEX® Healthcare Series, Thomson MICROMEDEX, Greenwood Village, CO. Copyright © 1974–2008.

21. Inturrisi CE, Max MB, Foley KM, et al. The pharmacokinetics of heroin in patients with chronic pain. *N Engl J Med.* 1984;310:1213–1217.

22. Rentsch KM, Kullak-Ublick GA, Reichel C, et al. Arterial and venous pharmacokinetics of intravenous heroin subjects who are addicted to narcotics. *Clin Pharm Ther.* 2001;70(3):237–246.

23. Heroin - MICROMEDEX® Healthcare Series, Thomson MICROMEDEX, Greenwood Village, CO.Copyright © 1974–2005.

24. McQuay HJ. Opioid problems, and morphine metabolism and excretion. Pain Research and Nuffield Department of Anaesthetics, University of Oxford, UK. 8 March 2005. Available at: http://www.jr2.ox.ac.uk/bandolier/booth/painpag/wisdom/c14.html#RTFToC44.

25. Yeh SY, McQuinn RL, Gorodetzky CW. Biotransformation of morphine to dihydromorphinone and normorphine in the mouse, rat, rabbit, guinea pig, cat, dog, and monkey. *Drug Metab Dispos.* 1977;5(4):335–342.

26. Lalovic B, Kharasch E, Hoffer C, Risler L, Liu-Chen LY, Shen DD. Pharmacokinetics and pharmacodynamics of oral oxycodone in healthy human subjects: Role of circulating active metabolites. *Clin Pharmaco Ther.* 2006;79(5):461–479.

27. Kalso E. Oxycodone. *J Pain Symptom Manage.* 2005;29(5Suppl):S47–56.

28. Darbari DS, Minniti CP, Rana S, van den Anker J. Pharmacogenetics of morphine: Potential implications in sickle cell disease. *Ame J Hematol.* 2008;83(3):233–236.

29. Cone EJ, Heit HA, Caplan YH, Gourlay D. Evidence of morphine metabolism to hydromorphone in pain patients chronically treated with morphine. *J Anal Toxicol.* 2006;30(1):1–5.

30. Murray A, Hagen NA. Hydromorphone. *J Pain Symptom Manage.* 2005;29(5 Suppl):S57–66.

31. Hutchinson MR, Menelaou A, Foster DJ, Coller JK, Somogyi AA. CYP2D6 and CYP3A4 involvement in the primary oxidative metabolism of hydrocodone by human liver microsomes. *Br J Clin Pharmacol.* 204;57(3):287–297.

32. Lugo RA, Satterfield KL, Kern SE. Pharmacokinetics of methadone. *J Pain Palliat Care Pharmacother.* 2005;19(4):13–24.

33. Prommer E. Oxymorphone. A review. *Support Care Cancer.* 2006;14(2):109–115.

34. Hydromorphone - MICROMEDEX® Healthcare Series, Thomson MICROMEDEX, Greenwood Village, CO. Copyright © 1974–2008.

35. Meperidine - MICROMEDEX® Healthcare Series, Thomson MICROMEDEX, Greenwood Village, CO. Copyright © 1974–2008.

36. Propoxyphene - MICROMEDEX® Healthcare Series, Thomson MICROMEDEX, Greenwood Village, CO. Copyright © 1974–2008

37. Latta, KS, Ginsberg B, Barkin, RL. Meperidine: A critical review. *Am J Ther.* 2002;9:53–68.

38. McNulty JP. Can levorphanol be used like methadone for intractable refractory pain? *J Palliat Med.* 2007;10:293–296.

39. Baselt RC. *Disposition of Toxic Drugs and Chemicals in Man*, 2nd ed. Davis, CA: Biomedical Publications, 1982.

40. *Physicians' Desk Reference*, 48th ed. Montvale, NJ: Medical Economics Data Production Company, 1994.

41. Goldberger BA. Opioids Abused Drugs Monograph Series. Ed. Caplan, Yale H. Irving, TX: Abbott Laboratories, 1994.

42. Endo professional [package insert]. Copyright © Endo Pharmaceuticals Inc. 2006.

43. morphine/naltrexone - MICROMEDEX® Healthcare Series, Thomson MICROMEDEX, Greenwood Village, CO. Copyright © 1974–2011.

44. buprenorphine/naloxone - MICROMEDEX® Healthcare Series, Thomson MICROMEDEX, Greenwood Village, CO. Copyright © 1974–2011.

45. Mendelson J, Upton RA, Evrhart ET, et al. Bioavailability of sublingual buprenorphine. *J Clin Pharmacol.* 1997;37:31–37.

46. Kuhlman JJ, Lalani S, Magiuilo J, et al. Human pharmacokinetics of intravenous, sublingual, and buccal buprenorphine. *J Anal Toxicol.* 1996;20:369–378.

47. Tapentadol - MICROMEDEX® Healthcare Series, Thomson MICROMEDEX, Greenwood Village, CO. Copyright © 1974–2011.

to form a depot. Afterwards, fentanyl is released into the systemic circulation slowly from small blood vessels within the dermis. Fentanyl exhibits wide tissue distribution to various organ systems, which is indicative of a high extravascular volume of distribution (3–8 L/kg). It takes about 17 hours to reach steady-state plasma concentrations after initiating fentanyl patch therapy.[18]

Following patch application, drug release occurs at a constant rate for up to 72 hours.[17] Neither the local blood supply nor the anatomical site affectively change the rate or extent of drug absorption. It may take 34 to 38 hours to reach a maximum serum concentration of fentanyl after patch application. Steady-state serum concentrations are typically reached by day 6 and can be maintained with regularly scheduled patch changes at 72-hour intervals.

Fentanyl is primarily metabolized by CYP 3A4 isoenzymes by N-dealkylation to norfentanyl, an inactive metabolite.[19] As previously described with methadone, potent inhibitors or inducers of 3A4 isoenzymes may significantly affect the metabolism of fentanyl.

CASES

Please note that the following cases may lend themselves to several therapeutic and clinical adjustment(s); however, discussion points will focus on opioid therapy pharmacokinetics and therapeutic interventions.

CASE 1: OXYCODONE SR AND ABERRANT BEHAVIOR

YE is a 47-year-old white male who recently moved to a new geographic location. He was referred to a new primary care provider (PCP) from his previous doctor. The referral indicated that the patient has chronic low back pain, is currently unemployed, and is seeking social security disability (SSI).

Problem List: DJD of Lumbar spine (L)4, L5, Sacral (S)1, status post (S/P) low back surgery for a herniated disc 6 years ago; magnetic resonance imaging (MRI) report finds no abnormalities other than mild arthritis and surgical evidence; no scar tissue present; hypertension controlled with medication; hyperchosterolemia; aberrant behavior; GERD; and history of substance abuse including heroin. The patient denies use of any recreational drugs at this time, including alcohol.

Current Medications:

OxyContin® 160 mg (2 × 80 mg tablets) PO q12h

oxycodone/acetaminophen/325, take 2 PO q4h prn pain

gabapentin 800 mg PO tid

simvastatin 40 mg PO qam

lisinopril 40 mg PO qam

ibuprofen 600 mg PO qid prn

omeprazole 20 mg PO qam

Height = 71 inches

Weight = 165 lbs

YE presents to his new PCP Dr. P. for a full exam and workup. The patient has 2 days left of OxyContin® and no more oxycodone/acetaminophen for breakthrough pain. He is requesting new prescriptions for these medications ASAP because he is fearful of pain and withdrawal symptoms should he not receive these medications promptly.

Dr. P. evaluates the patient and explains that all of his pain patients receiving chronic opioid therapy must agree to sign a "controlled substance treatment agreement," which includes consent for random urine drug screens (UDS) and serum analyses. Any

prescriptions on the first visit will require a baseline UDS. YE reluctantly agreed to these terms and provided a urine specimen and blood for a free serum oxycodone level. The initial UDS was positive for cannabinoids. The serum oxycodone analysis was expected to take approximately 10 days for the results.

Dr. P. contacted his collaborating pharmacist to discuss the case, as his policy is that if a patient is illegally using marijuana, opioids are not an option. The pharmacist is quick to point out that the UDS screen is an enzyme test and that it is possible to see a false positive from proton pump inhibitors, in this case, omeprazole.[20]

As the discussion unfolded, Dr. P. expressed concern for prescribing an opioid to this patient because of his substance abuse history and the positive preliminary finding of cannabinoids, but he also feels an obligation to provide opioids at least for the short term and to give the patient the benefit of doubt. He asks the pharmacist to make recommendations of a replacement medication that might reduce abuse liability in this patient. Dr. P. specifically inquired about use of a transdermal fentanyl patch with a requirement for the patient to return the used patches at a subsequent visit in 2 weeks.

QUESTION 1

What is a reasonable dose of transdermal fentanyl with which to replace OxyContin 160 mg PO q12h?

Answer:

No conversion between these two dosage forms is consistently reliable. A reasonable conservative starting point for an equivalent dose of oxycodone to transdermal fentanyl is 22.5–67 mg of oxycodone to 25 mcg/hr of transdermal fentanyl.[17] It is important to recognize that this equivalent is not bidirectional, as a conservative estimate in one direction could lead to an overdose when converting transdermal fentanyl back to oxycodone or another opioid.

Using the average of 22.5 mg and 67 mg, a reasonable equivalent dose of oxycodone to transdermal fentanyl is (22.5 mg + 67 mg)/2 = 44.75 mg. Rounded off, it is approximately 40 mg for each 25 mcg/hr of transdermal fentanyl. YE is currently prescribed 160 mg × 2 = 320 mg of oxycodone per 24 hours.

40 mg oxycodone/25 mcg per hour transdermal fentanyl
= 320 mg/x mcg per hour transdermal fentanyl
x = 200 mcg (2 × 100 mcg/hr patches) per hour
transdermal fentanyl

QUESTION 2

What issues of cross-tolerance need to be considered?
Because of potential for incomplete cross-tolerance, it is wise to reduce the converted opioid dose by 25 to 50 percent.[2,21]

The estimate for transdermal dosage calculation is conservative; therefore, a dose reduction of 30 percent might be unreasonable to the point of causing withdrawal, so a 25 percent reduction is chosen.

Transdermal fentanyl 200 mcg/hr × 75% = 150 mcg/hr
(2 × 75 mcg/hr patches)

The calculated dose is, therefore, 2 × 75 mcg/hr transdermal fentanyl with prescribed changes every 72 hours. Note that 15 to 20 percent of patients experience end-of-dose failure between 48 and 72 hours with transdermal fentanyl. In such patients, the patches should be changed every 48 hours because less than full-day changes often cause confusion and nonadherence.[22]

QUESTION 3

Dr. P. decided that he was uncomfortable prescribing breakthrough oxycodone/acetaminophen in addition to OxyContin and asks for you to include the equivalent of the short-acting dosage form in the conversion to transdermal fentanyl using the maximum allowable prescribed daily dosage of oxycodone 10 mg PO q4–6h prn.

Answer:

Rather than reducing this too for cross-tolerance, a reasonable approach is to use 10 mg × 4 doses (40 mg total) instead of the allowable 10 mg × 6 doses (60 mg).

Oxycodone 40 mg in 24 hours = approximately 25 mcg/hr of transdermal fentanyl

Therefore, the new calculated dose is transdermal fentanyl 175 mg per hour (1 × 100 mcg/hr and 1 × 25 mcg/hr patch) with q72h changes.

QUESTION 4

How do you transition from the oral to transdermal dosage form?

Answer:

Serum fentanyl levels increase gradually after initial application of a new transdermal patch, generally reaching a plateau 12–24 hours after application (mean time to steady-state serum levels). Levels will continually rise to a smaller degree over the next 72 hours. The peak concentration is generally achieved by hour 72, but steady state may not be reached until day 6 with q72h patch changes.[17]

Because of the large fentanyl dose required and variation in absorption, one might consider a lower fentanyl dose initially in combination with a lower dose of oxycodone. The rationale behind using these two extended-release dosage forms together lies strictly in using up a residual supply of the extended-release oxycodone in a case where the OxyContin had already been dispensed. This approach can be achieved by using half of each medication (i.e., OxyContin 80 mg PO q12h plus transdermal fentanyl 100 mcg/hr with q72h changes). Alternatively, the oxycodone could be given in the immediate-release form as 25 mg PO q4h using multiple-strength tablets.

For simplicity, we will use the theoretical equivalents established initially, that is, a complete replacement of all oxycodone using transdermal fentanyl 200 mcg/hr with q72h changes. Considering the pharmacokinetic parameters outlined earlier, we need to compensate for the initial absorption of fentanyl. Therefore, an oral oxycodone dose will be needed during the titration process at least on day 1. The easiest way to achieve this goal is to allow a single dose of OxyContin 160 mg PO when placing the first patch to allow the fentanyl time for uptake transdermally; the problem here is that we may have some dosage overlap or we may undershoot the mark. Therefore, it may be more practical to use an immediate-release formulation of oxycodone and allow the patient some leeway on the initial titration. OxyContin 160 mg PO q12h is equivalent to oxycodone IR 80 mg PO q6h, or 40 mg PO q3h. Using immediate-release plain oxycodone tablets (to avoid potential acetaminophen toxicity with combination products), we can achieve a reasonable titration schedule.

Recommendation: Place transdermal fentanyl patches 200 mcg/hr (2 × 100 mcg/hr) and change q72h. At the time of patch placement, the patient may take oxycodone 40 mg and repeat every 3 hours for three doses. If a fourth dose is needed, the patient should take half the dose of 20 mg to avoid another large oxycodone peak at the same time that fentanyl begins to become therapeutic. The fourth dose will be the last oxycodone dose.

QUESTION 5

What is the risk of replacing the currently prescribed OxyContin with transdermal fentanyl?

Answer:

Considering the previous aberrant history, caution should be used when replacing a fixed transdermal dose of fentanyl with oral oxycodone. If, for example, the patient was using half of the prescribed OxyContin, a replacement with the calculated dose of transdermal fentanyl could be fatal.

Recommendation: Consider a two-week supply of OxyContin until the previously pending results of serum oxycodone levels are available. Outcome: Two weeks later, the serum oxycodone level was reported at 124 ng/mL, and the quantified UDS was positive for cannabinoids. Upon review of Table 13-5, for each 20 mg of oxycodone we can expect a serum concentration of 15.1 ng/mL +/4.7. Setting up a ratio,

$$20 \text{ mg oxycodone}/15.1 \text{ ng/mL} = x \text{ mg}/124 \text{ ng/mL}$$
$$x = 164.24 \text{ mg per day}$$

Rounding this result off to 160 mg per day, it appears that this patient was using OxyContin 80 mg PO q12h, not the prescribed dose of 160 mg (2 × 80 mg) PO q12h. Therefore, the calculated fentanyl dose above could have been an overdose based on what was prescribed versus what was actually consumed.

QUESTION 6

Give an example of an opioid alternative that might mitigate abuse risk other than transdermal fentanyl, and explain why it might be a preferred prescription.

Answer:

Dr. P. decided that he will provide opioid treatment for this patient with a requirement to attend a substance abuse program. He asks you to recommend an opioid that may be less abusable, cannot be crushed for immediate release, and perhaps has a lesser street desirability. A reasonable alternative may be Embeda*, a formulation containing extended-release morphine surrounded by a naltrexone core. Crushing this dosage form results in immediate-release of naltrexone at a 4 percent ratio to morphine, the result of which would cause withdrawal symptoms in a regular user of opioids. But if used appropriately, less that 0.1 percent of naltrexone is released, which is not therapeutically significant in terms of mu-receptor blockade.[23]

QUESTION 7

What is a reasonable dose for the replacement chosen in question 3?

Using the calculated Embeda dose equivalent to the presumed intake of daily OxyContin actually consumed, 80 mg PO q12h and referring to Table 13-2, oral morphine 30 mg is equivalent to 20 mg of oxycodone. Setting up a ratio:

$$20 \text{ mg of oxycodone}/30 \text{ mg morphine sulfate} = 160 \text{ mg daily}$$
$$\text{oxycodone}/x \text{ mg morphine sulfate}$$
$$x = 240 \text{ mg morphine sulfate}$$

Reducing this dose by 25 percent for cross-tolerance:

$$240 \text{ mg} \times 75\% = 180 \text{ mg morphine sulfate}$$

The recommended prescription is Embeda 180 mg once daily (1 × 100 mg and 1 × 80 mg capsules).

CASE 2: CYP450 INTERACTION

HF is a 38-year-old Hispanic female who is well-known to her PCP. HF has trigeminal neuralgia to the left side of her face. She has been receiving tramadol 100 mg PO qid regularly for 6 years as a single agent, and her pain had been relatively stable for that time. Two years ago, topiramate was added for migraine prevention. Eight weeks ago she presented to her PCP with an elevated level of pain to her face, which she described as "getting worse over the past year." At that visit, she was placed on an escalating dose of carbamazepine, which she has been taking for 6 weeks at 200 mg PO bid. She receives Fioricet® prn for migraines and topiramate at bedtime for migraine prevention. This pain too has been relatively stable and her use of Fioricet has been minimal.

Problem List: Trigeminal neuralgia, migraine headaches, previous history of obesity (now at ideal body weight). Vital signs are within normal limits.

Current Medications:

Tramadol 100 mg PO qid

Fioricet Tablets, 1–2 PO qid prn headaches

topiramate 100 mg PO qhs

Height = 65 inches

Weight = 130 lbs.

HF presented to her PCP Dr. M. for an emergent flare-up of "burning pain" in her face that is now unbearable compared to her visit 8 weeks ago. She complained of a significant increase in the number of migraines and is using her Fioricet daily as compared to her previous usage of perhaps 8 tablets per month or less.

The patient has been previously stable on her topiramate and occasional Fioricet for headaches. Prior to initiating topiramate, the patient was quite obese. The topiramate served to prophylax against migraines and was attributable to significant weight reduction, which by the patient's report has resulted in an enhanced lifestyle, better diet, more exercise, and overall better health. Today she presents a bit panicked for fear that she is slipping back into her previous lifestyle because she is unable to exercise and carry out her daily routines because of increased face pain and increased frequency of migraines. She was hopeful that the carbamazepine would help, especially since for the first 2–3 weeks, the face pain clearly decreased to a livable level.

Dr. M. evaluated the patient and was concerned that HF was now on more medications than previous and the pain seems worse even though there was an initial benefit. Rather than adjusting dosages upwards and/or adding other medications, he decided to employ the expertise of his local pharmacist (RPH).

Upon review of the chart, RPH identified a number of potential issues.

QUESTION 1

Carbamazepine is a well-known potent 3A4 enzyme inducer. What medications in HF's profile are substrates to 3A4?

Answer:

tramadol

topiramate

butalbital (an autoinducer and active ingredient in Fioricet)

QUESTION 2

Trigeminal neuralgia was initially improved by the adding carbamazepine. Why?

Answer:

HF described an initial improvement to her facial pain for a few weeks following the initiation of carbamazepine. Following the initial improvement, her facial pain became unbearable and eventually her headaches progressed to a point where any relief by Fioricet only lasted up to 2 hours.

RPH made the following assessment:

a. The initial introduction of carbamazepine (an autoinducer) was likely beneficial for the trigeminal neuralgia.

b. Potent induction by carbamazepine can significantly diminish blood levels of tramadol and, because carbamazepine is an autoinducer, could likely diminish carbamazepine levels as well.[24]

c. Tramadol, topiramate, and butalbital are all 3A4 substrates, and serum levels of each may diminish significantly; therefore, it is feasible that the tramadol and topiramate became subtherapeutic. The butalbital levels may drop more rapidly than previous because of induced 3A4 isoenzymes.[25]

QUESTION 3

What therapeutic options exist so that tramadol and topiramate levels are maximized?

Answer:

- Increase dosages of tramadol and topiramate.
- Replace carbamazepine with an alternate anticonvulsant that minimally or doesn't affect 3A4 isoenzymes.

QUESTION 4

Given the options in question 3, what are the best therapeutic options?

Answer:

Rather than increasing the dosages of one or more medications, it is best to eliminate the culprit, which in this case is presumed to be carbamazepine. Recognizing that it was initially beneficial, one possibility is to use oxcarbazepine, which is most similar in activity and chemistry to carbamazepine. Oxcarbazepine is a mild 3A4 isoenzyme inducer compared to carbamazepine.[26] Another option is to raise the topiramate dose to ascertain whether significant therapeutic benefit to trigeminal neuralgia could be achieved; however, it is also a 3A4 inducer and may therefore have the potential to reduce serum tramadol levels.[27] Another option is to use a different anticonvulsant such as gabapentin, since it is not metabolized at all in humans and therefore does not affect any cytochrome P450 isoenzymes.

Recommendation: No answer is 100 percent correct. In the authors' experience, it would probably be best to use oxcarbazepine first because carbamazepine was initially beneficial. Elevate the oxcarbazepine dose gradually until benefit is seen. After the trigeminal neuralgia is under control and the migraines become stable, an attempt could be made to reduce the tramadol dose or even eliminate the tramadol.

CASE 3: METHADONE CONVERSION

Methadone is a synthetic mu receptor opioid with unique pharmacokinetic properties. It also has low affinity in the blockade of N-methyl-D-aspartate (NMDA) receptors. But the clinical importance of that effect is not clear. Methadone is highly bioavailable, and oral solid dosage forms may be crushed and/or dissolved without substantially affecting pharmacokinetics. It is protein bound to alpha-glycoprotein and widely distributed into body tissue. Methadone has a complex, long, and unpredictable elimination half-life requiring careful titration with washout time compared to other opioids. Equivalency ratios (although variable) are not bidirectional, because methadone remains behind for days, even after discontinuation. The average clearance time is 20–22 hours. Elimination half-life is variable with a range of 15–60 hours, with reported cases up to 120 hours. Inactive metabolites are eliminated by kidneys and minutely detectable in bile, feces, and sweat.

Methadone is FDA-approved for drug rehabilitation therapy and pain (malignant and nonmalignant). Methadone should not be administered for breakthrough pain due to its long half-life and resultant cumulative levels/effects.

Initial doses in opioid naïve patients should be 2.5 mg PO tid for pain, with titration as tolerated and/or until desired analgesia. All opioids have a biphasic elimination. Methadone has a uniquely long beta elimination resulting in subanalgesic levels accumulating over a period of 7–10 days with normal analgesic dosing. This long time to steady-state serum levels presents a real risk of accumulation toxicity if the drug is titrated up too rapidly or the patient takes extra doses. It is essential to strongly advise patients to take it only as directed, not to increase doses on their own, and to recognize that maximal analgesia may not occur for 7–10 days. Clinicians should always provide a short-acting, immediate-release opioid such as morphine or oxycodone for rescue doses during the first two weeks of therapy. If the patient is geriatric, renally or hepatically deficient, start at 2.5 mg every 12 hours or once daily and provide short-acting opioids for breakthrough pain.

In opioid-tolerant patients, the initial methadone dose must be individualized based on the previously prescribed opioid. Even though the methadone side effect profile is similar to that of other opioids, caution must be used to observe for latent opioid adverse effects or toxicities, varying from one-half hour to 7 days due to methadone's highly variable elimination half-life. When converting from other opioids to methadone, a complex conversion ratio is employed; several sources indicate that as the total daily dose of opioid increases, the amount of methadone needed to replace it decreases.[28,29]

Other important considerations include [an insignificant] QT prolongation in patients at high doses, especially in patients with concomitant pro-arrhythmic medications such as antidepressants. Use caution with CYP450 3A4 inducers, which may reduce methadone serum levels and/or analgesia, such as phenobarbital, phenytoin, carbamazepine, neveripine, and others. Methadone CYP 2B6 has recently been shown to have a major role. Previously, it was assumed that 2D6 was the major enzyme; now that does not appear to be true. In fact, (S)-methadone is primarily metabolized by CYP2B6, thus a poor metabolizer of CYP2B6 would be at increased risk for build up of the cardiotoxic S-enantiomer and is at higher risk for QTc prolongation, and Torsade de pointes arrhythmia which is associated with sudden death. Conversely, use caution with CYP and p-glycoprotein inhibitors, which may increase methadone serum levels, analgesia, and/or toxicity, such as erythromycin, clarithromycin, ketoconazole, and itraconazole.[30] When converting from methadone to another opioid, caution should be used to titrate the methadone downward by approximately 20 percent per day while slowly introducing the new agent to prevent overlap of methadone that will remain in the body tissue for days after discontinuation.

Methadone is inexpensive, available in several dosage forms, and requires generally only tid dosing for analgesia, although in rare cases qid dosing may be necessary. Theoretically, the weak NMDA inhibition may be helpful in neuropathic pain management, although evidence of a clinically useful advantage by virtue of robust controlled studies is lacking.

In short, while methadone offers many potential attributes over other opioids, it must be prescribed with extreme caution and only by those experienced and knowledgeable about the associated pharmacokinetics and potential adverse outcomes.[28-37]

Converting to Methadone from Morphine

LR is a 58-year-old white female who presents to her PCP with increased bilateral leg pain that has been diagnosed as diabetic neuropathy. She has tried several anticonvulsants previously, including gabapentin, pregabalin, and topiramate, but was unable to tolerate any of them. She was placed on venlafaxine with no benefit. She was eventually switched to duloxetine that was escalated to 60 mg PO qam with marginal efficacy. The duloxetine was eventually switched to amitriptyline 25 mg PO qhs, which has helped her sleep but had minimal if any benefit for her pain. After multiple trials with single and combined agents, she was placed on hydrocodone/acetaminophen. After more than a year of escalating doses, she eventually was switched to extended-release morphine with hydrocodone/APAP for breakthrough pain. Upon presentation to her PCP today, her vital signs are WNL

Height = 64 inches

Weight = 190 lbs.

Problem List: Type II diabetes mellitus, painful diabetic neuropathy, obesity, hypertension, hypercholesterolemia, hypothyroidism, osteopenia, and depression.

Current Medications:

Lortab® 10/325, 1–2 PO four times a day prn

Morphine SR 60 mg PO q8h

Calcium/Vit D (OTC)

Amitriptyline 25 mg PO qhs for sleep and depression

Levothyroxine 75 mcg PO qam

Pravastatin 40 mg PO qam

Alendronate 35 mg PO qam

Hydrochlorothiazide 25 mg PO qam

Acetaminophen 500 mg, 1–2 PO qid prn (maximum daily dose of acetaminophen combined with Lortab not to exceed 3,000 mg per day)

LR presents to her PCP, Dr. S., with a chief complaint of increased bilateral leg pain. Her most recent HgA1C was 8.3 percent. She has been using about 8 Lortabs per day in addition to her morphine, but she is not having benefit to her pain relief as previous. She is using all of her morphine exactly as prescribed and has never had a medication compliance issue. Dr. S. evaluated the patient and decided to initiate a trial of methadone.

Black Box Caveat

The authors caution and discourage endorsing any specific methadone conversion strategy. Although published strategies certainly provide starting points, none are definitive. Several authors have reported varying conversion formulae, all of which have been based on small sample sizes. A great deal of genetic polymorphism results in broadly varying interpatient responses to opioids,[4] particularly methadone.[35] For these reasons, we do not sanction any particular specific formula or authors' conversion guidelines due to lack of replicated data in good-sized controlled studies for which *a priori* power analyses have been done. Therefore, the authors recommend titration to response, recognizing that experience with one patient may not apply to others. The following case illustrates just one example of how to approach dosing with the provison that any calculations in this regard are only to give the clinician a general idea where the methadone conversion might fall. This example is not intended to work for all patients and may serve as a mathematical stepping stone only.

147

CHAPTER 13

Opioids

QUESTION

What is a plausible dose of methadone with which to replace the morphine and hydrocodone combined, assuming no opioid is offered for breakthrough pain?

Answer:

Using Ripamonti's 1998 conversion table.[24]

Dose Ranges	
Morphine (mg)	**Morphine to Methadone Ratio**
30–90	3.70 to 1
91–300	7.75 to 1
301 and higher 12.25 to 1	

If we choose a conservative conversion of hydrocodone to morphine, we can use a 1:1 ratio. This amount is below the equivalent dose of morphine; however, in this example, no dose reduction will be made for cross-tolerance in an effort to simplify the math. Therefore, we will use hydrocodone 80 mg = morphine 80 mg.

Morphine 180 mg + hydrocodone 80 mg
(equivalent to morphine 80 mg) = 260 mg morphine

260 mg morphine/*x* mg methadone = 7.75 mg morphine/
1 mg methadone

x = 33.548 methadone, rounded to 34 mg methadone

Alternatively, Fudin collaboratively developed the following formula, which he found useful in clinical practice.[38] This mathematical equation was based on Ripamonti's 1998 published methadone conversion table.

Many potential flaws exist with methadone conversions as outlined in the black box, but Ripamonti's approach is additionally significantly flawed at two data points where the formula changes. (See Figure 13-3.) Figure 13-4 is a mathematical attempt to smooth out Ripamonti's mathematical curve at each transition point and the formula eliminates those two flawed data points.

All calculations should be double-checked against traditional methods for methadone conversion and should be individually titrated.

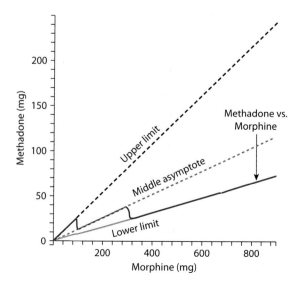

FIGURE 13-3. Relation between daily morphine and methadone dosages based on Ripamonti.

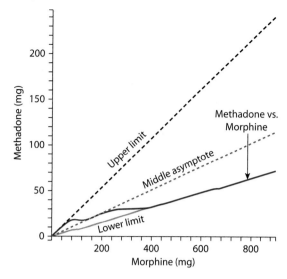

FIGURE 13-4. Relation between daily morphine and methadone dosages after smoothing.

Fudin Factor Copyright TXu 1-771-217

Fudin methadone conversion formula:

$$*\text{Oral methadone (mg)} = \frac{X}{21}\left\{5.7 - 3\sin\left(\frac{90}{\frac{110^5}{X}+1}\right) - \sin\left(\frac{90}{\frac{320^7}{X}+1}\right)\right\}$$

Using the derived equation to determine the dose:

Methadone equivalent dose (mg) = morphine 260 mg/21
× {5.7 – 3 sin [90/(110/260)5 + 1]
– sin [90/(320/260)7 + 1]}

Methadone equivalent dose (mg) = 12.38095 × 2.7 sin [88.8012]
– sin [17.0520]

Methadone equivalent dose (mg) = 12.38095 2.7[0.9997811]
– 0.293239

Methadone equivalent dose (mg) = 12.38095 × 2.6994 – 0.293239

Methadone equivalent dose (mg) = 33.421 – 0.293239 = 33.3916761,
rounded to **33 mg methadone**

Using the two methods, the final calculations are essentially the same (33 mg/day vs. 34 mg/day) in this example.

Because of patient variability, the morphine should be weaned as the methadone is introduced. Perhaps this patient will end up receiving around 30–35 mg of methadone after the titration.

Recommendation:

Continue morphine SR at 60 mg PO q8h.

Discontinue Lortabs 1–2 tablets PO four times a day.

Initiate methadone 2.5 mg PO q8h.

Each week, reduce the morphine gradually while slowly increasing the methadone dose. Monitor the patient for side effects and response during the titration process.

---

*Fudin J, Marcoux MD, Fudin JA. Mathematical model For methadone conversion examined. *Pract Pain Manag.* 2012;12(8):46–51.

CASES

CASE 1: SEROTONIN SYNDROME

SS is a 42-year-old female who presents to the hospital "just not feeling right." The patient has recently undergone detoxification about 8 weeks prior to admission and has been treated at a rehabilitation facility until about 4 weeks ago. During her stay at the rehab facility, the patient was started on suboxone 8 mg SL bid, paroxetine 25 mg PO daily, and quetiapine 50 mg PO tid. About one week prior to discharge, the paroxetine was increased to 50 mg PO daily and the quetiapine to 100 mg PO tid. The patient said that since she has been home, she was still feeling depressed, and the husband has noticed nightly tremors with shaking. For the past couple of days she has been having some difficulty breathing and she did not know who her children were yesterday. She thought one of the children was a radiator.

SS is currently complaining of a headache with some "foggy vision." She has had some muscle spasms and moments where she "feels like a lightening bolt is moving through her in waves."

Past medical history includes polysubstance abuse, chronic back pain (laminectomy surgery), depression, anxiety, smoker (about one pack per week), alcohol (prior to rehab) about 8–14 beers a day or one bottle of gin per night, and addiction to "prescription pain pills," with no know allergies to drug.

Medications:

Paroxetine 60 mg PO once daily

Quetiapine 100 mg PO tid

Suboxone (buprenorphine and naloxone) 8 mg SL bid

Ibuprofen 400–600 mg PO qid prn

SS was diagnosed with serotonin syndrome, admitted to the hospital, paroxetine and quetiapine were put on hold, suboxone was continued, and the patient was given IV hydration.

	Temperature	Blood pressure	Heart rate	Neurologic	TSH	Cr
Admission	100.3	101/63	106	Hyperreflexive, nystagmus, spontaneous clonus	1.36	1.3
Day 2	103	119/57	124	Agitated, disoriented		
Day 3	98.1	110/70	96	No twitching or myoclonus, somnolent		

QUESTION 1

Is the serotonin syndrome in this patient caused by a pharmacokinetic or pharmacodynamic drug interaction?

Answer:

Pharmacodynamic. The medications taken by this patient do not affect the absorption, distribution, metabolism, or excretion of each other to any significant extent.

QUESTION 2

Which of the following symptoms are suggestive of serotonin syndrome?

a. Tremor

b. Clonus

c. Hyperthermia

d. Altered mental status

e. All of the above

Answer:

e. All of the above. Serotonin syndrome can range from mild to severe and includes symptoms such as tremor, diaphoresis, restlessness, altered mental status, autonomic nervous system instability, and hyperreflexia.[39]

QUESTION 3

Which combination of medications most likely caused the development of serotonin syndrome?

a. Paroxetine + buprenorphine

b. Quetiapine + paroxetine

c. Buprenorphine + quetiapine + paroxetine

d. Quetiapine + buprenorphine

Answer:

c. Buprenorphine + quetiapine + paroxetine. Synthetic opioids have been shown to increase serotonin in animal models, and paroxetine is well known to cause serotonin syndrome due to its direct effects on serotonin reuptake.

QUESTION 4

Which of the following should be included in the differential diagnosis for this patient (taking into account medications and symptoms)?

a. Anticholinergic poisoning

b. Malignant hyperthermia

c. Neuroleptic malignant syndrome

d. None of the above

Answer:

c. Neuroleptic malignant syndrome. NMS should be considered in the differential diagnosis because the patient is taking quetiapine. Even though patients with NMS can have HTN, tachycardia, hyperthermia, and diaphoresis, they are usually bradyreflexic and present in a stupor or coma.

QUESTION 5

Which of the following vasoactive agents should not be used to control pulse and/or blood pressure in a patient with serotonin syndrome?

a. Norepinephrine

b. Dopamine

c. Phenylephrine

d. All of them may be used

Answer:

b. Dopamine. Dopamine should not be used because it is metabolized to norepinephrine and epinephrine. In cases of excess serotonin, monoamine oxidase cannot control the amounts of epinephrine and norepinephrine produced, which could lead to an exaggerated hemodynamic response.

QUESTION 6

Which of the following medications could be used to treat serotonin syndrome?

   a. Cyproheptadine 12 mg PT x1

   b. Benzodiazepines

   c. Both cyproheptadine and benzodiazepines may be used depending on severity of symptoms

   d. Neither of these agents is appropriate

Answer:

c. Both cyproheptadine and benzodiazepines may be used depending on severity of symptoms. In mild cases, supportive care, removal of precipitating drugs and benzodiazepines may enough to manage symptoms. For moderately to severely ill patients, 5-HT2A antagonists (i.e., cyproheptadine, mirtazapine, nefazodone, trazodone, and certain atypical antipsychotics), sedation, and even intubation may be necessary.

CASE 2: TRANSDERMAL FENTANYL CONVERSION DILEMMA

PK is a 91-year-old man who presents to a pain clinic with chief complaint of chronic low back pain. His problem list includes ocular hypertension, essential hypertension, osteoarthrosis of multiple sites, malignant neoplasm of the prostate, low back pain, CVA, peripheral neuropathy, pilonidal cyst without mention of abscess, sebaceous cyst, sensorineural hearing loss of combined types, nuclear sclerosis, primary open angle glaucoma, paroxysmal atrial fibrillation, onychomycosis, chronic kidney disease (Stage III, moderate), and anemia.

The following parameters are noted as of his last visit to the PCP.

HT: 69.5 in [176.5 cm] (03/28/2011 13:20)

WT: 182 lbs [82.7 kg] (03/28/2011 13:20)

BMI: 26.5 (3/28/2011 13:20:41)

BP: BP 118/58 (3/28/011 13:29:33) R ARM,STANDING,ADULT CUFF,CUFF-AUTOMATED

BP 124/64 (3/28/2011 13:20:41) R ARM,LYING,ADULT CUFF,CUFF-AUTOMATED

TEMP: 97.9 F [36.6 C] (03/28/2011 13:20)

RR: 20 (03/28/2011 13:20)

HR: 56 (03/28/2011 13:29)

Current medications:

aspirin 81 mg, 1 tablet daily

dibucaine 1% ointment, apply thin film rectally bid prn

docusate Na 50 mg/sennosides 8.6 mg, 1 capsule bid prn

dorzolamide 22.3 mg/timolol 6.8 mg/mL Oph Soln, instill 1 gtt OU bid

fentanyl transdermal matrix patch 75 mcg/hr, apply and change q72h for pain

gabapentin 60 mg PO qid

hypromellose 0.4% oph soln, instill 1 gtt OU qid

ketorolac tromethamine 0.5% oph soln, instill 1 gtt OD four times a day

lisinopril 20 mg PO qam

metoprolol tartrate 25 mg, 1½ tabs PO bid

moxifloxacin HCl 0.5% oph soln, instill 1 gtt OD four times a day

omeprazole 20 mg, 1 capsule PO before breakfast daily

prednisolone acetate 1% oph susp, instill 1 gtt OD four times a day

simvastatin 40 mg, 1 PO qhs

terazocin HCl 5 mg, 1 capsule qhs

travoprost Z 0.004% oph soln, instill 1 gtt OU qhs

The clinical pharmacist at the pain clinic evaluates the patient's medications following the patient's initial encounter with the physiatrist.

QUESTION 1

What findings in his profile might preclude this patient from receiving NSAIDs for maintenance therapy?

Answer:

Age, diagnosis of HTN, stage III kidney disease, a CVA with once daily ASA.

QUESTION 2

Assuming that your recommendation will be to switch this patient's opioid to another by the oral route, what must be considered in determining the dose conversion?

Answer:

Transdermal absorption of fentanyl in the elderly has been shown to be less predictable than the general population with reduced absorption.[12]

QUESTION 3

What are the risks of switching this patient to a theoretical equivalent oral dose of extended-release morphine 100 mg PO q12h?

Answer:

We don't know for certain that this patient is adequately absorbing fentanyl. If the morphine conversion is based on average absorptions, the calculated equivalent dose could be an overdose. With decreased kidney function, this patient is at risk to accumulate the active 6-glucuronide morphine metabolite, which could cause oversedation, fatal respiratory depression, and neurotoxicity.

Prior to making any changes, the clinical pharmacist ordered a serum fentanyl level in order to ascertain whether the fentanyl was significantly absorbed based on the average levels. As indicated in Table 13-5, an approximate expected fentanyl serum level for the 75 mcg/hr patch is 1.7 ng/mL +/− 0.7 ng/mL.

Ten days later, the report indicated fentanyl 0.3 ng/mL. As suspected, the reported fentanyl level is significantly lower than the predicted level based on his prescribed fentanyl dose. In fact, it is about half that of a fentanyl 25 mcg/hr patch.

The clinical pharmacist decides that a rational opioid alternative could be oxycodone, since this does not have the toxic 6-glucuonide metabolite associated with morphine.

QUESTION 4

Based on the serum fentanyl levels, what would be an equivalent dose of oral oxycodone with a calculated 25 percent dose reduction for cross-tolerance?

Answer:

If 0.6 ng/mL equates to a fentanyl 2.5 mg transdermal patch delivering 25 mcg/hr, then 0.3 ng/mL is approximately equal to fentanyl 1.25 mg transdermal patch delivering 12.5 mcg/hr. (See Table 13-5.)

Fentanyl 2.5 mg transdermal/oral oxycodone
40 mg = Fentanyl 1.25 mg transdermal/*x*
x = oral oxycodone 20 mg

Reducing this dosage by 25 percent for cross-tolerance, the oral oxycodone dose equals 15 mg orally per day, or oxycodone 5 mg PO tid.

QUESTION 5

What would have been the oxycodone dose prescribed if the clinical pharmacist had based her calculations on the prescribed fentanyl dose of 75 mcg/hr?

Answer:

Fentanyl 2.5 mg transdermal/oral oxycodone 40 mg
= Fentanyl 7.5 mg transdermal/x
x = oral oxycodone 120 mg.

DOUBLE-CHECKING:

Had the Clinical Pharmacist used the actual prescribed fentanyl 75 mcg/hr dose in this patient to convert to oxycodone, what percentage more oxycodone would the patient have received if in addition, a 25 percent reduction was not employed?

- If 30 mg represents a 100 percent increase over 15 mg, then 120 mg represents *x*% increase.

  30 mg/100% = 120 mg/*x*%
  x = 400% increase over actual dose

Had the pharmacist not calculated the fentanyl dose based on serum analysis, what would be the worst potential outcome of prescribing oral oxycodone at 400 percent above the actual prescribed fentanyl 75 mcg/hr dose with no reduction?

- Death

CASE 3: MORPHINE METABOLITES

MM is a 79-year-old male, hospice patient who has had his pain controlled with a continuous infusion of morphine (2 mg/mL) for the past several weeks. Prior to this past week, dosage increases have led to increased pain relief without significant side effects. Over the past 48 hours, the patient has been seeing cats on the wall, having uncontrolled movements, and his pain is worse with an increase in dose. His breathing is also worse, and the RN noted some pulmonary congestion. The nurses have also had trouble maintaining IV access. The patient's arms are bruised from all of the attempts to keep an IV going. Up until 48 hours ago, the morphine was infusing at a rate of 10 mg/hr. It is now at 12.5 mg/hr.

Height = 5′10″

Weight = 63 kg

Serum creatinine = 1.5 mg/dL

QUESTION 1

What is this patient's creatinine clearance using the Cockcroft-Gault equation?

Answer:

Approximately 35 mL/min.

QUESTION 2

Because this patient has decreased kidney function, he is at risk of accumulating morphine metabolites. Which [active] metabolite is most likely responsible for the new symptoms, especially considering the half-life?

a. Morphine – 3 – glucuronide

b. Morphine – 6 – glucuronide

c. 6 – acetylmorphine

d. Both a and b could be responsible

Answer: a

QUESTION 3

Which one of the following opioids is an equivalent total daily dose to the morphine that the patient is receiving?

a. Hydromorphone 45 mg IV

b. Fentanyl 3,000 mcg IV

c. Oxymorphone 30 mg IV

d. All are equivalent doses

Answer: d

QUESTION 4

Considering the patient's pulmonary congestion, decreased kidney function, and trouble with IV access, which one of the following opioids would be the best choice for transitioning this patient quickly?

a. Hydromorphone sc infusion

b. Fentanyl patches

c. Oxymorphone IV

d. All of the above would be good choices

Answer: a

QUESTION 5

What would be the best starting dose for this patient?

a. Hydromorphone sc infusion 1.3 mg/hr, with hydromorphone 0.5 mg sc q3h for breakthrough pain

b. Fentanyl patch 25 mcg/hr, apply q72h

c. Oxymorphone 1 mg/hr IV continuous infusion

d. None of the above are good alternatives

Answer: a

REFERENCES

1. Pasternak GW. Insights into mu opioid pharmacology: The role of mu opioid receptor subtypes. *Life Sciences.* 2001;68:19–20, 2213–2219.

2. Pasternak GW. Incomplete cross tolerance and multiple mu opioid peptide receptors. *Trends Pharmacol Sci.* 2001;22(2):67–70.

3. Xu J, Xu M, Hurd YL, Pasternak GW, Pan YX. Isolation and characterization of new exon 11-associated N-terminal splice variants of the human mu opioid receptor gene. *J Neurochem.* 2009;108(4):962–972.

4. Lötsch J, Skarke C, Grösch S, Darimont J, Schmidt H, Geisslinger G. The polymorphism A118G of the human mu-opioid receptor gene decreases the pupil constrictory effect of morphine-6-glucuronide but not that of morphine. *Pharmacogenetics.* 2002;12(1):3–9.

5. Violin JD, Lefkowitz RJ. β-arrestin-biased ligands at seven-transmembrane receptors. *Trends Pharmacol Sci.* 2007;28:416–422.

6. Blunk JA, Schmelz M, Zeck S, Skov P, Likar R, and Koppert W. Opioid-induced mast cell activation and vascular responses is not mediated by μ-opioid receptors: an in vivo microdialysis study in human skin. *Anesth Analg.* 2004;98:364–370.

7. Tuteja AK, Biskupiak J, Stoddard GJ, Lipman AG. Opioid-induced bowel disorders and narcotic bowel syndrome in patients with chronic non-cancer pain. *Neurogastroenterol Motil.* 2010;22(4):424–430.

8. Thomas J, Lipman AG, Slatkin N, et al. A phase III double-blind, controlled trial of methylnaltrexone (MNTX) for opioid-induced constipation in advanced medical illness, *J Clin Oncol.* 2005;23(16S Suppl).

9. Lipman AG, Karver S, Cooney GA, Stambler N, Israel RJ. Methylnaltrexone for opioid-induced constipation in patients with advanced illness: A three-month open-label treatment extension study. *J Pain Palliat Care Phamacother.* 2011;25(3):in press.

10. Chey WD, Webster L, Sostek M, Lappalainen J, Barker PN, Tack J. Naloxegol for Opioid-Induced Constipation in Patients with Noncancer Pain. *J Med.* 2014; 370:2387–2396.

11. Cook DS, Braithwaite RA, Hale KA. Estimating antemortem drug concentrations from postmortem blood samples: The influence of postmortem redistribution. *J Clin Pathol.* 2000;53:282–285.

12. Pounder DJ, Jones GR. Post-mortem drug redistribution—A toxicological nightmare. *Forensic Sci Int.* 1990;45:253–263.

13. Gourlay DL, Heit HA, Caplan YH. Urine Drug Testing in Clinical Practice: The Art and Science of Patient Care, 4th ed. California Academy of Family Physicians. Available at: http://www.familydocs.org/files/UDTMonograph_for_web.pdf (accessed April 25, 2011).

14. Collen M. The Fourth Amendment and random drug testing of people with chronic pain. *J Pain Palliat Care Pharmacother.* 2011;25:42–48.

15 Gerber JG et al. Stereoselective Metabolism of Methadone N-Demethylation by Cytochrome P4502B6 and 2C19. *Chirality* 2004;16:36–44.

16. Muijsers BBR, Wagstaff AJ. Transdermal fentanyl: An updated review of its pharmacological properties and therapeutic efficacy in chronic cancer pain control. *Drugs.* 2001;61:2289–2307.

17. Duragesic [package insert]. Janssen Pharmaceutica, April 2008.

18. Ashburn MA, Lipman AG. Management of pain in the cancer patient. *Anesth Analgesia.* 1993;76(2):402–416.

19. Labroo RB, Paine MF, Thummel KE, Kharasch ED. Fentanyl metabolism by human hepatic and intestingal cytochrome P450 3A4: Implications for interindividual variability in disposition, efficacy, and drug interactions. *Drug Metab Dispos.* 1997;25:1072–1080.

20. Moeller KE, Lee KC, Kissack JC. Urine drug screening: Practical guide for clinicians. *Mayo Clin Proc.* 2008;83(1):66–76.

21. Pereira J, Lawlor P, Vigano A, Dorgan M, Bruera E. Equianalgesic dose ratios for opioids: A critical review and proposals for long-term dosing. *J Pain Symptom Manage.* 2001;22(2):672–687.

22. Fudin J. Can fentanyl patches be replaced sooner to improve pain control? Available at: http://www.medscape.com/viewarticle/566115 (accessed April 25, 2011).

23. EMBEDA [package insert]. Bristol, TN: King Pharmaceuticals, Inc., 2009.

24. Gibson TP. Pharmacokinetics, efficacy, and safety of analgesia with a focus on tramadol HCl. *Am J Med.* 1996;101(Suppl. 1):S47–S53.

25. Tanaka, E. Clinically important pharmacokinetic drug–drug interactions: Role of cytochrome P450 enzymes. *J Clin Pharm Ther.* 1998;23:403–416.

26. French JA, Gidal EB. Antiepileptic drug interaction. *Epilepsia.* 2000;41(Suppl. 8):30–36.

27. Mula M. Anticonvulsants-antidepressants pharmacokinetic drug interactions: The role of the CYP450 system in psychopharmacology. *Curr Drug Metab.* 2008;9(8):730–737.

28. Ripamonti C, Groff L, Brunelli C, Polastri D, Stavrakis A, De Conno F. Switching from morphine to oral methadone in treating cancer pain: What is the equianalgesic dose ratio? *J Clin Oncol.* 1998;16:3216–3221.

29. Ayonrinde OT, Bridge DT. The rediscovery of methadone for cancer pain management. *Med J Aust.* 2000;173:536–540.

30. Fudin J, Fontenelle DV, Fudin HR, Carlyn C, Ashley CC, Hinden DA. Potential P-glycoprotein pharmacokinetic interaction of telaprevir with morphine or methadone. *J Pain Palliat Care Pharmacother.* 2013;27(3):261–267.

31. Utah opioid prescribing guidelines, Available at: http://health.utah.gov/prescription/pdf/Utah_guidelines_pdfs.pdf.

32. Cytochrome P450 Drug-Interaction Table. Indiana University Department of Medicine; Division of Clinical Pharmacology, updated May 16, 2006. Available at: http://medicine.iupui.edu/flockhart/table.htm. (accessed February 12, 2008).

33. Krantz MJ, Lowery CM, Martell BA, Gourevitch MN, Arnsten JH. Effects of methadone on QT-interval dispersion. *Pharmacother.* 2005;25(11):1523–1529.

34. Oda Y, Kharasch ED. Metabolism of methadone and levo-a-acetylmethadol (LAAM) by human intestinal cytochrome P450 3A4 (CYP3A4): Potential contribution of intestinal metabolism to presystemic clearance and bioactivation. *J Pharm Exp Ther.* 2001;298(3):1021–1032.

35. Toombs, JD, Kral LA. Methadone treatment for pain states. *Am Fam Physician.* 2005;71:1353–1358.

36. Goodman F, Jones WN, Glassman P. VA national guidelines: Methadone dosing recommendations for treatment of chronic pain. Available at: http://www.pbm.va.gov/monitoring/Methadone%20Dosing%20Final%20(Rev%20081103).pdf.

37. Li Y, Kantelip JP, Gerritsen-van Schieveen P, Davani S. Interindividual variability of methadone response: Impact of genetic polymorphism. *Mol Diagn Ther.* 2008;12(2):109–124.

38. Fudin J, Marcoux MD, Fudin JA. Mathematical model For methadone conversion examined. *Pract Pain Manag.* 2012;12(8):46–51.

39. Boyer EW, Shannon M. The serotonin syndrome. *N Engl J Med.* 2005;352:1112–1120.

CHAPTER

14

Phenobarbital and Primidone

DENISE H. RHONEY, PharmD, FCCP, FCCM, FNCS
KAREN J. McALLEN, PharmD
XI LIU-DeRYKE, PharmD
DENNIS PARKER JR., PharmD, BCPS

PHENOBARBITAL

Phenobarbital is a barbituric acid derivative with hypnotic activity and central nervous system (CNS) depressant effects. Phenobarbital is one of the oldest anticonvulsant agents still used in clinical practice. It is FDA-approved for short-term sedation/hypnosis and treatment of generalized or partial onset seizures and provides an alternative to treat refractory status epilepticus. It is less commonly used as the first-line anticonvulsant due to disadvantages such as cognitive impairment, respiratory depression, sedation, and significant drug interactions. The anticonvulsant activity of phenobarbital is thought to be due to its effect on postsynaptic GABA receptors, which increases seizure threshold but the full mechanism is not completely understood.[1] Phenobarbital has also been used off-label to treat alcohol withdrawal, neonatal seizures, febrile seizures, neonate hyperbilirubinemia, and adults with congenital nonhemolytic unconjugated hyperbilirubinemia or chronic cholestasis.

DOSING

Phenobarbital is available in an injectable formulation, which can be given intravenously or intramuscularly, and oral formulation (tablets and solution) (see Table 14-1). In adult patients, the recommended dose for sedation and hypnosis is 30–100 mg/day and titrated upward slowly to 400 mg/day. For epilepsy management, dosing is usually weight-based where an adult maintenance dose of 2 mg/kg/day would result in a predicted steady-state concentration of 20 mg/L. A case report suggests that dosing should be with total body weight.[2] If immediate therapeutic concentrations are required a loading dose of 15–20 mg/kg can be administered intravenously or orally in three divided doses every 2 to 3 hours. When phenobarbital is administered intravenously, a rate of no more than 50 mg/min is recommended to avoid toxicity with the propylene glycol diluent.[3] Maintenance dosing in children (1–15 years old) is usually 3–5 mg/kg/day and for neonates (<2 weeks of age) is 2–4 mg/kg/day.[4] Because phenobarbital has a long half-life, it can be dosed once daily; however, initially excessive sedation may limit the ability to use once-daily dosing. Excessive sedation can be minimized by gradually increasing the dose using the following schedule: Start with 25 percent of the final daily dose each evening for 5–7 days and if tolerated the dose can then be increased to 50 percent of the final recommended dose for the next 5–7 days and then 75 percent of the final recommended dose for the next 5–7 days. The titration to the final dose should be completed by the fourth week of therapy. Steady-state serum concentrations should be checked about 3–4 weeks after achieving the total maintenance dose. A serum phenobarbital concentration targeting between 10–40 mg/L is considered within optimum range for therapeutic drug monitoring (TDM).[5]

ADVERSE EVENTS

Adverse effects are listed in Table 14-2. The most common adverse effect of phenobarbital is related to CNS depression, which includes sedation, ataxia, fatigue, and confusion. However, in children and elderly a paradoxical effect may be seen producing insomnia and hyperkinetic activity.[6] Chronically, phenobarbital is associated with impairment of cognition, which is a major limitation for its use, especially a problem in children where memory impairment and compromised work/school performance may develop independent of the sedation properties. The intelligence quotient of children receiving phenobarbital was 8.4 points lower than other children, and these scores remained 5.2 points lower after the phenobarbital was discontinued.[7] Phenobarbital affects calcium and vitamin D metabolism leading to hypocalcemia, osteomalcia, osteopenia, osteoporosis, and fractures.[8-10] Although they are rare, dermatologic effects ranging from rash to Stevens-Johnson syndrome and thrombocytopenia/agranulocytosis have been reported with Phenobarbital and primidone. The rash is usually mild maculopapular, morbilliform, or scarlatiniform that disappears upon discontinuation of the drug. Hypersensitivity syndrome is rare (1 per 3,000 exposures, but fatal in 10% of cases) and can start with a severe rash that progresses into a purpuric or exfoliative dermatitis. Other signs of a hypersensitivity syndrome are lymphadenopathy, hepatitis, nephritis, carditis, and eosinophilia. This hypersensitivity is cross-reactive with other aromatic anticonvulsant agents like carbamazepine and phenytoin. Intravenous phenobarbital can also cause bradycardia, hypotension, and syncope. Phenobarbital is classified in Pregnancy Category D due to its propensity to cause serious fetal defects and neonatal hemorrhage and is not recommended during breast-feeding because it is excreted in the breast milk.

PRIMIDONE

Primidone is a 2-deoxy analogue of phenobarbital and was first synthesized in 1949. In the United States, primidone is approved for adjunctive and monotherapy use in generalized tonic-clonic seizures, simple partial seizures, complex partial seizures, and myoclonic seizures. Primidone is also considered to be a first-line therapy for essential tremor along with propranolol. Primidone rapidly converts to phenobarbital and phenylethylmalonamide (PEMA), which both possess anticonvulsant activity. The main anticonvulsant effects are thought to be derived from phenobarbital, but unchanged primidone also has anticonvulsant activity. It is thought that PEMA does not play a large role in the anticonvulsant effects based on its potency of only one-twentieth that of primidone, but PEMA does potentiate the activity of phenobarbital in experimental models.[11] The exact mechanism of primidone is unknown

TABLE 14-1	Dosage Formulations and Strengths	
	Phenobarbital (Luminal®)	Primidone (Mysoline®)
Injectable	30 mg/mL	—
	60 mg/mL	
	65 mg/mL	
	130 mg/mL	
Oral, Tablet	15 mg	50 mg
	16.2 mg	250 mg
	30 mg	
	32.4 mg	
	60 mg	
	97.2 mg	
	100 mg	
Oral, Elixir	20 mg/5 mL	—
Oral, Solution	20 mg/5 mL	—

but believed to work via interactions with voltage-gated sodium channels that inhibit high-frequency repetitive firing of action potentials.[12]

DOSING

Primidone is only available in an oral formulation. Patients 8 years of age and older may be started on primidone according to the following regimen:

Days 1 to 3: 100 to 125 mg at bedtime

Days 4 to 6: 100 to 125 mg bid

Days 7 to 9: 100 to 125 mg tid

Day 10 to maintenance: 250 mg tid

For most adults and children 8 years of age and over, the usual maintenance dosage is 250 mg tid or qid. If required, the dose may be increased but daily doses should not exceed 500 mg qid.

For children under 8 years of age, the following regimen of primidone may be used:

Days 1 to 3: 50 mg at bedtime

Days 4 to 6: 50 mg bid

Days 7 to 9: 100 mg bid

Day 10 to maintenance: 125 mg tid to 250 mg tid

TABLE 14-2	Adverse Effects Associated with Phenobarbital and Primidone
Concentration-Related	Idiosyncratic/Chronic
Sedation (≥5 mg/L)	Nausea/vomiting
Hyperactivity (≥5 mg/L)	Rash
Impaired cognition (≥20 mg/L)	Steven Johnson's syndrome
Ataxia (≥35 mg/L)	Toxic epidermal necrolysis
Coma/stupor (≥65 mg/L)	Megaloblastic anemia
Respiratory depression (≥85 mg/L)	Folate deficiency
	Aplastic anemia
	Hepatic failure
	Cognitive/memory impairment
	Intellectual blunting
	Attention deficit
	Passive-aggressive behavior (mood change)
	Connective tissue disorders
	Metabolic bone disease
	Fetal vitamin K deficit
	General joint pain
	Dupuytren's contracture
	Anticonvulsant hypersensitivity syndrome
	Suicidal behavior and ideation

For children under 8 years of age, the usual maintenance dosage is 125–250 mg three times daily or, 10–25 mg/kg/day in divided doses.

If serum concentration monitoring is required, then phenobarbital concentrations should be monitored instead of primidone.

ADVERSE EVENTS

The adverse effects of primidone are similar to phenobarbital, so please refer to the previous section. Upon initiation of therapy, primidone may be less well tolerated compared to phenobarbital due to intense dizziness, nausea, and sedation that may be related to high initial concentrations of the parent drug.

BIOAVAILABILITY

PHENOBARBITAL

All routes of administration (oral, intramuscular, or intravenous) of phenobarbital are readily and completely absorbed with an oral bioavailability ranging between 90 percent and 100 percent in adults and children.[13,14] In neonates, oral absorption may be variable and appears to be delayed and incomplete.[15] The injectable formulation of phenobarbital can be given rectally and is readily absorbed with >90 percent bioavailability.[16] The peak concentration following intravenous injection of phenobarbital is reached at 15–30 minutes post-administration, and >4 hours when given orally.[13,17] Phenobarbital is administered as the sodium salt, which is 91 percent phenobarbital acid (S = 0.91).

PRIMIDONE

Primidone is absorbed orally with a bioavailability approaching 100 percent. The bioavailability has significant intraindividual variability related to the different formulations/manufacturers. The time to peak concentrations in adults is 2.7 to 3.2 hours and in children 4 to 6 hours.[18]

VOLUME OF DISTRIBUTION

PHENOBARBITAL

Phenobarbital has a lower lipophilicity compared to other barbiturates, resulting in slower brain penetration, so an immediate onset of action is not expected. A few hours after administration, phenobarbital is found in near-equal concentrations in all tissues of the body. Phenobarbital is well distributed in the brain, and the concentration is in equilibrium with brain, cerebrospinal fluid, and free plasma drug.[19] Following intravenous administration, phenobarbital has a two-phase distribution with the early distribution to highly vascular organs including the kidney, liver, muscle, and heart (but not brain) and during the late phase a fairly equal distribution between all tissues except for fat.[20,21] Approximately 12–60 minutes are required for maximal entry into the adult brain with the rate of entry related to age; in younger patients, a more rapid entry may be observed.[22] The plasma volume of distribution of phenobarbital approximates 0.6–1.0 L/kg, depending on the age of the patient. Children and adults have a smaller volume of distribution (~0.7 L/kg) compared to neonates (~0.9 L/kg). Phenobarbital has minimal protein binding capacity of ~45 percent compared to other AEDs such as phenytoin and valproic acid (>90% protein-bound).[1,17,23,24] The drug is primarily bound to plasma albumin.

PRIMIDONE

The volume of distribution of the parent drug (primidone) approximates 0.6 L/kg. Protein binding of primidone the parent compound is approximately 25 percent. The distribution of primidone through tissues is similar to phenobarbital. Maximum brain concentrations occur 2 hours after drug administration. Primidone is also distributed to breast milk at concentrations of 40–96 percent of the maternal serum concentrations. Saliva concentrations seem to correlate with unbound plasma and cerebrospinal fluid concentrations.[18]

METABOLISM AND CLEARANCE/HALF-LIFE

PHENOBARBITAL

Phenobarbital is primarily metabolized through the liver via cytochrome P-450 and NADPH-cytochrome C reductase with <20 percent eliminated unchanged through the kidney.[25] The metabolite, p-hydroxyphenobarbital, is pharmacologically inactive and excreted in the urine in conjugated form. The total body clearance of phenobarbital in adults is 0.004 L/kg/hr (= 0.1 L/kg/day).[13,24] Therefore, it would be expected that for every 1 mg/kg/day of phenobarbital sodium administered a steady-state concentration of 10 mg/L would be achieved based upon the following equation:

$$C_{ss} = \frac{(S)(F)(Dose/\tau)}{Cl}$$

Phenobarbital has a long elimination half-life ranging from 50–160 hours (approximately 5 days) in adults. Therefore, it takes approximately 2–3 weeks for phenobarbital to reach steady state, and slow titration is important to avoid supratherapeutic levels.

PRIMIDONE

Primidone is metabolized by the cytochrome P-450 system (40–60%) and eliminated via renal excretion of the unchanged drug (40–60%), PEMA (50–70%), and phenobarbital (5–10%). Approximately 15–25 percent of an oral dose is metabolized to phenobarbital. The rate of metabolism of primidone into phenobarbital is inversely related to age; the highest rates in oldest patients (the maximum age being 55).[26] People aged 70–81, relative to people aged 18–26, have decreased renal clearance of primidone, phenobarbital, and PEMA, with a greater proportion of PEMA in the urine.[27] Primidone clearance following an initial dose varies from 0.012 to 0.070 L/kg/hr with a mean of 0.037 L/kg/hr.[28] Time-dependent changes in clearance necessitate an increase in dosage over time to maintain stable concentrations. The half-life of primidone ranges from 3 to 22 hours, with a mean half-life of 15.2 hours.[29] The half-life of PEMA ranges from 24 to 48 hours. Long-term dosing of primidone can alter its half-life potentially due to accumulation of phenobarbital, which can reduce the half-life of primidone. Thus, it may be necessary to shorten the dosing interval with chronic maintenance therapy.

Several factors can modify phenobarbital and primidone elimination:

- *Age*: The total body clearance of phenobarbital differs among age groups: the average clearance in neonates is similar to adults and is 0.004 L/kg/hr (0.1 L/kg/day), while clearance in children (1–18 years of age) is 0.008 L/kg/hr (0.2 L/kg/day).[24] The difference in the rate of clearance between neonates and children is a result of the maturation of the liver and production of the metabolizing enzymes. The elimination half-life of phenobarbital is therefore faster in children, with a range of 37–133 hours, compared to the adult and neonate ranges of 50–160 hours (approximately 5 days).[14,24] Limited information is available on any clearance alterations in elderly but it appears elderly patients require lower doses to achieve therapeutic concentrations.[30] The ability of neonates to metabolize primidone to phenobarbital is limited with a primidone half-life of 23 hours in neonates. In elderly patients both total and renal primidone clearance and half-life is similar to adult patients as a result a compensatory increase in nonrenal clearance due to a 30 percent decrease in renal clearance.[27] This result suggests a possible increase in the active metabolites of primidone.

- *Severe Liver Disease*: In severe liver disease, the metabolism of phenobarbital may be decreased where a 50 percent increase in the half-life of phenobarbital has been reported.[31] As expected, a lower dose should be considered in patients with liver dysfunction; however, no specific recommendations guide how dosage should be adjusted but should be related to the severity of the liver disease using the Child-Pugh score. A Child-Pugh score greater than 8 may represent a need to initiate therapy at 25–50 percent of the normal recommended dose and then monitor the patient closely for both response and toxicity with serum concentrations and clinical assessment.[4] A small study of primidone in patients with acute viral hepatitis did not find any alterations in pharmacokinetic parameters, although it was only a single dose study.[32]

- *Renal Impairment*: It is expected that renal dysfunction will increase the half-life of phenobarbital and primidone, and increased toxicity has been reported in patients with renal impairment.[33,34] Current data do not suggest empiric dosage adjustments are necessary for phenobarbital in patients with moderate-to-severe renal impairment (CrCl <30 mL/min) but they should be closely monitored.[3,35] Approximately 30 percent of phenobarbital and primidone is removed with hemodialysis, 7.5–15 percent is removed with peritoneal dialysis, and a significant amount is removed with hemoperfusion (sieving coefficient 0.86).[36-38] Clearance may be higher with high-efficiency hemodialyzers (up to 50%).[39] Supplemental dosing following dialysis is often required, but no clear guidelines indicate the amount required.[3] In adults on polytherapy and in children, approximately 40 percent of primidone is cleared via the kidney, with another 5–10 percent of an administered dose of primidone excreted via the kidney as phenobarbital.[40] Thus, the dosage of primidone should be reduced in patients with renal impairment, with a suggested 25–50 percent reduction in dosage in patients with creatinine clearance less than 30 mL/min.

- *Drug Interactions*: Drug interactions with phenobarbital have been described and are of varying clinical significance. Phenobarbital is a potent inducer of the cytochrome P-450 isoenzyme systems specifically CYP1A2, CYP2C9, and CYP3A4. Because phenobarbital is a metabolite of primidone, similar drug interactions are expected with primidone administration. In patients receiving concurrent enzyme-inducing anticonvulsant drugs, the half-life of primidone ranges from 3.3 to 11 hours. See Table 14-3 for a description of clinically significant drug interactions.

- *pH*: The elimination of phenobarbital is sensitive to body pH, where an increase in urine pH increases renal clearance of phenobarbital significantly.[41]

- *Nutritional State*: Patients with malnutrition may have increased clearance of phenobarbital and primidone, with a resulting decrease in half-life that can persist for long periods after refeeding.[42] These patients may need more aggressive dosing.[43]

TABLE 14-3 Phenobarbital Drug Interactions

Drugs Alter Phenobarbital and Primidone Serum Concentrations

Drug	Proposed Mechanism	Comment
Valproic acid Chloramphenicol Cimetidine	Enzyme-inhibition	Increases phenobarbital and primidone concentrations so doses may need to be reduced if these drugs are given concurrently. Serum concentration monitoring is necessary after starting or stopping therapy.
Phenytoin Carbamazepine Oxcarbazepine Rifampin	Enzyme-induction	Concomitant use of these medications enhances primidone conversion to phenobarbital, resulting an increase in the phenobarbital level.
Ethanol	Enzyme-induction	Chronic ethanol use may increase phenobarbital and primidone requirements.
Antacids	Reduction in absorption	May decrease concentrations.

Effect of Phenobarbital and Primidone on Serum Concentrations and Effects of Other Drugs Through Enzyme Induction

Drug	Comment
Atorvastatin Carbamazepine Clarithromycin/Erythromycin Corticosteroids Doxycycline Indinavir Itraconazole/Ketoconazole Lamotrigine Midazolam Olanzapine Omeprazole Oral contraceptives Phenytoin Risperidone Sertraline Sildenafil Simvastatin Theophylline Topiramate Tricyclic antidepressants Valproate Verapamil Warfarin Zidovudine Ziprasidone Zonisamide	Metabolism of these drugs is increased, which may necessitate higher dose rates to get adequate response. Close monitoring is recommended for evaluation of clinical significance.

CONCENTRATION MONITORING

PHENOBARBITAL

Several analytical methods can be used to assess phenobarbital concentrations. Gas-liquid chromatography may be performed to detect the unchanged drug or its alkylated metabolites; however, interference with the assay is significant. High-performance liquid chromatography can be used, but it is subject to interference with carbamazepine epoxide. Enzyme-multiplied immunoassay and fluorescence-polarization immunoassay are the most commonly used assay techniques because they have the advantage of rapid and accurate determination of concentrations in serum or plasma, but they also have a potential for cross-reaction with coadministered barbiturates.[5,44]

Phenobarbital exhibits linear pharmacokinetics where an increase in the dose results in a proportional increase in the serum concentration.[5,17] A minimum plasma level of 10 mg/L was found to be effective in controlling seizure activities. The upper limit of phenobarbital is controversial. Some patients exhibit toxic symptoms at a level above 30 mg/L where others tolerate a level greater than 40 mg/L. Common toxic signs and symptoms associated with a level >40–45 mcg/mL include sedation, nystagmus, ataxia, dysarthria, and seizure in severe cases. Concentrations above 100 mg/L may be considered to be potentially lethal.[45] Therefore, therapeutic level between 10–40 mg/L should be attained to ensure maximum efficacy and minimal toxicity.

Indications for serum concentration monitoring include loss of seizure control, possible toxicity, dosing changes, significant liver and/or renal impairment, dialysis, and addition or deletion of an interacting drug.[46] Ideally phenobarbital concentrations should be drawn immediately before the next dose to ensure a true trough. However, because of the long half-life, a random phenobarbital level can be obtained as long as levels are drawn consistently at similar time points to ensure correct interpretation.[5,23] Because steady state is not generally reached until 2–3 weeks, rechecking phenobarbital concentrations immediately following dosage adjustment will not accurately reflect the change. Routine monitoring of phenobarbital should only occur 2–3 weeks after dosing initiation or change; however, serum concentration monitoring may be necessary sooner to assess for the need of an additional loading dose or if toxicity is suspected. If concentrations are assessed following intravenous administration of phenobarbital, the sample should be drawn at least one hour after the end of the infusion to avoid the distribution phase.

PRIMIDONE

A poor correlation is found between serum primidone concentrations and the oral dose of primidone. A range of 5–12 mg/L of primidone has been suggested as therapeutic; however, only limited utility comes from using this guideline in using this clinically. It is recommended to measure phenobarbital concentrations to guide therapy; phenobarbital concentrations generally becomes detectable 24 hours after primidone initiation. A summary of the key pharmacokinetic parameters for phenobarbital and primidone can be found in Table 14-4.

TABLE 14-4 Key Pharmacokinetic Parameters of Phenobarbital and Primidone

	Phenobarbital	Primidone
Bioavailability	90–100%	~100%
Volume of distribution (L/kg)		
Adults and children	~0.7	0.6–1
Neonates	~0.9	
Protein binding	40–50%	25%
Clearance (L/kg/hr)		
Adults and neonates	0.004	0.035–0.052
Children	0.008	
Elimination half-life (hr)		
Adults and neonates	50–160	3–22
Children	37–133	(parent drug)
Plasma concentration (mg/L)	10–40	5–12 (parent drug) 10–40 (phenobarbital)

CASE STUDIES

CASE 1: LOADING DOSE AND ADMINISTRATION

JP is a 60-year-old female who presents to the emergency department with a diagnosis of intracerebral hemorrhage. She is 5′5″ and weighs 62 kg. Upon arrival in the intensive care unit, she is unresponsive. An EEG is obtained showing nonconvulsive status epilepticus. After administration of 6 mg of lorazepam and 1,000 mg of phenytoin, it is decided to start her on phenobarbital.

QUESTION 1

What loading dose of phenobarbital should be administered?

Answer:

Two methods can be used to calculate an initial loading dose of phenobarbital, the literature-based recommended dosing and the pharmacokinetic dosing method. Each method has advantages and disadvantages. The literature-based method is a popular method due to the ease of calculation, but it does not offer the flexibility of targeting a specific serum concentration. This method will generally achieve concentrations in the middle to lower portion of the therapeutic range. In addition, this method cannot be used if the patient presents with a subtherapeutic phenobarbital level and needs a loading dose to increase the serum level into the therapeutic range or if the patient has recently received a suboptimal loading dose. The pharmacokinetic dosing method is commonly based on population pharmacokinetic parameters and allows the flexibility of targeting a specific level.

If the literature-based recommended dosing method is chosen, it can be calculated in the following manner:

$$\text{Loading dose} = 15\text{--}20 \text{ mg/kg}$$
$$\text{Loading dose} = 62 \text{ kg} \times 20 \text{ mg}$$
$$\text{Loading dose} = 1,240 \text{ mg}$$

The targeted serum concentration dosing/pharmacokinetic dosing method can be calculated by using the following equation:

$$\text{Loading dose} = \frac{(C)(V_d)}{(S)(F)}$$

$$\text{Volume of distribution } (V_d) = 0.7 \text{ L/kg} \times \text{weight}$$

Because this dosage is given intravenously, the bioavailability F = 1.0 and the salt fraction S = 0.9 for phenobarbital sodium. In adults, the volume of distribution can be estimated at 0.7 L/kg. In most patients, a targeted serum concentration of 30 mg/L would be appropriate to achieve a serum level of 10–40 mg/L.

$$LD = \frac{30 \text{ mg/L} \times (0.7 \text{ L/kg} \times 62 \text{ kg})}{(1)(0.9)}$$

$$LD = 1,172 \text{ mg}$$

JP should receive a loading dose rounded up to 1,200 mg to achieve a serum concentration of 30 mg/L.

QUESTION 2

How should phenobarbital be administered?

Answer:

Phenobarbital can be administered either by intravenous push or diluted in an appropriate volume of fluid and given intravenously over a specific amount of time. The maximum infusion rate recommended to avoid toxicity (specifically hypotension) is 50 mg/min even though higher maximum rates may be found in the official product information. It is commonly divided into two or three portions and administered over several hours. This strategy can be used in patients to avoid cardiac toxicity from the propylene glycol diluents in the injectable dosage form. Phenobarbital loading doses can be rounded depending on the dosage forms available at each specific institution. It is important to monitor level of consciousness because higher doses of phenobarbital can produce somnolence and may require intubation of the patient. As mentioned earlier, phenobarbital is a cardiac depressant and likely will cause hypotension, particularly during infusion of the loading dose. Phenobarbital is stable in normal saline, dextrose 5 percent, and lactated ringers.[47]

In order to calculate the administration rate, you must first calculate the total administration time by using the following equation:

$$\text{Time of administration} = \frac{\text{Dose}}{50 \text{ mg/min}}$$

Next, the infusion rate in mL per hour should be calculated. The total volume to be infused is divided by the administration time. Because this calculation will give you the infusion rate in mL per minute, if the infusion pump is to be programmed in mL/hour, the rate should be multiplied by 60 minutes.

$$\text{Infusion rate (mL/hr)} = \frac{\text{Volume (mL)} \times 60 \text{ min}}{\text{Time of administration} \times 1 \text{ hr}}$$

$$\text{Time of administration} = 1,200 \text{ mg/50 mg/min}$$
$$\text{Time of administration} = 24 \text{ min}$$
$$\text{Infusion rate} = (100 \text{ mL/12 min}) \times 60 \text{ min}$$
$$\text{Infusion rate} = 8.3 \text{ mL/min} \times 60 \text{ min}$$
$$\text{Infusion rate} = 500 \text{ mL/hr}$$

Loading Dose Targeted to Increase to a Specific Serum Concentration

JP was given a loading dose of 500 mg over 10 minutes. A serum phenobarbital level was obtained and it was 10 mg/L.

QUESTION 3

What dose of phenobarbital should be given to achieve a therapeutic concentration of 30 mg/L?

Answer:

Using the pharmacokinetic dosing strategy, an additional loading dose can be calculated if a patient has a subtherapeutic phenobarbital level. The same principles are used as with initial loading doses, altering the targeted serum concentration to reflect the degree of increase desired. The additional loading dose to increase by a specific concentration can be calculated by the following equation:

$$LD = \Delta C \, (C_{desired} - C_{measured}) \times V_d$$
$$LD = (30 \text{ mg/L} - 10 \text{ mg/L}) \times (0.7 \text{ L/kg} \times 62 \text{ kg})$$
$$LD = 868 \text{ mg, rounded up to 900 mg}$$

Measurement of Serum Concentration

Although not yet at steady state, serum levels can be obtained following the loading dose of phenobarbital, which can determine whether an appropriate loading dose has been administered. As mentioned earlier, it is ideal to obtain serum phenobarbital levels immediately prior to giving the dose, but because of low fluctuation in levels between dosing intervals due to its long half-life, serum phenobarbital levels can be obtained at any time of the day.[5] When obtaining a serum concentration following the loading dose, it is important to allow enough time for distribution of the medication. In general, it is appropriate to wait 1 hour after IV administration to obtain a serum concentration and up to 2–5 hours for oral phenobarbital due to prolonged absorption.

CASE 2: MAINTENANCE DOSE WITH THE POPULATION PHARMACOKINETICS METHOD

SL, a 70-year-old male with a brain tumor, is being started on phenobarbital for seizures.

Height = 73″

Weight = 65 kg

QUESTION 1

What maintenance dose should he be started on to achieve a concentration of 30 mg/L?

Answer:

The maintenance dose is calculated by multiplying the desired concentration by the clearance (0.1 L/kg/day) and the dosing interval. Because oral phenobarbital is to be used for the maintenance dose, the bioavailability is approximately 100 percent (F = 1.0) and the salt factor is 0.9. The following equation is used to calculate the maintenance dose.

$$C = \frac{(F)(S)(D/\tau)}{Cl} \quad \text{where} \quad MD = \frac{(C)(Cl)(\tau)}{(F)(S)}$$

$$MD = \frac{(30 \text{ mg/L})(0.1 \text{ L/kg/day} \times 65 \text{ kg})(1 \text{ day})}{(1.0)(0.9)}$$

MD = 217 mg daily

Dose = 100 mg PO twice daily

QUESTION 2

If the patient does not receive a loading dose, how long will it take to achieve a level of 20 mg/L?

Answer:

To determine how long it will take to achieve a specific level, several equations must be used. The half-life of phenobarbital should first be calculated, followed by the elimination rate constant (k_e). Once this calculation is complete, the serum concentration after one half-life can be calculated by using the half-life and elimination rate constant. By dividing the desired concentration by the concentration estimated at one half-life, the time to achieve the desired concentration can be calculated using the following steps:

Step 1: Calculate half-life.

$$T_{1/2} = \frac{(0.693)(V_d)}{Cl}$$

$$T_{1/2} = \frac{(0.693)(0.7 \text{L/kg} \times 65 \text{ kg})}{(0.1 \text{ L/kg/day} \times 65 \text{ kg})}$$

$$T_{1/2} = 4.85 \text{ days}$$

Step 2: Calculate elimination rate constant.

$$K_e = \frac{0.693}{T_{1/2}}$$

$$K_e = \frac{0.693}{4.82}$$

$$K_e = 0.144 \text{ days}^{-1}$$

Step 3: Calculate concentration at end of one half-life.

$$C_p1 = \frac{(S)(F)\{dose/t\}}{Cl} \times (1 - e^{-ke \times t1/2})$$

$$C_p1 = \frac{(1.0)(1.0)\{200 \text{ mg/day}\}}{(0.1 \text{ L/kg/day} \times 65 \text{ kg})} \times (1 - e^{-0.144 \times 4.82})$$

$$C_p1 = 15 \text{ mg/L}$$

Step 4: Calculate number of half-lives to achieve desired concentration.

$$\text{Number of } T_{1/2} = \frac{20 \text{ mg/L}}{15 \text{ mg/L}}$$

$$\text{Number of } T_{1/2} = 1.3$$

Step 5: Calculate time to reach desired concentration.

$$\text{Time} = \text{Number of } T_{1/2} \times T_{1/2}$$

$$\text{Time} = 1.3 \times 4.82$$

It will take approximately 6 days to achieve a concentration of 20 mg/L if a loading dose is not given.

CASE 3: CALCULATION OF EXPECTED STEADY-STATE LEVEL

HR is a 50-year-old, 120 kg female receiving primidone 250 mg every 6 hours. It is recommended to obtain phenobarbital levels to assess dosing with primidone.

QUESTION

What concentration of phenobarbital would you expect to achieve at steady state?

Answer:

The phenobarbital concentration at steady state can be calculated by utilizing the following equation:

$$C_{SS} = \frac{(F)(S)(D/\tau)}{(Cl \times 24 \text{ hr})}$$

$$C_{SS} = \frac{(1.0)(1.0)(250 \text{ mg/6 hours})}{(0.1 \text{ mg/kg/day} \times 120 \text{ kg})}$$

$$C_{SS} = 83 \text{ mg/dL}$$

CASE 4: PATIENT SPECIFIC PHARMACOKINETICS

JJ is a 20-year-old male with a diagnosis of complex partial seizures who is being seen in the neurologist's office. He was discharged from the hospital on phenobarbital 60 mg twice daily and levetiracetam

500 mg orally twice daily. He had a serum phenobarbital level obtained this morning two hours after taking his morning dose, which was 9.8 mg/L. A target of 30 mg/L is desired.

Height = 71″

Weight = 95 kg

Serum creatinine = 1.2 mg/L

QUESTION

What new dosing regimen should be given for JJ's phenobarbital?

Answer:

Because phenobarbital and primidone concentrations increase linearly with dose, adjustment of the maintenance dose to achieve a specific concentration is relatively straightforward. The following equation is useful in determining a new dose. The new dose is equal to the desired new concentration (C_{SSnew}) divided by the measured concentration at steady state (C_{SSold}), then multiplied by the dose the patient was receiving when the steady state concentration was obtained (D_{old}).

$$D_{new} = (C_{SSnew}/C_{SSold})D_{old}$$
$$D_{new} = (30 \text{ mg/L}/9.8 \text{ mg/L})120 \text{ mg/L}$$
$$D_{new} = 367.3 \text{ mg, rounded to 350 mg}$$

Phenobarbital is available in several dosage forms, which should be considered when recommending the dose (see Table 14-1); therefore, the new dosage regimen should be 175 mg orally twice daily.

CASE 5: DRUG INTERACTIONS

XY, a 30-year-old female patient, has been receiving phenobarbital 60 mg bid for 6 years for the treatment of complex partial seizures after suffering a traumatic brain injury in a motor vehicle collision. The patient reports satisfactory seizure control over the past 2 years, but also reports that she has had drowsiness and difficulty concentrating at work in the past few weeks. Valproic acid 500 mg every 24 hours was added to her regimen for the prevention of migraine headaches 2 months ago. Phenobarbital concentrations were obtained 1 year ago and 1 week ago and were 22 mg/L and 32 mg/L, respectively. The patient, a mother of two children, has been using barrier methods for contraception and would like advice regarding the use of oral contraceptives (OCs) for birth control.

QUESTION

What recommendation would you make to XY?

Answer:

Phenobarbital is a potent inducer of cytochrome P450 (CYP) enzymes, particularly the CYP2C9 and CYP3A4 subfamily. It also can enhance uridine diphosphate-glucuronosyltransferase (UGTs). It is eliminated by renal excretion (25%) and is also a substrate for hepatic (75%) metabolism by CYP2C9 and to a smaller extent CYP2C19.[48] The effect of hepatic induction by phenobarbital results in a number of clinically significant drug interactions involving antiepileptic drugs such as carbamazepine, lamotrigine, and valproic acid, and a number of other drugs, including calcium channel blockers, oral contraceptives, and warfarin. Enzyme induction is a gradual process that involves protein synthesis, which may take several days or weeks to occur. The time-course of induction is dependent upon the half-life offending agent. Therefore, the effect of enzyme induction by phenobarbital may not be fully appreciated for several weeks based upon the prolonged half-life (~5 days) and time to reach steady state.[48]

Although other drugs can affect phenobarbital metabolism, few clinically significant interactions exist that alter phenobarbital metabolism because of the mixed nature (both hepatic and renal) of drug clearance and its low plasma protein binding.[49] Valproic acid is a potent inhibitor of CYP2C9 and is likely the agent involved in the most clinically important drug interaction altering phenobarbital metabolism. Clinical and experimental studies have demonstrated that coadministration with phenobarbital results in a 30–50 percent reduction in phenobarbital clearance with resultant elevation in serum concentrations.[50,51] Although not fully elucidated, this elevation may be the result of inhibition of both glucuronidation and glucosidation metabolic pathways by valproate.[52] The patient is complaining of an increase in cognitive and sedative side effects, and coupled with the reported elevation in phenobarbital serum concentrations, a significant drug interaction with valproic acid appears likely. Management strategies would include a reduction in phenobarbital dose to 30 mg bid or the use of an alternate agent for migraine headache prophylaxis devoid of an interaction such as nadolol. Phenobarbital may lower valproic acid levels but the significance of this interaction is less clear with reported reductions in plasma valproic acid levels of 10–76 percent.[53-55] Nonetheless, it would be prudent to monitor serum valproic acid concentrations if the two drugs are continued concomitantly.

Seizure disorders present a major concern for women of childbearing age. Women with epilepsy have a higher rate of pregnancy-associated complications such as eclampsia, preeclampsia, and spontaneous abortion.[56] Also, data from pregnancy registries suggest that several antiepileptic medications are associated with major congenital defects, particularly those receiving anticonvulsant polytherapy or valproic acid.[57,58] Antiepileptic drugs may have a substantial effect on therapeutic concentrations of oral contraceptives (OC), particularly enzyme-inducing agents such as carbamazepine, phenytoin, and phenobarbital. According to one population-based study examining the care of pregnant women with epilepsy, oral contraceptive failure was responsible for nearly 25 percent of pregnancies.[59] Both estrogen and progesterone are metabolized by CYP3A4, and enzyme-inducing AESs may reduce the concentration of OC by 50 percent.[60] Therefore, patients prescribed OC with concurrent administration of enzyme-inducing AEDs require at least 50 mcg of estrogen, and this dose should be increased if breakthrough bleeding occurs.[61] A more reliable option would be the use of a barrier method such as an intrauterine device (IUD).

CASE 6: DOSING IN PATIENTS WITH ALTERED VOLUME OF DISTRIBUTION: CRITICAL CARE CONSIDERATIONS

RY is a 50-year-old male who was admitted seven days ago with a 40 percent burn to the legs and abdomen after a house fire. Today, he has become hypotensive and started on norepinephrine and vasopressin most likely due to severe sepsis. He has a history of seizures and has received phenobarbital for several years prior to admission with consistent levels at 25–30 mg/L.

QUESTION

Would you expect any changes to RY's phenobarbital levels to occur during this admission?

Answer:

Critically ill patients can be challenging when dosing medications with a narrow therapeutic index. These patients commonly have alterations in volume of distribution, both increased as well as reduced. Acute changes in volume of distribution in critically ill patients are most commonly due to the movement of water from the intravascular to the extravascular space. Common disease states that can result in increases in volume of distribution include congestive heart failure, renal failure including patients on renal replacement therapy, liver failure with ascites, sepsis and major burns. Hypoproteinemia is common in critically ill patients and those with chronically reduced nutritional intake and can also reduce volume of distribution, especially in medications that are highly protein-bound.[62]

Little literature is available to direct practitioners in dosing of phenobarbital in patients with alterations of volume of distribution. In critically ill patients and those with suspected alterations in volume of distribution, therapeutic drug monitoring is essential. These patients should be regularly monitored to ensure changes of volume of distribution are recognized and adjustments made to prevent underdosing or toxicity.

In this case, because burns and sepsis may increase the phenobarbital volume of distribution, RY's phenobarbital levels may decrease and he may need to have his dose adjusted until the burns are healed and severe sepsis resolved. Closer monitoring of phenobarbital levels should be obtained during and immediately following RY's hospitalization.

CASE 7: DOSING IN OBESE/ UNDERWEIGHT PATIENTS

LK is a 16-year-old female (47 kg) who has been suffering from bulimia for several years. She presents to the emergency department after having a witnessed seizure and has an additional seizure once admitted to the neurology floor. She is hyponatremic and has low serum potassium, most likely due to vomiting. Her serum albumin is 1.1 g/dL.

QUESTION

What considerations need to be made when initiating maintenance dosing in this patient with severe malnutrition?

Answer:

Similar to patients with altered volumes of distribution, patients with extremes in weight can also be challenging, and little evidence is available to direct dosing for phenobarbital and primidone. Patients with malnutrition may have increased clearance of phenobarbital and primidone with a resulting decrease in half-life, which can persist for long periods after refeeding.[42] These patients may need more aggressive dosing.[43] One case report in the literature describes utilizing intravenous phenobarbital, which suggests morbidly obese patients should be dosed based on total body weight. This case reported a volume of distribution of 0.82 L/kg based on actual body weight, a clearance of 1.74 L/hr (0.22 L/kg/day), and a $T_{1/2}$ of 61 hours.[2] Although more evidence in this area is needed before dosing based on total body weight should be widely implemented, a strategy with dosing this patient population is to initially dose phenobarbital and primidone base on total body weight with close therapeutic drug monitoring.

LK should initially be given a loading dose of phenobarbital based on her actual body weight. Because LK's clearance may be increased, serum phenobarbital levels should be closely monitored to ensure therapeutic serum concentrations are maintained. From serum concentrations a calculated clearance for LK can be determined.

CASE 8: DOSING IN RENAL DYSFUNCTION WITHOUT DIALYSIS

BG is a 58-year-old female receiving phenobarbital 60 mg bid for her seizure disorder secondary to a stroke for the past 2 years. Since starting this regimen BG has developed renal impairment and her current serum creatinine is 2.5 mg/dL. A serum concentration has not been checked since initially starting therapy. The patient is in the clinic today complaining of difficulty in concentrating but has not experienced seizures during the past several months.

Height = 65″

Weight = 86 kg

QUESTION

Does this patient require dosage adjustment for renal impairment?

Answer:

Elimination of phenobarbital is through both metabolism and excretion unchanged in the urine. The exact amount excreted unchanged in the urine reported in the literature ranges from 10 to 50 percent.[63-65] The inter- and intraindividual variability in phenobarbital elimination require a cognizance of these discrepancies. The pH of the urine is an important consideration when assessing excretion, because alkaline urine facilitates excretion of unchanged phenobarbital, while acidic urine increases the reabsorption of phenobarbital leading to a prolonged half-life. In adults receiving primidone monotherapy, approximately 60 percent of primidone is cleared via the kidney.[40] In adults on polytherapy and in children, approximately 40 percent of primidone is cleared via the kidney. Another 5–10 percent of an administered dose of primidone is excreted via the kidney as phenobarbital.[40] These observations suggest that the dosage of primidone probably should be reduced in patients with renal impairment, with a 25–50 percent reduction in dosage in patients with creatinine clearance less than 30 mL/min. The amount of this reduction should be based on a determination of the plasma concentrations of primidone and phenobarbital. Current data do not suggest empiric dosage adjustments are necessary for phenobarbital in patients with moderate-to-severe renal impairment (CrCl <30 mL/min) but they should be closely monitored.[3,35] It is expected that renal dysfunction will increase the half-life of phenobarbital and primidone, and increased toxicity has been reported in patients with renal impairment.[33,34] Additionally no information is available on the impact of hepato-renal syndrome, although a reduction in clearance would be expected.

In this particular patient case, assessing a serum concentration is important when the patient is experiencing a side effect and likely has reduced clearance. BG's estimated creatinine clearance based upon the Cockcroft and Gault equation is 28 mL/min. Any dosage adjustments should be made based upon serum concentrations.

CASE 9: DOSING IN RENAL DYSFUNCTION WITH DIALYSIS

RU is a 65-year-old patient (72 kg) with chronic renal failure and a seizure disorder. He has been maintained on a phenobarbital regimen of 120 mg qpm for the past year. Recently his renal disease has progressed and now requires hemodialysis three times per week. Describe any alterations that may be necessary in his phenobarbital regimen and calculate the supplemental dosage that would be required if a measured postdialysis concentration is 7 mg/L and the desired concentration is 20 mg/L.

The extent of dialyzability of a particular drug is based on several characteristics of the drug including molecular size, protein binding, volume of distribution, water solubility, and plasma clearance. Drugs that are water-soluble, not highly protein-bound, and that have a small volume of distribution are readily removed by hemodialysis. Phenobarbital is sparingly soluble in water, is approximately 50 percent protein-bound, and has a modest volume of distribution, while primidone is poorly soluble in water, is minimally protein-bound, and has a modest volume of distribution, therefore both agents are at high risk for removal. Additionally the dialysis membrane, blood and dialysis flow rates, and type of dialysis/hemoperfusion will also determine the extent of drug removal. Approximately 30 percent of phenobarbital and primidone is removed with hemodialysis and 7.5–15 percent is removed with peritoneal dialysis. Clearance may be higher with high-efficiency hemodialyzers (up to 50%).[39] Supplemental dosing following dialysis is often required, but no clear guidelines indicate the amount required.[3] Phenobarbital is also significantly removed by hemoperfusion with a sieving coefficient of 0.86.[36,37] Supplemental dosing should be guided based on serum concentration monitoring.

To determine the amount of the one-time postdialysis supplemental dosing required the following equation can be utilized assuming a volume of distribution of 0.7 L/kg.

Supplemental loading dose

$$= (C_{desired} - C_{achieved}) \times V_d = (20 \text{ mg/L} - 7 \text{ mg/L})(50.4 \text{ L}) = 650 \text{ mg}$$

CASE 10: DOSING IN HEPATIC DYSFUNCTION

DZ is a 56-year-old (152 pounds) admitted to the hospital with a history of altered consciousness and irrelevant talking. His wife indicates that he has had abdominal "bloating" for the past 3 months that has been relieved with medication. He consumes approximately two bottles of alcohol everyday for the past 15 years. Examination revealed a drowsy but arousable patient with a flapping tremor, ascites, splenomegaly, and pitting edema. Vital signs were stable. Laboratory values include:

Na = 128 mEq/L

SCr = 1.5 mg/dL

albumin = 2.7 g/dL

total bilirubin = 2.8 mg/dL

platelets = 88,000 cells/μL

INR = 1.5

aspartate aminotransferase (AST) = 115 U/L

lactate dehydrogenase (LDH) =254 U/L

alkaline phosphatase (ALK) = 156 U/L

alanine aminotransferase (ALT) = 45 U/L

gamma-glutamyl transpeptidase (GGT) = 88 U/L

DZ develops tonic-clonic seizures while hospitalized and was given a loading dose of 1,200 mg intravenously of phenobarbital.

QUESTION

What maintenance dose of oral phenobarbital for DZ would achieve a concentration of 15 mg/L?

Answer:

Elevated serum concentrations of phenobarbital have been described in patients with severe liver disease.[33] Limited information is available; however, a 50 percent increase in the half-life of phenobarbital has been reported in patients with liver cirrhosis or acute viral hepatitis.[31] The difficulty in assessing these patients is that unlike renal dysfunction, no endogenous markers can be used to guide dosage adjustment. The Child-Pugh clinical classification can be used to determine the severity of the liver disease. The Child-Pugh accounts for various laboratory parameters as well as clinical symptoms and is scored as follows, where a score of 5 is considered normal liver.[66,67]

Assessment Parameter	Score 1 Point	Score 2 Points	Score 3 Points
Total bilirubin (mg/dL)	<2.0	2.0–3.0	>3.0
Serum albumin (g/dL)	>3.5	2.8–3.5	<2.8
INR	<1.7	1.71–2.20	>2.20
Ascites	absent	slight	moderate
Hepatic encephalopathy[a]	none (Grade 0)	Grade I–II (or suppressed with medication)	Grade III–IV (or refractory to medication)

[a]Grading: 0, fully conscious and aware; Grade I, drowsy/sleepy state (alert with stimulation); Grade II, stupor (semiconscious, drowsy, only responds to pain); Grade III, unconsciousness (no response to painful stimuli); Grade IV, coma (no response, but vital signs normal); Grade V, deep coma (unstable vital signs)

A Child-Pugh score of greater than 8 may represent a need to initiate therapy at 25–50 percent of the normal recommended dose and then monitor the patient closely for both response and toxicity with serum concentrations and clinical assessment.[4] This recommendation is the same for primidone. Alterations in protein binding or displacement from protein-binding sites may also be expected with severe liver disease, but because phenobarbital is not highly protein-bound (only 50% protein-bound in adults and children and 35% in neonates), dosing alterations is not necessary.

The first step is to estimate the maintenance dose for DZ assuming normal clearance since an estimate of clearance in liver impairment is unknown (0.1 L/kg/day). For the patient who is 152 pounds or 69 kg, clearance = 6.9 L/day.

$$\text{Maintenance dose} = \frac{(Cl)(C_{SSave})(\tau)}{(S)(F)}$$

$$= \frac{(6.9 \text{ L/day})(15 \text{ mg/L})(1 \text{ day})}{(1)(1)} = 104 \text{ mg/day}$$

Next determine the extent of liver failure for DZ using the Child-Pugh score.

Total bilirubin = 2 points

Serum albumin = 3 points

INR = 1 point

Ascites = 3 points

Hepatic encephalopathy = Grade I = 2 points

Total Score = 11 points

Because this patient has significant liver impairment, it would be expected that the clearance would be reduced, the calculated maintenance dose above should be decreased by 25–50 percent.

Adjusted dose for liver impairment

$$= (104 \text{ mg/day})(0.25) = 26 \text{ mg reduction at } 25\% = 78 \text{ mg/day}$$

$$= (104 \text{ mg/day})(0.5) = 52 \text{ mg reduction at } 50\% = 52 \text{ mg/day}$$

$$\text{Adjusted dose} = 52–78 \text{ mg/day}$$

To decide on the dose, you must consider the dosage formulation that you are going to use. Phenobarbital is available as an oral elixir, solution, or oral tablets (see Table 14-1). For ease of administration using oral tablets, a starting dose of 60 mg/day would be appropriate.

CASE 11: SPECIAL CONSIDERATIONS

Dosing in Neonates

SM is a two-day-old neonate born at 32 weeks' gestation (3.75 pounds, or 1,702 grams) with germinal matrix intraventricular hemorrhage. SM developed tonic seizure activity and it was decided to initiate intravenous phenobarbital after ruling out all other causes of the seizure activity.

QUESTION

Calculate a loading and maintenance dose for SM.

Answer:

Neonatal seizures by definition occur within the first 4 weeks of life in a full-term infant and up to 44 weeks from conception for premature infants. Seizures are most frequent during the first 10 days of life. Because of multiple etiologies for neonatal seizures, it is essential to rule out common metabolic and infectious causes prior to initiating anticonvulsant agents. Seizures due to intraventricular hemorrhage occur in preterm infants generally 2–7 days after delivery. Phenobarbital injection is commonly used in the treatment of neonatal seizures.

Phenobarbital volume of distribution varies, depending on age, with volumes relative to body weight largest at birth through infancy. The estimated volume of distribution for neonates is 0.96 ± 0.02 L/kg, which may be increased further with ECMO.[68] Protein binding in neonates is estimated at 36.8 ± 17.2 percent.[68] The clearance and half-life of phenobarbital is age dependent. Estimated values for neonates and infants include: Cl = 0.0047 ± 0.0002 L/hr/kg with about 0.2 to 0.6 fraction of the parent drug excreted in urine and half-life = 111 ± 34 hours with a correlated time to steady state of 16 to 30 days.[69,70] Due to the extended half-life, neonates may require lower maintenance doses. The recommended therapeutic concentration for neonatal seizures is 20–30 mg/L.

Dosing in these patients is commonly accomplished with standard weight-based dosing recommendations based upon previously published data. The standard dose is 20 mg/kg/IV slowly over 20 minutes (not faster than 1 mg/kg/min). If seizures persist after completion of this loading dose, repeat doses of phenobarbital 10 mg/kg may be used every 20–30 minutes until a total dose of 40 mg/kg has been given. The maintenance dose is 3–5 mg/kg/day in 1–2 divided doses, started 12 hours after the loading dose.[69-71] The expected response is 40 percent to the initial 20 mg/kg loading dose of phenobarbital and 70 percent to a total of 40 mg/kg of phenobarbital.[72] An intravenous loading dose has been shown to achieve therapeutic levels within 2 hours.[73] It is recommended to follow serum concentrations closely in neonates.

To calculate the dosage, use the following equations:

$$\text{Loading dose} = \frac{(C)(V)}{(S)(F)}$$

Because this dose is given intravenously, F = 1.0 and the salt fraction S = 0.9 for phenobarbital sodium. The volume of distribution can estimated at 0.9 L/kg and the desired concentration to achieve is 20 mg/L.

$$LD = \frac{(20 \text{ mg/L})(0.9 \text{ L/kg})(1.5 \text{ kg})}{(0.9)(1.0)} = 30 \text{ mg, which is also equivalent to } 20 \text{ mg/kg}$$

$$\text{Maintenance dose} = \frac{(Cl)(C_{SSave})(\tau)}{(S)(F)}$$

Clearance is a major determinant of phenobarbital maintenance dosing and can be estimated for preterm neonates as 0.0047 L/hr/kg, so for SM it would be 0.00705 L/hr, or 0.1692 L/day. The desired concentration to achieve is 20 mg/L. Because this dose is given intravenously, F = 1.0 and the S = 0.9 for phenobarbital sodium.

$$MD = \frac{(0.1692 \text{ L/day})(20 \text{ mg/L})(1 \text{ day})}{(0.9)(1.0)} = 3.76 \text{ mg/day (can be divided every 12 hours)}$$

Dosing in Elderly Patients

AG is an 82-year-old male receiving phenobarbital 150 mg PO qd for complex partial seizures that has been refractory to many other regimens. He has been on his current phenobarbital regimen for the past 3 months without any seizure activity. The first serum concentration that was obtained on this dosing regimen 2 months ago was 25 mg/L. He presented to the clinic today complaining of increasing sleepiness, which is significantly impairing his daily activities. A serum concentration of 45 mg/L was obtained. Because the patient is experiencing a concentration related adverse effect, it was decided to adjust his regimen to achieve a target concentration of 25 mg/L.

Height = 5′9″

Weight = 65 kg

QUESTION

Calculate a new maintenance regimen designed to achieve a phenobarbital concentration of 25 mg/L.

Answer:

The use of phenobarbital in elderly patients is limited due to the significant adverse effects this agent has on cognition, and decreased bone density increases the risk of fractures. Only limited data are available describing potential alterations in absorption, volume of distribution, plasma protein binding, and half-life of phenobarbital in elderly patients.[74] Therefore, estimates for adult patients should be used and include V_d = 0.61 L/kg, 51 percent protein binding, and half-life of 96 hours. The true impact of aging on phenobarbital metabolism is poorly described, however, and clearance appears to be significantly reduced in older versus younger patients with epilepsy (2.5 vs. 4.9 mL/kg/hr). This same study showed that total daily doses required to achieve a therapeutic concentration of 15 mg/L were also lower (0.9 vs. 1.75 mg/kg).[30] Because approximately 30 percent of phenobarbital is excreted unchanged in the urine, it may be expected that elderly patients will require lower doses to achieve therapeutic concentrations. Literature-based dosing recommendations for elderly patients (>65 years of age) include a loading dose of 10–20 mg/kg and maintenance dose of 1.1–2 mg/kg/day. Unlike phenobarbital, total clearance of primidone is similar for elderly and younger adult patients. However, the reduced ability of elderly patients to excrete unchanged primidone has led to increased PEMA formation.[27] Additionally, because primidone is metabolized to phenobarbital, it may be necessary to reduce the primidone dose to account for the reduced clearance of phenobarbital in elderly patients.

The first step to solving this problem is to calculate phenobarbital steady-state clearance. It would be expected to achieve steady state in 17–24 days in adult patients so the steady-state equation can be utilized.

$$CL = \frac{F(D/\tau)}{C_{SS}} = \frac{1(150 \text{ mg}/24 \text{ h})}{45 \text{ mg/L}} = 0.14 \text{ L/hr}$$

The next step is to calculate the new phenobarbital dose using the calculated clearance, assuming complete oral absorption (F = 1.0).

$$\text{Dose} = \frac{(C_{SS})(Cl)(\tau)}{F} = \frac{(25 \text{ mg/L})(0.14 \text{ L/hr})(24 \text{ hr})}{1} = 84 \text{ mg qd, or } 1.3 \text{ mg/kg/day}$$

The dose could be divided into twice-daily dosing to minimize any adverse effects; however, phenobarbital is typically given once daily due to its long half-life. If given once daily it is recommended to advise the patient to take it at bedtime to minimize daytime sedation. A steady-state trough concentration should be measured 3–4 weeks after the new dosing regimen is initiated.

CASE 12: MANAGEMENT OF OVERDOSE

KL is a 3-year-old (25 kg) male who ingested a bottle of his father's prescription of phenobarbital 100 mg tablets. The prescription was filled 15 days ago so it was estimated he ingested 30 pills equaling 3,000 mg. KL was taken by ambulance to the emergency department where his consciousness declined, became hypotensive, and was intubated. Upon examination, SL's deep tendon reflexes are intact, and he is able to respond to painful stimuli. A phenobarbital level was obtained, which was 98 mg/L. All other laboratory values are normal and his ABG does not indicated acidosis.

QUESTION

What treatment should be initiated for KL?

Answer:

Due to the prolonged half-life of phenobarbital, treatment of overdose can be challenging. Overdose in adults has become less common and is most often due to intentional ingestion. Mild intoxication can be a result of decreased clearance or alterations in protein binding, allowing increases in free drug. In children, overdose is most commonly accidental whereby the child ingests phenobarbital, or in the cases of medication errors where the child is unintentionally given a higher dose than prescribed. Due to the prolonged half-life, withdrawal reactions are uncommon following overdose.

Mild intoxications are typically non-life-threatening and usually are accompanied by somnolence, mild disorientation, impaired judgment, and nystagmus. However, these patients most commonly will remain arousable with normal vital signs and reflexes. Mild intoxication is treated with supportive therapy. Moderate intoxication results in depressed mental status, slowed respirations, and depressed reflexes, although corneal reflexes are not abnormal. Moderate intoxication is treated with closer observation and is associated with doses of five to ten times the normal dose of the medication.[75] Severe intoxication can be life threatening and requires intensive care management. Patients may become unresponsive, exhibit slow shallow respirations, with absent reflexes, absent gag reflex, hypothermia, hypotension, and the potential for severe brain damage from anoxia.

Grading scale of phenobarbital overdose[76]:

Grade 1   Serum levels 35–80 mg/L
          Lethargic but arousable
          Able to answer questions

Grade 2   Serum levels 65–117 mg/L
          Withdraws to painful stimuli
          Deep tendon reflexes intact

Grade 3   Unresponsive to pain
          Deep tendon reflexes absent

Grade 4   Serum levels above 100 mg/L
          Respiratory depression
          Cardiac depression

Activated charcoal can be used to enhance elimination. It is more effective in binding medications that are weak acids or bases, of which phenobarbital is a weak acid. Because the half-life of phenobarbital is prolonged, multiple doses of activated charcoal to enhance elimination are recommended. In a prospective evaluation, it was found that multiple doses of activated charcoal reduced the half-life of phenobarbital from 93 hours to 36 hours.[77] Activated charcoal is safer when used in patients with protected airways to reduce the chance of aspiration. In addition, a cathartic should be administered when using multiple doses of activated charcoal to reduce the risk of abdominal distention and bowel ischemia. The recommended regimen of activated charcoal is to give an initial dose of 50 grams with 250 mL magnesium citrate followed by 17 grams activated charcoal in 70 mL of 70 percent sorbitol every 4 hours.

Because resorption of phenobarbital occurs in the distal tubule, the half-life can also be reduced by hydration and diuresis. Phenobarbital is a weak acid, so alkalinization of the urine is a noninvasive strategy that may increase clearance by increasing ionization of the drug, slowing resorption in the distal tubule and enhancing elimination. The pH of the urine should be kept between 7.5 and 8.0.

Hemoperfusion against polymer-coated charcoal or against a resin is a useful strategy for eliminating phenobarbital but it will not correct acid-base or electrolyte disturbances. Barbiturates are cleared 2–4 times faster with hemoperfusion than with hemodialysis. Hemoperfusion is also associated with platelet consumption, hypothermia, hypotension, and decreases in serum calcium. This strategy should be reserved for the most severe cases of overdose.[75] Hemodialysis has been utilized in the treatment of many overdoses. Hemodialysis can be useful for enhancing the clearance of some medications as well as treatment of acid-base or electrolyte disturbances. Hemodialysis is usually ineffective for eliminating drugs that are highly protein-bound. Due to the adverse effects associated with hemoperfusion, hemodialysis is more commonly used and can enhance elimination of phenobarbital.[78]

KL is exhibiting symptoms of a Grade 2 coma and should therefore be managed with supportive therapy and enhanced elimination. Gastric lavage can be utilized because it has been less than 4 hours since ingestion. He should be given supportive therapy in the intensive care unit and observed closely for progression of coma. Repeated doses of activated charcoal should be administered until coma resolves and he can be extubated. Alkalinization of the urine may also be a useful strategy to enhance elimination. At this time, hemodialysis and hemoperfusion are not indicated.

PROBLEMS

1. *JG is a 3-year-old (35 lbs) who presented to the emergency department with complex febrile seizures. After reducing his temperature with acetaminophen, JG experienced another seizure. It was decided to begin JG on phenobarbital and you have been asked to calculate an appropriate maintenance dose. Calculate a maintenance dose using population-based pharmacokinetic parameters to a goal serum concentration of 20 mg/L and calculate a weight-based dose.*

Answer:

To calculate the maintenance dose using population-specific parameters, use the following equation with a clearance of 0.008 L/kg/hr in children:

$$\text{Maintenance dose} = \frac{(Cl)(C_{SSave})(\tau)}{(S)(F)}$$

$$= \frac{(0.008 \text{ L/kg/hr} \times 16 \text{ kg})(20 \text{ mg/L})(24 \text{ hours})}{(0.9)(1.0)} = 68 \text{ mg/day}$$

Maintenance dosing in children (1–15 years old) is usually 3–5 mg/kg/day, so for JG this dose would range from 48–80 mg/day. A dose of 60 mg/day would be appropriate for JG. When initiating therapy it is recommended to start with 25 percent of the final recommended dose each evening for the first 5–7 days. The dose can then be increased to 50 percent of the final recommended dose for the next 5–7 days and then 75 percent of the final recommended dose for the next 5–7 days. The titration to the final dose should be complete by the fourth week of therapy. Steady-state serum concentrations should be checked 3–4 weeks after achieving the total maintenance dose.

2. *AV is a 48-year-old (80 kg) patient who presents to the emergency department with status epilepticus due to noncompliance with his anticonvulsants. The patient received 1,300 mg of intravenous phenobarbital at an infusion rate of 25 mg/min. You have been asked to calculate the expected phenobarbital concentration AV would achieve after his loading dose. When would you recommend checking a serum concentration?*

Answer:

To calculate the predicted concentration achieved from a loading dose, the following equation can be used.

$$C = \frac{(S)(F)(\text{Loading dose})}{V_d} = \frac{(1)(1)(1,300 \text{ mg})}{(0.7 \text{ L/kg})(80 \text{ kg})} = 23 \text{ mg/L}$$

The serum concentration should be drawn at least one hour after the end of the infusion to avoid the distribution phase.

3. *BB is an 8-year-old patient with a history of asthma, allergic rhinitis, and complex partial seizures. The patient has no known drug allergies and weighs 30 kg. The patient's parents report satisfactory control of his seizures on phenobarbital 15 mg per day for 1 year. Unfortunately, BB has had poor control of his asthma over the past couple of years. Despite therapy with fluticasone MDI, salmeterol, and montelukast, he has had three emergency department (ED) visits in the past calendar year. Yesterday BB was discharged from the ED with a prescription for prednisone 20 mg PO daily for 14 days. Describe any expected drug interactions in this case.*

Phenobarbital is a potent inducer of CYP2C9 and CYP3A4 enzymes, which could contribute to worsened control of this patient's asthma. Because corticosteroids are metabolized by CYP3A4, lower systemic concentrations would be anticipated with concomitant use of phenobarbital. This consideration is particularly important with oral administration of prednisone. Several cases have indicated that phenobarbital can enhance metabolic clearance of steroids by ~80 percent, and worsening symptoms in asthmatics has been reported. This interaction has also been described in other patients receiving concurrent corticosteroids and phenobarbital or primidone, including renal transplant patients.[79-83] The clinical significance of this interaction on inhaled corticosteroids is unclear. Enzyme inhibitors such as ritonavir and itraconazole have been shown to substantially increase systemic concentrations and potentiate toxicity. It follows that an enzyme inducer would reduce serum levels, but the consequence of a reduction in efficacy has not been reported.

Inhaled corticosteroids provide the most effective therapy for patients with persistent asthma. In addition to encouraging compliance, proper inhaler technique, and avoidance of triggers, BB should use high dose (>352 mcg per day) fluticasone based on NHLBI guidelines. The patient has been prescribed prednisone 10 mg daily, which is at low end of the recommended dosing range (1–2 mg/kg/day) for this patient. Because BB is already taking an enzyme inducer, a higher dose of 40 mg daily would be seem more appropriate.

REFERENCES

1. Bruni J, Albright PS. The clinical pharmacology of antiepileptic drugs. *Clin Neuropharmacol.* 1984;7:1–34.
2. Wilkes L, Danziger LH, Rodvold KA. Phenobarbital pharmacokinetics in obesity. A case report. *Clin Pharmacokinet.* 1992;22:481–484.
3. Gal P. Phenobarbital and primidone. In: Taylor WJ, Diers Caviness MH, (Eds.). *A Textbook for the Clinical Application of Therapeutic Drug Monitoring.* Irving: Abbott Laboratories Diagnostics Division; 1986:237–252.
4. Thomson AH, Brodie MJ. Pharmacokinetic optimisation of anticonvulsant therapy. *Clin Pharmacokinet.* 1992;23:216–230.
5. Patsalos PN, Berry DJ, Bourgeois BF, et al. Antiepileptic drugs—Best practice guidelines for therapeutic drug monitoring: A position paper by the subcommission on therapeutic drug monitoring, ILAE Commission on Therapeutic Strategies. *Epilepsia.* 2008;49:1239–1276.
6. Ounsted C. The hyperkinetic syndrome in epileptic children. *Lancet.* 1955;269:303–311.
7. Farwell JR, Lee YJ, Hirtz DG, Sulzbacher SI, Ellenberg JH, Nelson KB. Phenobarbital for febrile seizures—Effects on intelligence and on seizure recurrence. *N Engl J Med.* 1990;322:364–369.
8. Christiansen C, Rodbro P, Lund M. Incidence of anticonvulsant osteomalacia and effect of vitamin D: Controlled therapeutic trial. *Br Med J.* 1973;4:695–701.
9. Valsamis HA, Arora SK, Labban B, McFarlane SI. Antiepileptic drugs and bone metabolism. *Nutr Metab (Lond).* 2006;3:36.
10. Pack AM, Morrell MJ. Adverse effects of antiepileptic drugs on bone structure: Epidemiology, mechanisms and therapeutic implications. *CNS Drugs.* 2001;15:633–642.
11. Frey HH. Primidone: Mechanism of action. In: Levy RH, Mattson RH, Meldrum BS, Perucca E (Eds.). *Antiepileptic Drugs.* New York: Raven Press; 2002:439–447.
12. Macdonald RL, Kelly KM. Antiepileptic drug mechanisms of action. *Epilepsia.* 1995;36(Suppl 2):S2– S12.
13. Wilensky AJ, Friel PN, Levy RH, Comfort CP, Kaluzny SP. Kinetics of phenobarbital in normal subjects and epileptic patients. *Eur J Clin Pharmacol.* 1982;23:87–92.
14. Nelson E, Powell JR, Conrad K, et al. Phenobarbital pharmacokinetics and bioavailability in adults. *J Clin Pharmacol.* 1982;22:141–148.
15. Yukawa E, Suematsu F, Yukawa M, Minemoto M. Population pharmacokinetic investigation of phenobarbital by mixed effect modelling using routine clinical pharmacokinetic data in Japanese neonates and infants. *J Clinical Pharm Ther.* 2005;30:159–163.
16. Graves NM, Holmes GB, Kriel RL, Jones-Saete C, Ong B, Ehresman DJ. Relative bioavailability of rectally administered phenobarbital sodium parenteral solution. *DICP.* 1989;23:565–568.
17. Porter RJ, Penry JK. Phenobarbital: Biopharmacology. *Adv Neurol.* 1980;27:493–500.
18. Cloyd JC, Leppik IE. Primidone: Absorption, distribuiton, and excretion. In: Levy RH, Mattson RH, Meldrum BS, Perucca E, (Eds.). *Antiepileptic Drugs.* New York: Raven Press; 2002:459–466.
19. Harvey CD, Sherwin AL, Van Der Kleijn E. Distribution of anticonvulsant drugs in gray and white matter of human brain. *Can J Neurol Sci.* 1977;4:89–92.
20. Butler TC. The rate of penetration of barbituric acid derivatives into the brain. *J Pharmacol Exp Ther.* 1950;100:219–226.

21. Engasser JM, Sarhan F, Falcoz C, Minier M, Letourneur P, Siest G. Distribution, metabolism, and elimination of phenobarbital in rats: Physiologically based pharmacokinetic model. *J Pharm Sci.* 1981;70:1233–1238.

22. Ferngren H. Brain and blood levels of phenobarbital-2-14C during postnatal development in the mouse. *Acta Pharm Suec.* 1969;6:331–338.

23. Morselli PL, Franco-Morselli R. Clinical pharmacokinetics of antiepileptic drugs in adults. *Pharmacol Ther.* 1980;10:65–101.

24. Hvidberg EF, Dam M. Clinical pharmacokinetics of anticonvulsants. *Clin Pharmacokinet.* 1976;1:161–188.

25. Linton AL, Luke RG, Briggs JD. Methods of forced diuresis and its application in barbiturate poisoning. *Lancet.* 1967;2:377–379.

26. Battino D, Avanzini G, Bossi L, et al. Plasma levels of primidone and its metabolite phenobarbital: Effect of age and associated therapy. *Ther Drug Monit.* 1983;5:73–79.

27. Martines C, Gatti G, Sasso E, Calzetti S, Perucca E. The disposition of primidone in elderly patients. *Br J Clin Pharmacol.* 1990;30:607–611.

28. Cloyd JC, Miller KW, Leppik IE. Primidone kinetics: Effects of concurrent drugs and duration of therapy. *Clin Pharmacol Ther.* 1981;29:402–407.

29. Booker HE, Hosokowa K, Burdette RD, Darcey B. A clinical study of serum primidone levels. *Epilepsia.* 1970;11:395–402.

30. Eadie MJ, Lander CM, Hooper WD, Tyrer JH. Factors influencing plasma phenobarbitone levels in epileptic patients. *Br J Clin Pharmacol.* 1977;4:541–547.

31. Alvin J, McHorse T, Hoyumpa A, Bush MT, Schenker S. The effect of liver disease in man on the disposition of phenobarbital. *J Pharmacol Exp Ther.* 1975;192:224–235.

32. Pisani F, Perucca E, Primerano G, et al. Single-dose kinetics of primidone in acute viral hepatitis. *Eur J Clin Pharmacol.* 1984;27:465–469.

33. Lous P. Elimination of Barbiturates. In: Johansen SH, (Ed.). *Barbiturate Poisoning and Tetanus.* Boston: Little Bron; 1966.

34. Asconape JJ, Penry JK. Use of antiepileptic drugs in the presence of liver and kidney diseases: A review. *Epilepsia.* 1982;23 Suppl 1:S65– S79.

35. Lacerda G, Krummel T, Sabourdy C, Ryvlin P, Hirsch E. Optimizing therapy of seizures in patients with renal or hepatic dysfunction. *Neurology.* 2006;67:S28– S33.

36. Golper TA. Update on drug sieving coefficients and dosing adjustments during continuous renal replacement therapies. *Contrib Nephrol.* 2001;349–353.

37. Golper TA, Marx MA. Drug dosing adjustments during continuous renal replacement therapies. *Kidney Int Suppl.* 1998;66:S165– S168.

38. Lee CS, Marbury TC, Perchalski RT, Wilder BJ. Pharmacokinetics of primidone elimination by uremic patients. *J Clin Pharmacol.* 1982;22:301–308.

39. Palmer BF. Effectiveness of hemodialysis in the extracorporeal therapy of phenobarbital overdose. *Am J Kidney Dis.* 2000;36:640–643.

40. Cloyd JC, Leppik IE. Primidone: Absorption, distribution, and excretion. In: Levy RH, Mattson RH, Meldrum BS, Perucca E (Eds.). *Antiepileptic Drugs.* New York: Raven Press; 1995:459–466.

41. Waddell WJ, Butler TC. The distribution and excretion of phenobarbital. *J Clin Invest.* 1957;36:1217–1226.

42. Wanwimolruk S, Levy G. Kinetics of drug action in disease states. XX. Effects of acute starvation on the pharmacodynamics of phenobarbital, ethanol and pentylenetetrazol in rats and effects of refeeding and diet composition. *J Pharmacol Exp Ther.* 1987;242:166–172.

43. Anderson GD. Phenobarbital and other barbiturates: Chemistry, biotransformation, and pharmacokinetics. In: Levy RH, Mattson RH, Meldrum BS, Perucca E (Eds.). *Antiepileptic Drugs.* New York: Raven Press; 2002:496–503.

44. Garnett WR, Anderson GD, Collins RJ. Antiepileptic drugs. In: Evans WE, Schentag JJ, Jusko WJ (Eds.). *Applied Pharmacokinetics and Pharmacodynamics: Principles of Therapeutic Drug Monitoring.* Philadelphia: Lippincott Williams & Wilkins, 2006:491–511.

45. Baselt RC, Wright JA, Cravey RH. Therapeutic and toxic concentrations of more than 100 toxicologically significant drugs in blood, plasma, or serum: A tabulation. *Clin Chem.* 1975;21:44–62.

46. Glauser TA, Pippenger CE. Controversies in blood-level monitoring: Reexamining its role in the treatment of epilepsy. *Epilepsia.* 2000;41 Suppl 8:S6– S15.

47. Trissel LA. Handbook of Injectable Drugs. Bethesda: American Society of Health-System Pharmacists, 2009.

48. French JA, Gidal BE. Antiepileptic drug interactions. *Epilepsia.* 2000;41 Suppl 8:S30–36.

49. Anderson GD. A mechanistic approach to antiepileptic drug interactions. *Ann Pharmacother.* 1998;32:554–563.

50. Kapetanovic IM, Kupferberg HJ, Porter RJ, Theodore W, Schulman E, Penry JK. Mechanism of valproate-phenobarbital interaction in epileptic patients. *Clin Pharmacol Ther.* 1981;29:480–486.

51. Patsalos PN, Perucca E. Clinically important drug interactions in epilepsy: Interactions between antiepileptic drugs and other drugs. *Lancet Neurol.* 2003;2:473–481.

52. Bernus I, Dickinson RG, Hooper WD, Eadie MJ. Inhibition of phenobarbitone N-glucosidation by valproate. *Br J Clin Pharmacol.* 1994;38:411–416.

53. May T, Rambeck B. Serum concentrations of valproic acid: Influence of dose and comedication. *Ther Drug Monit.* 1985;7:387–390.

54. Perucca E, Gatti G, Frigo GM, Crema A, Calzetti S, Visintini D. Disposition of sodium valproate in epileptic patients. *Br J Clin Pharmacol.* 1978;5:495–499.

55. Yukawa E, To H, Ohdo S, Higuchi S, Aoyama T. Population-based investigation of valproic acid relative clearance using nonlinear mixed effects modeling: influence of drug-drug interaction and patient characteristics. *J Clin Pharmacol.* 1997;37:1160–1167.

56. Kaplan PW, Norwitz ER, Ben-Menachem E, et al. Obstetric risks for women with epilepsy during pregnancy. *Epilepsy Behav.* 2007;11:283–291.

57. Pennell PB. Antiepileptic drugs during pregnancy: What is known and which AEDs seem to be safest? *Epilepsia.* 2008;49 Suppl 9:43–55.

58. Harden CL, Sethi NK. Epileptic disorders in pregnancy: An overview. *Curr Opin Obstet Gynecol.* 2008;20:557–562.

59. Fairgrieve SD, Jackson M, Jonas P, et al. Population-based, prospective study of the care of women with epilepsy in pregnancy. *BMJ.* 2000;321:674–675.

60. Reddy DS. Clinical pharmacokinetic interactions between antiepileptic drugs and hormonal contraceptives. *Expert Rev Clin Pharmacol.* 2010;3:183–192.

61. French JA, Pedley TA. Clinical practice. Initial management of epilepsy. *N Engl J Med.* 2008;359:166–176.

62. Uldemolins MJ, Roberts J, Rello J. Drug Distribution: Is it a more important determinant of drug dosing than clearance? In: Vincent JL (Ed.). *Yearbook of Intensive Care and Emergency Medicine.* New York: Springer, 2010:507–18.

63. Ravn-Jonsen A, Lunding M, Secher O. Excretion of phenobarbitone in urine after intake of large doses. *Acta Pharmacol Toxicol (Copenh).* 1969;27:193–201.

64. Butler TC, Mahaffee C, Waddell WJ. Phenobarbital: Studies of elimination, accumulation, tolerance, and dosage schedules. *J Pharmacol Exp Ther.* 1954;111:425–435.

65. Kallberg N, Agurell S, Ericsson O, Bucht E, Jalling B, Boreus LO. Quantitation of phenobarbital and its main metabolites in human urine. *Eur J Clin Pharmacol.* 1975;9:161–168.

66. Pugh RN, Murray-Lyon IM, Dawson JL, Pietroni MC, Williams R. Transection of the oesophagus for bleeding oesophageal varices. *Br J Surg.* 1973;60:646–649.

67. Child CG, Turcotte JG. Surgery and protal hypertension. In: Child CG (Ed.). *The Liver and Portal Hypertension.* Phildelphia: Saunders, 1964:50–64.

68. Elliott ES, Buck ML. Phenobarbital dosing and pharmacokinetics in a neonate receiving extracorporeal membrane oxygenation. *Ann Pharmacother.* 1999;33:419–422.

69. Lockman LA. Phenobarbital dosage for neonatal seizures. *Adv Neurol.* 1983;34:505–508.

70. Fischer JH, Lockman LA, Zaske D, Kriel R. Phenobarbital maintenance dose requirements in treating neonatal seizures. *Neurology.* 1981;31:1042–1044.

71. Painter MJ, Pippenger C, MacDonald H, Pitlick W. Phenobarbital and diphenylhydantoin levels in neonates with seizures. *J Pediatr.* 1978;92:315–319.

72. Volpe JJ. Neonatal seizures. In: *Neurology of the Newborn.* Phildelphia: WB Saunders, 1999.

73. Ouvrier RA, Goldsmith R. Phenobarbitone dosage in neonatal convulsions. *Arch Dis Child*. 1982;57:653–657.

74. Bernus I, Dickinson RG, Hooper WD, Eadie MJ. Anticonvulsant therapy in aged patients. Clinical pharmacokinetic considerations. *Drugs Aging*. 1997;10:278–289.

75. Lindberg MC, Cunningham A, Lindberg NH. Acute phenobarbital intoxication. *South Med J*. 1992;85:803–807.

76. Arieff AI, Friedman EA. Coma following nonnarcotic drug overdosage: Management of 208 adult patients. *Am J Med Sci*. 1973;266:405–426.

77. Pond SM, Olson KR, Osterloh JD, Tong TG. Randomized study of the treatment of phenobarbital overdose with repeated doses of activated charcoal. *JAMA*. 1984;251:3104–3108.

78. Zawada ET, Jr., Nappi J, Done G, Rollins D. Advances in the hemodialysis management of phenobarbital overdose. *South Med J*. 1983;76:6–8.

79. Brooks SM, Werk EE, Ackerman SJ, Sullivan I, Thrasher K. Adverse effects of phenobarbital on corticosteroid metabolism in patients with bronchial asthma. *N Engl J Med*. 1972;286:1125–1128.

80. Falliers CJ, Brooks SM, Werk EE, Jr. Corticosteroids and phenobarbital in asthma. *N Engl J Med*. 1972;287:201.

81. Gabrielsen J, Bendtsen A, Eriksen H, Andersen S. Methylprednisolone half-life during simultaneous barbiturate treatment and mechanical hyperventilation of neurosurgical patients. *J Neurosurg*. 1985;62:182–185.

82. Gambertoglio JG, Holford NH, Kapusnik JE, et al. Disposition of total and unbound prednisolone in renal transplant patients receiving anticonvulsants. *Kidney Int*. 1984;25:119–123.

83. Hancock KW, Levell MJ. Primidone/dexamethasone interaction. *Lancet*. 1978;2:97–98.

CATHERINE A. MILLARES-SIPIN, PharmD, CGP, BCPS, BCACP
ANTONIA ALAFRIS, BS, PharmD, CGP
HENRY COHEN, MS, PharmD, FCCM, BCPP, CGP

CHAPTER 15

Phenytoin and Fosphenytoin

OVERVIEW OF PHENYTOIN

Phenytoin (5,5-diphenylimidazolidine-2,4-dione, referred to as diphenylhydantoin) is an anticonvulsant medication that was first discovered in 1908 by Heinrich Biltz at the University of Kiel in Germany. In the 1920s, Arthur Dox, a chemist in Parke-Davis, compounded diphenylhydantoin in search of a hypnotic agent. Because the drug was not a hypnotic, he shelved it as "inactive." It was not until November 1936 that Tracy Putnam discovered the anticonvulsant activity of diphenylhydantoin, and in June 1938, Parke, Davis, and Company marketed sodium diphenylhydantoin (Dilantin®). In the 1970s, the generic name of Dilantin® was shortened to phenytoin.[1] Today, it is FDA-approved for the management of generalized tonic clonic (grand mal) seizures, complex partial seizures, and for the prevention of seizures after head trauma and neurosurgery.[2] Phenytoin also has multiple unlabeled indications including the management of trigeminal neuralgia, syndrome of inappropriate antidiuretic hormone (SIADH), torsade de pointes, and arrhythmias (as a Class IB antiarrhythmic). Topical phenytoin has also been used to heal multiple acute and chronic wounds.[3] As an anticonvulsant, phenytoin works by increasing the efflux and decreasing the influx of sodium ions in cell membranes of the motor cortex during the generation of nerve impulses.[2]

DOSING

Phenytoin is available in multiple dosage forms including an injectable formulation, extended-release capsule, oral suspension, and chewable tablet (Table 15-1).[2] Intramuscular (IM) administration of phenytoin is not recommended due to its erratic absorption and pain on injection. If IM administration is required, fosphenytoin is preferred. Intravenously (IV), phenytoin may be administered by IV push or IV piggyback using a 0.22 micron filter. The filter is used to remove crystals and minimize the incidence of phlebitis. The maximum rate of administration is 50 mg/min in adults and 0.5–1 mg/kg/min in neonates due to the risk of hypotension, as noted in a boxed warning in the drug package insert. In elderly or patients with preexisting cardiovascular conditions, phenytoin may be administered more slowly at 20 mg/minute.[4] It must be noted that the oral suspension and chewable tablets contain 8 percent more phenytoin than the other formulations (92 mg of phenytoin base is equivalent to 100 mg of phenytoin sodium). Therefore, when patients are being switched from one dosage formulation to another, dosage adjustments and closer serum monitoring are recommended.[2,4] The recommended dose for adult patients in status epilepticus is 15–20 mg/kg. For maintenance doses, adults may be loaded at 15–20 mg/kg. Due to the rate-limited gastrointestinal (GI) absorption of phenytoin, no more than 400 mg should be administered at a time. Hence, in order to ensure complete absorption and a decrease in GI side effects, a 1,000 mg loading dose may be administered in three

divided doses at 400 mg, 300 mg, and 300 mg every two hours. A target level is achieved within 6–10 hours. The maintenance dose is 300 mg/day or 5–6 mg/kg/day in three divided doses or once to twice daily if the extended-release formulation is being used. For obese patients, it is recommended to receive loading doses based on adjusted body weight with a correction factor of 1.33 for a maximum loading dose of 2,000 mg. For maintenance dosing, the ideal body weight may be used and be adjusted according to therapeutic drug monitoring and clinical effectiveness. A serum phenytoin concentration of 10–20 mg/L is considered within therapeutic range. Concentrations between 5 and 10 mg/L may be therapeutic for some patients; however, concentrations less than 5 mg/L are not recommended. The target free phenytoin concentration is 1–2 mg/L.

ADVERSE EVENTS

Phenytoin adverse effects can be common and chronic, and include hepatotoxicity, osteoporosis, megaloblastic anemia, gingival hyperplasia, hirsutism, and peripheral neuropathy. Phenytoin may cause gastrointestinal adverse effects such as nausea and vomiting; single doses above 100 mg increase the propensity of gastrointestinal intolerance. Phenytoin can cause central nervous system (CNS) adverse effects such as dizziness, confusion, drowsiness, and ataxia – although these usually occur at a greater frequency with high peak concentrations or toxic levels. Phenytoin-induced CNS adverse effects may be circumvented by administering a larger dose or the entire dose at bedtime. Phenytoin may cause cognitive dysfunction.

Phenytoin may cause a rash that presents as the *antiepileptic hypersensitivity syndrome* (AES). The onset of AES is generally within the first five weeks of initiating phenytoin therapy and presents with a symptom triad including rash, pruritus, and fever. AES presents with other nonspecific manifestations that can wax and wane including hepatotoxicity, blood dyscrasias, encephalitis, myositis, malaise, pulmonary infiltrates, and an acute respiratory distress syndrome. The rash may progress to life-threatening Steven–Johnsons syndrome or toxic epidermal necrolysis. Since it is difficult to discern if an isolated phenytoin-induced rash will be benign or progress to the AES, patients who develop rash should have phenytoin therapy discontinued. Patients who develop phenytoin-induced AES should avoid using other aromatic anticonvulsants that may cross-react, such as carbamazepine, oxcarbazepine, phenobarbital, lamotrigine, lacosamide, and zonisamide.

Acute phenytoin toxicity (levels above 20 mg/L) often exhibits concentration-dependent toxicities such as nystagmus and diplopia at levels between 20 and 30 mg/L; as the levels rise to 30–40 mg/L the nystagmus and diplopia dissipate and ataxia, nausea, and vomiting manifest. Intention tremor may persist at all phenytoin toxic levels. Some patients with phenytoin toxicity do present with cumulative symptomatology. Patients who present with chronic phenytoin toxicity may develop irreversible CNS effects such as

TABLE 15-1 Dosage Formulations and Strengths of Phenytoin

Injectable (phenytoin sodium)	50 mg/mL (2 mL, 5 mL)
Oral, Capsule (extended release) (phenytoin sodium)	100 mg, 200 mg, 300 mg
Dilantin®	30 mg, 100 mg
Phenytek®	200 mg, 300 mg
Oral, Suspension (phenytoin acid)	100 mg/4 mL (4 mL), 125 mg/5 mL (120 mL, 237 mL, 240 mL)
Dilantin-125®	125 mg/5 mL (240 mL; contains ethanol ≤0.6%, sodium benzoate; orange-vanilla flavor)
Oral, Tablet (chewable; phenytoin acid)	50 mg

Data from Lexi-Drugs Online: Phenytoin. Available at online.lexi.com (accessed June 12, 2011).

dysarthria, ataxia, and encephalopathy. A list of adverse effects associated with phenytoin is depicted in Table 15-2.[4,5] Hypotension is listed as a boxed warning in the package insert of phenytoin. It has been observed primarily in older adults and is associated with increased infusion rates. Monitoring of blood pressure and heart rate is recommended during IV administration and may be used to determine the safest rate for the patient. Due to the cardiotoxicity associated with phenytoin (e.g., bradycardia, hypotension, QRS prolongation, ventricular fibrillation), all patients receiving IV phenytoin must have continuous cardiac monitoring. Phenytoin is pregnancy category D because it crosses the placenta and has been associated with congenital malformations termed *fetal hydantoin syndrome* or *fetal anticonvulsant syndrome*. Isolated cases of malignancies and coagulation defects in the neonate have been reported. Phenytoin enters the breast milk and it is not recommended to be used by lactating women.

BIOAVAILABILITY

The bioavailability of phenytoin varies significantly among the different dosage forms.[6] Phenytoin is poorly soluble in water, but it readily dissolves in an alkali environment. Due to the acidity of the stomach, phenytoin sodium changes to free phenytoin acid that precipitates after it dissolves. Hence, the rate and extent of absorption are highly dependent on the size of the phenytoin particles entering the intestine. For this reason, the different dosage forms of phenytoin have widely different bioavailabilities. No systematic difference in bioavailability has been noted between phenytoin sodium and phenytoin acid. In fact, clinicians should be careful when switching patients whose seizures are controlled from one phenytoin preparation to another because even small increases or decreases in bioavailability can significantly change the steady-state plasma concentration during chronic therapy.[6-9] The evidence indicates that even changes in the excipient may result in phenytoin intoxication.[7] The rate of absorption after a single oral dose of a capsule or tablet can be anywhere from 3 to 12 hours. However, in some patients, it

may exceed 12 hours. The Food and Drug Administration recommends only the Dilantin Kapseals® to be administered once daily because many generic preparations are more rapidly absorbed and may produce fluctuations in the plasma phenytoin concentration.[4] Numerous case studies report a decrease in phenytoin absorption when it is coadministered with enteral feedings.[10] The exact mechanism is unknown; however, researchers speculate that phenytoin particles bind to certain components in the feeding formulas, such as calcium and dietary fiber. Others believe that phenytoin binds to the tube lumen, or the mechanism is pH dependent. Methods described to avoid this interaction include spacing the administration of the enteral feedings from that of phenytoin's without compromising the patient's dietary requirements. However, no consensus establishes the best method for avoiding this interaction.

VOLUME OF DISTRIBUTION

Phenytoin has an apparent volume of distribution of 0.6–0.7 L/kg adults and children and 1.2 L/kg in infants and neonates. Phenytoin distributes rapidly to the brain where plasma and brain concentrations achieve equilibrium within 20 minutes.[10]

PLASMA PROTEIN BINDING OF PHENYTOIN

Phenytoin is 92 percent bound to plasma albumin, and the free form (8%) is the pharmacologically active drug responsible for efficacy and toxicity.[10] A smaller portion is bound to alpha-1-acid glycoprotein.[11] When phenytoin levels are reported, they represent the unbound (free or active) and bound (inactive) phenytoin level, often referred to as phenytoin observed. In patients with normal albumin level and renal function, the fraction of unbound phenytoin (f_{up}) is 0.1. Hence, a *total* phenytoin concentration of 10–20 mg/L represents a f_{up} of 1–2 mg/L.

Conditions That Can Cause Hypoalbuminemia and the Effects on Free Phenytoin Concentration

Disease states or medications that can change the albumin concentration or phenytoin's binding affinity (K_a) to albumin can ultimately alter the concentration of free, fraction unbound of phenytoin (f_{up}). Disease states that can decrease the serum albumin concentration and eventually lead to increased free phenytoin concentrations include burns, hepatic cirrhosis, nephrotic syndrome, pregnancy, and cystic fibrosis.[2,4,12] In patients with hypoalbuminemia, the observed *total* phenytoin concentration can appear normal or low, even though the free phenytoin level is increased because of less albumin to bind to. As the free form increases, the total phenytoin level remains unchanged.[12] For example, a cachetic, hypoalbuminemic (albumin level <4.4 g/dL) patient has an observed *total* phenytoin level of 18 mg/L, which appears to be at target. However, the fraction of unbound phenytoin has increased from 0.1 to 0.2, resulting in a toxic free phenytoin level of 3.6 mg/L (normal free phenytoin is 1–2 mg/L).

TABLE 15-2 Adverse Effects Associated with Phenytoin[4,5]

Chronic Phenytoin Adverse Effects	Acute Phenytoin Toxicity	Chronic Phenytoin Toxicity
Megaloblastic anemia	Intention tremor at all concentrations	Confusional state (delirium, psychosis, encephalopathy)
Hepatotoxicity	>20 mg/L: nystagmus and diplopia	Irreversible cerebellar dysfunction (dysarthria, ataxia, intention tremor, muscular hypotonia)
Lymphadenopathy	>30 mg/L: ataxia and GI (nausea, vomiting, constipation)	Peripheral neuropathy
Osteoporosis	>40 mg/L: lethargy, confusion, combative, slurred speech	
Hirsutism	>50 mg/L: choreoathetoid movements and opisthotonic posturing	
Gingival hyperplasia		
Thickening of facial features		
Peripheral neuropathy		
Vitamin D deficiency		
Hyperglycemia		

The Sheiner-Tozer equation is a correction formula that uses the plasma albumin concentration to predict the free fraction of phenytoin using the total phenytoin observed[4,13]:

$$\text{Equation 1: Corrected phenytoin} = \frac{\text{Phenytoin observed}}{(\text{Albumin} \times 0.2) + 0.1}$$

This equation can empirically adjust the observed total phenytoin concentration in cases of decreased albumin. However, temperature plays a critical role in the application of the Sheiner-Tozer equation.[13] The formula was based on a free phenytoin assay, which was performed using a Centrifree micropartition filter for separation at a temperature of 37°C, resembling physiological body temperature. However, clinical laboratories routinely perform unbound phenytoin assays at room temperature of 25°C. In such cases, the Sheiner-Tozer equation must be changed to accommodate for the difference in room temperature by multiplying the albumin concentration by the constant 0.25[14]:

$$\text{Equation 2: Corrected phenytoin} = \frac{\text{Phenytoin observed}}{(\text{Albumin} \times 0.25) + 0.1}$$

Conditions That Can Decrease Phenytoin's Binding Affinity to Albumin and the Effects on Free Phenytoin Concentration

Certain disease states can decrease phenytoin's binding affinity (K_a) to serum albumin. Such disease states include, severe jaundice, hyperbilirubinemia (total bilirubin >15 mg/dL), and renal insufficiency or failure with a calculated creatinine clearance (CrCl) <25 mL/min (f_{up} increases two- to threefold in uremia).[2,4,12,13,15,16] The binding affinity of phenytoin decreases in these situations either because of low albumin or because of alterations in the albumin molecule leading to decreased binding, or due to the accumulation of a major metabolite of phenytoin [5-(p-hydroxyphenyl)-5-phenylhydantoin, or p-HPPH], which displaces phenytoin from albumin.[17] In addition, drugs like valproic acid, which has a high affinity for the same binding site as phenytoin, can easily displace phenytoin from albumin, resulting in increased amount of free phenytoin.[18,19] Whichever the mechanism for the decreased binding may be, the observed phenytoin concentration in these situations is a poor predictor of the patient's true phenytoin level.

Phenytoin's binding affinity to albumin (K_a) is less likely to be affected if the calculated creatinine CrCl is >25 mL/min. However, once the CrCl is 10–25 mL/min, K_a is likely to be decreased to an unknown extent. Patients with end-stage renal disease (ESRD), or CrCl <10 mL/min, have both decreased albumin level and K_a. In such situations, the Sheiner-Tozer equation must be changed where the albumin is multiplied by the constant 0.1[20,21]:

$$\text{Equation 3: Corrected phenytoin} = \frac{\text{Phenytoin observed}}{(\text{Albumin} \times 0.1) + 0.1}$$

CASE STUDIES

CASE 1: CALCULATING FOR THE CORRECTED PHENYTOIN LEVEL IN PATIENTS WITH HYPOALBUMINEMIA WHEN THE SERUM PHENYTOIN TEST IS PERFORMED AT 37°C

SP is a 72-year-old female (62 kg, 5′6″) with an observed phenytoin level of 6.2 mg/L at 37°C. Her recent albumin level was 2 g/dL, and her serum creatinine level was 0.6 mg/dL. Calculate for the corrected phenytoin level.

Step 1: Calculate her creatinine clearance. Since this patient is above the age of 65 y/o, round up the serum creatinine from 0.6 mg/dL to 1 mg/dL when calculating for her creatinine clearance.

$$\text{IBW}_{female} = 45.5 \text{ kg} + 2.3(\text{height in inches above 5 feet})$$

$$\text{IBW}_{female} = 45.5 + 2.3(6)$$

$$\text{IBW} = 59.3 \text{ kg}$$

$$\text{Creatinine clearance} = \frac{(140 - 72) \times 59.3}{72 \times 1} \times 0.85 = 47.6 \text{ mL/min}$$

Step 2: Calculate for the corrected phenytoin level. Because her creatinine clearance is >25 mL/min and the test is performed at 37°C, use Equation 1.

$$\text{Corrected phenytoin} = \frac{\text{Phenytoin observed}}{(\text{Albumin} \times 0.2) + 0.1}$$

$$= \frac{6.2 \text{ mg/L}}{(2 \times 0.2) + 0.1}$$

$$= 12.4 \text{ mg/L}$$

CASE 2: CALCULATING FOR THE CORRECTED PHENYTOIN LEVEL IN PATIENTS WITH HYPOALBUMINEMIA

A 26-year-old (52 kg, 5′5″) white female is receiving phenytoin 100 mg po tid for partial epilepsy. She has a steady-state phenytoin concentration of 14 mg/L. She is seizure free but has been complaining of daytime drowsiness and dizziness. An SMA-18 panel includes the following laboratory values: creatinine 0.5 mg/dL and albumin 2.8 g/dL. What is the corrected steady-state phenytoin concentration?

Step 1: It is not necessary to calculate the creatinine clearance in this case. This patient is 26 years old with a normal serum creatinine and, intuitively, will have a projected creatinine clearance above 25 mL/min.

Step 2. Calculate for the corrected phenytoin level. Although the temperature in which phenytoin was assayed is not mentioned, one can assume that phenytoin serum samples are maintained and assayed at room temperature at 25°C. Because her creatinine clearance is >25 mL/min and we are assuming that the phenytoin samples were maintained and assayed at room temperature at 25°C, use Equation 2.

$$\text{Corrected phenytoin} = \frac{\text{Phenytoin observed}}{(\text{Albumin} \times 0.25) + 0.1}$$

$$\text{Corrected phenytoin} = \frac{14 \text{ mg/L}}{(2.8 \text{ g/dL} \times 0.25) + 0.1}$$

$$\text{Corrected phenytoin} = 17.5 \text{ mg/L}$$

This patient has a corrected serum phenytoin concentration of 17.5 mg/L. Although this patient's corrected serum phenytoin concentration is within the target range of 10–20 mg/dL, she is experiencing phenytoin-induced CNS-adverse effects. The patient should be monitored for other CNS and non-CNS signs and symptoms of phenytoin toxicity. In order to mitigate the phenytoin-induced CNS-adverse effects, the medical team may consider administering the entire phenytoin dose at bedtime, or a reduced phenytoin daily dose.

CASE 3: CALCULATING FOR THE CORRECTED PHENYTOIN LEVEL IN PATIENTS WITH HYPOALBUMINEMIA WHEN THE SERUM PHENYTOIN TEST IS PERFORMED AT 25°C

TD is an 80-year-old male (59 kg, 5′2″) with an observed phenytoin level of 8.2 mg/L at 25°C. His recent albumin level was 3 g/dL, and his serum creatinine level was 0.8 mg/dL. Calculate for the corrected phenytoin level.

Step 1: Calculate his creatinine clearance.

$$IBW_{male} = 50 \text{ kg} + 2.3(\text{height in inches above 5 feet})$$

$$IBW_{male} = 50 \text{ kg} + 2.3(2)$$

$$IBW_{male} = 54.6 \text{ kg}$$

$$CrCl = \frac{(140 - 80) \times 54.6 \text{ kg}}{72 \times 1}$$

$$CrCl = 45.5 \text{ mL/min}$$

Step 2: Calculate for the corrected phenytoin level. Because his creatinine clearance is >25 mL/min and the test is performed at 25°C, use Equation 2.

$$\text{Corrected phenytoin} = \frac{\text{Phenytoin observed}}{(\text{Albumin} \times 0.25) + 0.1}$$

$$\text{Corrected phenytoin} = \frac{8.2 \text{ mg/L}}{(3 \text{ g/dL} \times 0.25) + 0.1}$$

$$\text{Corrected phenytoin} = 9.65 \text{ mg/L}$$

CASE 4: CALCULATING FOR THE CORRECTED PHENYTOIN LEVEL IN PATIENTS WITH HYPOALBUMINEMIA

A 67-year-old (50 kg, 5′2″) black female is receiving phenytoin 100 mg po tid for partial epilepsy. She has a steady-state phenytoin concentration of 6 mg/L and is seizure free. An SMA-18 panel includes the following laboratory values: creatinine 1 mg/dL and albumin 1.7 g/dL. What is the corrected steady-state phenytoin concentration?

Step 1: Calculate her creatinine clearance.

$$IBW_{female} = 45.5 \text{ kg} + 2.3(\text{height in inches above 5 feet})$$

$$IBW_{female} = 45.5 + 2.3(2)$$

$$IBW = 50.1 \text{ kg}$$

$$\text{Creatinine clearance} = \frac{(140 - 67) \times 50.1 \times 0.85}{72 \times 1} = 43.2 \text{ mL/min}$$

Step 2. Calculate for the corrected phenytoin level. Although the temperature in which phenytoin was assayed is not mentioned, one can assume that phenytoin serum samples are maintained and assayed at room temperature at 25°C. Because her creatinine clearance is >25 mL/min and we are assuming that the phenytoin samples were maintained and assayed at room temperature at 25°C, use Equation 2.

$$\text{Corrected phenytoin} = \frac{\text{Phenytoin observed}}{(\text{Albumin} \times 0.25) + 0.1}$$

$$\text{Corrected phenytoin} = \frac{6 \text{ mg/L}}{(1.7 \text{ g/dL} \times 0.25) + 0.1}$$

$$\text{Corrected phenytoin} = 11.4 \text{ mg/L}$$

This patient has a corrected serum phenytoin concentration of 11.4 mg/L. Because she is seizure free and her corrected serum phenytoin concentration is within the target range of 10–20 mg/L, no phenytoin dosage adjustments or heightened monitoring for toxicity is warranted.

CASE 5: CALCULATING FOR THE CORRECTED PHENYTOIN LEVEL IN PATIENTS WITH END-STAGE RENAL DISEASE

SM is an 88-year-old female with history of ESRD and receiving dialysis every Monday, Wednesday, and Friday. She has been receiving phenytoin suspension 125 mg every 12 hours for 8 months for seizure prophylaxis. Her observed phenytoin level was 5 mg/L and albumin was 3.6 g/dL. Calculate for the corrected phenytoin level assuming the phenytoin assay was performed at 37° C.

Step 1: No need to calculate for her creatinine clearance. For ESRD patients, always assume that the CrCl is going to be <10 mL/min.

Step 2: Calculate for the corrected phenytoin concentration using Equation 3.

$$\text{Corrected phenytoin} = \frac{\text{Phenytoin observed}}{(\text{Albumin} \times 0.1) + 0.1}$$

$$\text{Corrected phenytoin} = \frac{5 \text{ mg/L}}{(3.6 \text{ g/dL} \times 0.1) + 0.1}$$

$$\text{Corrected phenytoin} = 10.9 \text{ mg/L}$$

CASE 6: CALCULATING FOR THE CORRECTED PHENYTOIN LEVEL IN PATIENTS WITH END-STAGE RENAL DISEASE AND HYPOALBUMINEMIA

A 28-year-old (85 kg, 6′1″) black male is receiving phenytoin capsule 100 mg po twice daily and at bedtime for epilepsy. He has a steady-state phenytoin concentration of 12 mg/L. He has a history of chronic kidney disease with a creatinine clearance of 8 mL/min. An SMA-18 panel includes the following laboratory values: BUN = 66 mg/dL, albumin 3 g/dL, and globulin 2.7 g/dL. What is the corrected steady-state phenytoin concentration?

Step 1: It is not necessary to calculate the creatinine clearance in this case; this patient has CKD with a CrCl of 8 mL/min.

Step 2: Calculate for the corrected phenytoin concentration using Equation 3. Be careful to use the serum albumin in the equation and not the serum globulin, since phenytoin is a weak acid and is highly bound to the albumin portion [not globulin] of the plasma protein binding sites.

$$\text{Corrected phenytoin} = \frac{\text{Phenytoin observed}}{(\text{Albumin} \times 0.1) + 0.1}$$

$$\text{Corrected phenytoin} = \frac{12 \text{ mg/L}}{(3 \text{ g/dL} \times 0.1) + 0.1}$$

$$\text{Corrected phenytoin} = 30 \text{ mg/L}$$

This patient has a toxic corrected serum phenytoin concentration of 30 mg/L. The patient should be monitored for signs and symptoms of phenytoin toxicity, the phenytoin dose should be held and a new reduced dosing regimen should be considered.

CASE 7: CALCULATING FOR THE CORRECTED PHENYTOIN LEVEL IN PATIENTS WITH END-STAGE RENAL DISEASE AND HYPOALBUMINEMIA

A 65-year-old (55 kg, 5′7″) white male is receiving phenytoin capsule 100 mg po bid for epilepsy. He has a steady-state phenytoin concentration of 9 mg/L. He has a history of chronic kidney disease with a creatinine clearance of 10 mL/min. An SMA-18 panel includes the following laboratory values: BUN = 66 mg/dL, albumin 1.5 g/dL, and globulin 1.9 g/dL. What is the corrected steady-state phenytoin concentration?

Step 1: It is not necessary to calculate the creatinine clearance in this case; this patient has CKD with a CrCl of 10 mL/min.

Step 2: Calculate for the corrected phenytoin concentration using Equation 3. Be careful to use the serum albumin in the equation and not the serum globulin, since phenytoin is a weak acid and is highly bound to the albumin portion [not globulin] of the plasma protein binding sites.

$$\text{Corrected phenytoin} = \frac{\text{Phenytoin observed}}{(\text{Albumin} \times 0.1) + 0.1}$$

$$\text{Corrected phenytoin} = \frac{9 \text{ mg/L}}{(1.5 \text{ g/dL} \times 0.1) + 0.1}$$

$$\text{Corrected phenytoin} = 36 \text{ mg/L}$$

This patient has a toxic corrected serum phenytoin concentration of 36 mg/L. The patient should be monitored for signs and symptoms of phenytoin toxicity, the phenytoin dose should be held and a new reduced dosing regimen should be considered.

CASE 8: CALCULATING FOR THE CORRECTED PHENYTOIN LEVEL IN PATIENTS WITH END-STAGE RENAL DISEASE AND A NORMAL ALBUMIN

A 47-year-old (65 kg, 5′10″) Hispanic male is receiving phenytoin 100 mg po tid for epilepsy. He has a steady-state phenytoin concentration of 15 mg/L. He has a history of chronic kidney disease with a creatinine clearance of 5 mL/min. An SMA-18 panel includes the following laboratory values: albumin 4.6 g/dL and globulin 1.9 g/dL. What is the corrected steady-state phenytoin concentration?

Step 1: It is not necessary to calculate the creatinine clearance in this case; this patient has CKD with a CrCl of 5 mL/min.

Step 2: Calculate for the corrected phenytoin concentration using Equation 3. Be careful to use the serum albumin in the equation and not the serum globulin, since phenytoin is a weak acid and is highly bound to the albumin portion [not globulin] of the plasma protein binding sites. Although the patient's albumin is 4.6 g/dL, be sure to use an albumin of 4.4 g/dL as the Sheiner Tozer equation is only designed to correct for hypoalbuminemia at less than 4.4 g/dL.

$$\text{Corrected phenytoin} = \frac{\text{Phenytoin observed}}{(\text{Albumin} \times 0.1) + 0.1}$$

$$\text{Corrected phenytoin} = \frac{15 \text{ mg/L}}{(4.4 \text{ g/dL} \times 0.1) + 0.1}$$

$$\text{Corrected phenytoin} = 27.8 \text{ mg/L}$$

This patient has a toxic corrected serum phenytoin concentration of 27.8 mg/L. The patient should be monitored for signs and symptoms of phenytoin toxicity, and the phenytoin dose should be held and a new reduced dosing regimen should be considered.

CASE 9: CALCULATING FOR THE CORRECTED PHENYTOIN LEVEL IN PATIENTS WITH END-STAGE RENAL DISEASE AND A NORMAL ALBUMIN

A 36-year-old (75 kg, 5′11″) white male is receiving phenytoin 100 mg po qid for epilepsy. He has a steady-state phenytoin concentration of 22 mg/L. He has a history of chronic kidney disease with a creatinine clearance of 8 mL/min. An SMA-18 panel includes the following laboratory values: albumin 5.2 g/dL and globulin 3 g/dL. What is the corrected steady-state phenytoin concentration?

Step 1: It is not necessary to calculate the creatinine clearance in this case; this patient has CKD with a CrCl of 8 mL/min.

Step 2: Calculate for the corrected phenytoin concentration using Equation 3. Be careful to use the serum albumin in the equation and not the serum globulin, since phenytoin is a weak acid and is highly bound to the albumin portion [not globulin] of the plasma protein binding sites. Although the patient's albumin is 5.2 g/dL, be sure to use an albumin 4.4 g/dL as the Sheiner Tozer equation is only designed to correct for hypoalbuminemia at less than 4.4 g/dL.

$$\text{Corrected phenytoin} = \frac{\text{Phenytoin observed}}{(\text{Albumin} \times 0.1) + 0.1}$$

$$\text{Corrected phenytoin} = \frac{22 \text{ mg/L}}{(4.4 \text{ g/dL} \times 0.1) + 0.1}$$

$$\text{Corrected phenytoin} = 40.7 \text{ mg/L}$$

This patient has a toxic corrected serum phenytoin concentration of 40.7 mg/L. The patient should be monitored for signs and symptoms of phenytoin toxicity, the phenytoin dose should be held and a new reduced dosing regimen should be designed.

CASE 10: CALCULATING FOR THE CORRECTED PHENYTOIN LEVEL IN PATIENTS WITH RENAL FAILURE

JZ is a 75-year-old male (62 kg, 5′6″) who recently developed acute renal failure secondary to intravenous vancomycin. He has a history of seizure disorder and has been on phenytoin 200 mg capsule twice a day with previous phenytoin levels within normal limits. The most recent laboratory levels revealed a phenytoin level of 7.9 mg/L, albumin of 4 g/dL, and SCr of 3.2 mg/dL. No seizure activity was reported in the last week. Calculate for the corrected phenytoin level for this patient assuming that the test was performed at temperature of 37°C.

Step 1: Calculate his creatinine clearance.

$$\text{IBW}_{male} = 50 \text{ kg} + 2.3(\text{height in inches above 5 feet})$$
$$\text{IBW} = 50 \text{ kg} + 2.3(6)$$
$$\text{IBW} = 63.8 \text{ kg}$$

$$\text{Creatinine clearance} = \frac{(140 - 75) \times 63.8 \text{ kg}}{72 \times 3.2} = 18 \text{ mL/min}$$

Because the calculated creatinine clearance of this patient falls between 10 and 25 mL/min, our corrected phenytoin formulas cannot be used (Equations 1 and 3). Instead, take the average of Equation 1 and Equation 3 to calculate an estimated corrected phenytoin.

Step 2: Calculate the corrected phenytoin levels as if the creatinine clearance was below 10 mL/min using Equation 3.

$$\text{Corrected phenytoin} = \frac{\text{Phenytoin observed}}{(\text{Albumin} \times 0.1) + 0.1}$$

$$\text{Corrected phenytoin} = \frac{7.9 \text{ mg/L}}{(4 \text{ g/dL} \times 0.1) + 0.1}$$

$$\text{Corrected phenytoin} = 15.8 \text{ mg/L}$$

Step 3: Calculate the corrected phenytoin level concentration as if the creatinine clearance was >25 mL/min using Equation 1.

$$\text{Corrected phenytoin} = \frac{\text{Phenytoin observed}}{(\text{Albumin} \times 0.2) + 0.1}$$

$$\text{Corrected phenytoin} = \frac{7.9 \text{ mg/L}}{(4 \text{ g/dL} \times 0.2) + 0.1}$$

$$\text{Corrected phenytoin} = 8.8 \text{ mg/L}$$

Step 4: Take the average of the calculated corrected phenytoin levels from Steps 2 and 3 to estimate the overall corrected phenytoin level for JZ.

$$(15.8 \text{ mg/L} + 8.8 \text{ mg/L})/2 = 12.3 \text{ mg/L}$$

Based on the corrected phenytoin concentrations above, JZ's corrected phenytoin concentration falls between 8.8 mg/L and 15.8 mg/L, which averaged to 12.3 mg/L.

LOADING DOSE OF PHENYTOIN

There are two scenarios whereby loading dose of phenytoin is required. First, when a newly diagnosed patient who is phenytoin-naïve is to be started on phenytoin, and second, when a patient who is already receiving phenytoin has a phenytoin level that is below the desired concentration. Loading doses allow such patients to achieve target levels quickly.

When calculating for a loading dose, it is important to determine the target peak phenytoin concentration (C_p) and the formulation of phenytoin that is to be used for the loading. Typically, for phenytoin-naïve patients, the target C_p is 20 mg/L. The oral suspension and the intravenous formulations are the most commonly used dosage forms for loading phenytoin because they have been associated with the most rapid increase in serum concentration as compared to the tablet and capsule formulations.[9]

The following formula is used when calculating the loading dose in phenytoin-naïve patients.

$$\text{Equation 4: } \text{Loading dose} = \frac{(V_d)(\text{Actual body weight})(\text{Target } C_p)}{(F)(S)}$$

Under normal K_a and f_{up}, the estimated volume of distribution (V_d) falls between 0.6 and 0.7 L/kg, with an average of 0.65 L/kg. All phenytoin formulation has a bioavailability (F) of 1. Phenytoin sodium, available as interavenous and as capsule, has a salt factor (S) of 0.92. Phenytoin acid on the other hand is available as suspension and chewable tablets, and has a salt factor of 1.

The phenytoin loading dose equation (Equation 4) must be changed for patients who are currently on phenytoin and the observed phenytoin level is below target. The newly revised formulation accounts for the presence of the phenytoin already in the patient's plasma.

Equation 5: Loading dose

$$= \frac{(V_d)(\text{Actual body weight})(\text{Target } C_p - \text{Phenytoin Observed})}{(F)(S)}$$

In cases where K_a or f_{up} are altered (e.g., hypoalbuminemia, renal failure, ESRD), it is not necessary to substitute the "phenytoin observed" with the "corrected phenytoin" in the loading dose equations because the V_d and the target peak concentration are inversely related. A decrease in serum albumin or albumin affinity results in an opposite increase in the calculated V_d, and a subsequent decrease in the target concentration by almost the same factor. Hence, these changes negate each other, having little or insignificant effect on the final loading dose calculation.[22]

For obese patients, defined as actual body weight 20 percent above the ideal body weight, the excess adipose tissue can increase the V_d of phenytoin, thus resulting in a higher loading dose. To adjust for the increase in V_d, instead of calculating for the V_d by using the actual body weight, multiply the excess weight by a factor of 1.33 and add this to the IBW. Use this *adjusted* weight to determine the new V_d.[23,24]

Equation 6: $V_{d \text{ obese}} = 0.65 \text{ L/kg} \times [\text{IBW} + 1.33 (\text{Actual body weight} - \text{IBW})]$

CASE 11: CALCULATE THE PHENYTOIN LOADING DOSE IN PHENYTOIN-NAÏVE PATIENTS

JT is a 60-year-old male (75 kg) newly diagnosed with seizure disorder. He has normal renal function and albumin level. His physician wants to load him with phenytoin. Calculate a loading dose using phenytoin suspension and intravenous, and recommend appropriate dosing administration for both.

Answer:

Calculate a loading dose for JT if phenytoin suspension is to be administered.

$$\text{Loading dose} = \frac{(0.65 \text{ L/kg})(75 \text{ kg})(20 \text{ mg/L})}{(1)(1)}$$

$$= 975 \text{ mg of phenytoin suspension}$$

Calculate a loading dose for JT if phenytoin IV is to be administered.

$$\text{Loading dose} = \frac{(0.65 \text{ L/kg})(75 \text{ kg})(20 \text{ mg/L})}{(1)(0.92)}$$

$$= 1,060 \text{ mg or } \sim 1,000 \text{ mg of phenytoin IV}$$

For oral loading doses, due to the slow rate of gastrointestinal absorption,[25,26] it is recommended to administer the loading dose of phenytoin in smaller incremental doses rather than give the entire loading dose at one time. Furthermore, due to phenytoin's limited gastrointestinal absorption, dose increases may result in longer times to reach peak plasma concentration.[27] Remember, the goal of giving a loading dose is to achieve the target peak concentration quickly. As a general rule, oral loading doses should be given at increments of no more than 400 mg every 2 hours. Thus, for JT, the total oral loading dose of 975 mg can be administered as 400 mg, 400 mg, and 175 mg, with a 2-hour interval between each dose. Another option is to administer the 975 mg oral loading dose as 400 mg, 300 mg, and 275 mg with a 2-hour interval between each dose. No published studies prove that either approach is better than the other. However, one can surmise that giving higher doses at the beginning of the loading process may shorten the time to reach target concentration, but it may increase the incidence of gastrointestinal side effects. While dividing doses equally and not using the maximum dose at each interval may decrease the incidence of such side effects. Either one of these approaches is acceptable.

If a more rapid peak plasma concentration must be achieved, it is be best to administer the loading dose of phenytoin via the IV route. As mentioned earlier in the chapter, the IV formulation of phenytoin contains propylene glycol, which has been associated with cardiovascular events when administered rapidly. Therefore, when the IV formulation must be used for loading phenytoin, it must be administered at a rate no more than 50 mg/min.[28] For JT, an IV loading dose of 1,000 mg can be administered no faster than 20 minutes. It may be advisable to extend or lower the rate of infusion to 20–25 mg/min to further lower the risk of cardiovascular toxicity, especially in the elderly (>65 years old) and those with a history of cardiac disease.[29] Cardiac monitoring and the use of a 0.22 micron filter are necessary during intravenous phenytoin administration.

CASE 12: CALCULATE THE IV PHENYTOIN LOADING DOSE IN PHENYTOIN-NAÏVE PATIENTS

A 33-year-old white male (100 kg) is to be placed on phenytoin for generalized tonic-clonic status epilepticus. The patient has already received two doses of IV lorazepam without a response. An SMA-18 panel includes the following laboratory values: creatinine 0.5 mg/dL and albumin 5 g/dL. Calculate an IV phenytoin loading dose to achieve a target of 18 mg/L.

Answer:

Use Equation 5 to calculate the IV phenytoin loading dose for this patient. Because this patient has a normal albumin and a creatinine clearance above 25 mL/minute, it is not necesarry to determine the loading dose based on the corrected phenytoin level.

$$\text{Loading dose} = \frac{(V_d)(\text{Actual body weight})(\text{Target C}_p)}{(F)(S)}$$

$$\text{Loading dose} = \frac{(0.65 \text{ L/kg})(100 \text{ kg})(18 \text{ mg/L})}{(1)(0.92)}$$

$$= 1{,}272 \text{ mg of phenytoin suspension}$$

The IV phenytoin loading dose for this patient may be rounded up to 1,300 mg. Because this patient is in status epilepticus and is yet to respond to lorazepam, the rate of IV phenytoin administration should be 50 mg/min. Additionally, young patients tend to be at lower risk of developing phenytoin-induced hypotension and bradycardia during rapid IV administration at 50 mg/min. Continuous cardiac monitoring and the use of a 0.22 micron filter are necessary during intravenous phenytoin administration.

CASE 13: CALCULATING PHENYTOIN LOADING DOSE IN PATIENTS WHO ARE ALREADY ON PHENYTOIN

PC is a 62-year-old male patient (75 kg) who has been receiving phenytoin for the past 12 months for the management of grand mal seizures. He returned to the doctor's office for a follow up. His latest laboratory test revealed an observed phenytoin concentration of 6 mg/L. His albumin and renal function were normal. Calculate a loading dose for PC using phenytoin suspension.

Answer:

Loading dose

$$= \frac{(V_d)(\text{Actual body weight})(\text{Target C}_p - \text{Phenytoin observed})}{(F)(S)}$$

$$= \frac{(0.65 \text{ L/kg})(75 \text{ kg})(20 \text{ mg/L} - 6 \text{ mg/L})}{(1)(1)}$$

$$= 683 \text{ mg, or} \sim 675 \text{ mg of phenytoin suspension}$$

It is important to round off the final phenytoin loading dose to the nearest measurable volume available. Phenytoin suspension is available in 100 mg/4 mL or 25 mg/mL concentration. Therefore, 675 mg will be equivalent to 27 milliliters. Because no more than 400 mg can be administered at a time, the loading dose for PC can be administered as 375 mg followed by 300 mg, administered 2 hours apart.

CASE 14: CALCULATING FOR PHENYTOIN LOADING DOSE IN PATIENTS WHO ARE ALREADY ON PHENYTOIN WITH HYPOALBUMINEMIA

JR is a 37-year-old male (80 kg) with history of seizure disorder, who returns to the clinic complaining of breakthrough seizures. His most recent phenytoin observed level was 5 mg/L and his albumin was 3.1 g/dL. His renal function was normal. Calculate a loading dose for JR using phenytoin suspension. Assume test for phenytoin level was performed at 37°C.

Step 1: Calculate for the corrected phenytoin level to determine whether a loading dose is needed.

$$\text{Corrected phenytoin} = \frac{\text{Phenytoin observed}}{(\text{Albumin} \times 0.2) + 0.1}$$

$$\text{Corrected phenytoin} = \frac{5 \text{ mg/L}}{(3.1 \times 0.2) + 0.1}$$

$$\text{Corrected phenytoin} = 6.9 \text{ mg/L}$$

Because the corrected phenytoin level is below the target range of 10–20 mg/L, a loading dose is required.

Step 2: Calculate the loading dose accounting for the phenytoin observed. Remember, *do not* use the corrected phenytoin level in this formula; rather use the phenytoin observed.

Loading dose

$$= \frac{(V_d)(\text{Actual body weight})(\text{Target C}_p - \text{Phenytoin observed})}{(F)(S)}$$

$$\text{Loading dose} = \frac{(0.65 \text{ L/kg})(80 \text{ kg})(20 \text{ mg/L} - 5 \text{ mg/L})}{(1)(1)}$$

Loading dose = 780 mg, or 800 mg of phenytoin suspension

The loading dose for JR is 800 mg, which can be given as 400 mg, and 400 mg administered 2 hours apart.

CASE 15: CALCULATING PHENYTOIN LOADING DOSE IN PATIENTS WHO ARE OBESE

PH is a 62-year-old female (92 kg, 5′2″) who was admitted in the ED for seizure breakthrough. Her observed phenytoin level was found to be 2.2 mg/L due to noncompliance. After receiving two doses of lorazepam, her seizures abated. Her albumin level was 4.6 g/dL, and SCr was 0.8 mg/dL. Her physician wants to load her with IV phenytoin. Calculate the appropriate loading dose and recommend a rate of infusion.

Step 1: Calculate for the IBW.

$$\text{IBW}_{female} = 45.5 + (2.3 \times 2)$$
$$\text{IBW}_{female} = 50.1 \text{ kg}$$

Step 2: Determine whether patient is obese.

$$\frac{(\text{Actual body weight} - \text{IBW})}{\text{IBW}} \times 100\%$$

$$\frac{(92 \text{ kg} - 50.1 \text{ kg})}{50.1 \text{ kg}} \times 100\% = 84\%$$

Because the patient's actual body weight is 92 kg, which is greater than 20 percent over the ideal weight, we need to calculate for the V_d using the factor of 1.33 (Equation 6).

Step 3: Calculate for $V_{d \text{ obese}}$.

$$V_{d \text{ obese}} = 0.65 \text{ L/kg} \times [\text{IBW} + 1.33(\text{Actual body weight} - \text{IBW})]$$
$$= 0.65 \text{ L/kg} \times [50.1 \text{ kg} + 1.33(92 \text{ kg} - 50.1 \text{ kg})]$$
$$= 68.8 \text{ L}$$

Step 4: Calculate for the loading dose using the new adjusted V_d for obese patients.

$$\text{Loading dose} = \frac{(V_d)(\text{Target } C_p - \text{Phenytoin observed})}{(F)(S)}$$

$$= \frac{(68.8 \text{ L})(20 \text{ mg/L} - 2.2 \text{ mg/L})}{(1)(0.92)}$$

$$= 1331 \text{ mg, or } 1,300 \text{ mg of phenytoin IV}$$

Step 5: Calculate the rate of infusion.

Rate of infusion should be no more than 50 mg/min.

$$\frac{1,300 \text{ mg}}{x} = \frac{50 \text{ mg}}{\text{min}}$$

$$x = 26 \text{ minutes}$$

Recommendation is to infuse 1,300 mg of phenytoin IV no faster than 26 minutes. To further decrease the risk of cardiotoxicity, extend the infusion time to 30–45 minutes. In addition, ensure the patient is on a cardiac monitor and a 0.22 micron filter is used for the drug administration.

METABOLISM AND CLEARANCE/HALF-LIFE

Phenytoin is primarily metabolized in the liver by para-hydroxylation to the inactive metabolite, HPPH [5-(p-hydroxyphenyl)-5-phenylhydantoin], which is further conjugated in the liver with glucuronic acid and eventually eliminated in the urine. Approximately 5 percent of phenytoin is eliminated unchanged in the urine.[8] Phenytoin follows Michaelis-Menten kinetics or capacity-limited metabolism. For most medications, as the dose increases, the rate of metabolism increases proportionally, and the rate of metabolism is not maximized at therapeutic doses. However, for phenytoin, as the dose increases, at a given point in time the liver metabolism is maximized or saturated. As a result, even small increases in dosage can lead to toxic plasma concentrations because the liver can no longer metabolize the phenytoin fast enough. Medications that follow Michaelis-Menten kinetics are said to go from first-order to zero-order kinetics (nonlinear kinetics). Unfortunately, it is unknown at which dose the liver metabolism of phenytoin is maximized or saturated. Therefore, small differences may separate the therapeutic from the toxic dose of phenytoin for a patient. It is recommended that as a patient approaches the target phenytoin concentration, small increments in dosage are implemented in order to avoid toxic levels when the liver metabolism saturation is unknown.[4,8,30,31]

For most patients the maximum metabolic capacity of phenytoin (V_{max}) is between 5 and 15 mg/kg/day, with an average of 7 mg/kg/day. Meanwhile, the K_m is the substrate concentration at which the velocity or rate of metabolism is half of V_{max}. Therefore, K_m for most patients is approximately 4 mg/L. The population-based average K_m and V_{max} can be used to calculate the phenytoin maintenance dose in patients who are phenytoin-naïve.

$$\text{Equation 7: Maintenance dose}_{\text{population-based}} = \frac{(V_{max})(C_{pSS})}{(C_{pSS} + K_m)(F)(S)}$$

where V_{max} = 7 mg/kg/day, K_m = 4 mg/L, and C_{pSS} = Target steady state peak concentration of 15 mg/L.

If the patient is already taking phenytoin and a phenytoin plasma level is available, then calculate for the patient's own maximum rate of metabolism or patient specific V_{max} ($V_{max,ptspecific}$) using Equation 8, assuming that the C_{pSS} is at steady state.

$$\text{Equation 8: } V_{max,ptspecific} = \frac{(\text{Total dose/day})(F)(S)(C_{pSS} + K_{max})}{(C_{pSS})}$$

In the setting of decreased K_a or increased f_{up}, C_{pSS} must be adjusted to reflect the normal plasma binding when calculating for the $V_{max,ptspecific}$.

Using patient-specific V_{max}, a new maintenance dose can then be calculated using the following equation:

$$\text{Equation 9: Maintenance dose}_{\text{ptspecific}} = \frac{(V_{max,ptspecific})(C_{pSS})}{(C_{pSS} + K_m)(F)(S)}$$

CASE 16: CALCULATING MAINTENANCE DOSE OF PHENYTOIN IN PHENYTOIN-NAÏVE PATIENTS

KC is a 35-year-old female (62 kg) who was admitted in the emergency room for new-onset seizures. She received a dose of lorazepam 6 mg and was loaded on phenytoin. Now, she is to be admitted to the internal medicine floor where she is to be started on a maintenance dose of phenytoin. Calculate a maintenance dose for KC if phenytoin capsules are to be given.

Step 1: Calculate for the V_{max} using the patient's actual weight.

$$V_{max} = (7 \text{ mg/kg/day})(62 \text{ kg})$$
$$V_{max} = 434 \text{ mg/day}$$

Step 2: Calculate the maintenance dose using Equation 7.

$$\text{Maintenance dose} = \frac{(V_{max})(C_{pSS})}{(C_{pSS} + K_m)(F)(S)}$$

$$\text{Maintenance dose} = \frac{(434 \text{ mg/day})(15 \text{ mg/L})}{(15 \text{ mg/L} + 4 \text{ mg/L})(1)(0.92)}$$

$$= 372 \text{ mg, or } \sim 360 \text{ mg capsules per day}$$

CASE 17: CALCULATING FOR THE PATIENT-SPECIFIC V_{max} AND NEW MAINTENANCE DOSE

SC is a 44-year-old male receiving phenytoin suspension 125 mg q8h for the past two years. His phenytoin level was found to be 2.6 mg/L at 37°C and albumin 2.3 g/dL. He has ESRD and receiving HD on M/W/F. Calculate for this patient's V_{max} and new maintenance dose using phenytoin suspension.

Step 1: Because this patient has low albumin and has ESRD, calculate for the corrected phenytoin level first.

$$\text{Corrected phenytoin} = \frac{\text{Phenytoin observed}}{(\text{Albumin} \times 0.1) + 0.1}$$

$$= \frac{2.6 \text{ mg/L}}{(2.3 \text{ g/dL} \times 0.1) + 0.1}$$

$$= 7.9 \text{ mg/L}$$

Step 2: Calculate the V_{max} using the corrected phenytoin level. We can assume that the C_{pSS} is at steady state since this patient has been taking the same dose of phenytoin for the past 2 years.

$$V_{max,ptspecific} = \frac{(\text{Total dose/day})(F)(S)(C_{pSS} + K_m)}{(C_{pSS})}$$

$$= \frac{(375 \text{ mg/day})(1)(1)(7.9 \text{ mg/L} + 4 \text{ mg/L})}{(7.9 \text{ mg/L})}$$

$$= 565 \text{ mg/day}$$

Step 3: Calculate for a new maintenance dose using the patient-specific V_{max}.

$$\text{New maintenance dose} = \frac{(V_{max,ptspecific})(C_{pSS})}{(C_{pSS} + K_M)(F)(S)}$$

$$= \frac{(565 \text{ mg/day})(15 \text{ mg/L})}{(15 \text{ mg/L} + 4 \text{ mg/L})(1)(1)}$$

$$= 446 \text{ mg/day, or 450 mg per day of}$$
phenytoin suspension, administered
at 150 mg every 8 hours

PHENYTOIN HALF-LIFE AND STEADY STATE

The unique metabolism/elimination of phenytoin makes half-life measurements inaccurate with little utility. In capacity-limited metabolism, the half-life of the drug depends on the drug's serum concentration. As the phenytoin concentration increases, the half-life increases, and vice versa. Phenytoin therefore does not have a constant half-life.

Due to phenytoin's capacity-limited metabolism, the application of half-life to estimate time to achieve steady state and time to eliminate the drug from the body in settings of toxicity can be challenging. The half-life of drugs that follow linear kinetics shows the time that it takes to metabolize 50 percent of the drug. Because phenytoin follows nonlinear kinetics, the exact half-life is difficult to predict. In fact, multiple studies have shown great variability in phenytoin's half-life ranging from 10 to 95 hours in adults.[4,8,32]

In order to calculate a patient's specific V_{max}, one must first determine whether the phenytoin plasma concentration observed has reached steady state. To determine if the phenytoin level drawn is at steady state, one can use the $t_{90\%}$ formula that represents the time required for the phenytoin to reach 90 percent of its steady-state value.

$$\text{Equation 10: } t_{90\%} = \frac{[115 + 35 \times (C_p)](C_p)}{(S)(F)(\text{dose/day})}$$

This equation was based on a 70 kg patient; thus, the dose of phenytoin must first be converted to an equivalent dose as it would apply to a 70 kg patient. In addition, in the presence of decreased albumin or renal function, the phenytoin observed (C_p) must be corrected.

If the serum phenytoin observed is not at steady state based on the $t_{90\%}$ formula, then the phenytoin observed cannot be used to calculate the patient's specific V_{max}, and no new maintenance dose can be calculated either. Instead, you must estimate the amount of phenytoin metabolism over time using two different phenytoin concentrations drawn at two separate occasions.

Equation 11:

$$\text{Amount eliminated/t} = (S)(F)(\text{dose/day}) - \frac{[(C2 - C1) \times (V_d)]}{t}$$

In this formula, C1 represents the initial phenytoin level and C2 represents the second phenytoin level. Both C1 and C2 need to be corrected in the setting of altered plasma binding. t is the time interval (in days) between C2 and C1. However, in order for this formula

to accurately calculate the patient-specific V_{max}, a few criteria need to be met:

1. The time between C1 and C2 must be ≥ 3 days.
2. C2 must be $\leq$ twice C1 if the plasma concentration is rising, OR
3. C2 must be $\geq \frac{1}{2}$ of C1 if the plasma concentration is declining.
4. Phenytoin dose, route, and formulation must be consistent.

Once the amount eliminated per time (amount eliminated/t) is determined, calculate for the V_{max} by making a few key substitutions to the $V_{max,ptspecific}$ formula (Equation 8). Substitute total dose/day with the amount eliminated/t, and C_{pSS} with the average of C1 and C2, resulting in a new equation for $V_{max,CpNSS}$, whereby phenytoin observed (C_p) is not at steady state:

Equation 12:

$$V_{max,CpNSS} = \frac{(\text{Amount eliminated/day}) \times ([\text{average of C1 + C2}] + K_M)}{(\text{Average of C1 + C2})}$$

A new maintenance dose (Equation 9) can then be calculated using the answer to the $V_{max,CpNSS}$.

CASE 18: CALCULATING TIME REQUIRED BEFORE REACHING STEADY STATE

DN is a 72-year-old male (98 kg) who was started on phenytoin suspension 250 mg every 12 hours for the past 17 days. His observed phenytoin level is 11 mg/L. His albumin level was 4.9 g/dL, and SCr was 1 mg/dL. Determine whether the phenytoin observed is likely to be at steady state.

Step 1: Adjust dosing based on a 70 kg patient.

$$\frac{500 \text{ mg}}{98 \text{ kg}} = \frac{x}{70 \text{ kg}}$$

$$x = 357 \text{ mg}$$

Step 2: Calculate for $t_{90\%}$ using the dose based on a 70 kg patient.

$$t_{90\%} = \frac{[115 + 35 \times (C_p)](C_p)}{(S)(F)(\text{dose/day})}$$

$$t_{90\%} = \frac{[115 + 35 \times (11 \text{ mg/L})](11 \text{ mg/L})}{(1)(1)(357 \text{ mg/day})}$$

$$t_{90\%} = 15 \text{ days}$$

Based on the calculated $t_{90\%}$, the estimated time to reached steady state is approximately 15 days. Because the serum phenytoin level was drawn on day 17, this level is considered to be at steady state.

CASE 19: CALCULATING V_{max} IF PHENYTOIN OBSERVED IS NOT AT STEADY STATE

AC is a 52-year-old female (82 kg) who received an 800 mg loading dose of phenytoin suspension and was started on a maintenance dose of phenytoin 225 mg suspension every 12 hours for 5 days. Her follow-up serum phenytoin level was found to be subtherapeutic at 8 mg/L at 37°C. Albumin and renal function were within normal. Assuming that the level is not at steady state, calculate for a new maintenance dose:

Step 1: Calculate for initial concentration (C1) of PHT after the loading dose of 800 mg suspension.

$$C1 = \frac{(S)(F)(\text{Loading dose})}{V_d}$$

$$C1 = \frac{(1)(1)(800 \text{ mg})}{(0.65 \text{ L/kg})(82 \text{ kg})}$$

$$C1 = 15 \text{ mg/L}$$

Step 2: Calculate the amount eliminated over time.

$$\text{Amount eliminated/t} = (S)(F)(\text{dose/day}) - \frac{[(C2 - C1) \times (V_d)]}{t}$$

Amount eliminated/t

$$= (1)(1)(450 \text{ mg/day}) - \frac{[(8 \text{ mg/L} - 15 \text{ mg/L})(53.3 \text{ L})]}{5 \text{ days}}$$

Amount eliminated/t = 524.6 mg/day

The amount eliminated over time gives an average range of the amount of phenytoin that is eliminated per day for this patient. Use this information to calculate for the $V_{max,CpNSS}$. In this case, patient AC has an average phenytoin elimination of 524.6 mg/day, which should provide a phenytoin concentration average between C1 (15 mg/L) and C2 (8 mg/L), which in this case is 11.5 mg/L.

Step 3: Calculate a new dose using the amount eliminated/t as the Total dose/day, and the average phenytoin concentration between C1 and C2 as C_{pSSavg}.

$$V_{max,CpNSS} = \frac{(\text{Total dose/day})(F)(S)(C_{pSS} + K_M)}{(C_{pSS})}$$

$$V_{max,CpNSS} = \frac{(524.6 \text{ mg/day})(1)(1)(11.5 \text{ mg/L} + 4 \text{ mg/L})}{11.5 \text{ mg/L}}$$

$$V_{max,CpNSS} = 707 \text{ mg/day}$$

Step 4: Calculate a new maintenance dose using $V_{max,CpNSS}$.

$$\text{New maintenance dose} = \frac{(V_{max,CpNSS})(C_{pSS})}{(C_{pSS} + K_M)(F)(S)}$$

$$\text{New maintenance dose} = \frac{(707 \text{ mg/day})(15 \text{ mg/L})}{(15 \text{ mg/L} + 4 \text{ mg/L})(1)(1)}$$

New maintenance dose = 558 mg/day or ~ 550 mg/day of phenytoin suspension given in divided doses of 275 mg Q12 hours

CALCULATING THE RATE OF DECLINE OF PHENYTOIN IF LEVELS ARE TOXIC

Due to the unpredictability of phenytoin kinetics, it is often difficult to determine when toxic phenytoin levels are expected to decline to target levels. Once again, the nonlinear kinetics of phenytoin's half-life make the practice of using half-lives to calculate the time needed for the drug level to decline (e.g., one half-life decreases serum drug by 50%, two half-lives by 75%, three half-lives by 87.5%, and so on) inapplicable. Often, clinicians are forced to obtain frequent or even unnecessary drug levels that can be time-consuming, costly, and may affect patient's quality of life due to frequent blood draws. In other cases, frequent blood work may not be feasible, such as an outpatient setting or in patients with poor venous access.

To circumvent frequent and unnecessary blood work, one can calculate the rate of phenytoin decline over time. The rate of phenytoin decline can provide us with an estimated time of decay or decline to desired phenytoin level. Using the phenytoin observed, desired, or target phenytoin concentration, patient-specific V_{max}, and V_d, we can calculate the time it would take for a toxic phenytoin level to decline to the target or desired level.

Equation 13:

$$\text{Time to decline, days (t)} = \frac{[K_M \times (\text{Ln}\,(C1/C2))] + (C1 - C2)}{V_{max}/V_d}$$

In this formula, time to decline (t) is represented in days. C1 is the initial phenytoin concentration, while C2 is the final or desired concentration. C1 must be corrected in the setting of altered protein binding prior to being applied in this formula.

In the setting of an oral phenytoin overdose, this formula is rendered ineffective in determining the time it will take for the drug to decline to normal levels because the initial phenytoin concentration may not be an accurate representation of the peak phenytoin concentration after the overdose. Remember, the rate of GI absorption is increased with higher dose administration, which also means that the time to reach the peak concentration is prolonged. The initial phenytoin concentration may not be the true peak concentration if enough time has not elapsed between the time of ingestion and the time of phenytoin blood draw to allow for complete GI absorption of phenytoin. However, this formula is valid in the setting of an intravenous phenytoin overdose because GI absorption is bypassed.

CASE 20: CALCULATING THE RATE OF DECLINE OF PHENYTOIN IN TOXIC PHENYTOIN LEVELS

TR is a 43-year-old male (72 kg) who has been on phenytoin 200 mg capsule every 12 hours for the past 6 months. His phenytoin levels in the past have been therapeutic. However, during his most recent physician visit, he was found to have CNS symptoms consistent of phenytoin toxicity, his phenytoin level was found to be 22 mg/L, albumin 3.4 g/dL, and renal function was normal. Overdose and non-compliance were ruled out. Calculate what the correct phenytoin level would be and determine how long it will take for the phenytoin levels to return at target (15 mg/L), assuming steady state has been achieved and test was performed at 37°C.

Step 1: Calculate the corrected phenytoin level.

$$\text{Corrected phenytoin} = \frac{\text{Phenytoin observed}}{(\text{Albumin} \times 0.2) + 0.1}$$

$$\text{Corrected phenytoin} = \frac{22 \text{ mg/L}}{(3.4 \text{ g/dL} \times 0.2) + 0.1}$$

Corrected phenytoin = 28.2 mg/L

Step 2: Calculate for the V_{max} (assuming C_{pss} is at steady state).

$$V_{max,ptspecific} = \frac{(400 \text{ mg/day})(1)(0.92)(28.2 \text{ mg/L} + 4 \text{ mg/L})}{(28.2 \text{ mg/L})}$$

$$V_{max,ptspecific} = 420 \text{ mg/day}$$

Step 3: Calculate the rate of decline of phenytoin.

$$t = \frac{[4 \text{ mg/L} \times (\text{Ln}\,(28.2/15))] + (28.2 - 15)}{420 \text{ mg/day} \div (72 \text{ kg})(0.65 \text{ L/kg})}$$

$$t = 15.73/9$$

$$t = 1.7 \text{ days}$$

The phenytoin level should return to 15 mg/L after 1.7 days. In practice, it would mean that the phenytoin dose should be held for 1 day, and phenytoin levels to be repeated on the following day, rather than drawing daily phenytoin levels.

PATIENT-SPECIFIC K_M

So far, the K_M used in the previous formulas is assumed to be 4 mg/L. For the most part, this approach is acceptable. However, in cases where conservative dosage adjustments are needed, the patient-specific K_M can be valuable. In order to calculate for the patient-specific

K_M, two steady-state concentrations and doses must be available. Patient-specific K_M can be calculated using this formula:

$$\text{Equation 14: } -K_{M,ptspecific} = \frac{R1 - R2}{(R1/C_{SS1}) - (R2/C_{SS2})}$$

In this formula, R1 and C_{SS1} represent the first dose and steady-state concentration, respectively, and R2 and C_{SS2} represent the second dose and steady-state concentration. It is important that both phenytoin levels are at steady state.

CASE 21: CALCULATING A NEW DOSE USING PATIENT-SPECIFIC K_M

UR is a 62-year-old female (48 kg) with a history of traumatic brain injury 20 years ago. She has been taking phenytoin 375 mg PO suspension twice daily for 6 months and has an observed phenytoin level of 22 mg/L. A year ago, she was taking 300 mg of phenytoin suspension twice daily for 6 months, but her level was found to be too low at 8 mg/L and having breakthrough seizures every 2–3 weeks. As a result, the phenytoin dose was increased to 375 mg bid. Both phenytoin levels were performed at the hospital laboratory at 37°C. Her albumin level has been steady at 4.6 g/dL for the past year. Her SCr is 1 mg/dL. Her physician wants to make another dose adjustment, but would like to be more conservative in lowering the dose as to decrease the risk of subtherapeutic level and subsequent seizure breakthroughs. Calculate the patient-specific K_M and a new dose.

Step 1: Calculate for patient-specific K_M.

$$-K_{M,ptspecific} = \frac{R1 - R2}{(R1/C_{SS1}) - (R2/C_{SS2})}$$

$$-K_{M,ptspecific} = \frac{600 \text{ mg} - 750 \text{ mg}}{(600 \text{ mg}/8 \text{ mg/L}) - (750 \text{ mg}/22 \text{ mg/L})}$$

$$-K_{M,ptspecific} = \frac{-150 \text{ mg}}{75 \text{ L} - 34.1 \text{ L}}$$

$$K_{M,ptspecific} = 3.67 \text{ mg/L}$$

Step 2: Calculate for the patient-specific V_{max} using patient-specific K_M

$$V_{max,ptspecific} = \frac{(\text{Total dose/day}) \times (F) \times (S) \times (C_{pSS} + K_{M,ptspecific})}{(C_{pSS})}$$

$$V_{max,ptspecific} = \frac{(750 \text{ mg/day}) \times (1) \times (1) \times (22 \text{ mg/L} + 3.67 \text{ mg/L})}{(22 \text{ mg/L})}$$

$$V_{max,ptspecific} = 875 \text{ mg/day}$$

Step 3: Calculate for the new maintenance dose using both patient-specific V_{max} and K_M.

$$\text{New maintenance dose} = \frac{(V_{max,ptspecific})(C_{pSS})}{(C_{pSS} + K_{M,ptspecific})(F)(S)}$$

$$\text{New maintenance dose} = \frac{(875 \text{ mg/day})(15 \text{ mg/L})}{(15 \text{ mg/L} + 3.67 \text{ mg/L})(1)(1)}$$

New maintenance dose = 703 mg/day, or ~700 mg/day of phenytoin suspension in divided doses of 350 mg twice a day.

CASE 22: CALCULATING TIME TO DECLINE USING PATIENT-SPECIFIC K_M AND V_{max}

The physician accepted the recommendation to lower patient UR's phenytoin dose to 350 mg suspension bid. When can this new maintenance dose be initiated?

Answer:

It would be best to start the new dose of phenytoin once the phenytoin level falls to 10–20 mg/L. The best way to determine the time it would take for the phenytoin level to decrease to the desired concentration is by using the time to decline formula (Equation 13). Notice that the patient's specific V_{max} and K_M are now being used, and the target desired level (C2) is 15 mg/L.

$$\text{Time to decline (t)} = \frac{[K_{M,ptspecific} \times (\text{Ln }(C1/C2))] + (C1 - C2)}{V_{max,ptspecific}/V_d}$$

Time to decline (t)

$$= \frac{[3.67 \text{ mg/L} \times (\text{Ln }(22 \text{ mg/L}/15 \text{ mg/L})] + (22 \text{ mg/L} - 15 \text{ mg/dL})}{875 \text{ mg/day} \div (0.65 \text{ L/kg} \times 48 \text{ kg})}$$

Time to decline (t) = 8.41/28

Time to decline (t) = 0.3 days, or ~7 hours

Therefore, the new phenytoin dose can be restarted at least 7 hours after the last dose.

DRUG INTERACTIONS

Phenytoin's drug interactions can result from any of the following mechanisms:

- *Extensive plasma protein binding* The extensive plasma protein binding of phenytoin and the effects of disease states that can cause changes in albumin concentration have already been discussed in a previous section. Valproic acid (VPA) is an anticonvulsant that has a higher affinity than phenytoin for albumin's binding sites, which becomes evident at VPA levels approaching 100 mg/L where phenytoin's unbound concentration can be increased by 50 percent or more.[4,33,34] Valproic acid also can inhibit phenytoin's oxidation. It is recommended that unbound phenytoin levels be monitored in patients where both anticonvulsants must be prescribed.

- *Hepatic metabolism* Phenytoin undergoes extensive metabolism in the liver and, as noted earlier, less than 5 percent is eliminated unchanged in the urine. It is a substrate for CYP2C9 (primarily), 2C19, and 3A4 while it induces CYP2B6, 2C8, 2C9, 2C19, and 3A4.[2,34,35] Hence, it is no surprise that phenytoin interacts with a number of other medications as listed in Table 15-3.[34,35] Drugs that inhibit CYP2C9 and 2C19 have been shown to increase phenytoin's serum levels leading to toxicities and side effects from the anticonvulsant, while drugs that induce the isoenzymes decrease phenytoin's concentration and place the patient at risk for developing seizures. In the last decade, it has also been shown that CYP2C9 and 2C19 are polymorphic, and population genetic polymorphisms play an important role in the pharmacokinetics of phenytoin. Defective genes in CYP2C9 and 2C19 can lead to decreased phenytoin metabolism and subsequent toxic levels. Careful monitoring of phenytoin is recommended, especially at higher doses. Others also suggest that rare polymorphisms of the drug-transporting p-glycoprotein (pGP) may play a role.[35]

  Carbamazepine (CBZ) has been shown to decrease phenytoin's clearance in about half of patients.[34,36] In such cases, patients have exhibited signs of neurotoxicity. It is not clear at what point in therapy after the addition of CBZ patients are at risk for toxic phenytoin levels. To complicate matters further, it has also been shown that phenytoin has the ability to decrease CBZ's levels by about 30 percent, possibly by phenytoin's induction of the CYP3A4 isoenzyme system.

TABLE 15-3	Phenytoin Drug Interactions[2,42]

Drugs That Decrease Phenytoin's Concentration

Drugs	Comment
Antacids	Phenytoin levels must be monitored during concomitant therapy and dose adjustments made accordingly. Alternatively, if possible, other medications can be prescribed in lieu of the interacting ones.
Charcoal	
Diazoxide	
Primidone	
Pyridoxine	
Rifampin	
Sucralfate	

Drugs That Increase Phenytoin's Concentration

Drugs	Comment
Allopurinol	Phenytoin levels must be monitored during concomitant therapy and dose adjustments made accordingly. Alternatively, if possible, other medications can be prescribed in lieu of the interacting ones.
Amiodarone	
Carmustine	
Chloramphenicol	
Chloridazepoxide	
Chlorpheniramine	
Cimetidine	
Clarithromycin	
Dexamethasone	
Dicumarol	
Disulfiram	
Felbamate	
Fluconazole	
Fluoxetine	
Ibuprofen	
Isoniazid	
Methotrexate	
Nifedipine	
Omeprazole	
Phenylbutazone	
Salicylates	
Sulfamethizole	
Ticlodipine	
Trimethoprim	
Tolbutamide	
Valproic acid	

Phenytoin's Effect on Other Drugs: Decrease of Other Drugs' Concentration

Drugs	Comment
Acetaminophen	Where applicable alternative agents for these medications may be chosen or higher doses may be used in concomitant administration with phenytoin as necessary.
Chloramphenicol	
Cyclophosphamide	
Cyclosporine	
Dicoumarol	
Digitoxin	
Digoxin	
Doxycycline	
Furosemide	
Itraconazole	
Meperidine	
Methadone	
Mexiletine	
Misonidazole	
Oral contraceptives	
Praziquantel	
Prednisone	
Prednisolone	
Quetiapine	
Quinidine	
Theophylline	
Vecuronium	

(Continued)

TABLE 15-3	Phenytoin Drug Interactions[2,42] *(Continued)*

Mixed Effects on Drug Concentrations

Drugs	Comments
Carbamazepine	• May decrease phenytoin's concentration • May increase phenytoin's concentration • Phenytoin may decrease carbamazepine's concentration • The mechanism of this drug interaction may be due to the competitive inhibition at sites of metabolism
Diazepam	• May increase phenytoin's levels • Short-term exposure to diazepam may not present an interaction
Warfarin	• Phenytoin may increase the anticoagulant effects of warfarin • Warfarin may increase phenytoin's levels • Monitor INR levels closely

As a general rule, it is recommended that if an interacting antiepileptic drug is to be used concomitantly with phenytoin the levels of the initial antiepileptic be monitored and doses be adjusted accordingly.

• *Phenytoin dosing in patients taking interacting drugs or having disease states that may increase or decrease free phenytoin levels* In patients taking medications that interact with phenytoin or having disease states that decrease the amount of phenytoin bound to albumin, taking free phenytoin levels can be useful. The target free phenytoin (fu) level is 1–2 mg/L. Using the free phenytoin level, one can estimate the total phenytoin concentration as if the patient were not on any medications that can alter phenytoin's binding affinity using the following formula:

Total phenytoin = Free phenytoin/Percent unbound (10%)

Using the estimated total phenytoin level from the preceding equation, V_{max}, new maintenance, time to decline, and so on can be calculated.

CASE 23: CALCULATING PHENYTOIN DOSE IN PATIENT ON DRUGS THAT INCREASE FREE PHENYTOIN LEVELS

BR is a 62-year-old female (55 kg) who has been on phenytoin 100 mg tid capsules for the past 10 years. She recently was started on valproic acid 500 mg bid by her neurologist due to poor seizure control with phenytoin despite having phenytoin levels of 10–20 mg/L. Today during her follow-up physician visit, her phenytoin level was found to be 13.4 mg/L @ 37°C, but free phenytoin level was 2.6 mg/L. Her albumin level was 4.6 g/dL, and her calculated CrCl was 45 mL/min. Calculate the time to decline, and recommend a new phenytoin maintenance dose using phenytoin capsules.

Step 1: Calculate the estimated total phenytoin level if $K_a(\alpha)$ were = 0.1.

Total phenytoin = Free phenytoin/Percent unbound (10%)

Total phenytoin = 2.6 mg/L ÷ 0.10

Total phenytoin = 26 mg/L

The estimated total phenytoin level is 26 mg/L for BR.

Step 2: Calculate for patient-specific V_{max} (assuming that 26 mg/L is already at steady state since patient has been on the same dose of phenytoin for the past 10 years).

$$V_{max,ptspecific} = \frac{(\text{Total dose/day})(F)(S)(C_{pSS} + K_M)}{C_{pSS}}$$

$$V_{max,ptspecific} = \frac{(300 \text{ mg/day})(1)(0.92)(26 \text{ mg/L} + 4 \text{ mg/L})}{26 \text{ mg/L}}$$

$$V_{max} = 318 \text{ mg/day}$$

Step 3: Calculate how long it will take for phenytoin to fall within the target serum concentration (10–20 mg/L). In this case you can use an average of 15 mg/L as your target.

$$\text{Time to decline (t)} = \frac{[K_M \times (Ln (C1/C2))] + (C1 - C2)}{V_{max,ptspecific}/V_d}$$

Time to decline (t)

$$= \frac{[4 \text{ mg/L} \times (Ln (26 \text{ mg/L} \div 15 \text{ mg/L}))] + (26 \text{ mg/L} - 15 \text{ mg/L})}{318 \text{ mg/day} \div (0.65 \text{ L/kg} \times 55 \text{ kg})}$$

Time to decline (t) = ~1.5 days

Based on the time to decline, it appears that it will take 1.5 days before the phenytoin level returns to an acceptable level of about 15 mg/L. It means that the phenytoin dose must be held at least one and half days before repeating levels. A new free phenytoin level is still warranted in this scenario because the total or observed phenytoin level may appear normal.

Step 4: Calculate for the new maintenance dose using the previously calculated $V_{max,ptspecific}$.

$$\text{New maintenance dose} = \frac{(V_{max,ptspecific})(C_{pSS})}{(C_{pSS} + K_M)(F)(S)}$$

$$\text{New maintenance dose} = \frac{(318 \text{ mg/day})(15 \text{ mg/L})}{(15 \text{ mg/L} + 4 \text{ mg/L})(1)(0.92)}$$

Maintenance dose = 273 mg/day or ~280 mg/day of phenytoin capsule (can be given as one 100 mg capsule and six 30 mg capsules).

OVERVIEW OF FOSPHENYTOIN

Fosphenytoin (Cerebyx®) is the phosphate ester prodrug of phenytoin. It was developed as a replacement for the IV formulation of phenytoin.[2,37,38] Intravenous phenytoin is associated with many infusion-related (>50 mg/min) side effects such as cardiac (e.g., hypotension, arrhythmias) and injection site–related side effects (e.g., venous irritation, tissue damage, purple glove syndrome) due to its sodium hydroxide, 40 percent propylene glycol, and 10 percent alcohol content. Local toxicity is much less with fosphenytoin when it is administered via the IV or IM routes. Systemic toxicity is similar between the two medications, except that paresthesias and pruritus are more common with fosphenytoin.

Fosphenytoin is a water-soluble prodrug of phenytoin. After absorption, phenytoin is cleaved off fosphenytoin (conversion half-life 8–15 minutes) by phosphatases in the liver, red blood cells, and other tissues.[37,39] The more rapid conversion has been observed in patients with renal or hepatic diseases, due to the decreased protein binding of fosphenytoin. Because it is water soluble (unlike phenytoin), it is rapidly absorbed by the IM route. It can take up to 15 minutes for fosphenytoin to be converted to phenytoin, so it is inappropriate for the *initial* treatment of status epilepticus.[40] It is FDA-approved for the management of status epilepticus of the tonic-clonic (grand mal) seizures and for the prevention and treatment of seizures in those patients having neurosurgery and/or head trauma. It is also approved as an alternative to oral phenytoin if oral administration is not possible and/or contraindicated.

DOSING, ADMINISTRATION, AND MONITORING

It is imperative to remember that the dose, concentration in solutions, and infusion rates for fosphenytoin are expressed as phenytoin sodium equivalents (PE). Fosphenytoin must always be prescribed and dispensed in PE.[40] In fact, 1.5 mg of fosphenytoin is equivalent to 1 mg of phenytoin equivalents (150 mg of fosphenytoin for 100 mg of phenytoin equivalent). The recommended loading dose of IV fosphenytoin is 15–20 mg PE/kg administered at 100–150 mg PE/min. The target concentration can be achieved within 1 minute via the IV route and by 24 minutes by the IM route. For nonemergent loading and maintenance dosing, 10–20 mg PE/kg can be given. The IV dose can be infused over 30 minutes at a maximum rate of 150 mg PE/min. The initial daily maintenance dose is 4–6 mg PE/kg/day.[2,40] The IM route of fosphenytoin can be administered as a single daily dose on one or two injection sites. A 0.22 micron filter during IV administration is not needed; however, the patient must still be observed via a cardiac monitor.

Overdoses are a concern with the use of fosphenytoin due to a confusion between the mg/mL concentration of fosphenytoin expressed in PE (50 mg PE/mL) and the total drug content per vial (either 100 mg PE/2 mL vial or 500 mg PE/10 mL vial). It is recommended to indicate on the containers the *total* drug content rather than the concentration in mg/mL. For pediatric use, it is advised to carry only the 2 mL vial.[2,41]

Cross-reactivity between fosphenytoin and phenytoin immunoassays has been reported. Fosphenytoin displaces phenytoin from albumin binding sites and transient high phenytoin levels have been reported. It is recommended to monitor phenytoin levels at least 4 hours after the IM administration of fosphenytoin and at least 2 hours after the IV administration of fosphenytoin.[39] The most accurate assay is high-performance liquid chromatography (HPLC).

The pharmacokinetic dosing calculations for fosphenytoin are essentially the same as phenytoin. The only difference is an added step of converting fosphenytoin to a PE. To convert fosphenytoin to PE, use the following formula, using a factor of 1.5:

Phenytoin sodium equivalent dose = Fosphenytoin dose/1.5

Once the phenytoin sodium equivalent dose has been determined, it can be used to calculate for the V_{max}, K_M, and the new maintenance dose.

CASE 24: CALCULATING V_{max}, AND NEW MAINTENANCE DOSE OF FOSPHENYTOIN

WR is a 34-year-old male (62 kg) who was admitted to the ICU after a motor vehicle accident that resulted in traumatic brain injury. His neurologist started him on fosphenytoin loading dose of 1,200 mg, followed by 450 mg IV infusion every 12 hours for seizure prophylaxis 5 days ago. His albumin level was 3 g/dL, and SCr was 0.6 mg/dL. His phenytoin level was 4 mg/L @ 37°C. Determine if this patient's phenytoin level is at steady state and calculate for a new maintenance dose.

Step 1: Calculate for the phenytoin sodium equivalent dose.

Phenytoin sodium equivalent dose = Fosphenytoin dose ÷ 1.5 mg

Phenytoin sodium equivalent dose = 900 mg/day ÷ 1.5 mg

Phenytoin sodium equivalent dose = 600 mg/day

Step 2: Determine whether the phenytoin level was drawn at steady state using the $t_{90\%}$ formula before calculating for the patient-specific V_{max}. Since this patient has low albumin, the phenytoin observed must be corrected first.

$$\text{Corrected phenytoin} = \frac{\text{Phenytoin observed}}{(\text{Albumin} \times 0.2) + 0.1}$$

$$\text{Corrected phenytoin} = \frac{4\ \text{mg/L}}{(3\ \text{g/dL} \times 0.2) + 0.1}$$

$$\text{Corrected phenytoin} = 5.71\ \text{mg/L}$$

The $t_{90\%}$ formula is based on a 70 kg patient, so the total daily dose must also be converted to an equivalent dose. Using phenytoin sodium equivalent maintenance dose, calculate for the equivalent dose for a 70 kg patient:

$$\frac{600\ \text{mg}}{62\ \text{kg}} = \frac{x}{70\ \text{kg}}$$

$$x = 677\ \text{mg}$$

Using the equivalent dose of phenytoin sodium for a 70 kg patient, calculate for the $t_{90\%}$:

$$t_{90\%} = \frac{[115 + 35 \times (C_p)](C_p)}{(S)(F)(\text{Dose/Day})}$$

$$t_{90\%} = \frac{[115 + 35 \times (5.71\ \text{mg/L})](5.71\ \text{mg/L})}{(0.92)(1)(677\ \text{mg/Day})}$$

$$t_{90\%} = 2.89\ \text{days}$$

Step 3: If the phenytoin level was drawn 5 days after starting the maintenance dose and the $t_{90\%}$ is achieved in 2.89 days, then the phenytoin level is considered to be at steady state. The patient-specific V_{max} can now be calculated. Again, the phenytoin sodium equivalent dose and corrected phenytoin must be used in this formula.

$$V_{max,ptspecific} = \frac{(\text{Total dose/day})(F)(S)(C_{pSS} + K_M)}{C_{pSS}}$$

$$V_{max,ptspecific} = \frac{(600\ \text{mg/day})(1)(0.92)(5.71\ \text{mg/L} + 4\ \text{mg/L})}{(5.71\ \text{mg/L})}$$

$$V_{max,ptspecific} = 939\ \text{mg/day}$$

Step 4: Using the patient-specific V_{max}, calculate the new maintenance dose. Note that the salt factor used in this equation is 0.92 because we are calculating for the phenytoin sodium equivalent dose.

$$\text{New maintenance dose} = \frac{(V_{max,ptspecific})(C_{pSS})}{(C_{pSS} + K_M)(F)(S)}$$

$$\text{New maintenance dose} = \frac{(939\ \text{mg/day})(15\ \text{mg/L})}{(15\ \text{mg/L} + 4\ \text{mg/L})(1)(0.92)}$$

$$\text{New maintenance dose} = 806\ \text{mg of phenytoin sodium}$$

Step 5: Convert the phenytoin sodium to fosphenytoin equivalent dose.

Fosphenytoin equivalent dose = Phenytoin sodium × 1.5

Fosphenytoin equivalent dose = 806 mg × 1.5

Fosphenytoin equivalent dose = 1,209 mg or ~ 1,200 mg of fosphenytoin given in divided doses of 600 mg every 12 hours

Step 6: Determine the rate of infusion of the new maintenance dose.

The recommended rate of infusion of fosphenytoin is based on its phenytoin sodium equivalent of 100–150 mg/min. The new maintenance dose of 600 mg every 12 hours of fosphenytoin is equivalent to 400 mg of phenytoin sodium every 12 hours. Therefore, 600 mg of fosphenytoin can be infused intravenously over 3–4 minutes.

REFERENCES

1. Anderson RJ. The little compound that could: how phenytoin changed drug discovery and development. *Mol Interventions*. 2009;9:208–214.
2. Lexi-Drugs Online: Phenytoin. Available at online.lexi.com (accessed June 12, 2011).
3. Rhodes RS, Heyneman CA, Culbertson VL, et al. Topical phenytoin treatment of stage II decubitus ulcers in the elderly. *Ann Pharmacother*. 2001;35:675–681.
4. Tozer TN, Winter ME. Phenytoin. In: Evans WE, Schentag JJ, Jusko WJ et al., eds. *Applied Pharmacokinetics: Principles of Therapeutic Drug Monitoring*. 3rd ed. Vancouver, WA: Applied Therapeutics, Inc.; 1992.
5. Graves NM, Garnett WR. Epilepsy. In: Dipiro JT, Talbert RL, Yee GC, et al., eds. *Pharmacotherapy: A Pathophysiologic Approach*. 4th ed. Stamford, CT: Appleton & Lange; 1999.
6. Neuvonen PJ. Bioavailability of phenytoin: clinical pharmacokinetic and therapeutic implications. *Clin Pharmacokin*. 1979;4:91–103.
7. Smith TC, Kinkel A. Absorption and metabolism of phenytoin from tablets and capsules. *Clin Pharmacol Ther*. 1976;20:738–742.
8. Olanow CW, Finn AL. Phenytoin: pharmacokinetics and clinical therapeutics. *Neurosurg*. 1981;8:112–117.
9. Sanson LN, O'Reilly WJ, Wiseman CW, et al. Plasma phenytoin levels produced by various phenytoin concentrations. *Med J Aust*. 1975;2:593–595.
10. Yeung SCA, Ensom MHH. Phenytoin and enteral feedings: does evidence support an interaction? *Ann Pharmacother*. 2000;34:896–905.
11. Hong JM, Choi YC, Kim WJ. Differences between the measured and calculated free serum phenytoin concentrations in epileptic patients. *Yonsei Med J*. 2009;50:517–520.
12. Lindow J, Wijdicks EF. Pheytoin toxicity associated with hypoalbuminemia in critically ill patients. *Chest*. 1994;105:602–604.
13. Dager WE, Inciardi JF, Howe TL. Estimating phenytoin concentrations by the Sheiner-Tozer method in adults with pronounced hypoalbuminemia. *Ann Pharmacother*. 1995;29:667–670.
14. Anderson GD, Pak C, Doane KW, et al. Revised Winter-Tozer equation for normalized phenytoin concentrations in trauma and elderly patients with hypoalbuminemia. *Ann Pharmacother*. 1997;31:279–284.
15. Hooper WE, Bochner F, Eadie MJ, et al. Plasma protein binding of diphenylhydantoin: effects of sex hormones, renal and hepatic disease. *Clin Pharmacol Ther*. 1974;15:276–282.
16. Odar-Cedarlof I, Borga O, et al. Kinetics of diphenylhydantoin in uremic patients: consequences of reduced protein binding. *Euro J Clin Pharmacol*. 1974;7:31.
17. Reichen A. Clinical pharmacokinetics of phenytoin. *Clin Pharmacokinet*. 1979;4:153–169.
18. Perucca E, Hebdige S, Frigo GM, et al. Interaction between phenytoin and valproic acid: plasma protein binding and metabolic effects. *Clin Pharmacol Ther*. 1980;28:779–789.
19. Bruni J, Gallo JM, Lee CS, et al. Interactions of valproic acid with phenytoin. *Neurology*. 1980;30:1233.
20. Liponi DE, Winter ME, Tozer TN. Renal function and therapeutic concentration of phenytoin. *Neurology*. 1984;34:395–397.
21. Reynolds F, Ziroyanis PN, Jones NP, Smith SE. Salivary phenytoin concentrations in epilepsy and chronic renal failure. *Lancet*. 1976;2:384–386.
22. Winter ME, Tozer TN. Phenytoin. In: Burton ME, Shaw LM, Schentag JJ, eds. *Applied Pharmacokinetics and Pharmacodynamics: Principles of Therapeutic Drug Monitoring*. 4th ed. Baltimore MD: Lippincott; 2006:463–490.
23. Cheymol G. Effects of obesity on pharmacokinetics: implications for drug therapy. *Clin Pharmacokinet*. 2000;39:215–231.

24. Abernethy DR, Greenblatt DJ. Phenytoin disposition in obesity: determination of loading dose. *Arch Neurol.* 1985;42:468–471.

25. Gugler R, Manion CV, Azarnoff DL. Phenytoin: pharmacokinetics and bioavailability. *Clin Pharmacol Ther.* 1976;19:135–142.

26. Jung D, Powell JR, Walson P, et al. Effect of dose on phenytoin absorption. *Clin Pharmacol Ther.* 1980;28(4):479–485.

27. McCauley DL, Tozer TN, Winter ME. Time for phenytoin concentration to peak: consequences of first-order and zero-order absorption. *Ther Drug Monit.* 1989;11(5):540–542.

28. Phenytoin sodium injection, phenytoin sodium injection [package insert]. Hospira, Inc., Lake Forest, IL, 2004.

29. Donovan PJ, Cline D. Phenytoin administration by constant intravenous infusion: selective rates of administration. *Ann Emerg Med.* 1991;20(2):139–142.

30. Richens A. A study of the pharmacokinetics of phenytoin (diphenylhydantoin) in epileptic patients, and the development of a nomogram for making dose increments. *Epilepsia.* 1975;16:627–646.

31. Bauer LA, Blouin A. Phenytoin Michaelis-Menten pharmacokinetics in Caucasian pediatric patients. *Clin Pharmacokinet.* 1983;8:545–549.

32. Valodia PN, Seymour MA, McFadyen ML, et al. Validation of population pharmacokinetic parameters of phenytoin using the parallel Michaelis-Menten and first-order elimination model. *Ther Drug Monit.* 2000;22:313–319.

33. Nation RL, Evans AM, Milne RW. Pharmacokinetic drug interactions with phenytoin. *Clin Pharmacokinet.* 1990;18:37–60.

34. Bachmann KA, Belloto RJ. Differential kinetics of phenytoin in elderly patients. *Drugs & Aging.* 1999;15:235–250.

35. Kerb R, Aynacioglu AS, Brockmoller J, et al. The predictive value of MDR1, CYP2C9, and CYP2C19 polymorphisms for phenytoin plasma concentrations. *Pharmacogenomics J.* 2001;1:204–210.

36. Zielinski JJ, Haidukewych D. Dual effects of carbamazepine-phenytoin interaction. *Ther Drug Monit.* 1987;9:21–23.

37. Browne TR. Fosphenytoin (Cerebyx). *Clin Neuropharmacol.* 1997;20: 1–12.

38. Department of Surgical Education, Orlando Regional Medical Center. Use of fosphenytoin (Cerebyx) and intravenous phenytoin (Dilantin) in adult patients. 2003.

39. Roberts WL, De BK, Coleman JP, et al. Falsely increased immunoassay measurements of total and unbound phenytoin in critically ill uremic patients receiving fosphenytoin. *Clin Chem.* 1999;45:829–837.

40. UK Drug Information Pharmacists Group. Fosphenytoin. 1999; Monograph number 4/99/04.

41. Pellock JM. Fosphenytoin use in children. *Neurology.* 1996;46:14–16.

42. Miller RF. Phenytoin (Dilantin®, Phenytek®). A service of the Epilepsy Therapy Project. 2007. Available at: epilepsy.com (accessed on July 9, 2011).

CHAPTER

16

Extended-Spectrum Triazole Antifungals: Posaconazole and Voriconazole

KELLY E. MARTIN, PharmD, BCPS
MAURICE ALEXANDER, PharmD, BCOP, CPP
BENYAM MULUNEH, PharmD, BCOP, CPP

OVERVIEW

Voriconazole and posaconazole are broad-spectrum triazole antifungal agents. They decrease ergosterol synthesis by interfering with the lanosterol-14α-demethylase (P450 enzyme) activity leading to a malformation of the fungal cell membrane. These agents have activity against most yeasts, such as fluconazole-resistant *Candida* spp. and molds, such as *Aspergillus* spp. and *Fusarium* spp. Unlike voriconazole, posaconazole has activity against the Mucorales order.[1,2] Posaconazole and voriconazole play a significant role in both the prevention and treatment of opportunistic invasive fungal infections, especially in immunocompromised patients. Because of its wide spectrum of activity, posaconazole is indicated for prophylaxis of invasive *Aspergillus* and *Candida* infections in patients who are at high risk of developing these infections due to prolonged immunosuppression after stem cell transplant or prolonged neutropenia after chemotherapy for a hematologic malignancy.[1,3] Voriconazole is considered the drug of choice for treatment of most invasive aspergillosis infections.[2,4] Voriconazole is also approved for use in nonneutropenic candidemia and as salvage therapy for *Scedosporium apiospermum* and *Fusarium* spp. infections.[2] Although posaconazole is FDA-indicated for the treatment of refractory oropharyngeal candididasis, the suspension formulation also has positive data to support its use at higher doses for the treatment of other invasive fungal infections including mucormycosis and cryptococcal infections.[5,6] Refer to Table 16-1 for FDA-approved treatment and prophylactic dosing recommendations for voriconazole and posaconazole. To date, the data for posaconazole delayed-release (DR) tablets and intravenous formulations are limited to prophylactic indications.[1] Voriconazole and posaconazole therapeutic drug monitoring (TDM) can be utilized to improve patient outcomes and, in the case of voriconazole, to limit toxicity.

BIOAVAILABILITY (F)

Posaconazole oral suspension has variable bioavailability that is significantly influenced by dose and food intake. This formulation has saturable absorption requiring a smaller, multiple daily dosing schedule despite the drug's long half-life. For example, dosing posaconazole 400 mg every 12 hours versus 800 mg once doubles the bioavailability and dosing it 200 mg every 6 hours increases it by nearly threefold. These evaluations, however, were done in patients in the fasted state.[7] Administration of posaconazole oral suspension with a high-fat meal has been shown to increase the bioavailability fourfold leading to the current recommendation to take posaconazole oral suspension with a fatty meal.[8] Of note, the absorption of posaconazole oral suspension is also influenced by suppression of gastric acid secretion by proton-pump inhibitors and prokinetic agents such as metoclopramide.[1] In 2013, the FDA approved a delayed-release tablet formulation of posaconazole. While there is less variability compared to the suspension, the tablets should also be taken with food. Pharmacokinetic studies have shown that a high-fat meal increases the AUC by 51%. Unlike the suspension, the tablet formulation absorption is not affected by gastric acid suppressors or gastrointestinal motility agents.[1,9] Of note, an intravenous formulation of posaconazole was approved by the FDA in 2014.

Voriconazole is also available in both oral and intravenous formulations. In healthy subjects, voriconazole has 96 percent oral bioavailability with the time to maximum plasma concentration (C_{max}) ranging from 1–2 hours after administration.[2] Oral voriconazole should be administered in the fasting state.[2,10] Ingestion of voriconazole following a high-fat meal resulted in a mean decrease in C_{max} of 34 percent and 58 percent with the tablet and oral suspension, respectively.[2] Unlike posaconazole, medications that increase gastric pH have not been found to impact voriconazole absorption.

VOLUME OF DISTRIBUTION (V)

Both voriconazole and posaconazole have a large volume of distribution, with extensive distribution from the plasma into tissues. After absorption, posaconazole has a volume of distribution that ranges from 5 L/kg to 25 L/kg, allowing substantial tissue penetration.[8] Cerebrospinal fluid (CSF) drug levels are low compared to serum levels (CSF to plasma ratio of 0.004–0.009), suggesting poor penetration into the central nervous system (CNS). However, it is postulated that patients with CNS fungal infections have a potentially compromised blood-brain barrier leading to increased posaconazole penetration and positive clinical outcomes.[11]

At steady state, voriconazole has a volume of distribution estimated to range from 2 L/kg to 4.6 L/kg, suggesting extensive tissue distribution.[2,12] Voriconazole is able to penetrate the blood-brain barrier and achieve concentrations in the CSF of approximately 50 percent of the plasma concentrations.[12] However, voriconazole concentrations in the brain may be even higher than the CSF as shown in an autopsy study of eight patients.[13] Animal studies have shown voriconazole concentrations to be significant in the pulmonary epithelial lining fluid, which may be of importance for the treatment of pulmonary fungal infections. Voriconazole also distributes into intracellular components including the polymorphonuclear leukocytes (PMNs). It has been demonstrated that concentrations within the PMNs may be up to 8.5 times greater than the concentrations found in the plasma.[12]

CLEARANCE (CL)

Posaconazole and voriconazole differ substantially in how they are cleared from the body. About 15 percent of posaconazole is metabolized through glucoronidation, avoiding the cytochrome

TABLE 16-1	Pharmacokinetic Parameters of Voriconazole and Posaconazole[1,2,8,12,15,31,46,47]	
Parameter	**Voriconazole**	**Posaconazole**
Pharmacokinetics	Linear in children; nonlinear in adults	Linear
Absorption (impact of food)	Decreased by high-fat content meals	Increased by high-fat content meals[a]
Volume of distribution (L/kg)	4.6	20–66 (S)
Plasma protein binding (%)	58	26-31 (T)
$T_{1/2}$ (hr)	Dose-dependent	27 (IV)
Time to reach steady state	7–10 days (S)	6 days (T)
Elimination	CYP2C19 (primary), CYP2C9, CYP3A4	Hepatic (glucoronidation to inactive metabolites) Renal: <1% excreted unchanged in urine Fecal: 66% excreted unchanged in feces

[a]Posaconazole suspension, 4-fold increase in Cmax and AUC; Posaconazole tablets, 16% increase in Cmax and 51% increase in AUC

S, suspension; T, tablets: IV, intravenous

TABLE 16-2	Voriconazole and Posaconazole Dosing[1,2]
Posaconazole Dosing	
Prophylaxis	Oral Suspension: 200 mg PO three times daily
	Tablets: 300 mg PO q12h for the first 24 hours, followed by 300 mg PO daily
	Intravenous: 300 mg IV q12h for the first 24 hours, followed by 300 mg IV daily
Treatment (suspension only)	Oropharyngeal Candidiasis: 100 mg bid × 1 day then 100 mg once daily × 13 days
	Invasive aspergillosis: 200 mg four times daily (may transition to 400 mg bid at steady state)
Voriconazole Dosing	
Loading Dose (IV)	6 mg/kg q12h for the first 24 hours
Maintenance Dose (IV)	4 mg/kg q12h
Maintenance Dose (PO)	200 mg q12h

P450 (CYP) pathway. Although posaconazole is not metabolized by the P450 (CYP) pathway it is a potent inhibitor of CYP3A4.[11,14] P-glycoprotein has also been implicated in the excretion of posaconazole because of the increased drug concentrations observed with inhibition of this enzyme.[8] Fecal excretion of the parent drug accounts for 77 percent of the drug's elimination, with renal excretion playing a minor role (metabolites: 13–14%; parent: negligible).

Voriconazole is both a substrate and inhibitor of the CYP enzyme system. It is primarily metabolized by CYP2C19, and to a lesser extent metabolized by CYP3A4 and CYP2C9.[2] Voriconazole displays nonlinear pharmacokinetics likely due to saturable metabolism, meaning that an increase in dose results in a disproportionate increase in plasma concentration.[12,15] The major metabolite of voriconazole, which accounts for almost three-quarters of all voriconazole metabolites, is N-oxide. N-oxide has minimal antifungal activity and an unknown impact on toxicity.[2,12,16]

The CYP2C19 isoenzyme exhibits genetic polymorphism, which results in poor and extensive metabolizer phenotypes and may account for almost 50 percent of the variability in voriconazole clearance[2,12,16,17] The poor metabolizer phenotype is found in 15–20 percent of Asian populations and 3–5 percent of Caucasian and Black populations. Those with the poor metabolizer phenotype can have up to fourfold higher voriconazole concentrations compared to the homozygous extensive metabolizer phenotype.[2,16] Despite this known variability, no current specific dosing recommendations are based on CYP2C19 genotype.[2]

Less than 2 percent of voriconazole is excreted in the urine and no dose adjustments are required in renal dysfunction. However, in both posaconazole and voriconazole IV formulations, the vehicle, sulfobutyl ether beta-cyclodextrin sodium (SBECD), can accumulate in patients with creatinine clearance (CrCl) <50 mL/min.[1,2,18]

ELIMINATION HALF-LIFE (T1/2)

Due to the nonlinear pharmacokinetics, voriconazole has dose-dependent elimination. The mean elimination is estimated to range 6–9 hours and increases after multiple doses compared to single dose administration.[2,12,15]

Posaconazole also had a dose-dependent half-life, ranging 20-66 hours, which is decreased by prior hematopoietic stem cell transplantation and varies based on formulation administered.[1,7,11,19] Table 16-2 summarizes the pharmacokinetic parameters of voriconazole and posaconazole.

THERAPEUTIC CONCENTRATIONS

A voriconazole exposure-response relationship has been established through studies in which lower serum concentrations were associated with a lack of clinical response, progression of fungal infection, or increased breakthrough fungal infections. Although no consensus sets an exact lower limit of the therapeutic range, studies have targeted voriconazole concentrations based on the minimum inhibitory concentrations (MIC) of clinically relevant fungal pathogens. Most *Candida* and *Aspergillus* species have an MIC_{90} of 0.25–1 mg/L.[20,21] In general, treatment success has been associated with voriconazole trough concentrations >1 mg/L, although some studies suggest targeting troughs ≥2 mg/L for maximal efficacy.[22-24]

Because of the erratic absorption and variable half-life, determining a serum concentration-to-effect relationship is important for posaconazole. In patients who are critically ill or have undergone stem cell transplantation, absorption can be decreased, leading to variability in serum concentrations secondary to altered gastric mucosa and/or decreased appetite.[15] A number of studies have attempted to characterize the concentration-efficacy relationship. The authors of one study that evaluated posaconazole in the treatment of invasive aspergillosis found 75 percent of patients responded with an average serum concentration (C_{avg}) of 1,250 ng/mL compared with only 24 percent that responded with a C_{avg} of 134 ng/mL.[25] Based on these findings, it is recommended to target a concentration greater than 1,000–1,250 ng/mL when treating invasive fungal infections.[26,27]

Studies looking at the prophylactic effects of posaconazole in immunocompromised patients have not found a similar concentration-effect relationship.[3,28] However, a clinical pharmacology review and logistic regression by the Food and Drug Administration (FDA) found achieving a C_{avg} of less than 700 ng/mL was strongly predictive of an invasive fungal infection.[29]

TOXIC CONCENTRATIONS

Voriconazole trough concentrations should be maintained below an upper limit of 5–5.5 mg/L to minimize adverse events including hepatotoxicity and neurotoxicity.[22-24]

A posaconazole exposure-toxicity relationship remains to be established. A logistic regression of two separate trials by the FDA found that patients with lower serum concentrations (C_{avg} = 205 ± 105 ng/mL) developed fewer toxicities compared to patients with higher concentrations (C_{avg} = 1,751 ng/mL ± 538 ng/mL). However, no statistical difference or definitive conclusion was made regarding a concentration beyond which posaconazole would be considered toxic.[29]

DRUG LEVEL MONITORING

Monitoring of voriconazole concentrations is recommended for assessment of both efficacy and toxicity. Variability in voriconazole concentrations is multifactorial due to nonlinear pharmacokinetics, CYP2C19 genotype polymorphisms, underlying hepatic dysfunction, drug-drug interactions as well as still undefined factors. For example, a recent study suggested that oral voriconazole doses are not equivalent to IV voriconazole doses despite the high bioavailability initially described in the package insert.[30] In clinical practice, most patients should receive voriconazole therapeutic drug monitoring.

Because of the interpatient variability in absorption in most patients—including those with graft-versus-host disease, diarrhea, compromised mucosal barriers, decreased oral intake limiting administration with food, and gastric acid suppression—checking plasma concentrations of posaconazole is recommended to assess for efficacy. This is particularly true of the posaconazole suspension for which absorption is most variable. It is theorized that serum concentrations may not always be accurate in predicting the therapeutic efficacy of posaconazole because of the high volume of distribution leading to a higher concentration in tissues rather than in plasma.[15] Although not incorporated in clinical practice, concentrations in isolated alveolar cells and intracellular measurements of neutrophils and monocytes are 22–67 times larger than plasma concentrations.[26]

TIME TO DRAW LEVELS AND FREQUENCY, MONITORING

Voriconazole trough concentrations are used clinically to monitor for efficacy and toxicity. Due to the nonlinear kinetics, it is important that voriconazole trough concentrations are measured at the end of the 12-hour dosing interval (30 minutes to 1 hour prior to the next dose). No mathematical equations are available to extrapolate a random serum concentration that is drawn during the middle of the dosing interval. Concentrations should be measured once steady state is reached 5–7 days after the maintenance dose has been initiated.[15] Although steady-state concentrations can be reached in 1–2 days following a loading dose, it is generally considered prudent to wait at least 5 days to measure a trough concentration because of variability in the elimination half-life that also requires time to reach steady-state. As mentioned earlier, voriconazole has saturable metabolism and the mean elimination half-life increases after multiple doses.[12,15] It is also recommended to obtain a voriconazole trough concentration at any time during therapy if clinical failure is suspected or signs of toxicity are exhibited.

Due to posaconazole's long half-life, the frequent dosing of the oral suspension, and the delayed-release properties of the tablet formulation, serum concentrations can be drawn at any time after the drug has reached steady state (7–10 days). Some limited evidence suggests that measuring levels earlier (at 3 days) may be predictive of steady-state concentrations.[26] Because it takes about one week to reach steady state and several more days for most institutions to report level results, it may be beneficial to assess a level earlier to prevent delay in responding to a level that is subtherapeutic. However, levels should be reassessed once steady state is reached.

CASES

CASE 1: VORICONAZOLE INTRAVENOUS (IV) LOADING DOSE AND MAINTENANCE DOSE

JS is a 53-year-old African American male with a history of HIV (most recent CD4 count <20 cells/mm³) who was admitted for right-sided flank pain. He was found to have a renal abscess that was drained and sent for culture. The microbiology lab reported Aspergillus fumigatus. *The patient is not currently compliant with their antiretroviral (ARV) regimen. Calculate a voriconazole IV loading dose followed by a maintenance dose.*

Height = 6′

Weight = 185 lbs

Step 1: Calculate IV loading dose.

The package insert recommends administration of an IV loading dose of 6 mg/kg for 2 doses given 12 hours apart.

$$Weight = 185\ lbs/2.2 = 84.1\ kg$$
$$Dose = 84.1\ kg \times 6\ mg/kg = 504.6\ mg$$

For ease of IV preparation, the dose can be rounded to 500 mg every 12 hours for the first 24 hours.

Step 2: Calculate the IV maintenance dose.

After 24 hours, the dose should be reduced to the maintenance dose of 4 mg/kg every 12 hours administered intravenously.

$$Dose = 84.1\ kg \times 4\ mg/kg = 336.4\ mg$$

The dose can be rounded to voriconazole 300 mg IV every 12 hours with the recommendation to check a trough concentration on day 5-7.

CASE 2: VORICONAZOLE IV TO ORAL (PO) CONVERSION

SM is a 48-year-old Caucasian female with chronic graft-versus-host disease on prolonged prednisone treatment who is admitted to the hospital for a productive cough for the past two weeks. Chest CT and galactomannan antigen testing suggest possible invasive pulmonary aspergillosis.

Height = 5′1″

Weight = 83 lbs

She is initially given a loading dose of IV voriconazole 6 mg/kg on day 1 and then started on voriconazole 150 mg IV every 12 hours. Determine an oral maintenance dose of voriconazole for this patient.

Step 1: Calculate weight in kilograms

$$Weight = 83\ lbs/2.2 = 37.7\ kg$$

Weight is important for oral dosing despite the fact that the FDA approved dosing is only weight-based when dosing intravenous voriconazole. The package insert recommends that adult patients who weigh less than 40 kg should receive half of the oral maintenance dose.

Step 2: Determine an oral maintenance dosing regimen for treatment of invasive aspergillosis infection

Two different methods may be used to determine a voriconazole regimen for the treatment of invasive aspergillosis using the oral formulation. The regimen can be determined using the FDA-approved fixed dosing or using weight based dosing (similar to the dosing for the IV formulation).

Although the FDA-approved recommendation is to utilize standardized doses of 200 mg every 12 hours when administering oral voriconazole, data show that this dose provides similar exposure to a 3 mg/kg IV dose. To achieve similar exposure to a 4 mg/kg IV dose, the equivalent oral dose is 300 mg.[2,32] One concern with using the 200 mg oral dose is the possibility that this dose will not achieve steady-state concentrations greater than the MIC of *Aspergillus* species in most patients. In a pharmacokinetic study of 42 healthy male subjects, the 200 mg oral dose did not maintain troughs greater than 1 mg/L and thus fell within subtherapeutic concentrations.[32] Additionally, a study using pharmacokinetic modeling demonstrated that oral voriconazole doses result in lower trough concentrations when compared to equivalent intravenous doses.[30] For example, the likelihood of achieving a voriconazole trough concentration >1 mg/L with a 200 mg intravenous dose and 200 mg oral dose was 86 percent and 60 percent, respectively.[30] Interestingly, this study suggests a lower oral bioavailability of about 60 percent than what has been reported in the package insert. Because this patient is being treated for an invasive fungal infection, it is necessary to achieve adequate trough concentrations for maximum efficacy. Based on the literature, concentrations are most likely achieved with an oral voriconazole dose of 300 mg every 12 hours.[2,30,32] However, this patient is less than 40 kg and thus the dose should be reduced by 50 percent to 150 mg PO every 12 hours.[2]

Alternatively, many practitioners utilize oral weight-based dosing for treatment of invasive fungal infections. For this patient who weighs 37.7 kg, a 4 mg/kg oral dose would also result in dosing voriconazole at 150 mg PO every 12 hours. After 5–7 days of oral dosing, a trough voriconazole plasma concentration should be measured.

CASE 3: SUPRATHERAPEUTIC VORICONAZOLE TROUGH CONCENTRATIONS

DP is a 31-year-old Asian male who was admitted for an autologous hematopoietic stem cell transplant (HSCT). On day 3 following HSCT, he developed febrile neutropenia and was started on broad-spectrum empiric antibiotics with cefepime and vancomycin. After 96 hours, DP remained febrile at which time empiric antifungal treatment was initiated. He was given a loading dose of voriconazole 6 mg/kg IV every 12 hours for two doses and then started on voriconazole 200 mg PO every 12 hours. On day 6 of voriconazole therapy, a trough plasma concentration was drawn 30 minutes before the next dose was to be given. The patient denied any visual changes or disturbances. Determine how to interpret and respond to the voriconazole plasma trough concentration.

Height = 5′10″

Weight = 77 kg

Pertinent medications: omeprazole 40 mg PO daily

Voriconazole trough: 7.2 mg/L (therapeutic range: 1.0–5.5 mg/L)

AST: 20 IU/L

ALT: 15 IU/L

Total bilirubin: 0.8 mg/dL

Step 1: Identify possible factors that may have resulted in a supratherapeutic trough concentration.

Voriconazole has significant inter- and intrapatient variability, and several factors may contribute to trough concentrations that fall outside of the therapeutic range. It is important to consider CYP2C19 genotype polymorphisms, drug-drug interactions, timing of the trough concentration, and liver function.

- **CYP2C19 Genotype**: In clinical practice, the CYP2C19 genotype is often unknown and not a test that is routinely ordered prior to initiation of voriconazole therapy. However, this patient is known to be of Asian descent, which means a 15–20 percent likelihood he carries the CYP2C19 polymorphism that results in the "poor metabolizer" phenotype. As discussed earlier, this phenotype could result in voriconazole concentrations fourfold greater than the "wild type" phenotype.

- **Drug-Drug Interactions**: Medications that are CYP2C19 inhibitors, such as oral contraceptives containing ethinyl estradiol, can result in increased voriconazole plasma concentrations. In this case, the patient is receiving omeprazole 40 mg PO daily, which is a known CYP2C19 inhibitor. Studies conflict regarding the clinical impact of this drug-drug interaction.[2,22,30,33-35] With the supratherapeutic trough, it would be prudent to change therapy from omeprazole to an H2-receptor antagonist, if the omeprazole is not specifically indicated. Of note, the package insert does not recommend any initial adjustments to voriconazole dose when coadministered with omeprazole.[2] Therefore, omeprazole does not need to be discontinued when voriconazole is coadministered, unless it is suspected the drug-drug interaction is leading to supratherapeutic voriconazole concentrations or voriconazole toxicities.

- **Liver function:** In this case, the patient has normal liver function tests (LFTs), making it unlikely to be a factor contributing to the supratherapeutic voriconazole concentration. As voriconazole is hepatically metabolized, diminished liver function can result in reduced clearance of the drug.

Step 2: Determine an appropriate voriconazole dose adjustment based on the plasma trough concentration.

Voriconazole dose adjustments based on therapeutic drug monitoring have not been well-defined. With a supratherapeutic concentration, the first thing to consider is whether the patient is experiencing any toxicity. In this case, the patient does not have visual disturbances and LFTs are within normal limits. Due to the nonlinear pharmacokinetics and other potential factors that may be affecting the plasma concentrations such as CYP2C19 polymorphisms, it is difficult to predict the impact of a dose adjustment on the resulting concentration. The package insert recommends reducing the dose by 50 mg increments.[2] A decrease to oral voriconazole 150 mg every 12 hours followed by another trough concentration in 5–7 days would be appropriate. Studies have shown significant intrapatient variability, so some practitioners, in the absence of toxicities, would consider repeating the trough concentration or waiting 5–7 days following discontinuation of the omeprazole and then repeating the trough concentration.

CASE 4: VORICONAZOLE DOSING IN AN OBESE PATIENT

EK is a 63-year-old Caucasian female who was admitted for erythematous nodules on her left knee, which worsened in the last four weeks and have not responded to outpatient oral antibiotics. The patient reports falling and scraping her left knee about seven months ago. The skin lesions are biopsied and sent for bacterial and fungal culture. The microbiology lab reports the cultures grew Scedosporium apiospermum. *Past medical history includes rheumatoid arthritis, hypertension, and hyperlipidemia. Her medications include etanercept 50 mg subcutaneously once weekly, hydrochlorothiazide 25 mg daily, and simvastatin 10 mg every evening.*

Height = 5′3″

Weight = 84 kg

Step 1: Determine the patient's body mass index (BMI) and whether the patient is clinically obese.

BMI = weight (kg)/[height (m)]²

Convert inches to meters: 63 inches × 2.54 = 160.02 cm = 1.6 m

BMI = 84 kg/(1.6 m)² = 32.8 kg/m²

This patient is considered to be obese with a BMI ≥30. Alternatively, a second method is sometimes used to determine whether a patient is overweight. Clinically, it may be considered that a patient is obese if the actual body weight is >130 percent of the ideal body weight (IBW).

Ideal body weight (female) = 45.5 kg + (2.3 × inches greater than 5′)

IBW = 45.5 kg + (2.3 × 3) = 52.4 kg

130% IBW = 52.4 kg × 1.3 = 68.1 kg

Actual body weight/IBW = 84 kg/52.4 kg = 1.6

The patient weighs 84 kg, which is 160 percent of her ideal body weight and thus the patient can be considered clinically obese using this method.

Step 2: Calculate a weight-based intravenous voriconazole dosing regimen.

The manufacturer does not make any recommendations regarding the use of oral or IV voriconazole in obese patients, and only limited studies have been done.[2,36-38] A pharmacokinetic study conducted in obese volunteers (median BMI = 46.2 kg/m²) found the volume of distribution and clearance of oral voriconazole was similar in obese and nonobese individuals.[36] This finding suggests that using weight-based doses calculated using actual body weight in obese individuals could result in supratherapeutic concentrations. Studies in obese patients have shown that IV doses result in significantly higher voriconazole concentrations when compared to nonobese patients.[37,38] With the current information available, it would be prudent to use adjusted body weight when dosing voriconazole in obese patients.[36-38]

Calculate adjusted body weight: IBW + 0.4 (TBW − IBW)

Adjusted body weight: 52.4 kg + 0.4 (84 kg − 52.4 kg) = 65.04 kg

Using an adjusted body weight of 65 kg, calculate the loading and maintenance dose:

Loading dose = 6 mg/kg (65 kg) = 390 mg, rounded to voriconazole 400 mg IV q12h × 2 doses

Maintenance dose = 4 mg/kg (65 kg) = 260 mg

Administer 260 mg IV q12h.

CASE 5: INTRAVENOUS VORICONAZOLE DOSING IN RENAL DYSFUNCTION

TK is a 62-year-old Hispanic female with uncontrolled type 2 diabetes mellitus and rheumatoid arthritis on chronic steroids who presented with a two-month history of right ear pain and purulent nasal discharge. Over the past week, the pain has become progressively worse and she has begun to develop severe headaches. A CT scan of the sinuses showed enhanced soft tissue density in the left maxillary sinus and biopsies were obtained from the nasal and sinus walls. Bacterial cultures were negative. Fungal cultures grew Aspergillus fumigatus. The patient was taken to surgery for debridement and started on IV voriconazole.

Past medical history includes uncontrolled diabetes mellitus (HgbA1C on admission: 12.4%), rheumatoid arthritis, chronic kidney disease, and hypertension. Her serum creatinine is 1.4 (baseline 1.3–1.5).

Height = 5′4″

Weight = 60 kg

IBW = 54.7 kg

Step 1: Calculate the patient's creatinine clearance using the Cockcroft-Gault equation.

Cl_{Cr} = [(140 − Age)(Weight)]/[(72)(SCr)] × (0.85, if female)

The patient's creatinine clearance is 36 mL/minute, using ideal body weight.

Step 2: Determine a therapeutic regimen that includes an IV voriconazole loading dose and maintenance dose that will minimize toxicity in this patient.

Voriconazole is metabolized through the cytochrome P450 enzyme system, and concentrations are unaffected by renal insufficiency. However, the solubilizing vehicle for IV voriconazole, called sulfobutyl ether beta-cyclodextrin sodium (SBECD), is cleared at the same rate as glomerular filtration, and therefore, is known to accumulate during renal insufficiency.[39] The toxicity of SBECD in animal models has been found to be low. In rats, borderline renal toxicity occurred due to massive cellular vacuolation at extremely large SBECD doses of 3,000 mg/kg. In dogs, SBECD doses up to 1,500 mg/kg did not produce histopathological signs of nephrotoxicity. Of note, for a 70 kg person receiving a 200 mg intravenous dose of voriconazole, the exposure of SBECD is approximately 45 mg/kg (which is 55 times less than the SBECD dose found to be toxic in rats).[39,40] The prescribing information suggests that patients with a creatinine clearance <50 mL/minute should receive maintenance therapy with oral voriconazole to avoid potential nephrotoxicity from SBECD accumulation.[2,40] Several recent retrospective studies in patients receiving intravenous voriconazole for a course of approximately 7 days found no significant incidence of renal toxicity.[41-43] Of note, intravenous posaconazole also contains SBECD.[1,18] Using actual body weight, this patient should receive voriconazole 360 mg IV (6 mg/kg) loading dose every 12 hours for the first 2 doses and then voriconazole 240 mg IV (4 mg/kg) every 12 hours. Once the patient recovers from surgery and has good oral intake, the voriconazole should be changed from IV to PO with a trough concentration measured at steady state.

CASE 6: VORICONAZOLE DOSING IN HEPATIC DYSFUNCTION

ME is a 53-year-old male admitted for recurrent brain abscess on MRI. He has a known history of CNS aspergillosis following a traumatic brain injury resulting in a craniotomy and VP shunt. It is determined the patient will require another course of voriconazole. He has some underlying hepatic dysfunction due to chronic alcohol abuse. He has no ascites or hepatic encephalopathy.

Pertinent labs:

AST: 34 IU/L   ALT: 43 IU/L   Total bilirubin: 2.3 mg/dL

Albumin: 2.8 g/dL   INR 1.2

Step 1: Calculate the Child-Pugh score.

	1 point	2 points	3 points
Total bilirubin (mg/dL)	<2	2–3	>3
Serum albumin (g/dL)	>3.5	2.8–3.5	<2.8
INR	<1.7	1.71–2.20	>2.2
Ascites	None	Mild–Moderate	Severe
Hepatic encephalopathy	None	Grade I–II	Grade III–IV

Explanation of Result: Class A: 5–6 points, Class B: 7–9 points, Class C: 10–15 points

This patient would receive 2 points for a total bilirubin between 2–3 mg/dL, 2 points for serum albumin between 2.8–3.5 g/dL, 1 point for an INR <1.7, 1 point for the absence of ascites, and 1 point for the absence of hepatic encephalopathy. The total score is 7, which means the patient falls into Child-Pugh Class B.

Step 2: Determine a voriconazole dosing regimen based on the Child-Pugh classification.

The prescribing information recommends a standard loading dose followed by a 50 percent reduction in the maintenance dose.[2] Therefore, this patient should receive a maintenance dose of 2 mg/kg IV every 12 hours. Liver function tests and voriconazole trough concentrations should be carefully monitored.

CASE 7: POSACONAZOLE DOSE ADJUSTMENT BASED ON LOW PLASMA LEVELS

DT is a 49-year-old female with a history of chronic kidney disease who underwent hematopoietic stem cell transplantation for acute myeloid leukemia three months ago and is admitted to the inpatient transplant service with progressive hypoxia and a temperature of 102°F. On admission, medications included tacrolimus, prednisone for graft-versus-host disease of the gastrointestinal tract, posaconazole 200 mg every 8 hours for prophylaxis of invasive fungal infections, and phenytoin for a history of seizures. A computed tomography (CT) scan of her chest revealed new multifocal patchy opacities involving all lobes of the right lung and the left lower lobe. The radiology report also noted adjacent tree-in-bud opacities in the right upper lobe likely representing endobronchial spread of infection or mucoid impaction. Based on this probable fungal aspergillosis, the inpatient team increases the posaconazole dose to 400 mg every 12 hours. The physician team asks the following questions:

QUESTION 1

Should serum concentrations be drawn for this patient? If so, when are they to be drawn?

Answer:

Compromised integrity of the mucosal barrier, diarrhea, poor oral intake, or concomitant medications that interfere with absorption or clearance contribute to inter- and intrapatient differences in serum concentrations of posaconazole. Although not definitive, a relationship has been established between posaconazole serum concentrations and efficacy in the treatment of invasive aspergillosis. This relationship was best characterized by Walsh and colleagues who, through a logistic regression model, concluded the lower efficacy quartile of patients had lower concentrations compared to the upper quartile (1st quartile, 24% responders: C_{avg} = 134 ng/mL vs. 4th quartile, 75% responders: C_{avg} = 1,250 ng/mL).[25] Although the data for checking serum concentrations are less clear for prophylaxis, it is recommended in the treatment setting.[26,27]

Because of posaconazole's long half-life (15–35 hours), it takes roughly one week to reach steady state.[8] Therefore, levels should be drawn 7–10 days after initiation of therapy or a dose change. Levels can be drawn at any time during the dosing interval given the repeated dosing and long half-life of posaconazole. It has been suggested that early monitoring of levels can be predictive of steady-state concentrations and would allow for earlier interventions to help increase or decrease serum concentrations, but would not replace serum concentration monitoring after the patient has reached steady state.[26]

QUESTION 2

What posaconazole serum concentration should be targeted?

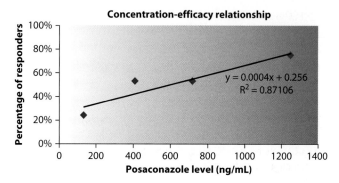

FIGURE 16-1. Logistic regression indicating a relatively strong concentration-efficacy relationship.

Answer:

Based on the study by Walsh and colleagues, a logistic regression can be plotted (Figure 16-1). An R^2 of 0.87 indicates a relatively strong concentration-efficacy relationship. A target posaconazole concentration of at least 1,000–1,250 ng/mL would be expected to be efficacious in about 65–75 percent of patients.[25-27]

QUESTION 3

If the level is found to be subtherapeutic, how should the team proceed?

Answer:

Step 1: Switch the antifungal agent.

In this case, the patient is being treated for invasive aspergillosis and the first step should be to consider switching the antifungal agent. Amphotericin B and voriconazole are both options for treatment of invasive aspergillosis; however, voriconazole would be preferred in this patient based on superior efficacy and tolerability data.[4] In addition, the patient has a history of chronic kidney disease, making amphotericin B an unfavorable option.

Step 2: Consider switching to posaconazole delayed-release tablets or intravenous formulations.

In November 2013, the FDA approved a tablet formulation of posaconazole based on pharmacokinetic data which showed higher plasma concentrations compared to the oral suspension. Duarte and colleagues evaluated posaconazole levels in high-risk patients who were given posaconazole tablets (taken without regard to food) for prophylaxis of invasive fungal infections. The authors found that patients who took posaconazole tablets at doses of 200 mg and 300 mg orally once daily had steady state concentrations of 951 and 1,460 ng/ml respectively. Of note, patients did receive a loading dose of 200-300 mg twice daily for two doses.[44] Another option would be to consider switching to IV posaconazole to avoid issues of absorption, particularly in this patient with GVHD of the gastrointestinal tract. It is important to highlight that the FDA approval of the delayed-release tablets and IV formulations and the available data in patients is for prophylaxis of invasive fungal infection and not treatment. Because this patient has probable fungal aspergillosis, switching to voriconazole would be the preferred approach until further data supporting the use of posaconazole DR tablets or IV infusion for the *treatment* invasive fungal infections is available.

Step 3: Ensure administration with a high-fat meal and inspect for drug-drug interactions.

Several medications that induce the uridine diphosphate glucuronidation (UDP) pathway, such as phenytoin, rifampin, and efavirenz, result in increased excretion of posaconazole.[1] Because this patient is on phenytoin, the clinician should consider an alternative antiepileptic.

Step 4: Fractionate the posaconazole suspension dose.

Dosing posaconazole suspension at 200 mg every 6 hours instead of 400 mg every 12 hours has been shown to result in increased serum concentrations.[10] All patients being treated for invasive aspergillosis should be dosed at 200 mg every 6 hours until they reach steady state, after which the 12-hour dosing can be used.[27]

Step 5: Increase the dose of posaconazole suspension.

If posaconazole has to be used (i.e., in the setting of mucormycosis with a contraindication to amphotericin B), careful thought must be given to dose escalation in response to a low serum concentration. Based on the available literature, only poor evidence suggests that increasing the dose of posaconazole would lead to higher serum concentrations. The absorption of posaconazole beyond 800 mg per day is believed to reach saturation. One small study in solid organ-transplant patients found that although increasing the daily dose of posaconazole to 1,200 mg per day resulted in no subsequent increase in concentrations, a daily dose of 1,600 mg in three patients resulted in serum concentrations >1,000 ng/mL. It should be noted, however, that these patients experienced gastrointestinal toxicity and hepatic enzyme elevation.[45] Because of the poor data, increasing the dose of posaconazole suspension beyond the recommended dosing of 200 mg every 6 hours should be considered a last resort.

CASE 8: POSACONAZOLE ADMINISTRATION WITH FOOD

IB is a 59-year-old Caucasian female who is admitted for complaints of spontaneous nose bleeds and unexplained upper extremity ecchymosis. A workup reveals a new diagnosis of acute myeloid leukemia, and induction chemotherapy is emergently started. She completes a course of 7 days of chemotherapy, including 3 days of idarubicin and 7 days of cytarabine. She completes her course of chemotherapy without complication and is started on routine antibacterial, antifungal, and antiviral prophylaxis with levofloxacin 500 mg PO daily, posaconazole 200 mg PO tid, and valacyclovir 500 mg PO daily. Twelve days after the initiation of chemotherapy, her absolute neutrophil count (ANC) nadirs at 0.0/mm³ and IB begins to complain of mild mucositis and mild respiratory symptoms. One week after starting antifungal prophylaxis, a posaconazole level is checked and comes back at 735 ng/mL. You resume therapy with no changes. However, a couple of days later, IB complains of worsening mouth pain. Upon examination you notice worsened mouth sores and IB reports that she has not been able to maintain the same oral intake. Given her worsening mucositis and mild respiratory symptoms, you decide to check another posaconazole level to ensure it remains therapeutic. The level results back at 589 ng/mL. Her ANC remains 0.0/mm³.

QUESTION

What is your assessment of this level, and what recommendations do you have at this time?

Answer:

IB's posaconazole was initially appropriate for the prophylactic indication (>700 ng/mL), but has now become subtherapeutic. It should be noted that IB has developed progressively worsening mucositis that is compromising her oral intake. Posaconazole absorption and systemic exposure, particularly with the oral suspension, is largely dependent upon administration with or following food, particularly food of high-fat content.[1,31]

Step 1:

One should consider switching this patient to posaconazole delayed-release tablets. Based on pharmacokinetic studies available to date, adequate absorption of the tablets is less dependent on the administration with food. The package labeling recommends administering with food as there was a 16% and 51% increase in Cmax and AUC, respectively when the tablet was administered with a high-fat content meal. However, this impact is far less than the 3-4-fold increase in Cmax and AUC seen when posaconazole oral suspension is administered with food. Additionally, there are data that suggest increased plasma concentrations with the tablet, even when administered without regard to food, compared to the oral suspension.[44] Thus, the tablet formulation would be an attractive alternative for IB. Posaconazole plasma concentration should be obtained at least 6 days after the switch to the tablet formulation to ensure adequate drug levels.

Step 2:

If IB's mucositis impairs her ability to swallow pills making administration of tablets challenging, then factors influencing absorption of the suspension should be addressed.

A study evaluating exposure of the posaconazole oral suspension under various gastric conditions compared posaconazole alone or in combination with a nutritional supplement (Boost®). When administered with the supplement, the C_{max} and AUC of a single 200 or 400 mg dose increased by 65 percent and 66 percent, respectively. Exposure was also assessed when posaconazole was administered before, with, or after a high-fat meal. While C_{max} and AUC were both increased with administration prior to meals, the greatest increase occurred during or after meals by up to 339 percent and 387 percent, respectively.[46]

Another randomized single-dose study had consistent findings. Oral posaconazole suspension was administered after a 10-hour fast, with a nonfat breakfast, or with a high-fat meal. Relative to the fasting state, administration with a nonfat meal enhanced exposure. However, increases in exposure were greatest when administered with a high-fat meal, with mean increases in AUC and C_{max} of about 400 percent.[47]

IB's oral intake should be assessed. Encouraging meals as tolerated will aid in absorption of posaconazole. Ideally, she should be encouraged to consume food of high-fat content with each meal. If unable to tolerate a solid diet, nutritional supplementation (e.g., Boost, Ensure, etc.) with each dose of posaconazole should be recommended. Posaconazole levels should continue to be followed to assess for adequate exposure. Mucositis has also been shown to reduce posaconazole exposure, but was not found to significantly affect mean total posaconazole exposure (AUC and C_{max}) at steady state. The reduction in exposure from mucositis was overcome by increasing the total dose and dosing frequency of posaconazole.[48] Since IB's mucositis will likely not improve until her ANC begins to recover, its severity should be assessed. Thus, increasing posaconazole to 200 mg PO qid would be a reasonable option to achieve adequate levels in the setting of mucositis and persistently subtherapeutic levels. Posaconazole plasma concentration should be drawn in 7–10 days after the dose increase to assess achievement of a therapeutic level.

Step 3:

If IB's mucositis continues to compromise her oral intake to the point that subsequent posaconazole levels continue to be subtherapeutic with oral therapy, switching to IV posaconazole would be an appropriate intervention.[1]

CASE 9: POSACONAZOLE AND DRUG-DRUG INTERACTIONS

KL is a 63-year-old Caucasian male with a past medical history significant for poorly controlled diabetes mellitus complicated by diabetic gastroparesis and neuropathy, hypertension, and rheumatoid arthritis requiring chronic steroids. He presents to the ED complaining of a 3-day history of progressive shortness of breath and cough. He reports that he finally made a decision to come in after having two episodes of hemoptysis in the last 24 hours. A chest CT revealed a right upper lobe consolidation and lobar cavitary lesion concerning for fungal pneumonia. Respiratory cultures were sent and broad-spectrum antimicrobials were initiated including voriconazole. However, after 48 hours without clinical improvement, a bronchoscopy was performed and bronchoalveolar lavage (BAL) cultures grew Mucor spp. A diagnosis of pulmonary mucormycosis was made, and KL was switched to posaconzole oral suspension 200 mg PO qid for treatment. KL's other medications include:

Omeprazole 20 mg PO daily

Methotrexate 7.5 mg PO weekly

Prednisone 10 mg PO daily

Metformin 1,000 mg PO twice daily

Lantus 40 units sq at bedtime

Lisinopril 20 mg PO daily

Hydrochlorothiazide 25 mg PO daily

Metoclopramide with 10 mg PO each meal and at bedtime

Gabapentin 300 mg PO three times daily

QUESTION 1

A level after 96 hours of posaconazole therapy is reported as 735 ng/mL. What is your assessment of this level?

Answer:

The level is subtherapeutic given the previously discussed target concentration of 1,000 – 1,250 ng/mL for treatment doses of posaconazole. However, posaconazole achieves steady state after approximately 7–10 days of therapy. Therefore, the level drawn after only 4 days of therapy is premature for accurate steady-state interpretation.[1,31] As previously mentioned, levels drawn prior to steady state may be predictive of steady-state concentrations.[26] In this case, clinical judgment would be necessary to assess the trend of the posaconazole level. KL's level is indicative of accumulation of some drug, but has not necessarily reached a therapeutic concentration for treatment. An appropriate assessment here would be that given an additional 72–96 hours of posaconazole therapy, KL's levels could potentially continue to accumulate to a therapeutic concentration. Thus, a modification to KL's regimen at this point in time is not necessary. However, in the case that levels return profoundly subtherapeutic (e.g., 200–300 ng/mL) after 72–96 hours of dosing, a fair assessment would be that the patient is not on an appropriate trajectory to reach therapeutic concentrations at steady state and a modification to the regimen would potentially be warranted after ensuring the absence of other contributing factors that could account for such low levels (e.g., interacting medications and poor oral intake as discussed later). In either case, one should repeat a level after at least 7 days of therapy to assess steady-state concentrations.[1,31]

QUESTION 2

Another level is drawn one week after initiation of posaconazole and is 873 ng/mL. What is your assessment of this level?

Answer:

The posaconazole level is still subtherapeutic. However, it should be noted that KL is on concomitant medications that could account for persistently subtherapeutic levels and suboptimal treatment.

The absorption of posaconazole suspension is highly dependent on maintaining an acidic gastric pH. Thus, omeprazole therapy as GI protection from chronic steroid therapy in KL presents an interaction that can lead to decreased serum concentrations of posaconazole when using the oral suspension.[1,49] However, gastric acid reducers and gastric motility agents do not have a significant impact on the absorption of posaconazole delayed-release tablets. Thus, if acid-suppressing and gastric motility therapy is indicated, switching KL to the posaconazole tablets 300 mg PO BID for the first day followed by 300 mg PO daily would potentially enhance posaconazole absorption, and facilitate achievement of a therapeutic level. A posaconaozle concentration should be drawn at least 6 days after the switch to the tablets.

If acid-suppressing therapy is not warranted, then the suspension could remain a reasonable option with appropriate adjustments made to concomitant therapies. When administered with a PPI, posaconazole C_{max} and AUC can be reduced by as much as 46 percent and 32 percent, respectively.[46] Histamine-2 receptor antagonists (H2RAs), particularly cimetidine, have a similar effect on posaconazole exposure, reducing both the C_{max} and AUC by 39 percent.[1] Administration of posaconazole with an acidic carbonated beverage has been shown to increase the C_{max} by 92 percent and the AUC by 70 percent.[46] If possible, KL's omeprazole should be discontinued and PPIs and H2RAs should be avoided. Another level should be evaluated approximately 1 week after discontinuation of the acid-suppressing agent to assess for adequate posaconazole absorption and serum concentrations. If acid-suppressing therapy is necessary while a patient is on posaconazole oral suspension, an antacid can be considered as reductions in posaconazole systemic exposure with concomitant antacids has been shown to be clinically insignificant.[50] If acid-suppressing therapy must be administered with posaconazole oral suspension, close monitoring is recommended to ensure adequate serum levels and antifungal efficacy. A switch to oral delayed-release tablets is encouraged if this acid-suppressing therapy proves to impair the patient's ability to achieve a therapeutic concentration.

Systemic exposure of posaconazole suspension is also reduced with increased gastric motility. Concomitant use of metoclopramide reduced the C_{max} of posaconazole by 21 percent and the AUC by 19 percent. Contrastingly, gastric slowing agents (i.e., loperamide) have no significant effect on posaconazole serum concentrations.[46] Posaconazole, delayed-release tablets are not affected by gastric promotility agents, thus it would be preferred with such therapy. If a patient cannot be switched to posaconazole tablets, and the oral suspension must be used with gastric promotility agents, routine therapeutic drug monitoring is recommended to ensure adequate levels and effective therapy. Metoclopramide use should be minimized in KL, if possible, to maximize posaconazole absorption and systemic exposure.

CASE 10: POSACONAZOLE AND QT-INTERVAL PROLONGATION

PJ is a 47-year-old African American male with HIV. He has a medical history significant for invasive pulmonary aspergillosis, coronary artery disease, and HSV encephalitis. He was originally initiated on voriconazole for his aspergillosis, but was switched to posaconazole DR tablets 300 mg PO bid × 1 day, followed by 300 mg PO daily due to visual hallucinations with voriconazole. He has continued on maintenance therapy for six weeks. His CD4+ count is 133 cells/mm³ and the posaconazole is to be continued until the CD4+ count is at least ≥200 cells/mm³. He continues on highly active antiretroviral therapy. He is admitted to the hospital for severe diarrhea resulting in fluid loss and acute kidney injury. During his admission, PJ developed atrial fibrillation despite aggressive fluid and electrolyte repletion. Upon consulting cardiology, they decide to initiate an IV load of amiodarone with a subsequent transition to oral maintenance amiodarone.

QUESTION

What is your recommendation regarding this therapy for PJ's atrial fibrillation?

Answer:

Rare cases of QTc interval prolongation and torsades de pointes (TdP) have been reported with posaconazole therapy. A study evaluating the safety of long-term oral posaconazole use for treatment of refractory invasive fungal infections in 428 patients found a 1 percent incidence of treatment-related QTc interval prolongation.[51] Because of this rare but serious risk, administration of posaconazole with other medications with a known risk of prolonging the QTc interval and causing TdP should be done with caution, and the QTc interval should be closely monitored.

Amiodarone is also associated with the risk of QTc interval prolongation and TdP. However, risk is heightened in this case because amiodarone is also a CYP3A4 substrate. Posaconazole is a strong inhibitor of CYP3A4 and, thus, inhibits CYP3A4-mediated amiodarone metabolism. Decreased metabolism results in increased amiodarone plasma concentrations and can lead to an increased risk of QTc interval prolongation and TdP. Thus, concomitant use of posaconazole and CYP3A4 substrates that prolong the QTc interval (e.g., terfenadine, cisapride, pimozide, quinidine, amiodarone) is contraindicated.[1,31]

Voriconazole is not an option given his history of visual hallucinations and the drug's associated risk of QTc interval prolongation. A lack of feasibility of administering amphotericin B for maintenance therapy as an outpatient makes it an impractical option. Echinocandins have inferior activity against *Aspergillus* sp. along with a lack of oral availability for outpatient administration. Therefore, posaconazole remains most optimal for PJ as maintenance for aspergillosis. Prioritization of posaconazole therapy is important given his infection history and HIV status (CD4+ count of 133 cells/mm³). Therefore, an alternative to amiodarone should be considered.

Aggressive electrolyte and fluid replacement should continue. If amiodarone becomes the agent of choice for management of PJ's atrial fibrillation, potential methods for echinocandin maintenance therapy (e.g., caspofungin or micafungin) should be explored as an alternative to posaconazole. A dose reduction of posaconazole is not ideal and could result in subtherapeutic serum concentrations and ineffective antifungal treatment.

CASE 11: SPECIAL POPULATIONS: POSACONAZOLE IN HEMATOPOIETIC STEM CELL TRANSPLANT AND GVHD

JK is a 65-year-old Caucasian male who is 45 days post–allogeneic stem cell transplant with myeloablative conditioning for chronic myeloid leukemia (CML). He has engrafted and his hematocrit, WBC/ANC, and platelets have recovered. To date, he has done well on levofloxacin, fluconazole, and valacyclovir for posttransplant prophylaxis and has not experienced any infectious complications, but has begun to develop diarrhea. Testing for C.difficile infection has been negative. A colon biopsy performed confirms gastrointestinal graft vs. host disease (GVHD). Prednisone 1 mg/kg is initiated and the fluconazole is switched to posaconazole for expanded antifungal coverage while on steroid therapy. The bone marrow transplant attending expresses concerns regarding adequate exposure of posaconazole in JK given his diarrhea and GVHD.

QUESTION

What are your recommendations to him regarding antifungal prophylaxis for JK in the setting of his GVHD?

Answer:

Posaconazole has an established role in the prevention of invasive fungal infections in the hematopoietic stem cell population, especially those with GVHD. Ullman and colleagues evaluated the use of posaconazole versus fluconazole in this population in a phase III, randomized fashion. Posaconazole was shown to be noninferior to fluconazole in preventing invasive fungal infections. Notable in this trial was that more than 50 percent of the invasive fungal infections were invasive aspergillosis and that posaconazole was superior in preventing aspergillosis (2.3% with posaconazole vs. 7.0% with fluconazole developed invasive aspergillosis; p = 0.006). Furthermore, while overall mortality was similar, posaconazole significantly reduced the rate of death from invasive fungal infections (1% vs. 4%; p = 0.046).[28]

As a result of posaconazole being considered as an option for prophylaxis in stem cell transplant patients with GVHD, it was necessary to evaluate the pharmacokinetics of posaconazole in this population. Krishna and others completed a pharmacokinetic analysis of 246 patients from the evaluation by Ullman and colleagues that had pharmacokinetic data available.[52] Of these, five patients developed invasive fungal infections and had significantly lower average (median C_{avg} 611 ng/mL) and maximum (median C_{max} 635 ng/ml) posaconazole concentrations compared to those that did not develop invasive fungal infections (median C_{avg} 922 ng/mL; median C_{max} 1,360 ng/mL). Median plasma concentrations were also higher in patients with chronic GVHD compared to those with acute GVHD. Extensive gastrointestinal compromise is a pathophysiologic feature of acute GVHD and could possibly account for the lower serum concentrations in these patients.[52] However, observed posaconazole plasma concentrations were adequate to prevent invasive fungal infections in patients with both acute (C_{avg} 814 ± 650 ng/mL; C_{max} 1,130 ± 858 ng/mL) and chronic (C_{avg} 1,413 ± 842 ng/mL; C_{max} 1,785 ± 1,030 ng/mL) GVHD.[52]

Given the aforementioned data, it is possible to achieve adequate serum concentrations of posaconazole in patients with GVHD to effectively prevent invasive fungal infections. JK should have steady-state levels of posaconazole measured (after at least 7 days of therapy) and treatment decisions should be dictated by ability to achieve therapeutic concentrations. Lack of examination of variables such as vomiting, dysphagia, mucositis, and changes in GVHD status were acknowledged to be limitations of the pharmacokinetic evaluation by Krishna and colleagues.[52] These factors could potentially affect the exposure of posaconazole due to an injury to the gastrointestinal lining. Therefore, the recommendation is to assess these variables in JK and consider them when interpreting monitored levels. While this data for posaconazole prophylaxis in stem cell transplant patients with GVHD is with the oral suspension, the oral delayed-release tablets are certainly a reasonable therapy for fungal prophylaxis in this population. Pharmacokinetic data evaluating concentrations with the tablet including stem cell transplant patients with GVHD.[1]

CASE 12: SPECIAL POPULATIONS: POSACONAZOLE IN CRITICALLY ILL WITH LARGE Vd

NN is a 29-year-old male admitted to the surgical intensive care unit after complications of abdominal surgery. He is discovered to have biopsy-proven invasive cutaneous mucormycosis at the site of surgery and is initiated on posaconazole 200 mg every 6 hours administered via nasogastric tube. NN is receiving appropriate stress-ulcer prophylaxis.

QUESTION 1

What factors can impact posaconazole serum concentrations in critically ill patients?

Answer:

In critically ill patients, volume of distribution for posaconazole is increased to about 3,300–5,300 liters (compared to 2–3 times less in non-ICU patients).[53,54] This increased V_d occurs because of capillary leak syndrome and edema, which causes fluid shift from the intravascular compartment to the interstitial space, which in turn causes decreased plasma concentrations.[55] This effect is most profound on hydrophilic medications with low V_d. Although posaconazole is known to be lipophilic, a pharmacokinetic analysis of posaconazole in ICU patients found a maximum serum concentration of 531 ng/mL. None of the patients in this ICU cohort were able to achieve therapeutic concentrations greater than 700 ng/mL.[53] In addition to the increased volume of distribution, patients in the ICU setting are also on stress-ulcer prophylaxis with proton-pump inhibitors, decreasing absorption of posaconazole suspension. The hypermetabolic state of critically ill patients contributes to increased clearance of posaconazole and potentially decreased serum concentrations.[53] In addition, nasogastric administration of posaconazole, even in healthy patient volunteers, results in about 20 percent decreased AUC and C_{max}.[19]

QUESTION 2

How should posaconazole be monitored? Is this treatment the preferred regimen for the patient?

Answer:

Posaconazole serum levels should be drawn after 2–3 days of therapy to assess the trajectory of the serum concentration. Because posaconazole pharmacokinetics can be characterized in a one-compartment model, early monitoring of serum levels can be a surrogate to steady-state concentrations.[26,53] An additional level after 7 days of therapy is also required to ensure adequate serum concentration levels are reached. In general, due to the complex pharmacokinetic and pharmacodynamic alterations in critically ill patients, posaconazole should be avoided. Changing NN's therapy to amphotericin B would be the best intervention. Alternatively, intravenous posaconazole may be considered which avoids issues related to absorption.

REFERENCES

1. Noxafil (posaconazole) oral suspension, delayed-release tablets, injection [package insert]. Whitehouse Station, NJ: Merck & Co, 2014.
2. Vfend (Voriconazole) Tablets, Oral Suspension, and IV [package insert]. New York: Pfizier, 2011.
3. Cornely OA, Maertens J, Winston DJ, Perfect J, Ullman AJ, Walsh TJ, et al. Posaconazole vs. fluconazole or itraconazole prophylaxis in patients with neutropenia. *N Engl J Med.* 2007;356:348–359.
4. Herbrecht R, Denning DW, Patterson TF, Bennett JE, Greene RE, Oestmann JW, et al. Voriconazole versus amphotericin B for primary therapy of invasive aspergillosis. *N Engl J Med.* 2002;347(6):408–415.
5. Vehreschild JJ, Birtel A, Vehreschild MJ, Liss B, Farowski F, Kochanek M, et al. Mucormycosis treated with posaconazole: Review of 96 case reports. *Crit Rev Microbiol.* 2012:1–15.
6. Flores VG, Tovar RM, Zaldivar PG, Martinez EA. Meningitis due to Cryptococcus neoformans: Treatment with posaconazole. *Curr HIV Res.* 2012;10(7):620–623.
7. Ezzet F, Wexler D, Courtney R, Krishna G, Lim J, Laughlin M. Oral bioavailability of posaconazole in fasted healthy subjects: Comparison between three regimens and basis for clinical dosage recommendations. *Clin Pharmacokinet.* 2005;44(2):211–220.
8. Li Y, Theuretzbacher U, Clancy CJ, Nguyen MH, Derendorf H. Pharmacokinetic/Pharmacodynamic profile of posaconazole. *Clin Pharmacokinet.* 2010;49(6):379–396.
9. Krishna G, Ma L, Martinho M, O'Mara E. Single-dose phase I study to evaluate the pharmacokinetics of posaconazole in new tablet and capsule formulations relative to oral suspension. *Antimicrob Agents Chemother.* 2012;56(8):4196–4201.
10. Purkins L, Wood N, Kleinermans D, Greenhalgh K, Nichols D. Effect of food on the pharmacokinetics of multiple-dose oral voriconazole. *Br J Clin Pharmacol.* 2003;56:17–23.
11. Lipp HP. Posaconazole: Clinical pharmacokinetics and drug interactions. *Mycoses.* 2011;54(Suppl 1):32–38.
12. Theuretzbacher U, Ihle F, Derendorf H. Pharmacokinetic/Pharmacodynamic profile of voriconazole. *Clin Pharmacokinet.* 2006;45(7):649–663.
13. Weiler S, Fiegl D, MacFarland R, Stienecke E, Bellmann-Weiler R, Dunzendorfer S, et al. Human tissue distribution of voriconazole. *Antimicrob Agents Chemother.* 2011;55(2):925–928.
14. Ghosal A, Hapangama N, Yuan Y, Achanfuo-Yeboah J, Iannucci R, Chowdhury S, et al. Identification of human UDP-glucuronosyltransferase enzyme(s) responsible for the glucuronidation of posaconazole (Noxafil). *Drug Metab Dispos.* 2004;32(2):267–271.
15. Hussaini T, Ruping M, Faroski F, Vehreschild JJ, Cornely OA. Therapeutic drug monitoring of voriconazole and posaconazole. *Pharmacother.* 2011;31(2):214–225.
16. Mikus G, Scholz IM, Weiss J. Pharmacogenomics of the triazole antifungal agent voriconazole. *Pharmacogenomics.* 2011;12(6):861–872.
17. Weiss J, Ten Hoevel MM, Burhenne J, Walter-Sack I, Hoffmann MM, Rengelshausen J, et al. CYP2C19 genotype is a major factor contributing to the highly variable pharmacokinetics of voriconazole. *J Clin Pharmacol.* 2009;49(2):196–204.
18. Maertens J, Cornely OA, Ullmann AJ, Heinz WJ, Krishna G, Patino H, et al. Phase 1b study of the pharmacokinetics and safety of posaconazole intravenous solution in patients at risk for invasive fungal disease. *Antimicrob Agents Chemother.* 2014;58(7):3610–3617.
19. Dodds Ashley ES, Varkey JB, Krishna G, Vickery D, Ma L, Yu X, et al. Pharmacokinetics of posaconazole administered orally or by nasogastric tube in healthy volunteers. *Antimicrob Agents Chemother.* 2009;53(7):2960–2964.
20. Pfaller MA, Diekema DJ, Rex JH, Espinel-Ingroff A, Johnson EM, Andes D, Chatuvedi V, et al. Correlation of MIC with outcome for *Candida* species tested against voriconazole: Analysis and proposal for interpretive breakpoints. *J Clin Microbiol.* 2006;44:819–826.
21. Hope WW, Cuenca-Estrella M, Lass-Florl C, Arendrup MC, and The European Committee on Antimicrobial Susceptibility Testing-Subcommittee on Antifungal Susceptibility Testing. EUCAST technical note on voriconazole and Aspergillus spp. *Clin Microbiol Infect.* 2013:1–3.

22. Pascual A, Calandra T, Thierry B, Bille J, Marchetti O. Voriconazole therapeutic drug monitoring in patients with invasive mycoses improves efficacy and safety outcomes. *Clin Infect Dis.* 2008;46:201–211.

23. Troke PF, Hockey HP, Hope WW. Observational study of the clinical efficacy of voriconazole and its relationship to plasma concentrations in patients. *Antimicrob Agents Chemother.* 2011;55(10):4782–4788.

24. Ueda K, Nannya Y, Kumano K, Hangaishi A, Takahashi T, Imai Y, et al. Monitoring trough concentration of voriconazole is important to ensure successful antifungal therapy and to avoid hepatic damage in patients with hematologic disorders. *Int J Hematol.* 2009;89(5):592–599.

25. Walsh TJ, Raad I, Patterson TF, Chandrasekar P, Donowitz GR, Graybill R, et al. Treatment of invasive aspergillosis with posaconazole in patients who are refractory to or intolerant of conventional therapy: An externally controlled trial. *Clin Infect Dis.* 2007;44(1):2–12. Epub 2006 Nov 28.

26. Ananda-Rajah MR, Grigg A, Slavin MA. Making sense of posaconazole therapeutic drug monitoring: A practical approach. *Curr Opin Infect Dis.* 2012;25(6):605–611.

27. Howard SJ, Felton TW, Gomez-Lopez A, Hope WW. Posaconazole: The case for therapeutic drug monitoring. *Ther Drug Monit.* 2012;34(1):72–76.

28. Ullmann AJ, Lipton JH, Vesole DH, Chandrasekar P, Langston A, Tarantolo SR. Posaconazole or fluconazole for prophylaxis in severe graft-versus-host disease. *N Engl J Med.* 2007;356(4):335–347.

29. Jang SH, Colangelo PM, Gobburu JV. Exposure-response of posaconazole used for prophylaxis against invasive fungal infections: Evaluating the need to adjust doses based on drug concentrations in plasma. *Clin Pharmacol Ther.* 2010;88(1):115–119.

30. Pascual A, Csajka C, Buclin T, Bolay S, Bille J, Calandra T, et al. Challenging recommended oral and intravenous voriconazole doses for improved efficacy and safety: Population pharmacokinetics-based analysis of adult patients with invasive fungal infections. *Clin Infect Dis.* 2012;55(3):381–390.

31. Nagappan V, Deresinski S. Posaconazole: A broad-spectrum triazole antifungal agent. *Clin Infect Dis.* 2007;45:1610–1617.

32. Purkins L, Wood N, Ghahramani P, Greenhalgh K, Allen MJ, Kleinermans. Pharmacokinetics and safety of voriconazole following intravenous- to oral-dose escalation regimens. *Antimicrob Agents Chemother.* 2002;46(8):2546–2553.

33. Kim S-H, Yim D-S, Choi S-M, Kwon J-C, Han S, Lee D-G, et al. Voriconazole-related severe adverse events: Clinical application of therapeutic drug monitoring in Korean patients. *Int J Infect Dis.* 2011. doi:10.1016/j.ijid.2011.06.004.

34. Wood N, Tan K, Purkins I, Layton G, Hamlin J, Kleinermans D, et al. Effect of omeprazole on the steady state pharmacokinetics of voriconazole. *Br J Clin Pharmacol.* 2003;56(Suppl 1):56–61.

35. Dolton MJ, Ray JE, Chen S, Ng K, Pont LG, McLachlan AJ. Multicenter study of voriconazole pharmacokinetics and therapeutic drug monitoring. *Antimicrob Agents Chemother.* 2012;56(9):4793–4799.

36. Pai MP, Lodise TP. Steady-state plasma pharmacokinetics of oral voriconazole in obese adults. *Antimicrob Agents Chemother.* 2011;55(6):2601–2605.

37. Davies-Vorbrodt S, Ito JI, Tegtmeier BR, Dadwal SS, Kriengkauykiat J. Voriconazole serum concentrations in obese and overweight immunocompromised patients: A retrospective review. *Pharmacother.* 2013;33(1):22–30.

38. Koselke E, Kraft S, Smith J, Nagel J. Evaluation of the effect of obesity on voriconazole serum concentrations. *J Antimicrob Chemother.* 2012;67(12):2957–2962.

39. Luke DR, Tomaszewski, Damle B, Schlamm HT. Review of the basic and clinical pharmacology of sulfobutylether-b-cyclodextrin (SBECD). *J Pharm Sci.* 2010;99(8):3291–3301.

40. Food and Drug Administration. Antiviral Drugs Advisory Committee briefing document for voriconazole (oral and intravenous formulations). Available at: http://www.fda.gov/ohrms/dockets/ac/01/briefing/3792b2_01_Pfizer.pdf (accessed February 11, 2013).

41. Oude Lashof AML, Sobel JD, Ruhnke M, Pappas PG, Viscoli C, Schlamm HT. Safety and tolerability of voriconazole in patients with renal insufficiency and candidemia. *Antimicrob Agents Chemother.* 2012;56(6):3133–3137.

42. Neofytos D, Lombardi LR, Shields RK, Ostrander D, Warren L, Nguyen MH. Administration of voriconazole in patients with renal dysfunction. *Clin Infect Dis.* 2012;54(7):913–921.

43. Alvarez-Lerma F, Allepuz-Palau A, Garcia MP, Angeles Leon M, Navarro A, Sanchez-Ruiz H, et al. Impact of intravenous administration of voriconazole in critically ill patients with impaired renal function. *J Chemother.* 2008;20(1):93–100.

44. Duarte RF, López-Jiménez J, Cornely OA, Laverdiere M, et al. Phase 1b study of new posaconazole tablet for prevention of invasive fungal infections in high-risk patients with neutropenia. *Antimicrob Agents Chemother.* 2014;58(10):5758–5765.

45. Shields RK, Clancy CJ, Vadnerkar A, Kwak EJ, Silveira FP, Massih RC, et al. Posaconazole serum concentrations among cardiothoracic transplant recipients: Factors impacting trough levels and correlation with clinical response to therapy. *Antimicrob Agents Chemother.* 2011;55(3):1308–1311.

46. Krishna G, Moton A, Ma L, et al. Pharmacokinetics and absorption of posaconazole oral suspension under various gastric conditions in healthy volunteers. *Antimicrob Agents Chemother.* 2009;53(3):958–966.

47. Courtney R, Wexler D, Radwanski E, et al. Effect of food on the relative bioavailability of two oral formulations of posaconazole in healthy adults. *Br J Clin Pharmacol.* 2004;57(2):218–222.

48. Gubbins P, Krishna G, Sansone-Parsons A, et al. Pharmacokinetics and safety of oral posaconazole in neutropenic stem cell transplant recipients. *Antimicrob Agents Chemother.* 2006;50(6):1993–1999.

49. Alffenaar, J, van Assen S, van der Werf T, et al. Omeprazole significant reduces posaconazole serum trough level. *Clin Infect Dis.* 2009;48:839.

50. Courtney R, Radwanski E, Lim J, et al. Pharmacokinetics of posaconazole coadministered with antacid in fasting and nonfasting healthy men. *Antimicrob Agents Chemother.* 2004;48(3):804–808.

51. Raad I, Graybill J, Bustamante A, et al. Safety of long-term oral posaconazole use in the treatment of refractory invasive fungal infections. *Clin Infect Dis.* 2006;42:1726–1734.

52. Krishna G, Martinho M, Chandrasekar P, et al. Pharmacokinetics of oral posaconazole in allogeneic hematopoietic stem cell transplant recipients with graft-vs-host disease. *Pharmacother.* 2007;27(12):1627–1636.

53. Störzinger D, Borghorst S, Hofer S, Busch CJ, Lichtenstern C, Hempel G, et al. Plasma concentrations of posaconazole administered via nasogastric tube in patients in a surgical intensive care unit. *Antimicrob Agents Chemother.* 2012;56(8):4468–4470.

54. AbuTarif MA, Krishna G, Statkevich P. Population pharmacokinetics of posaconazole in neutropenic patients receiving chemotherapy for acute myelogenous leukemia or myelodysplastic syndrome. *Curr Med Res Opin.* 2010;26(2):397–405.

55. Roberts JA, Lipman J. Pharmacokinetic issues for antibiotics in the critically ill patient. *Crit Care Med.* 2009;37(3):840–851.

CHAPTER 17

Procainamide

VICTOR COHEN, BS, PharmD, BCPS, CGP
SAMANTHA P. JELLINEK-COHEN, PharmD, BCPS, CGP

OVERVIEW

Procainamide was introduced in 1951 as a Class 1a antiarrhythmic agent. Class 1a antiarrythmics, the oldest class of antiarrythmics on the market, are considered membrane-stabilizing agents that work by blocking sodium channels. Agents in this class include quinidine, procainamide, and disopyramide. Although these agents are quite effective in suppressing both atrial and ventricular ectopy, they are associated with significant toxicity, and thus, their use has fallen out of favor. Procainamide is indicated for the treatment of life-threatening ventricular arrhythmias, such as sustained ventricular tachycardia.[1] Off-label uses of procainamide include conversion of atrial fibrillation/flutter to sinus rhythm.[1,2]

Procainamide decreases the ability of incompletely repolarized fibers to generate an active response and delays completion of repolarization. These actions increase the effective refractory period of atrial and ventricular fibers, thereby accounting for its antifibrillatory effects.[3] Converting from a unidirectional to a bidirectional block, procainamide decreases reentrant arrhythmias. Procainamide has been proven to be safe and effective against ventricular arrhythmias when administered orally and intramuscularly. Historically, the oral formulation was preferred for less urgent arrhythmias and for long-term maintenance after initial parenteral therapy. Intramuscular administration was reserved for patients unable to tolerate the oral formulation secondary to gastrointestinal toxicity (nausea and vomiting). In addition to the intolerable gastrointestinal adverse effects associated with oral procainamide, other extracardiac effects, including central nervous system symptoms (headache, dizziness, psychosis, hallucinations, and depression), fever, agranulocytosis, rash, myalgias, digital vasculitis, Raynaud's phenomenon, and a systemic lupus-like syndrome, have been reported.[3] Toxicity associated with oral formulations of procainamide, availability of alternative antiarrhythmic agents, and the lack of necessity of the drug led to the eventual discontinuation of this dosage form in the mid to late 2000s. Parenteral formulations 500 mg/1 ml in a 2 ml vial remain periodically available. Although undesirable infusion rate related cardiovascular side effects associated with the use of intravenous infusions of procainamide have made this mode of administration unpopular, the use of procainamide as an intravenous bolus remains a viable option. Procainamide exerts electrophysiological effects similar to those of quinidine. However, procainamide lacks quinidine's vagolytic and alpha-adrenergic blocking activity, and as a result, is better tolerated when given intravenously.[4]

ELECTROPHYSIOLOGICAL EFFECTS

Procainamide produces increases in the QT_c interval and widening of the QRS complex in a concentration-dependent manner, usually starting at concentrations >12 mg/mL. Procainamide has been associated with life-threatening arrhythmias such as torsades de pointes

and has resulted in sudden cardiac death. N-acetylprocainamide (NAPA), the acetyled metabolite of procainamide, which has been shown to have antiarrhythmic actions of its own, prolongs only the QT_c interval.[4-6] Because NAPA has Class III antiarrhythmic properties, it is of clinical importance to use the total concentrations of both procainamide and NAPA to assess pharmacological activity and toxicity; solely reviewing the procainamide level may be misleading.[6]

AVAILABILITY

Procainamide is available in an injectable formulation, which can be given intravenously for rapid control of serious arrhythmias. Dosage strengths include 100 mg/mL and 500 mg/mL.[7] The oral formulation of procainamide is no longer available in the United States.

DOSING

The American Heart Association guidelines for cardiopulmonary resuscitation and emergency cardiovascular care recommend that adult patients with atrial fibrillation/flutter or stable monomorphic ventricular tachycardia receive 20–50 mg procainamide per minute intravenously until the arrhythmia is suppressed, hypotension ensues, or QRS complex is prolonged by 50 percent from its original duration, or a total cumulative dose of 17 mg/kg has been given. The maintenance infusion rate is 1–4 mg/min. Alternatively, 100 mg procainamide can be administered intravenously every 5 minutes until the arrhythmia is controlled or the other conditions already described are met.[8] Manufacturer recommendations suggest that initial arrhythmia control can be accomplished by administering repeated bolus injections to be infused at a rate of no faster than 50 mg/min to a maximum advisable dose of 1 gram.[1] Once 500 mg has been administered, it is advisable to wait 10 minutes or longer before resuming treatment to allow for greater distribution into the tissues. Alternatively, a loading infusion containing procainamide 20 mg/mL (1 gram diluted to 50 mL with dextrose 5% injection) may be administered at a constant rate of 1 mL/min for 25–30 minutes to deliver 500–600 mg of procainamide. Some effects may be seen after infusion of the first 100 or 200 mg. It is unusual that more than 600 mg is needed to achieve satisfactory antiarrhythmic effects. To achieve maintenance of therapeutic procainamide levels, a diluted intravenous infusion of 2 mg/mL may be administered at 1–3 mL/min. The infusion rate will deliver 2–6 mg/min. In fluid-restricted patients, a 4 mg/mL concentration may be used. In a patient with normal renal function, a maintenance infusion of 50 mcg/kg/min will produce a procainamide plasma level of 6.5 mcg/mL. Procainamide loading and maintenance doses should be based on ideal body weight in morbidly obese patients.[9,10] Procainamide is not approved by the Food and Drug Administration for use in children.

BIOAVAILABILITY

The absorption of intravenous procainamide is immediate with a bioavailability of 100 percent. Following intravenous administration, peak levels are reached within 20–30 minutes and are maintained for 1–2 hours.[11]

VOLUME OF DISTRIBUTION

Approximately 10–20 percent of procainamide is protein bound, and the apparent volume of distribution is large (about 1.5–2.5 L/kg body weight).[4,12] However, the volume of distribution can be significantly reduced under conditions such as congestive heart failure or cardiogenic shock, resulting in higher concentrations from a dose.[3] Procainamide has an octanol-to-water partition coefficient that would indicate a high lipid affinity; however, its volume of distribution is not influenced by obesity because the partition coefficient remains low enough to limit distribution into adipose tissue.[13] Intravenous procainamide follows a two-compartment model. Initially after the loading dose, the concentration decreases rapidly as the drug is distributed, which is then followed by the elimination phase.

METABOLISM AND CLEARANCE/HALF-LIFE

Approximately 50 percent of procainamide is eliminated unchanged in the urine and the average half-life is approximately 3 hours in healthy subjects.[14] Procainamide also undergoes hepatic metabolism. The major pathway for hepatic metabolism is conjugation of N-acetyl transferase, polymorphically distributed cytosolic enzyme, to form NAPA, which is renally eliminated and has an elimination half-life of approximately 7.5–10 hours in individuals with normal renal function.[4] In cardiac patients with renal failure, NAPA can accumulate in the plasma and produce signs of clinical toxicity. Age also appears to affect both procainamide clearance and the NAPA:Procainamide concentration ratio, independent of the decline in renal function that occurs in elderly patients.[4,15] Increased urine pH can decrease renal elimination of procainamide.[6] Both procainamide and NAPA are actively secreted by the proximal tubules of the kidney and competition between the two for renal secretion results in decreased elimination of procainamide.[6]

HEART FAILURE

In patients with heart failure, procainamide is not cleared as well, and therefore, a dose reduction of 30–50 percent in initial therapy is recommended for patients with severely compromised cardiac function.[16] In patients with uncompensated heart failure, a reduction in hepatic blood flow decreases the clearance of procainamide. Furthermore, the volume of distribution is decreased. The half-life of procainamide may not be drastically increased because both the clearance and volume of distribution are decreasing ($t_{1/2} = 0.693V/Cl$); however, a dose reduction of 25–50 percent may be necessary. Patients with compensated heart failure do not require dose adjustments.

LIVER DISEASE

N-acetyltransferase 2 (NAT2) is a liver enzyme responsible for the conversion of procainamide to NAPA. Despite limited data on the pharmacokinetics of procainamide in patients with liver disease, it is suggested that a dose reduction might be warranted in patients with liver disease. In patients with a Child-Pugh score of 8–10, most recommend a 25 percent reduction in the initial dosage. Those with a score >10, a 50 percent reduction is recommended. From there, doses may be titrated as needed.

RENAL FAILURE AND END-STAGE RENAL DISEASE

As creatinine clearance decreases, the clearance of procainamide is reduced proportionally. The half-life of procainamide in renal failure is approximately 6 hours.[14] In end-stage renal disease, the half-life of procainamide is prolonged to about 14 hours. The volume of distribution of procainamide in end-stage renal disease has been calculated to be about 1.4 L/kg.[16]

NAPA

NAPA, the acetylated metabolite of PA, has been shown to have antiarrhythmic actions of its own. It is 85 percent eliminated by the kidneys, and the half-life in patients with normal renal function is about twice that of PA (6–8 hours).[17] The expected half-life in patients with renal failure is 35 hours.[14] Hepatic conjugation of procainamide to NAPA exhibits genetic polymorphism. The fast acetylator phenotype occurs in 10–20 percent of Asians; 50 percent of Americans; and 60–70 percent of Northern Europeans. In fast acetylators, NAPA may accumulate and exceed that of procainamide. The impairment of acetylation in chronic liver disease also seems to be phenotype specific, with a more prominent effect in fast acetylators than in slow acetylators.[18] A fast acetylator is considered a patient without renal impairment who has a NAPA concentration equal to or greater than procainamide three hours after dosing.[2,6] A lower incidence of lupus-like syndrome occurs or a higher dose is needed for this adverse event to occur in patients who are fast acetylators. In patients with normal renal function, the steady-state concentration ratio, or acetylator ratio, of NAPA:PA can be used to possibly determine those who are slow or fast acetylators. A ratio ≥1.2 can be considered a fast acetylator, while a ratio of ≤0.8 a slow acetylator.

ADVERSE EVENTS

The frequency of toxic manifestations, such as depression of cardiac output and blood pressure, vascular collapse, depression of cardiac impulse formation and conduction, prolongation of the QRS and QT intervals, and induction of ventricular arrhythmias has been identified with intravenous administration of procainamide. Toxicity typically occurs at infusion rates of 100 mg or more per minute and is likely secondary to inadequate drug distribution. It is generally accepted that infusion rates of 25–50 mg/min are safe and associated with a low incidence of toxicity.[19] Such undesirable effects have led to the recommendation that during intravenous procainamide therapy, the blood pressure be continually monitored and phenylephrine or norepinephrine either be readily available or actually given. Furthermore, to avert potentially dangerous drug-induced alterations in the ECG, constant electrocardiographic monitoring and equipment to treat ventricular asystole, fibrillation, or both has been advised.[20] The small molecular size and low protein binding of procainamide and NAPA are desirable attributes for extracorporeal drug removal. Procainamide toxicity has been treated, with varying degrees of efficiency, by several modalities, including peritoneal dialysis, hemodialysis, hemoperfusion, and continuous arteriovenous hemofiltration/hemodiafiltration.[16]

THERAPEUTIC DRUG MONITORING

Plasma levels of procainamide correlate well with the clinical effects of the drug.[21] When monitoring procainamide therapy, it is customary to measure serum levels of both procainamide and NAPA, which has significant antiarrhythmic action, particularly Class III activity (prolongation of the action potential via potassium channel blockade).[22] Serum concentrations of procainamide should not be assessed alone. NAPA should also be analyzed (on the same sample), and each analyte should be quantified with reference to its own reference range. The common practice of summing their concentrations should be avoided.[6] The therapeutic plasma concentration of procainamide is generally thought to be in the range of 4–10 mg/L. However, this range varies up to a maximum of 32 mg/L and is controversial and poorly determined from small-scale studies that lacked standardized sampling procedures.[4,23] Therapeutic plasma levels of less than 4 mg/L suppress arrhythmias in only a minority of patients. Toxic manifestations are common with concentrations greater than 10 mg/L. At levels >10 mg/L, procainamide produces hypotension and reductions in efferent vasoconstrictor sympathetic outflow that are thought to be the result of ganglionic blockade and/or central nervous system sympathetic inhibition.[4] The clinical importance of toxic effects on circulatory function depends largely on the patient's previous cardiovascular status. Most patients can easily compensate for some depression of myocardial contractility by toxic concentrations of procainamide, but the same is not true for patients with preexisting circulatory depression.[21] The fluorescence polarization immunoassay and enzyme immunoassays are used most commonly for therapeutic drug monitoring of procainamide and of the active metabolite NAPA.[22] Measurement of plasma concentrations is helpful in all patients with cardiac or renal failure and in critically ill patients.[21] When the desired antiarrhythmic effect is not achieved or when toxic effects are suspected, knowledge of the plasma level can greatly clarify the situation.[21] In routine therapeutic monitoring, a sample collected one hour before the next dose (trough) is recommended for determination of both procainamide and NAPA. The effective range of concentrations of NAPA is 2–22 mg/L, and levels as high as 40 mg/L appear to be well tolerated.[16] Typically, lupus-like syndrome is one of the adverse events not seen with NAPA. (See Table 17-1)

TABLE 17-1	Drug Interactions[24-26]	
Drug	**Proposed Mechanism**	**Comment**
Amiodarone	Decreases clearance and increases elimination half-life of procainamide	• Plasma concentrations of procainamide and NAPA may be increased • Concomitant use may produce additive electrophysiological effects • May decrease procainamide dose by 20%
Trimethoprim	Decreased renal tubular secretion of procainamide by competitive inhibition with trimethoprim	• Results in an increase of the AUC of procainamide and NAPA
Ofloxacin Levofloxacin Ciprofloxacin	Renal tubular secretion competition resulting in a decrease in procainamide tubular secretion	• Results in increases of AUC and peak plasma concentration of procainamide and a decrease in plasma clearance • NAPA pharmacokinetics are not altered
Propranolol	Unknown	• Increases the elimination half-life of procainamide by 56% • Close monitoring of procainamide concentrations is recommended
Cimetidine	Inhibits active tubular secretion in the kidney	• Increases plasma concentrations of procainamide and NAPA

PHARMACOKINETIC DOSING METHOD VERSES LITERATURE-BASED RECOMMENDED DOSING

Pharmacokinetic Dosing Method

By utilizing this method to dose procainamide, population as well as patient-specific parameters can be used. The patient-specific parameters allow dosing to be individualized and adjusted based on disease states.

Because procainamide is eliminated by tubular secretion, rather than glomerular filtration, creatinine clearance cannot be used to estimate renal elimination. Different disease states result in various clearance rates as discussed previously under metabolism and clearance. The estimated half-life for each disease state should be utilized. For example, in renal failure the half-life is approximately 14 hours. Utilize this half-life rather than the normal 5.5 hours when calculating a dose. In order to avoid overdoses in patients with multiple disease states, utilize the disease state with the longest half-life, which can then be computed to determine the elimination rate constant.

Similar to the half-life, volume of distribution varies based on disease states. Normally, Vd is 1.5–2.7 L/kg. It is suggested that for renal failure patients Vd is 1.7 L/kg and 1.6L/kg for uncompensated heart failure patients. All other patients, a Vd of 2.7 L/kg can be used. For obese patients, ideal body weight should be substituted for actual body weight.

Literature-Based Dosing Method

Literature-based dosing method is a way to standardize procainamide dosing. Often a patient will have multiple disease states and conditions, making it difficult to determine the appropriate pharmacokinetic parameters. For this reason, it is feasible and sometimes preferable to use the literature-based dosing method. A steady-state concentration of 4–10 μg/mL should be maintained. In patients with moderate-to-severe liver disease, having a Child-Pugh score ≥8 and/or heart failure classified as NYHA class II or higher, a 25–50 percent dose decrease is recommended. Renal dysfunction patient should receive a 25–75 percent dose decrease.

CASE STUDIES

CASE 1: LOADING DOSE

AK is a 45-year-old male who presents to the ED with a chief complaint of palpitations. Patient stated that he started to get palpitations overnight and was brought from home by an ambulance. Patient's PMH includes HTN, DM2, CVA, hypercholesterolemia, and kidney stones. Patient's past surgical history includes cardiac stents, CABG, and internal cardiac defibrillator. Social and family history was noncontributory. Physical exam of patient is within normal limits. ECG revealed a PR interval of 0.75 ms, QRS interval of 103 ms, and heart rate of 161 bpm. Patient is tachycardic.

Vital signs:

HR 163 bpm

RR 21 breaths/min

BP 150/113 mm Hg

O₂ saturation is 98%

Medical impression is significant for a rule/out Wolff-Parkinson-White rhythm with observed delta waves; the prescriber wants to avoid calcium channel blockers because they may worsen the tachycardia and instead had ordered a procainamide drip. Calculate a loading dose for this 80 kg patient. The desired concentration is 8 mg/L.

Answer:

Use the following loading dose equation. The volume of distribution (V) is 2 L/kg and the concentration desired (8) is 8 mg/L. The salt factor (S) is 0.87 for the hydrochloride salt. The bioavailability (F) is 100 percent or 1.0 for the parental administration.

$$\text{Loading dose} = \frac{(Vd)(C)}{(S)(F)}$$

$$\text{Loading dose} = \frac{(2\ \text{L/kg})(80\ \text{kg})(8\ \text{mg/L})}{(0.87)(1)}$$

$$\text{Loading dose} = 1{,}471\ \text{mg}$$

CASE 2: MAINTENANCE DOSE USING POPULATION PHARMACOKINETICS

Calculate the maintenance dose in mg/min for the 80 kg patient in the preceding case. Patient's creatinine clearance is 70 mL/min (4.2 L/hr), average acetylation clearance as 0.13 L/kg/hr, and clearance other is 0.1 L/kg/hr.

Answer:

Use the following maintenance dose equation:

$$\text{Maintenance dose} = \frac{(Cl)(C_{ss\,ave})(\tau)}{(S)(F)}$$

Cl_{total} must be calculated before calculating the maintenance dose because maintenance dose is dependent on clearance.

$$Cl_{total} = Cl_{renal} + Cl_{acetylation} + Cl_{other}$$

$$Cl_{renal} = (3)(CrCl)$$

$$Cl_{renal} = (3)(4.2\ \text{L/hr})$$

$$Cl_{renal} = 12.6\ \text{L/hr}$$

$$Cl_{acetylation} = (0.13\ \text{L/kg/hr})(80\ \text{kg})$$

$$Cl_{acetylation} = 10.4\ \text{L/hr}$$

$$Cl_{other} = (0.1\ \text{L/kg/hr})(80\ \text{kg})$$

$$Cl_{other} = 8\ \text{L/hr}$$

$$Cl_{total} = Cl_{renal} + Cl_{acetylation} + Cl_{other}$$

$$Cl_{total} = 12.6\ \text{L/hr} + 10.4\ \text{L/hr} + 8\ \text{L/hr}$$

$$Cl_{total} = 31\ \text{L/hr}$$

$$\text{Maintenance dose} = \frac{(31\ \text{L/hr})(6\ \text{mg/L})(1\ \text{hr})}{(0.87)(1)}$$

$$\text{Maintenance dose} = 214\ \text{mg/hr}$$

$$(214\ \text{mg/hr})(1\ \text{hr/60 min}) = 3.6\ \text{mg/min}$$

The infusion rate of 3.6 mg/min is within the usual range of 1–4 mg/min.

CASE 3: MAINTENANCE DOSE USING PATIENT'S ACTUAL PHARMACOKINETIC PARAMETERS (ITERATION MAY BE USED)

AK has been receiving a procainamide infusion of 214 mg/hr or 3.6 mg/min. The patient's steady-state plasma procainamide concentration is 4 mg/L. Calculate a maintenance dose using patient's actual pharmacokinetic parameters with a target concentration of 6 mg/L.

Answer:

Use the following formula. The new clearance formula is based on the maintenance dose formula.

$$\text{New Cl} = \frac{(S)(F)(Dose/\tau)}{C_{ss\,ave}}$$

$$\text{New Cl} = \frac{(0.87)(1)(214\ \text{mg/hr})}{(4\ \text{mg/L})}$$

$$\text{New Cl} = 46\ \text{L/hr}$$

$$\text{New maintenance dose} = \frac{(Cl)(C_{ss\,ave})(\tau)}{(S)(F)}$$

$$\text{New maintenance dose} = \frac{(46\ \text{L/hr})(6\ \text{mg/L})(1\ \text{hr})}{(0.87)(1)}$$

$$\text{New maintenance dose} = 317\ \text{mg/hr}$$

$$(317\ \text{mg/hr})(1\ \text{hr/60 min}) = 5.2\ \text{mg/min}$$

CASE 4: DRUG INTERACTION THAT INCREASES LEVELS*

AK has received a maintenance infusion of procainamide. The physician would like to initiate another antiarrhythmic, quinidine or amiodarone; an H2 receptor antagonist, ranitidine, cimetidine, famotidine, or a PPI pantoprazole for stress ulcer prophylaxis; antibiotics for CA-MRSA, sulfamethoxazole/trimethoprim, clindamycin or doxycycline; and insulin glargine for diabetes. The physician wants to hold the patient's blood pressure medications for now and wants to know if any of these medications will interact with procainamide.

List the drug interactions that will increase the procainamide level and explain the mechanism.

Answers:

- Quinidine sulfate and procainamide

  According to the package insert for quinidine sulfate, quinidine may compete for renal clearance with procainamide and may decrease the excretion of procainamide resulting in increased serum levels of procainamide.[28] Quinidine and procainamide may compete for renal tubular secretion.[29,30]

  Monitor for blood pressure and ECG in patients receiving procainamide and another Class 1a antiarrhythmic agent.[29,30] Procainamide doses may need to be reduced. Closely observe patients for signs of procainamide toxicity, especially in patients with cardiac decompensation.[29,30]

  Hughes and colleagues report an incident of a significant increase in procainamide and NAPA concentration in a 53-year-old male with ventricular arrhythmias on concurrent quinidine.[31] The clearance of procainamide decreased by 41 percent and the half-life increased 95 percent. It is hypothesized that quinidine interferes with the renal elimination of procainamide.

- Trimethoprim and procainamide

  Trimethoprim may increase the concentration of the active metabolites of procainamide, thus increasing the serum concentration of procainamide.[29,30]

---

*Note that none of the literature indicates any drugs interact to decrease procainamide levels.

Monitor for toxic effects of procainamide including QTc intervals, ECG, and drug serum concentrations of procainamide.

The clearance of procainamide was decreased by 42 percent in eight participants when administered with trimethoprim for 8 days.[32]

- Amiodarone and procainamide

The addition of amiodarone to procainamide therapy has been reported to significantly increase single-dose and steady-state procainamide plasma concentrations, decrease clearance, and increase elimination half-life, with evidence of clinical toxicity.[33,34,35] A 20 percent reduction in procainamide dose normalized the procainamide steady-state plasma concentrations with concurrent use of amiodarone.[34]

When amiodarone is taken concomitantly with procainamide for less than seven days, the plasma concentrations of procainamide and n-acetyl procainamide increase by 55 percent and 33 percent, respectively. Procainamide dose should be reduced by one-third when administered with amiodarone.[34]

The addition of amiodarone to procainamide therapy has been reported to increase steady-state procainamide plasma concentrations by 57 percent, with evidence of clinical toxicity. A 20 percent reduction in procainamide dose normalized the procainamide steady-state plasma concentrations with concurrent use of amiodarone.[34]

Concurrent amiodarone and procainamide administration result in a 23 percent decrease in single-dose procainamide clearance and a 38 percent increase in procainamide elimination half-life.[35]

If amiodarone and procainamide are to be administered concurrently, decrease the procainamide dose by one-third to one-half, and monitor procainamide levels and electrophysiological evidence of toxicity (QT prolongation, torsades de pointes, cardiac arrest).[29]

Amiodarone may enhance the QTc prolonging effect when administered with procainamide.[29]

Monitor for decrease cardiac conduction and prolonged QTc.

The physician decided on using amiodarone over quinidine for AK. The physician orders amiodarone 150 mg infusion over 20 minutes followed by an infusion at 1 mg/min. Calculate the new hourly and minute infusion rates after the making the dosage adjustment that is needed for the concomitant administration of amiodarone and procainamide.

The calculations for the preceding situation are as follows:

$$\text{Maintenance dose} = \frac{(Cl)(C_{ss\,ave})(\tau)}{(S)(F)}$$

Maintenance dose = 317 mg/hr

Adjusted hourly infusion rate

= (Amiodarone adjustment (50%)) (Maintenance infusion rate)

Adjusted hourly infusion rate = (0.50) (317 mg/hr)**

Adjusted hourly infusion rate = 158.5 mg/hr

Adjusted minute infusion rate = 2.64 mg/min

- Cimetidine and procainamide

Cimetidine may decrease the excretion of procainamide resulting in an increase in procainamide concentration. This effect has been suggested from cimetidine's renal tubular secretion.

**Recommendation is 33–50 percent dose reduction.[29] Decrease the dose by 50 percent for this problem.

Concomitant cimetidine and procainamide administration has been reported to reduce procainamide elimination, possibly by competition for active tubular secretion.[36-42]

The plasma concentration-time curve and elimination half-life of procainamide were increased significantly during concomitant cimetidine therapy.[37] The renal clearance of procainamide was reduced from 347 to 196 mL/min. In addition, the area under the plasma concentration-time curve for N-acetylprocainamide (NAPA) was increased by a mean of 25 percent during cimetidine therapy, due to a reduction in renal clearance from 258 to 197 mL/min. These data indicate that cimetidine inhibits the tubular secretion of both procainamide and NAPA. In another reported case, cimetidine administration was associated with increases in procainamide and NAPA serum concentrations and potential signs and symptoms of procainamide toxicity. Following discontinuation of cimetidine, the concentrations decreased to pretreatment levels.[38]

Concomitant administration of sustained-release procainamide (at steady state) and cimetidine was reported to result in significant increases in the AUC, and decreases in renal clearance, of procainamide and NAPA. It is suggested that monitoring of both procainamide and NAPA levels be undertaken in patients receiving combined cimetidine therapy.[43]

The mean steady-state concentration of procainamide increased by 55 percent and N-acetylprocainamide increased by 36 percent in 36 patients following three days of cimetidine therapy.[44]

- Famotidine did not decrease the excretion of procainamide.[45]

- Ranitidine and procainamide

Ranitidine may result in the increase in procainamide concentration and its metabolite, N-acetyl-procainamide (NAPA).[30]

Coadministration of procainamide and high doses of ranitidine may result in increased serum concentrations of procainamide due to competition for active tubular secretion, thereby decreasing renal clearance of procainamide.[29,30] Monitor for potentially increased adverse effects of procainamide (cardiac arrhythmias, hypotension, CNS depression) when procainamide and ranitidine at doses greater than 300 mg/day are coadministered.[46]

CASE 5: DISEASE STATE INTERACTIONS

JL is a 70-year-old female with a PMH of renal insufficiency, HTN, CHF, CVA, type 2 diabetes, and obesity. Doctor wants to start a loading dose of procainamide for ventricular arrhythmia. Please state the disease state interactions with procainamide on volume of distribution, clearance, and half-life.

Answer:

- Renal insufficiency

Renal insufficiency may lead to an accumulation of procainamide because procainamide is eliminated renally. Clearance of procainamide may be decreased in patients with renal insufficiency. The half-life is increased in patients with renal insufficiency. In patients with mild renal impairment, decrease the maintenance infusion rate by one-third. In patients with severe renal impairment, decrease the maintenance infusion rate by two-thirds.[47]

- Chronic heart failure (CHF) and low cardiac output

In patients with CHF or acute ischemic heart disease, use procainamide with caution because decreased myocardial contractility can further reduce cardiac output. In patients with normal cardiac output and cardiac function, the volume of distribution is 2 L/kg.[46] The volume of distribution is decreased approximately 25 percent in patients with decreased cardiac output. Clearance of procainamide in a patient with CHF is half the clearance of a patient with normal cardiac output.[30]

- Obesity

In patients who are obese, the volume of distribution is best correlated with ideal body weight (IBW). Also, the clearance of procainamide in obese patients is increased. Thus, in obese patients, the renal clearance of procainamide should be based on total body weight (TBW) and the metabolic clearance on the patient's ideal body weight.

CASE 6: DOSING IN RENAL DYSFUNCTION (NO HEMODIALYSIS)

HK is a 75-year-old male admitted to the cardiac intensive care unit. Patient has a creatinine clearance of 40 mL/min (mild renal impairment). Patient is 70 kg and has normal acetylation. Calculate a loading dose of procainamide to achieve a concentration of 8 mg/L. Then calculate a maintenance infusion in mg/min.

Answer:

$$\text{Loading dose} = \frac{(V)(C)}{(S)(F)}$$

$$\text{Loading dose} = \frac{(2 \text{ L/kg})(70 \text{ kg})(8 \text{ mg/L})}{(0.87)(1)}$$

$$\text{Loading dose} = 1{,}287 \text{ mg}$$

$$Cl_{total} = Cl_{renal} + Cl_{acetylation} + Cl_{other}$$

$$Cl_{renal} = 3(2.4 \text{ L/hr})$$

$$Cl_{renal} = 7.2 \text{ L/hr}$$

$$Cl_{acetylation} = (0.13 \text{ L/kg/hr})(70 \text{ kg})$$

$$Cl_{acetylation} = 9.1 \text{ L/hr}$$

$$Cl_{other} = (0.1 \text{ L/kg/hr})(70 \text{ kg})$$

$$Cl_{other} = 7 \text{ L/hr}$$

$$Cl_{total} = 7.2 \text{ L/hr} + 9.1 \text{ L/hr} + 7 \text{ L/hr}$$

$$Cl_{total} = 23.3 \text{ L/hr}$$

$$\text{Maintenance dose} = \frac{(Cl)(C_{ss\,ave})(\tau)}{(S)(F)}$$

$$\text{Maintenance dose} = \frac{(23.3 \text{ L/hr})(8 \text{ mg/L})(1 \text{ hr})}{(0.87)(1)}$$

$$\text{Maintenance dose} = 214 \text{ mg/hr}$$

Decrease the maintenance infusion rate by one-third because patient has mild renal impairment. The maintenance dose reduced by one-third is 143 mg/hr.

(143 mg/hr)(1 hr/60 min) = 2.4 mg/min (within the range of 1–4 mg/min as per package insert)

For a patient on hemodialysis, the maintenance dose in severe renal impairment is administered after dialysis sessions.

CASE 7: DOSING IN HEPATIC DYSFUNCTION

MS is a 72-year-old, 90-kg male with ventricular tachycardia requiring therapy with intravenous procainamide. MS has liver cirrhosis with a Child-Pugh score of 11. Recommend an initial intravenous procainamide dosing regimen in order to achieve a steady-state level of 5 g/mL.

Because no pharmacokinetic studies have been performed in patients with severe liver disease, the literature-based dosing must be applied. The appropriate dose should be chosen based on the patient's disease states.

Administer a loading dose of 500 mg. The usual rate of infusion is 2–6 mg/min; however, this patient has a Child-Pugh score of 11 and the dose should be decreased by 50 percent. The rate of infusion for MS is 1–3 mg/min.

MS needs to be monitored continuously. A steady-state procainamide and NAPA level should be obtained after steady state (3–5 half-lives).

CASE 8: DOSING IN OBESE PATIENTS

LB is a 40-year-old male. The patient's ideal body weight (IBW) is 63.6 kg. Patient has an Scr of 1 mg/dL and an average acetylation clearance. The target concentration is 6 mg/L. Patient has a history of HTN, hyperlipidemia, and ventricular arrhythmias. Recommend a procainamide loading dose and maintenance dose in mg/min for this patient.

Height = 5′6″

Weight = 100 kg

Answer:

$$\text{Loading dose} = \frac{(V)(C)}{(S)(F)}$$

The volume of distribution is based on IBW because the patient is obese.

$$\text{Loading dose} = \frac{(2 \text{ L/kg})(63.6 \text{ kg})(6 \text{ mg/L})}{(0.87)(1)}$$

$$\text{Loading dose} = 877 \text{ mg}$$

$$CrCl = \frac{(140 - \text{Age})(\text{Weight})}{(72)(\text{Scr})}$$

The CrCl is based on total body weight because the patient is obese.

$$CrCl = \frac{(140 - 40)(100 \text{ kg})}{(72)(1)}$$

$$CrCl = 134 \text{ mL/min}$$

$$CrCl = 8 \text{ L/hr}$$

$$Cl_{renal} = (3)(CrCl)$$

$$Cl_{renal} = 24 \text{ L/hr}$$

Because the patient is obese, his Cl acetylation is based on IBW.

$$Cl_{acetylation} = (0.13 \text{ L/kg/hr})(\text{Weight})$$

$$Cl_{acetylation} = (0.13 \text{ L/kg/hr})(63.6 \text{ kg})$$

$$Cl_{acetylation} = 8.3 \text{ L/hr}$$

In obese patients, Cl_{other} is based on IBW.

$$Cl_{other} = (0.1 \text{ L/kg/hr})(\text{weight})$$

$$Cl_{other} = (0.1 \text{ L/kg/hr})(63.6 \text{ kg})$$

$$Cl_{other} = 6.3 \text{ L/hr}$$

$$Cl_{total} = Cl_{renal} + Cl_{acetylation} + Cl_{other}$$

$$Cl_{total} = 24 \text{ L/hr} + 8.3 \text{ L/hr} + 6.3 \text{ L/hr}$$

$$Cl_{total} = 38.6 \text{ L/hr}$$

$$\text{Maintenance dose} = \frac{(\text{Cl})(C_{ss\,ave})(\tau)}{(S)(F)}$$

$$\text{Maintenance dose} = \frac{(38.6\ \text{L/hr})(6\ \text{mg/L})(1\ \text{hr})}{(0.87)(1)}$$

$$\text{Maintenance dose} = 266\ \text{mg/hr}$$

$$(266\ \text{mg/hr})(1\ \text{hr/60 min}) = 4.4\ \text{mg/min}$$

CASE 9: DOSING IN PATIENTS WITH SPECIAL CONSIDERATIONS

JS is a 55-year-old male admitted to the emergency room for ventricular arrhythmia. JS has a PMH of HTN, hyperlipidemia, and CHF. Patient is 60 kg and IBW is also 60 kg. JS has a serum creatinine of 1 mg/dL. Patient also has an average acetylation clearance of 0.13 L/kg/hr.

Calculate a loading dose in mg and maintenance dose in mg/min for JS with a target concentration of 8 mg/L.

Answer:

$$\text{Loading dose} = \frac{(V)(C)}{(S)(F)}$$

The volume of distribution needs to be reduced by 25 percent because the patient has CHF (Vd is 1.5 L/kg).

$$\text{Loading dose} = \frac{(1.5\ \text{L/kg})(60\ \text{kg})(8\ \text{mg/L})}{(0.87)(1)}$$

$$\text{Loading dose} = 828\ \text{mg}$$

Because the maintenance dose is dependent on the Cl_{total}, the Cl_{total} must be calculated first.

$$\text{CrCl} = \frac{(140 - \text{Age})(\text{IBW})}{(72)(\text{Scr})}$$

$$\text{CrCl} = \frac{(140 - 55)(60\ \text{kg})}{(72)(1)}$$

$$\text{CrCl} = 71\ \text{mL/min}$$

CrCl needs to be in the units L/hr, so the 71 mL/min needs to be converted to L/hr by multiplying by 0.06.

$$\text{CrCl} = 4.3\ \text{L/hr}$$

$$Cl_{renal} = (3)(\text{CrCl})$$
$$Cl_{renal} = (3)(4.3\ \text{L/hr})$$
$$Cl_{renal} = 12.9\ \text{L/hr}$$

$$Cl_{acetylation} = (0.13\ \text{L/kg/hr})(60\ \text{kg})$$
$$Cl_{acetylation} = 7.8\ \text{L/hr}$$

$$Cl_{other} = (0.1\ \text{L/kg/hr})(60\ \text{kg})$$
$$Cl_{other} = 6\ \text{L/hr}$$

$$Cl_{total} = Cl_{renal} + Cl_{acetylation} + Cl_{other}$$
$$Cl_{total} = 12.9\ \text{L/hr} + 7.8\ \text{L/hr} + 6\ \text{L/hr}$$
$$Cl_{total} = 26.7\ \text{L/hr}$$

Because the patient has CHF, the total clearance is decreased by half, so the patient's total clearance is 13.35 L/hr.

$$\text{Maintenance dose} = \frac{(\text{Cl})(C_{ss\,ave})(\tau)}{(S)(F)}$$

$$\text{Maintenance dose} = \frac{(13.35\ \text{L/hr})(8\ \text{mg/L})(1)}{(0.87)(1)}$$

$$\text{Maintenance dose} = 122.8\ \text{mg/hr}$$

$$(122.8\ \text{mg/hr})(1\ \text{hr/60 min}) = 2\ \text{mg/min}$$

Tau (τ) is 1 hour because the infusion rate is per hour.

The infusion rate of 2 mg/min is within the recommended infusion rate of 1–4 mg/min as stated in the package insert.

ACKNOWLEDGMENTS

The author acknowledges Pharmacy Interns Sherman Liao, Irina Hopkins, Jessica Sexton, Maria Sobrera for their research and development of this chapter.

REFERENCES

1. Procainamide hydrochloride injection solution [package insert]. Lake Forest, IL: Hospira Inc. 2007.
2. Stiell IG, Clement CM, Symington C, et al. Emergency department use of intravenous procainamide for patients with acute atrial fibrillation or flutter. *Acad Emerg Med.* 2007;14(12):1158–1164.
3. Giardina EV. Procainamide: Clinical pharmacology and efficacy against ventricular arrhythmias. *Ann NY Acad Sci.* 1984;432:177–188.
4. Nolan PE Jr. Pharmacokinetics and pharmacodynamics of intravenous agents for ventricular arrhythmias. *Pharmacotherapy.* 1997;17(2 Pt 2): 65S–75S.
5. Funck-Brentano C, Light RT, Lineberry MD, et al. Pharmacokinetic and pharmacodynamic interaction of n-acetyl procainamide and procainamide in humans. *J Cardiovasc Pharmacol.* 1989;14:364–373.
6. Valdes Jr. R, Jortani SA, Gheorghiade M. Standards of laboratory practice: Cardiac drug monitoring. *Clin Chem.* 1998;44(5):1096–1109.
7. Red Book Online. http://www.thomsonhc.com.cwplib.proxy.liu.edu/ micromedex2/librarian. Accessed January 4, 2013.
8. Neumar RW, Otto CW, Link MS, et al: 2010 American Heart Association guidelines for cardiopulmonary resuscitation and emergency cardiovascular care. Part 8: adult advanced cardiovascular life support. *Circulation.* 2010;122(18 Suppl.3):S729–S767.
9. Erstad BL. Dosing of medications in morbidly obese patients in the intensive care unit setting. *Intensive Care Med.* 2004;30:18–32.
10. Brunette DD. Resuscitation of the morbidly obese patient. *Am J Emerg Med.* 2004;22:40–47.
11. Brittain HG. Procainamide hydrochloride. *Analytical Profiles of Drug Substances and Excipients.* Volume 28.
12. Koch-Weser J. Pharmacokinetics of procainamide in man. *Ann NY Acad Sci.* 1971;179(1):370–382.
13. Macgregor AMC, Boggs L. Drug distribution in obesity and following bariatric surgery: A literature review. *Obes Surg.* 1996;6:17–27.
14. Gibson TP, Atkinson Jr AJ, Matusik E, et al. Kinetics of procainamide and N-acetylprocainamide in renal failure. *Kidney Int.* 1977;12:422–429.
15. Reidenberg MM, Camacho M, Kluger J, et al. Aging and renal clearance of procainamide and acetylprocainamide. *Clin Pharmacol Ther.* 1980; 28(6):732–735.
16. Low CL, Phelps KR, Bailie GR. Relative efficacy of haemoperfusion, haemodialysis, and CAPD in the removal of procainamide and NAPA in a patient with severe procainamide toxicity. *Nephrol Dial Transplant.* 1996;11:881–884.
17. Woosley RL, Shand DG. Pharmacokinetics of antiarrhythmic drugs. *Am J Cardiol.* 1978(41):986–995.
18. Klotz U. Antiarrhythmics. Elimination and dosage considerations in hepatic impairment. *Clin Pharmacokinet.* 2007;46(12):985–996.
19. Halpern SW, Ellrodt G, Singh BN, et al. Efficacy of intravenous procainamide infusion in converting atrial fibrillation to sinus rhythm. Relation to left atrial size. *Br Heart J.* 1980;44:589–595.
20. Giardina EV, Heissenbuttel RH, Bigger JT. Correlation of plasma concentration with effect on arrhythmia, electrocardiogram, and blood pressure. *Ann Intern Med.* 1973;78:183–193.
21. Koch-Weser J, Klein SW. Procainamide dosage schedules, plasma concentrations, and clinical effects. *JAMA.* 1971;215(9):1454–1460.

22. Campbell TJ, Williams KM. Therapeutic drug monitoring: Antiarrhythmic drugs. *Br J Clin Pharmacol.* 2001;52:21S–34S.

23. Jurgerns G, Graudal NA, Kampmann JP. Therapeutic drug monitoring of antiarrhythmic drugs. *Clin Pharmacokinet.* 2003;42(7):647–663.

24. Yamreudeewong W, DeBisschop M, Martin LG, et al. Potentially significant drug interactions of class III antiarrhythmic drugs. *Drug Safety.* 2003;26(6):421–438.

25. Trujillo TC, Nolan PE. Antiarrhythmic agents. Drug interactions of clinical significance. *Drug Safety.* 2000;23(6):509–532.

26. Christian Jr CD, Meredith CG, Speeg Jr KV. Cimetidine inhibits renal procainamide clearance. *Clin Pharmacol Ther.* 1984;36(2):221–227.

27. Bauer LA. Cardiovascular agents: Procainamide/n–acetyl procainamide. *Appl Clin Pharmacokin.* 2008;3(8).

28. Quinidine Sulfate [package insert]. Corona, CA: Watson Pharma, Inc., 2009.

29. DRUGDEX® System [Internet database]. Greenwood Village, CO: Thomson Reuters (Healthcare) Inc.

30. Lexi-Comp Online. http://www.uptodate.com/crlsql/interact/frameset.jsp. Accessed December 26, 2012.

31. Hughes B, Dyer JE, Schwartz AB. Increased procainamide plasma concentrations caused by quinidine: A new drug interaction. *Am Heart J.* 1897;114(4):908–909

32. Kosoglou T, Rocci ML, Vlasses PH. Trimethoprim alters the disposition of procainamide and N-acetylprocainamide. *Clin Pharmcol Ther.* 1988;44:467–477.

33. Cordarone® IV [package insert]. Philadelphia, PA: Wyeth Laboratories, 2002.

34. Saal AK, Werner JA, Greene HL, et al. Effect of amiodarone of serum quinidine and procainamide levels. *Am J Cardiol.* 1984;53:1264–1267.

35. Windle J, Prystowsky EN, Miles WM, et al. Pharmacokinetic and electrophysiological interactions of amiodarone and procainamide. *Clin Pharmacol Ther.* 1987;41:603–610.

36. Somogyi A, Heinzow B. Cimetidine reduces procainamide elimination. *N Engl J Med.* 1982;307:1080.

37. Somogyi A, McLean A, Heinzow B. Cimetidine-procainamide pharmacokinetic interaction in man: Evidence of competition for tubular secretion of basic drugs. *Eur J Clin Pharmacol.* 1983;25:339–345.

38. Higbee MD, Wood JS, Mead RA. Procainamide-cimetidine interaction: A potential toxic interaction in the elderly. *J Am Geriatr Soc.* 1984;32:162–164.

39. Christian CD, Meredith CG, Speeg KV. Cimetidine inhibits renal procainamide clearance. *Clin Pharmacol Ther.* 1984;36:221–227.

40. Lai MY, Jiang FM, Chung CH, et al. Dose dependent effect of cimetidine on procainamide disposition in man. *Int J Clin Pharmacol Ther Toxicol.* 1988;26:118–121.

41. Baciewicz AM, Baciewicz FA. Effect of cimetidine and ranitidine on cardiovascular drugs. *Am Heart J.* 1989;118:144–154.

42. Smith SR, Kendall MJ. Ranitidine versus cimetidine: A comparison of their potential to cause clinically important drug interactions. *Clin Pharmacokinet.* 1988;15:44–56.

43. Rodvold KA, Paloucek FP, Jung D, et al. Interaction of steady-state procainamide with H(2)-receptor antagonists cimetidine and ranitidine. *Ther Drug Monit.* 1987;9:378–383.

44. Bauer LA, Black D, Gensler A, Procainamide-Cimetidine Interaction in Elderly Male Patients, *J Am Geriatr Soc.* 1990;38:467–469. [PubMed 2329253]

45. Klotz U, Arvela P, Rosenkranz B. Famotidine, a new H$_2$-receptor antagonist, does not affect hepatic elimination of diazepam or tubular secretion of procainamide. *Eur J Clin Pharmacol.*1985;28:671–675.

46. Zantac® injection [package insert]. Research Triangle Park, NC: GlaxoSmithKline, 2009.

47. Procainamide hydrochloride injection solution [package insert]. Lake Forest, IL: Hospira Inc., 2011.

EDGAR R. GONZALEZ, PharmD, FASHP, FASCP
REBECCA B. GONZALEZ, PharmD

CHAPTER 18

Quinidine

OVERVIEW

The medicinal effects of the bark of the cinchona tree have been known for over 350 years. The tree is indigenous to South America and is known as Peruvian, Jesuit's, or Cardinal Bark. During the 1600s and 1700s, Jesuit priests imported cinchona bark from South America to Europe where it was used as a powder, extract, or infusion to treat fevers as well as "rebellious palpitation."[1,2] In the early 1800s, Pelletier and Caventou worked to isolate the more than 20 structurally related alkaloids found in the bark of the cinchona tree, quinine and quinidine being the most important ones.[1-3] Pelletier and Caventou successfully isolated quinine in 1820 (see Figure 18-1).[2,3]

In 1918, Walter von Frey of Berlin reported that quinidine was the most effective of the four principal cinchona alkaloids in controlling atrial arrhythmias.[2-4] Quinidine, the d-isomer of quinine, is both more potent and more toxic than quinine (see Figure 18-2).[5] By the 1920s, quinidine became the drug of choice for maintaining normal sinus rhythm (NSR) in patient with atrial fibrillation or atrial flutter (Afib/flutter) and to prevent the recurrence of ventricular tachycardia (VT) or ventricular fibrillation; albeit, quinidine was known to produce a potentially lethal idiosyncratic pro-arrhythmic effect.[4] In 1998, quinidine was the most frequently prescribed antiarrhythmic agent to maintain NSR in after conversion from Afib/flutter.[4] Today, quinidine is used infrequently because studies show that quinidine therapy is associated with a threefold increase in the risk of sudden cardiac death when compared with placebo or other antiarrhythmic agents, especially in patients with structural heart disease, including left ventricular dysfunction.[6,7]

CLINICAL PHARMACOLOGY[9,10]

ANTIMALARIAL ACTIVITY

Quinidine is an intraerythrocytic schizonticide; it is gametocidal to Plasmodium vivax and P. malariae, but not to P. falciparum. Quinidine has minimal effects on sporozites or preerythrocytic parasites.

ANTIARRHYTHMIC ACTIVITY

Quinidine is a Class 1A antiarrhythmic agent that is devoid of negative inotropism. In cardiac muscle and in Purkinje fibers, quinidine depresses the rapid inward depolarizing sodium current, thereby slowing phase-0 depolarization and reducing the amplitude of the action potential without affecting the resting potential.[10] In normal Purkinje fibers, it reduces the slope of phase-4 depolarization, shifting the threshold voltage upward toward zero. The result is slowed conduction and reduced automaticity in all parts of the heart, with increase of the effective refractory period relative to the duration of the action potential in the atria, ventricles, and Purkinje tissues.

Quinidine also raises the fibrillation thresholds of the atria and ventricles, and it raises the ventricular defibrillation threshold as well.

By slowing conduction and prolonging the effective refractory period, quinidine can interrupt or prevent reentrant arrhythmias and arrhythmias due to increased automaticity, including atrial flutter, atrial fibrillation, and paroxysmal supraventricular tachycardia. In patients with the sick sinus syndrome, quinidine can cause marked sinus node depression and bradycardia. In most patients, however, use of quinidine is associated with an increase in the sinus rate secondary to quinidine's vagolytic effects.

Quinidine prolongs the QT interval in a dose-related fashion, which may lead to increased ventricular automaticity and polymorphic ventricular tachycardias, including torsades de pointes (TdP).[4-11] Intravenous quinidine is a potent α-adrenergic blocker that can precipitously lower blood pressure. These three effects can adversely affect clinical outcome in patient with cardiac arrhythmias requiring treatment with quinidine.

INDICATIONS

Today, the range of indications for quinidine is curtailed by the increased reliance on radiofrequency ablative surgery and implantable devices to correct or control cardiac rhythm disturbances; by the awareness that treatment with quinidine can increase paradoxically the risk of sudden cardiac death; and by the evolution of more effective and potentially safer antiarrhythmic compounds (e.g., sotalol and amiodarone).[4,11] Quinidine may still play a useful role for patients in whom more advanced therapeutic modalities are not acceptable or contraindicated (Table 18-1). However, the use of quinidine must follow clear instruction to the patient that quinidine therapy is associated with a threefold increase in the risk of sudden cardiac death when compared with placebo or other antiarrhythmic agents, especially in patients with structural heart disease including left ventricular dysfunction as described in the FDA boxed warning (Table 18-2).[6-11]

CURRENTLY AVAILABLE DOSAGE FORMULATIONS[8,9]

Quinidine is formulated as either the gluconate salt or the sulfate salt. On a molar basis, 267 mg of quinidine gluconate (QG) is equivalent to 200 mg of quinidine sulfate (QS). The gluconate salt is available for oral or parenteral administration; whereas, the sulfate salt comes only in oral formulations (Table 18-3).

Quinidine formulations must be dispensed in well-closed, light-resistant container with child-resistant closure. Formulations of quinidine should be stored at ambient temperature (i.e., 20° to 25°C or 68° to 77°F) and should be protected from light and moisture. Parenteral quinidine gluconate is stable for 24 hours at ambient temperature and for 48 hours under refrigeration at 4°C. Approximately 3 percent of quinidine is lost to adsorption with a

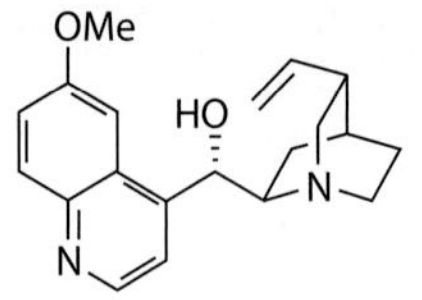

FIGURE 18-1. Chemical structure of quinine.

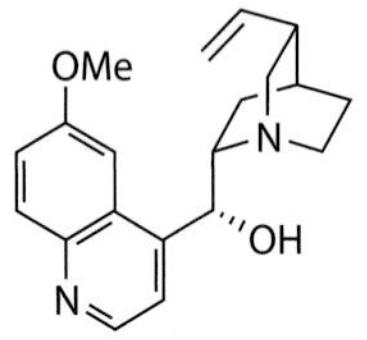

FIGURE 18-2. Structure of quinidine.

12-inch polyvinyl chloride (PVC) catheter, and 30 percent of drug is lost to adsorption with a 112-inch PVC catheter.

DOSING AND ADMINISTRATION

The initial dosing and administration of quinidine require careful monitoring to safeguard against the potential for an idiosyncratic fall in blood pressure and/or pro-arrhythmic effect (i.e., quinidine syncope).[12] Therefore, therapy should be initiated only when the patient can be hospitalized and adequate measures are in place for continuous monitoring of vital signs and the electrocardiogram.[4,13] The response to therapy should be guided by electrophysiologic testing, evaluation of the serum quinidine concentration, and assessment of the patient's tolerance to quinidine (e.g., acute gastric distress, diarrhea). Table 18-4 lists the recommended initial dosing regimens for the various commercially available formulations of quinidine. Dosage adjustment for renal failure, liver failure, advanced age, or obesity will be discussed elsewhere in this chapter.

SAFETY

Cinchonism

The most common side effects of quinidine are gastrointestinal complaints or the occurrence of "cinchonism" (e.g., tinnitus, headache, vertigo, fever, visual disturbances, or tremor).[4] These effects occur in susceptible patients and result from localized gastric irritation and central nervous system effects of cinchona alkaloids. Table 18-5 lists side effects of quinidine that may be encountered in the clinical setting.

Pro-arrhythmogenicity

Quinidine-induced, concentration-dependent prolongation of the QT interval and alpha-adrenergic blockade, especially with

TABLE 18-2	FDA Boxed Warning for Quinidine

Trials of antiarrhythmic therapy for non-life-threatening arrhythmias, active antiarrhythmic therapy resulted in increased mortality; the risk of active therapy is probably greatest in patients with structural heart disease.

In the case of quinidine used to prevent or defer recurrence of atrial flutter/fibrillation, the best available data come from meta-analysis that show mortality associated with the use of quinidine was more than three times greater than the mortality associated with the use of placebo.

Meta-analysis of data from patients with non-life-threatening ventricular arrhythmias show mortality associated with quinidine was consistently greater than that associated with the use of any of a variety of alternative antiarrhythmics.

intravenous administration, can precipitate syncope and sudden cardiac death. These effects are commonly referred to as "quinidine syncope" or quinidine associated TdP. The frequency of TdP is approximately 4.5 percent per patient year.[4,11] While initially thought to be an idiosyncratic reaction, we now know that the occurrence of quinidine syncope is highest among patients who meet any of the following criteria: (1) impaired left ventricular function; (2) preexisting cardiac conduction abnormalities, such as familial QT prolongation syndromes; (3) female gender; (4) hypokalemia; or (5) underlying Afib.[4,11-14] In these patients, quinidine should be used only if the benefits outweigh the risks.

PHARMACOKINETICS[8,9]

The pharmacokinetics and pharmacodynamics of quinidine have been studies extensively over the past 30 years.[4,10,15] Quinidine exhibits linear pharmacokinetics in most patients.[4,15,16] Table 18-6 lists the pertinent pharmacokinetic parameter for quinidine

BIOAVAILABILITY

The absolute bioavailability (F) of quinidine ranges from 70 percent to 80 percent because the drug undergoes considerable first pass extraction in the liver.[15] The presence of a strong first pass effect explains the wide-ranging (i.e., 45%–100%) interindividual variability in F observed with quinidine.[4] The F value is unaffected by the formulation of quinidine with respect to either the salt or the use of IRT or EXT formulations. Oral absorption of quinidine following administration of IRTs is complete within two hours after administration. Serum quinidine concentrations peak approximately two hours after administration of IRTs; whereas, it takes approximately three to six hours to reach peak serum quinidine concentrations following the administration of ERT formulations. Food decreases the rate of absorption for quinidine without altering the amount of drug absorbed over time. Most importantly, F is unchanged by the presence of congestive heart failure (CHF).[17]

TABLE 18-1	Use of Quinidine in Clinical Practice

FDA-Approved Indications	Other Clinical Indications
Conversion of Afib/flutter	Paroxysmal atrial tachycardia
Reduction of frequency of relapse into Afib/flutter	Paroxysmal AV junctional rhythm
Suppression of ventricular arrhythmias	Atrial premature complexes
Treatment of malaria	Ventricular premature complexes
	Paroxysmal ventricular tachycardia
	Short-QT syndrome
	Brugada syndrome

TABLE 18-3	Commercially Available Formulations of Quinidine

Salt	Route	Dosage Form	Strength	Quinidine Base
Gluconate	IV	Injection	80 mg/mL	50 mg
Gluconate	Oral	Extended-release tablet (ERT)	324 mg	200 mg
Sulfate	Oral	Immediate-release tablet (IRT)	200 mg	166 mg
Sulfate	Oral	IRT	300 mg	249 mg
Sulfate	Oral	ERT	300 mg	249 mg

TABLE 18-4 Recommended Initial Dosing Regimens for Quinidine

Indication	QG Injection 80 mg/mL	QG ERT 324 mg Tab	QS IRT 200 mg Tab 300 mg Tab	QS ERT 300 mg Tab
Arrhythmias (adult)	30 mg/kg/day in 5 divided daily doses	20–60 mg/kg/day in 3 divided daily doses	15–60 mg/kg/day in 4–5 divided daily doses	Do not recommend
Malaria (adult)	10 mg/kg diluted to 16 mg/mL to run over 1–2 hr; then 20 mcg/kg/min for 24 hr or until parasitemia is reduced to <1% and oral QS is tolerated (for life-threatening malaria only)		300–600 mg every 8 hr for 5–7 days	
Arrhythmias (pediatrics)		1–2 tablets every 8–12 hr	1–2 tablets every 4–6 hr	1–2 tablets every 8–12 hr
Life-threatening malaria (pediatrics)	10 mg/kg (16 mg/mL concentration); run over 1–2 hr; then 20 mcg/kg/min for 24 hr or until parasitemia is reduced to <1% and oral QS is tolerated	Do not recommend	Do not recommend	Do not recommend

VOLUME OF DISTRIBUTION

Quinidine is distributed rapidly to most organs except the brain. The volume of distribution of quinidine (V_dQ) ranges from 2 to 3.5 L/kg and is unchanged by age.[16,17] However, the presence of CHF can reduce V_dQ to 1.8 L/kg because of decreased perfusion of body tissues, with an associated increase in the amount of drug remaining in plasma.[17] Renal disease may also decrease V_dQ because of an increase in plasma protein binding (PPB) that keeps quinidine in the intravascular space.[16] In contrast, liver failure and hypoalbuminemia reduce PPB and increase V_dQ up to 5 L/kg. Smoking does not appear to alter V_dQ.

PLASMA PROTEIN BINDING

Quinidine binds avidly to α1-acid glycoprotein and to albumin. Within the serum quinidine concentration range of 2–6 mg/L, quinidine is 80–88 percent plasma protein bound in adults and older children. Quinidine PPB falls to between 50 percent and 70 percent in neonates and infants as well as during pregnancy. Because α1-acid glycoprotein levels are increased in response to stress, the total amount of quinidine in the intravascular space will increase, but the free fraction or active fraction of quinidine (i.e., which exerts its pharmacologic effect may fall in acute stress states such a circulatory shock or acute myocardial infarction. The PPB of quinidine is increased in chronic renal failure, but binding abruptly falls toward or below normal when heparin is administered for hemodialysis because of displacement of quinidine at PPB sites by heparin. Quinidine readily crosses the placenta and is found in

breast milk.[18] The administration of quinidine during pregnancy can cause damage to the eighth cranial nerve in utero as well as posing a risk for transient neonatal thrombocytopenia.[19]

TOTAL BODY CLEARANCE AND PLASMA HALF-LIFE

Hepatic Metabolism

Approximately 60–85 percent of an administered dose of quinidine undergoes biotransformation via hepatic CYP3A4.[15,16] Total body clearance for quinidine (ClQ) is 3–5 mL/min/kg in adults, and 6–15 mL/min/kg in children. The elimination half-life for quinidine ($T_{1/2}Q$) is 6–8 hours in adults and 3–4 hours in children. Quinidine clearance is not reduced by hepatic cirrhosis.[16] The hepatic metabolism of quinidine gives rise to two, pharmacologically active metabolites (i.e., 3-hydroxyquinidine (3HQ) and 2-oxyquinidinone).[4] The 3HQ metabolite is of clinical importance because 3HQ is 50 percent as potent as quinidine and accumulates during chronic therapy.[20] Metabolite 3HQ contributes to the prolongation of the QT interval observed during treatment with quinidine.[4,10,15,20] The volume of distribution of 3HQ appears to be larger than that of quinidine, and the elimination half-life of 3HQ is about 12 hours.[10,15]

Renal Elimination of Unchanged Quinidine

Approximately 15–40 percent of the administered dose of quinidine is eliminated unchanged via glomerular filtration and active tubular secretion.[4] The renal elimination of quinidine is moderated by pH-dependent, renal tubular reabsorption. Quinidine is a basic alkaloid; therefore, urinary acidification increases the quantity of ionized

TABLE 18-5 Adverse Effects of Quinidine

Adverse Event	Occurrence
Diarrhea	35%
Dyspepsia	22%
Lightheadedness	15%
Headache	7%
Fatigue	7%
Palpitations	7%
Angina	6%
Weakness	5%
Rash	5%
Visual changes	3%
Insomnia	3%
Tremors	2%
Nervousness	2%
In coordination	1%

TABLE 18-6 Quinidine Pharmacokinetics

Parameter	Population Value	Factors That May Alter Value
Bioavailability	70–80%	Extent of first pass metabolism
Volume of distribution	2–3.5 L/kg	Heart failure, hepatic failure
Plasma protein binding	80–88%	Age, pregnancy, stress
Total body clearance	3–5 mL/min/kg 6–15 mL/min/kg in children	Reduced by advanced age, heart failure, renal failure, or hepatic failure
Hepatic metabolism	60–85%	CYP3A4; 3HQ active metabolite
Quinidine renal clearance	1 mL/min/kg	Age and renal function
Renal elimination of unchanged drug	15–40%	Inversely proportional to urinary pH
Half-life of elimination	6–8 hr	3–4 hr in children
Therapeutic range	2–6 mg/L	Assay specific

TABLE 18-7 Quinidine-Related Pharmacodynamic Drug-Drug Interactions

Interacting Agent	Mechanism of Interaction	Clinical Relevance
Flecainide, propafenone	Potentiation of antiarrhythmic action, increased intraventricular conduction block, and prolongation of QT interval	Increased risk of quinidine toxicity and TdP **Avoid concomitant therapy.**
Warfarin	Quinidine's hypoprothrombinemic effects potentate the actions of warfarin	Increased risk of warfarin-induced bleeding at any given dose of warfarin **Monitor**
Anticholinergic agents	Potentiation of vagolytic action	Predispose to anticholinergic toxicity; may accelerate AV nodal conduction and ventricular response rate **Monitor**
Cholinergic agents, cholinesterase inhibitors	Quinidine antagonizes the action of cholinergic agent and cholinesterase inhibitors	Diminished clinical response to cholinergic stimulation (e.g., neostigmine); avoid quinidine in patients with Myesthenia gravis **Monitor**
Alpha-adrenergic blocking agent and ganglionic blockers	Quinidine potentiates the hypotensive action of peripheral alpha-adrenergic blocking agents	Increased hypotensive response to phentolamine, antidepressants, and phenothiazines **Monitor**
Neuromuscular blockers	Quinidine potentiates action of all neuromuscular blockers	Prolonged paralysis refractory to neostigmine **Avoid quinidine**
Mefloquine	Both agents prolong the QT interval	Increase risk of TdP **Avoid concurrent use**

quinidine in the urine. Because only unionized drug can be reabsorbed via the renal tubules, acidified urine decreases the amount of quinidine reabsorbed by the renal tubules and increases the amount of quinidine excreted unchanged in urine.[21] Conversely, urinary alkalinization allows quinidine to become unionized and readily reabsorbed by the renal tubules. Thus, an alkaline urine increase the tubular reabsorption of quinidine thereby increasing the amount of quinidine retained in the circulation and reducing the amount of unchanged drug recovered in urine.[21] The net renal clearance of quinidine is about only about 1 mL/min/kg in healthy adults.

QUINIDINE ASSAYS

The serum quinidine concentration measured in blood varies, depending on the assay used thus creating a source of confusion.[4,10,15,20] If a laboratory uses a nonspecific assay for quinidine, then the values reported for the serum quinidine concentration will include the sum of quinidine plus its two metabolites. The therapeutic range for quinidine when measured by nonspecific assay is usually reported to be 2–6 mg/L. If the serum quinidine concentration is measured via high-pressure liquid chromatography, an assay specific for quinidine, then the therapeutic range for quinidine is 1–3 mg/L. Clinicians should contact their clinical laboratory to become informed about the assay used to measure the serum quinidine concentration in their patients.

CONDITIONS OF ALTERED PHARMACOKINETICS

The clinical conditions described in this section contribute to a reduction in ClQ. Patients who exhibit any of the conditions warrant a reduction in their total daily dose of quinidine and require careful monitoring for signs and symptoms of cinchonism, as well as monitoring of their serum potassium concentrations, their electrocardiograms, and their serum quinidine concentrations to prevent the occurrence of quinidine toxicity.

Hepatic or Renal Failure

Hepatic and renal impairment decrease ClQ and increase $T_{1/2}Q$.[4] The dosing interval for IRT of quinidine should be reduced to no more than twice daily when creatinine clearance drops below 50 mL/min.[16]

Age

Age also affects the pharmacokinetics of quinidine. Studies show that ClQ falls and $T_{1/2}Q$ increases in patients 60 years of age or older.[4,15,16] The changes reflect age-dependent reductions in renal function.

Heart Failure

The presence of left ventricular dysfunction (ejection fraction below 30%) reduces ClQ and increases $T_{1/2}Q$; however, F is unchanged.[4,15,17] Although quinidine is not a negative inotrope, accumulation of the drug in the setting of heart failure will increase the risk of TdP.

DRUG INTERACTIONS[4,8,9]

Quinidine interacts with many drugs to produce clinically relevant interactions that must be considered if concurrent therapy is to be administered.[4] Drug interactions with quinidine can be divided into pharmacodynamic interactions (Table 18-7) or pharmacokinetic interactions (Table 18-8). Pharmacodynamic interactions produce changes in the intensity of the pharmacologic effects of one of the interacting drug pairs without changing the serum concentration of either medication. Pharmacokinetic drug interactions occur as the result of quinidine-induced inhibition of hepatic cytochrome CYP2D6 to either increase the concentration of those medications metabolized by CYP2D6 or decrease the formation of active moieties from prodrugs that require CYP2D6-dependent activation in-vivo (see Table 18-8). Quinidine is a substrate for CYP3A4 albeit no significant drug-drug interactions are observed as the result of inhibition or induction of CYP3A4 (see Table 18-8). Agents that alkalinize the urine reduce the renal elimination of quinidine and increase the serum quinidine concentration.

CASE STUDIES

CASE 1: LOADING DOSE AND ADMINISTRATION

RG is a 72-year-old female with new onset Afib. She is anticoagulated with warfarin (INR 2.2) and is admitted to the hospital for initiation of quinidine therapy. The patient is also receiving digoxin 0.25 mg daily (serum digoxin concentration is 1.1 ng/mL). Her past medical history is remarkable for heart failure (ejection fraction 35%), ischemic heart disease, elevated lipids, and hypertension. RG does not smoke or drink. Her medications include lisinopril 40 mg daily; furosemide 40 mg twice daily; spironolactone 25 mg daily; carvedilol 12.5 mg twice daily; aspirin 81 mg daily; pravastatin 40 mg daily; digoxin 0.25 mg daily; warfarin 5 mg daily; one multivitamin with iron.

Height = 5′7″

Weight = 70 kg

Serum creatinine = 0.92

TABLE 18-8 Quinidine-Related Pharmacokinetic Drug-Drug Interactions

Interacting Agent	Mechanism of Interaction	Clinical Relevance
Antacids, carbonic anhydrase inhibitors, bicarbonate	Urinary alkalinization reduces renal quinidine clearance	Increased serum quinidine concentration and pharmacologic effects **Monitor**
Amiodarone	Increased serum quinidine concentration; potentiates antiarrhythmic action of quinidine	Increased risk of quinidine toxicity and TdP; reduce dose of quinidine by 33–50% **Avoid concomitant therapy**
Verapamil	Decreases clearance of quinidine and potentiation of hypotensive effects of quinidine	Increased risk of quinidine toxicity and TdP **Avoid concomitant therapy**
Clarithromycin; IV erythromycin	Reduced hepatic clearance of quinidine and QT prolongation	Increased risk of quinidine toxicity and TdP **Avoid concomitant therapy**
Digoxin	Quinidine reduces renal digoxin clearance and produces a 2.5-fold increase in serum digoxin concentration	In the absence of atrial fibrillation, reduce dose of digoxin by 50% upon the addition of quinidine therapy to prevent digitalis toxicity **Monitor**
Azole antifungals	Reduced quinidine clearance and subsequent toxicity	Increased risk of TdP **Avoid concurrent use**
Bosutinib	May increase bosutinib concentrations and produce toxicity	Increase risk of bosutinib toxicity **Avoid concurrent use**
Conivaptan	Reduced quinidine clearance with subsequent toxicity	Increased risk of TdP **Avoid concurrent use**
Crizotinib	Reduced quinidine clearance with subsequent toxicity	Increased risk of TdP **Avoid concurrent use**
Protease inhibitors	Reduced quinidine clearance with subsequent toxicity	Increased risk of TdP **Avoid concurrent use**
Silodosin	May reduce silodosin clearance with subsequent toxicity	Increase risk of silodosin toxicity **Avoid concurrent use**
Tamoxifen	Reduced formation of tamoxifen's active metabolites	Failed tamoxifen therapy **Avoid concurrent use**
Vincristine	May reduce vincrisitine clearance with subsequent toxicity	Increase risk of vincristine toxicity **Avoid concurrent use**
Mifepristone	Reduced quinidine clearance	Increase risk of TdP **Avoid concurrent use**

Calculate a loading dose and maintenance dose regimen of quinidine sulfate IRT to achieve a peak serum quinidine concentration (C_pQ) of 3 mg/L.

Loading Dose

To calculate the loading use the following formula:

Loading dose (LD) =

$$\frac{\text{Concentration } (C_p)(mg/L) \times \text{Volume of distribution } (V_d)\ (L/kg) \times \text{Weight (kg)}}{\text{Salt fraction (S)} \times \text{Bioavailability (F)}}$$

Volume of distribution of quinidine in heart failure = 1.8L/kg × Actual body weight

The bioavailability of quinidine sulfate IRT = 0.7 and the salt fraction (S) = 0.83 for quinidine sulfate.

$$LD = \frac{3\ mg/L \times 1.8L/kg \times 70\ kg}{(0.83)(0.7)} = \frac{378\ mg}{0.581} = 650\ mg$$

LD = 600 mg

RG should receive 600 mg of quinidine sulfate IRT (i.e., 300 mg IRT; quantity = 2) orally as one-time dose.

Measurement of Serum Concentration

Although not yet at steady state, a peak serum quinidine concentration obtained following the loading dose of quinidine can help determine whether an appropriate loading dose was administered. A serum quinidine concentration should be ordered at the peak of the oral absorption of IRT of the sulfate salt. The oral absorption of quinidine sulfate is complete within two hour after the administration of IRT of the sulfate salt. Therefore, the correct time to obtain a blood sample to measure the peak serum quinidine concentration is two hours after the administration of IRT of quinidine sulfate.

Loading Dose Targeted to a Specific Serum Concentration

RG's peak serum quinidine concentration was only 1.7 mg/L following the initial 600 mg oral loading dose. What dose of IRT oral quinidine sulfate should be given to achieve a therapeutic concentration of 3 mg/L? Using the pharmacokinetic dosing strategy, an additional loading dose can be calculated if a patient has a subtherapeutic peak serum quinidine concentration. The same principles are used as with initial loading doses, altering the targeted serum concentration to reflect the degree of increase desired. The additional loading dose to increase by a specific concentration can be calculated by the following equation:

$$LD = \frac{\Delta C\ (C_{desired} - C_{measured}) \times V_d}{S \times F}$$

$$LD = \frac{(3mg/L - 1.7\ mg/L) \times (1.8L/kg \times 70kg)}{(0.83)(0.7)}$$

$$LD = \frac{2.3\ mg/L \times 126\ L}{(0.83)(0.7)} = \frac{290\ mg}{0.581} = 490\ mg,\ \text{rounded up to 500 mg}$$

CASE 2: MAINTENANCE DOSE OF QUINIDINE GLUCONATE USING POPULATION PHARMACOKINETICS METHOD

EG is a 55-year-old male (125 kg) with recurrent, sustained monomorphic ventricular tachycardia documented by electrophysiologic testing, suppressed by quinidine at peak serum quinidine concentration of 5 mg/L following oral administration of quinidine gluconate.

QUESTION 1

What oral maintenance dose (MD) of quinidine gluconate should EG receive to achieve a peak serum quinidine concentration of 2.5 mg/L?

Answer:

The oral MD of quinidine gluconate is calculated by multiplying the desired peak serum quinidine concentration by the total body clearance of quinidine (4 mL/min/kg, or 0.24 L/kg/hr) and the dosing interval. Since we selected quinidine gluconate ERT for the MD, the bioavailability is approximately 70 percent (F = 0.7) and the salt fraction (S) is 0.62. The following equation is used to calculate MD for EG:

$$C = \frac{(F)(S)(D/\tau)}{Cl} \quad \text{where MD} = \frac{(C)(Cl)(\tau)}{(F)(S)}$$

$$MD = \frac{(2.5 \text{ mg/L})(0.24 \text{ L/kg/hr} \times 125 \text{ kg})(6 \text{ hr})}{(0.7)(0.62)}$$

$$MD = \frac{(2.5 \text{ mg/L})(30 \text{ L/hr})(6 \text{ hr})}{(0.7)(0.62)}$$

$$MD = \frac{(2.5 \text{ mg/L})(180 \text{ L})}{(0.7)(0.62)} = \frac{450 \text{ mg}}{0.434}$$

MD = 1,036 mg = Quinidine gluconate 324 mg ERT, quantity 3 tabs, PO every 6 hours

QUESTION 2

If the patient does not receive a loading dose, how long will it take to achieve a serum quinidine concentration of 2.5 mg/L?

Answer:

To determine how much time it will take for EG to achieve a serum quinidine concentration of 2.5 mg/L, you must perform several calculations. First you must determine the half-life of quinidine in EG. From the half-life you will derive the elimination rate constant with the following steps:

Step 1: Calculate half-life ($T_{1/2}$).

$$T_{1/2} = \frac{(0.693)(V_d)}{Cl}$$

$$T_{1/2} = \frac{(0.693)(2.75 \text{L/kg} \times 125 \text{ kg})}{(0.24 \text{ L/kg/hr} \times 125 \text{ kg})} = \frac{(0.693)(344 \text{ L})}{30 \text{ L/hr}}$$

$$T_{1/2} = 7.95 \text{ hr}$$

Step 2: Calculate elimination rate constant (K_e).

$$K_e = \frac{0.693}{T_{1/2}}$$

$$K_e = \frac{0.693}{7.95 \text{ hr}}$$

$$K_e = 0.087 \text{ hr}^{-1}$$

Step 3: Calculate concentration at end of one half-life (C_p at T1).

$$C_p \text{ at T1} = \frac{(S)(F)(\text{dose}/t)}{Cl} \times (1 - e^{-ke \times T1/2})$$

Convert total daily dose to mg/hr = 324 mg/ERT × 3 tabs/dose × 4 doses/24 hr = 162 mg/hr

$$C_p \text{ at T1} = \frac{(0.62)(0.7)(162 \text{ mg/hr}) \times (1 - e^{-0.087})(e^{-0.087 \times 7.95})}{(0.24 \text{ L/kg/hr} \times 125 \text{ kg})}$$

$$C_p \text{ at T1} = \frac{70 \text{ mg/hr} \times (1 - e^{-0.087})(e^{-0.087 \times 7.95})}{30 \text{ L/hr}}$$

$$C_p \text{ at T1} = 2.3 \text{ mg/L} \times 0.083 \times 7.29$$

$$C_p \text{ at T1} = 1.41 \text{ mg/L}$$

Step 4: Calculate time to achieve a serum quinidine concentration of 2.5 mg/L (T2).

$$T2 = \frac{7.95 \text{ hr} \times 2.5 \text{ mg/L}}{1.4 \text{ mg/L}}$$

$$T2 = \frac{19.87 \text{ hr/mg/L}}{1.4 \text{ mg/L}}$$

$$T2 = 14.1 \text{ hr}$$

CASE 3: CALCULATION OF EXPECTED STEADY-STATE LEVEL

BK is a 70-year-old male (105 kg) receiving quinidine sulfate ERT 600 mg every 8 hours for the treatment of Afib/flutter.

QUESTION 1

What would be the expected steady-state serum quinidine concentration in BT at the end of each dosing interval?

Answer:

The trough steady-state serum quinidine concentration in BK is calculated by utilizing the following equation:

$$C_{SSmin} = \frac{(F)(S)(D)}{V_d} \frac{(e^{-KeT})}{(1 - e^{-KeT})}$$

$$C_{SSmin} = \frac{(0.7)(0.83)(600 \text{ mg})}{(2.75 \text{ L/kg} \times 105 \text{ kg})} \frac{(e^{-0.087(8)})}{(1 - e^{-0.087(8)})}$$

$$C_{SSmin} = 349 \text{ mg} \frac{(289 \text{ L})}{0.501} 0.498$$

$$C_{SSmin} = \frac{1.21 \text{ mg/L}}{0.501} 0.498$$

$$C_{SSmin} = 2.41 \text{ mg/L} (0.498)$$

$$C_{SSmin} = 1.20 \text{ mg/L}$$

From C_{SSmin}, you can calculate the steady-state peak serum quinidine concentration for BT by using the following equation:

$$C_{SSmax} = C_{SSmin} + \frac{(S)(F)(\text{Dose})}{V_d}$$

$$C_{SSmax} = 1.2 \text{ mg/L} + \frac{(0.83)(0.7)(600 \text{ mg})}{(2.75 \text{ L/kg})(105 \text{ kg})}$$

$$C_{SSmax} = 1.2 \text{ mg/L} + \frac{(349 \text{ mg})}{(289 \text{ L})}$$

$$C_{SSmax} = 1.2 \text{ mg/L} + 1.21 \text{ mg/L}$$

$$C_{SSmax} = 2.41 \text{ mg/L}$$

Alternatively, the following equations may be used to calculate C_{SSmax} and C_{SSmin}:

$$C_{SSmax} = \frac{(S)(F)(Dose)}{V_d \underline{}}$$
$$\phantom{C_{SSmax} = xxxxx} (1 - e^{-KeT})$$

$$C_{SSmin} = C_{SSmax}(e^{-KeT})$$

QUESTION 2

Therefore, if asked to calculate C_{SSmin} and C_{SSmax} for BG, an 80-year-old female (60 kg) taking quinidine gluconate 324 mg ERT once every 8 hours and who has coexisting end-stage renal failure (creatinine clearance = 20 mL/min) and severe congestive heart failure (Kilip Class III, ejection fraction = 20%), you would perform the following calculations:

Answer:

Step 1. Calculate the total body clearance of quinidine using the following equation:

Total body clearance of quinidine = 2 mL/min/kg

Convert clearance to L/kg/hr = 0.12 L/kg/hr

Total body clearance of quinidine = 0.12 L/kg/hr × 60 kg

Total clearance of quinidine = 7.2 L/hr

Step 2. Derive K_e quinidine (hr^{-1}) from total body clearance of quinidine using the following equation:

Total clearance of quinidine = $K_e \times V_d$

Total clearance of quinidine = 7.2 L/hr = $[K_e (hr^{-1})] \times [2 \text{ L/kg} \times 60 \text{ kg}]$

Total clearance of quinidine = 7.2 L/hr = $[K_e (hr^{-1})] \times [102 \text{ L}]$

$$K_e = \frac{7.2 \text{ L/hr}}{120 \text{ L}}$$

$$K_e = 0.06 \text{ hr}^{-1}$$

Step 3. Solve for C_{SSmax} using the following equation:

$$C_{SSmax} = \frac{(S)(F)(Dose)}{V_d \underline{}}$$
$$\phantom{C_{SSmax} = xxxxx} (1 - e^{-KeT})$$

$$C_{SSmax} = \frac{(0.62)(0.7)(324)}{\dfrac{(2 \text{ L/kg})(60 \text{ kg})}{(1 - e^{-(0.06)(8)})}}$$

$$C_{SSmax} = \frac{141 \text{ mg}}{\dfrac{120 \text{ L}}{0.381}}$$

$$C_{SSmax} = \frac{1.17 \text{ mg/L}}{0.381}$$

$$C_{SSmax} = 3.1 \text{ mg/L}$$

Step 4. Solve for C_{SSmin} using the following formula:

$$C_{SSmin} = C_{SSmax}(e^{-KeT})$$
$$C_{SSmin} = 3.1 \text{ mg/L}(e^{-(0.06)(8)})$$
$$C_{SSmin} = 3.1 \text{ mg/L}(0.619)$$
$$C_{SSmin} = 1.92 \text{ mg/L}$$

CASE 4: PATIENT-SPECIFIC PHARMACOKINETICS

TJ is a 65-year-old former baseball star who has developed AFib/flutter that is resistant to other medical therapies, and he is not a candidate for surgical intervention, radiofrequency ablation, or implantable devices to control his Afib/flutter. He currently takes digoxin 0.25 mg/day (serum digoxin concentration 0.9 ng/mL) and warfarin 2.5 mg every other day (INR 2.5). He is referred to your pharmacokinetic consult service because his cardiologist want to change his quinidine sulfate IRT 300 mg, 2 tablets PO five times daily to quinidine sulfate ERT PO tid regiment to help TJ with his medication compliance. TJ weighs 90 kg and his steady-state serum quinidine concentration measured just prior to his afternoon dose today was 3.95 mg/L.

QUESTION 1

How would you convert TJ's current quinidine sulfate regimen to a quinidine gluconate ERT regimen as requested by the cardiologist?

Answer:

Step 1. You must first determine the total daily dose quinidine base currently prescribed based on his current quinidine sulfate IRT regimen by using the following equation:

Total daily dose of quinidine base = Total daily dose of quinidine sulfate (mg/day) × (Salt fraction) × (Bioavailability)

Total daily dose of quinidine base = (300 mg/tab × 10 tabs/day) × [(0.83)(0.7)]

Total daily dose of quinidine base = (3,000 mg/day) × 0.581

Total daily dose of quinidine base = 1,743 mg/day

Step 2. Convert 1,743 mg/day quinidine base to equivalent daily dose of quinidine gluconate administered in three divided daily doses using the following equation:

$$\text{Total daily dose of quinidine gluconate} = \frac{\text{Total daily dose of quinidine base}}{(S) \times (F) \text{ for quinidine gluconate}}$$

$$\text{Total daily dose of quinidine gluconate} = \frac{1,743 \text{ mg/day}}{(0.62) \times (0.7)}$$

$$\text{Total daily dose of quinidine gluconate} = \frac{1,743 \text{ mg/day}}{0.434}$$

Total daily dose of quinidine gluconate = 4,016 mg/day

Step 3. Determine the number of tablets per dose to administer quinidine gluconate ERT three times daily by using the following equation:

Number of tablets per dose

$$= \frac{\text{Total daily dose of quinidine gluconate}}{\text{(Doses per day) (mg of quinidine gluconate salt in 1 tab)}}$$

Number of tablets per dose $= \dfrac{4{,}016 \text{ mg}}{(3) \times (324 \text{ mg/tab})}$

Number of tablets per dose $= \dfrac{4{,}016 \text{ mg}}{972 \text{ mg/dose}}$

Number of tablets per dose $= 4$

QUESTION 2

TJ's cardiologist wishes to know how soon after the start of the quinidine gluconate can he obtain a steady-state peak serum quinidine concentration?

Answer:

As a clinical pharmacokineticist, you know that a medication reaches steady state after approximately five half-lives. To determine the amount of time required for quinidine to reach steady state after the start of the quinidine gluconate ERT oral regimen, you must calculate the half-life of quinidine in TJ by using the following equation:

$$\text{Half-life } (T_{1/2}) = \frac{0.693}{\text{Elimination rate constant } (K_e)}$$

You can extrapolate K_e for quinidine in TJ by using his last known steady-state serum quinidine concentration and the corresponding oral quinidine sulfate ERT (i.e., 600 mg (2 tabs) five times daily) using the formula for the steady-state serum quinidine concentration as follows:

Step 1.

Quinidine steady-state concentration (C_{ss})

$$= \frac{(S) \times (F) \times (\text{Dose/dose interval})}{\text{Clearance} = (V_d \times K_e)}$$

Please note that you are using the steady-state concentration obtained from the quinidine sulfate IRT data so the value for (S) must reflect the sulfate salt and not the gluconate salt.

Therefore, the preceding equation is set up as follows:

Quinidine steady-state concentration (3.9 mg/L)

$$= \frac{(0.83)(0.7)(600 \text{ mg Dose/5 hr})}{(2.75 \text{ L/kg} \times 90 \text{ kg})(K_e)}$$

Quinidine steady-state concentration (3.9 mg/L) $= \dfrac{70 \text{ mg/hr}}{247 \text{ L} \times (K_e)}$

$$K_e = \frac{70 \text{ mg/hr}}{247 \text{ L} \times 3.9 \text{ mg/L}}$$

$$K_e = \frac{70 \text{ mg/hr}}{963 \text{ mg}}$$

$$K_e = 0.072 \text{ hr}^{-1}$$

Step 2. Use the following formula to solve for $T_{1/2}$ for quinidine in hours.

Quinidine half-life (hr) $= 0.693/ K_e$

Quinidine half-life (hr) $= 0.693/0.072 \text{ hr}^{-1}$

Quinidine half-life (hr) $= 9.6 \text{ hr}$

Step 3. Time to steady state = 5 half-lives; 5×9.6 hr = 48 hr

QUESTION 3

Lastly, TJ's cardiologist wishes to know what can he estimate the new steady-state serum quinidine concentration will be on TJ's quinidine gluconate ERT (972 mg every 8 hours)?

Answer:

You can determine the new steady-state quinidine concentration using the following formula:

Quinidine steady-state concentration $(C_{ss}) = \dfrac{(S)(F)(\text{Dose/dose interval})}{\text{Clearance} = (V_d \times K_e)}$

Quinidine steady-state concentration (C_{ss})

$$= \frac{(0.62)(0.7)(972 \text{ mg/8 hr})}{\text{Clearance} = (247 \text{ L} \times 0.072)}$$

Quinidine steady-state concentration $(C_{ss}) = \dfrac{53 \text{ mg/hr}}{18 \text{ L/hr}}$

Quinidine steady-state concentration $(C_{ss}) = 2.94 \text{ mg/L}$

CASE 5: DRUG INTERACTIONS

JK is a 69-year-old female with congestive heart failure (Kilip Class III; ejection fraction of 22%), sustained monomorphic ventricular tachycardia treated with quinidine gluconate 324 mg (2 tablets) PO every 8 hours, and COPD treated with inhaled ipratropium bromide combined with albuterol (Combivent) 2 puffs every 6 hours. Last week the patient suffered an exacerbation of chronic bronchitis and was prescribed clarithromycin 500 mg PO bid for 10 days. JK takes warfarin 5 mg daily for recurrent DVTs. Her INR last week was 1.9. Today, she presents to the emergency department (ED) with complaints of tinnitus, palpitations, nausea, vomiting, and diarrhea. The ED physicians requested the old medical records from clinic and obtained a 12-lead EKG as well as a STAT serum quinidine concentration. The EKG showed new onset QT prolongation and a U wave. Her serum potassium concentration was 4.2 mEq/L; and her serum quinidine concentration was 7.9 mg/L. up from 4.1 mg/L measured in clinic when JK was seen for her COPD exacerbation and she was prescribed clarithromycin. Of interest, JK's INR today in the ED was 2.9, from 1.9 during the same time frame as the change in serum quinidine concentration; she shows no objective evidence of warfarin-induced bleeding or other warfarin-induced side effects at this time. JK's weight today was 80 kg. The ED physicians stops all medications and requests a pharmacokinetic STAT consult to address the following questions.

QUESTION 1

What is the patient's current clearance of quinidine?

Answer:

You must first determine the clearance of quinidine in JK before and after the initiation of clarithromycin, which can be accomplished by means of the following equation:

$$\text{Quinidine steady-state concentration } (C_{ss}) = \frac{(S)(F)(\text{Dose/dose interval})}{\text{Clearance}}$$

Quinidine steady-state concentration (4.1 mg/L)

$$= \frac{(0.62)(0.7)(648 \text{ mg/8 hr})}{\text{Clearance}}$$

$$\text{Quinidine steady-state concentration } (4.1 \text{ mg/L}) = \frac{35 \text{ mg/hr}}{\text{Clearance}}$$

$$\text{Quinidine clearance } (Cl) = \frac{35 \text{ mg/hr}}{4.1 \text{ mg/L}}$$

$$\text{Quinidine clearance } (Cl) = 8.57 \text{ L/hr}$$

QUESTION 2

What was the quinidine clearance prior to the start of clarithromycin?

Answer:

Now you must determine the clearance of quinidine from the body after the initiation of clarithromycin 500 mg tid by solving for quinidine steady-state concentration with the following equation:

$$\text{Quinidine steady-state concentration } (C_{ss}) = \frac{(S)(F)(\text{Dose/dose interval})}{\text{Clearance}}$$

Quinidine steady-state concentration (7.9 mg/L)

$$= \frac{(0.62)(0.7)(648 \text{ mg/8 hr})}{\text{Clearance}}$$

$$\text{Quinidine steady-state concentration } (7.9 \text{ mg/L}) = \frac{35 \text{ mg/hr}}{\text{Clearance}}$$

$$\text{Quinidine clearance } (Cl) = \frac{35 \text{ mg/hr}}{7.9 \text{ mg/L}}$$

$$\text{Quinidine clearance } (Cl) = 4.43 \text{ L/hr}$$

QUESTION 3

How long before JK's serum quinidine concentration returns to a baseline value of 4.1 mg/L?

Answer:

To determine the time it will take from now to obtain a steady-state serum quinidine concentration of 4.1 mg/L, you can use the following equation:

$$\text{Time (hr)} = \frac{\ln (\text{concentration 1/concentration 2})}{K_e (\text{hr}^{-1})}$$

$$\text{Time (hr)} = \frac{\ln (7.9 \text{ mg/L}/4.1 \text{ mg/L})}{0.03 \text{ hr}^{-1}}$$

$$\text{Time (hr)} = \frac{0.656}{0.03 \text{ hr}^{-1}}$$

$$\text{Time (hr)} = 21.7 \text{ hr}$$

QUESTION 4

What factors caused the INR to rise from 1.9 to 2.9 without a change in dose of warfarin?

Answer:

In this patient, the addition of clarithromycin, a potent inhibitor of hepatic cytochrome P450 enzyme produces a significant reduction in the metabolism of both quinidine and warfarin such that each of the agents produced exaggerated pharmacologic responses. Notably, JK presented to the ED with signs and symptoms of quinidine toxicity (i.e., QT prolongation with prominent U wave and cinchonism). Furthermore, the increased amount of quinidine in JK produced an increased hypoprothombonemic effect that accentuated the clarithromycin-induced increase in warfarin response observed in JK. Fortunately, no evidence of warfarin-induced bleeding was present.

CASE 6: MANAGEMENT OF OVERDOSE

RW is a 53-year-old female (75 kg) who ingested approximately 15 tablets from a bottle of #90 tablets quinidine sulfate 300 mg IRT in an attempted suicide. She presents to the ED approximately 3 hours after ingestion obtunded, diaphoretic, tachycardic, and delirious. Her vital sighs show that she has a temperature of 100.8°F; a pulse of 115 beats per minutes and it is regular; her respirations are 24; and her systemic arterial pressure is 88/40 mm Hg. The serum quinidine concentration on admission to the ED was 9.7 mg/L. The EKG shows impaired intraventricular conduction (QRS 140 msec.), and the QT interval corrected for a heart rate of 115 beats per minute measured 500 msec. The patient is receiving physiologic saline at a rate of 250 mL/hr. The physicians in the ED wish to know if quinidine can be removed by any form of dialysis or hemoperfusion. They wish to know your recommendations regarding the treatment of an acute overdose of quinidine.

QUESTION 1

Is quinidine removed from the body by extracorporeal removal mechanisms?

Answer:

No. Quinidine is minimally removed by any form of dialysis or hemoperfusion.

QUESTION 2

What is the appropriate treatment in this case?

Answer:

Patients with quinidine overdose should always be admitted to an intensive care unit. Because cardiovascular shock may occur rapidly, intravenous access lines, oxygen, and monitoring of ECG and vital signs are the first priorities. Treatment depends on the dose ingested and on the severity. It includes gastric lavage and supportive treatment with artificial ventilation, inotropic and vasopressor drugs, and hypertonic sodium solutions. EKG monitoring is required to detect cardiotoxicity. The patient should have a complete metabolic panel drawn on admission. Measurement of serum quinidine concentrations may be helpful in diagnosis but is not useful for clinical management. Levels over 8 mg/l may be associated with toxic symptoms and levels over 12 to 14 mg/l are usually seen in patients with severe cardiotoxicity. Systematically monitor vital signs, EKG, blood pressure, and central venous pressure. Repeated noninvasive blood pressure monitoring is essential for the detection of circulatory arrest due to electromechanical dissociation.

Reversal of the quinidine-induced sodium channel blockade is induced can be accomplished either with molar sodium lactate (100–250 mL over 15–45 minutes) or molar sodium bicarbonate—100–250 mL of molar sodium bicarbonate solution (8.4 g/L) over 15–45 minutes. Consider adding 2 g potassium chloride per 250 mL of these solutions in order to avoid hypokalemia. Repeated monitoring of electrolytes is necessary because hypernatremia and hypokalemia may appear. Antiarrhythmic drugs, especially those with quinidine-like effects, are contraindicated. Electric counter-shock is indicated for ventricular fibrillation, sustained ventricular tachycardia, or torsade de pointes. Convulsions may be treated by intravenous diazepam. Initial hypokalemia should be corrected cautiously. Hypokalemia persisting beyond 8 hours after the ingestion may promote ventricular dysrhythmia and should be corrected. Administer potassium continuously with frequent monitoring of plasma potassium levels (every 4 hours). Add 5 g KCl to 500 mL of dextrose 5 percent and do not exceed infusion of more than 1–1.5 g KCl per hour. No antidote for quinidine is available.

REFERENCES

1. Lévy S, Azoulay S. Stories about the origin of quinquina and quinidine. *J Cardiovasc Electrophysiol.* 1994;5:635–636.

2. Hollman A. Plants in cardiology: Quinine and quinidine. *Br Heart J.* 1991;66:301.

3. Quinine. *Wikipedia: The Free Encyclopedia.* Available at: http://en.wikipedia.org/wiki/Quinine (accessed January 2, 2013).

4. Grace AA, Camm J. Quinidine. *N Engl J Med.* 1998;338:35–45.

5. Quinidine. *Wikipedia: The Free Encyclopedia.* Available at: http://en.wikipedia.org/wiki/Quinidine. Internet (accessed January 2, 2013).

6. The Cardiac Arrhythmia Suppression Trial (CAST) Investigators. Preliminary report of encainide and flecainide on mortality in a randomized trial of arrhythmia suppression after myocardial infarction. *N Engl J Med.* 1989;321:406–412.

7. Morganroth J, Goin JE. Quinidine-related mortality in the short- to medium-term treatment of ventricular arrhythmias. *Circulation.* 1991;84:1977–1983.

8. Quinidine sulfate tablet USP prescribing information. Corona, CA: Watson Laboratories, 2009.

9. Quinidine gluconate tablet, extended-release prescribing information. Corona, CA: Watson Laboratories, 2009.

10. Gonzalez ER, Meyers DG. Correlation of electrocardiographic changes with plasma quinidine concentration. *Nebraska Med J.* 1985;70:87–91.

11. Roden DM, Thompson KA, Hoffman BF, Woosley RL. Clinical features and basic mechanisms of quinidine-induced arrhythmias. *J Am Coll Cardiol.* 1986;8(Suppl A):73A–78A.

12. Swerdlow CD, Yu JO, Jacobson E. Safety and efficacy of intravenous quinidine. *Am J Med.* 1983;75:36–41.

13. Roden DM, Woosley RL, Primm RK. Incidence and clinical features of the quinidine associated long QT syndrome: Implications for patient care. *Am Heart J.* 1986;111:1088–1098.

14. Makkar RR, Fromm BS, Steinmann RT, Meissner MD, Lehmann MH. Female gender as a risk factor for torsades de pointes associated with cardiovascular drugs. *JAMA.* 1993;270:2590–2595.

15. Ueda CT. Quinidine. In: Evans WF, Schentag JJ, Jusko WJ (Eds.). *Applied Pharmacokinetics: Principles of Therapeutic Drug Monitoring.* Vancouver, WA: Applied Therapeutics, 1992:23–32.

16. Nolan PE. Pharmacokinetics and pharmacodynamics of intravenous agents for ventricular arrhythmias. *Pharmacother.* 1997;17:65S–75S.

17. Woosley RL. Pharmacokinetics and pharmacodynamics of antiarrhythmic agents in patients with congestive heart failure. *Am Heart J.* 1987;114:1280–1291.

18. Hill LM. Malkasian GD. The use of quinidine sulfate throughout pregnancy. *Obstet Gynecol.* 1979;54:36–39.

19. Maur AM, DeVaus W, Lahey ME. Neonatal and maternal thrombocytopenia purpura due to quinine. *Pediatrics.* 1957;19:84–85.

20. Holford NHG, Coates PE, Guentert TW, Riegelman S, Sheiner LB. The effects of quinidine and its metabolites on the EKG and systolic time intervals: Concentration-effect relationships. *Br J Clin Pharmacol.* 1981;11:187–195.

21. Gerhardt RE, Knouss RF, Thyrum PT. Quinidine excretion in aciduria and alkaluria. *Ann Intern Med.* 1969;71:97–101.

CHAPTER

19

Valproic Acid

ELJIM P. TESORO, PharmD, BCPS
GRETCHEN M. BROPHY, PharmD, BCPS, FCCP, FCCM, FNCS
HENRY COHEN, MS, PharmD, FCCM, BCPP, CGP

Valproic acid (VPA) is a broad-spectrum, carboxylic acid-derived anticonvulsant that has been used in the treatment of epilepsy, bipolar disease, schizophrenia, and migraine headache. Its main mechanism of action is not well understood, but it is thought that it increases the amount of the inhibitory neurotransmitter, gamma-aminobutyric acid (GABA), in the central nervous system (CNS). It comes in several different preparations and salt forms (Table 19-1). Divalproex sodium is a mixture of equal parts of the acid and sodium salts of valproic acid. The delayed-release (Depakote) and extended-release (Depakote ER) formulations are not bioequivalent.[1] A 20 percent increase in the daily dose is recommended when switching from Depakote to Depakote ER to account for the differences in rate and extent of absorption.

DOSING

Dosing is done in terms of valproic acid content. For seizure disorders, initial oral dosing for patients 10 years of age and older is 10–15 mg/kg/day. Dosing intervals for the oral and parenteral preparations are typically every 8–12 hours (although dosing every 6 hours may be needed in some patients), with the exception of the extended-release formulation, which can be administered once or twice daily. The daily dose can be titrated weekly by 5–10 mg/kg/day to a maximum recommended dose of 60 mg/kg/day. Loading doses are not recommended for the oral VPA formulations due to intolerable gastrointestinal side effects; however, intravenous loading doses of valproate sodium 25 mg/kg are commonly given for patients in status epilepticus. Intravenous loading doses can be given at a rate of 1.5–3 mg/kg/min, but faster rates of up to 6 mg/kg/min appear to be safe.[2,3,4] Therapeutic drug monitoring (TDM) is used in conjunction with the clinical exam to optimize seizure control and minimize toxicity. Measuring serum concentrations is routinely performed via immunoassay, and the therapeutic range is reported as 50–100 mcg/mL, although individual patients may have optimal responses outside these ranges. Concentrations higher than 150 mcg/mL are associated with a high incidence of CNS side effects. Free (unbound) concentrations are also available with a therapeutic range reported to be 6–22 mcg/mL with toxicity occurring above 50 mcg/mL. Trough levels (obtained prior to a dose) are preferred to assure that minimum therapeutic concentrations are maintained. Diurnal variations in the serum concentration of VPA have been reported, so it is important to be consistent when sampling in order to properly compare levels and adjust dosing regimens. Clearance tends to be higher in the evening compared to the morning times[5] in both young adults and elderly subjects,[6] so trough levels are recommended before the morning dose.

BIOAVAILABILITY

All of the formulations of valproic acid have bioavailabilities near 100 percent (F = 1), reflecting the absence of a first-pass effect in the liver. The enteric-coated formulation has a bioavailability of approximately 90 percent (F = 0.9).[7] Valproate sodium is rapidly converted to valproic acid in the stomach and then readily absorbed via the gastrointestinal tract. Peak concentrations are achieved within 0.5–2 hours after oral administration.[8] The presence of food will delay the peak concentration but not the extent of absorption.[9] The volume of distribution in adults is reported to range from 0.1 to 0.4 L/kg,[10] indicating that VPA remains primarily within the intravascular and extracellular space. The volume of distribution tends to increase with higher doses due to saturable protein binding.[11] VPA has been isolated from cerebrospinal fluid (10% of serum concentrations), breast milk (1–10% of serum concentrations), and saliva (1% of serum concentrations, although correlation is poor).[12] It readily crosses the placenta[13] and can increase the risk of neural tube defects if given in pregnant women.

PLASMA PROTEIN BINDING

VPA is approximately 90–95 percent protein bound, primarily to serum albumin. The free fraction of VPA ranges from 6 to 10 percent, and its protein binding depends on serum concentration, serum albumin, age, and end-organ failure. The free fraction has been reported to be increased in elderly patients (10.7%) versus younger adults (6.4%).[6] At concentrations above 70 mcg/mL, VPA displays a higher free fraction with minimal changes in total concentration. Renal failure may increase the free fraction to 18 percent while cirrhosis can increase it to 29 percent. Caution must be used when interpreting total VPA serum levels in these patients because they can be falsely low while their free levels may be therapeutic or higher.[14] In addition, VPA may displace other highly protein-bound drugs, such as phenytoin; therefore, free phenytoin levels should be monitored when these drugs are given concomitantly.[15]

METABOLISM

VPA is primarily metabolized in the liver via glucuronidation (40%), β-oxidation, and ω-oxidation (20%) and then eliminated via the kidneys, with less than 3 percent of the drug excreted in the urine unchanged. VPA is characterized as a low-extraction drug with its clearance being independent of hepatic blood flow. Many of the metabolites are thought to be responsible for anticonvulsant activity as well as toxicity.[16] VPA has an average elimination half-life

TABLE 19-1	Valproic Acid Formulations	
Valproic Acid		
Depakene®	Liquid-filled oral capsules: 250 mg	
Stavzor®	Delayed-release oral capsules: 125 mg, 250 mg, 500 mg	
Valproate Sodium		
Depakene Syrup®	Oral solution: 250 mg per 5 mL	
Depacon®	Parenteral injection: 100 mg per mL	
Divalproex Sodium		
Depakote Sprinkle®	Oral capsules: 125 mg	
Depakote®	Delayed-release tablets: 125 mg, 250 mg, 500 mg	
Depakote® ER	Extended-release tablets: 250 mg, 500 mg	

of 11 hours and follows first-order kinetics. The mean plasma clearance for total VPA is reported to be approximately 6–7 mL/hr/kg in adults[6] (range 5–10 mL/hr/kg),[8] which may be decreased in patients with renal or hepatic failure, and increased in patients taking concomitant hepatic enzyme-inducing agents. Total clearance increases with higher doses due to saturable protein binding, which leads to a higher free fraction and more unbound drug available for metabolism (assuming normal hepatic function).[10] VPA acts as a substrate and inhibitor of various cytochrome P450 enzymes, reflecting a high potential for drug interactions (Table 19-2).

CASE STUDIES

CASE 1: VALPROIC ACID LOADING DOSE/ MAINTENANCE DOSE

A 43-year-old female is admitted with status epilepticus. She has a history of coronary artery disease, hyperlipidemia, and asthma. Her medications prior to admission include aspirin 81 mg PO daily, amlodipine 10 mg PO daily, simvastatin 20 mg PO qhs, and Advair 250/50 ii puffs BID. She has no known drug allergies. Her vital signs are:

HR: 107   BP: 100/56   RR: 20   T: 38.8°C

Height = 63 inches

Weight = 80 kg

QUESTION

What is the best approach for loading and maintenance doses for this patient?

Answer:

Intravenous (IV) loading doses will ensure rapid achievement of therapeutic serum levels and increase the likelihood of seizure control in emergent cases of status epilepticus. Valproate sodium (Depacon) can be given as an IV load in cases of status epilepticus, especially when concern for hemodynamic or pulmonary compromise is present. One study reported a series of patients receiving 21–28 mg/kg of IV valproate sodium at a rate of 3–6 mg/kg/min (the recommended rate for nonemergent administration is listed at 20 mg/min).[17] Peak

TABLE 19-2	Cytochrome P450 Enzymes Associated with Valproic Acid	
Enzymes That Metabolize VPA	**Enzymes That VPA Inhibits**	**Enzymes That VPA Induces**
CYP2A6, 2B6, 2C9, 2C19, 2E1	CYP2C9 (weak), 2C19 (weak), 2D6 (weak), 3A4 (weak)	CYP2A6 (weak)

serum levels 20 minutes after the end of the infusion were 105–204 mcg/mL, with no reports of hemodynamic or CNS side effects. This loading dose would provide therapeutic serum levels until a maintenance dosing regimen could be initiated 8–12 hours later.

For this patient, a dose of 30 mg/kg (~2,400 mg) given at 400 mg/min would be reasonable to attain rapid therapeutic levels. Maintenance doses would be calculated the traditional way: 10–15 mg/kg/day or 800–1,200 mg/day, or valproate sodium 500 mg PO q12h with the first dose starting 12 hours after the IV load. A postload serum level may be collected to document achievement of the therapeutic range, but clinical cessation of seizure activity should take precedence. Postload levels should be obtained no sooner than one hour after the loading dose to assure complete distribution and an accurate reading.

Another way to calculate the maintenance dose is by using population-based pharmacokinetic parameters. Using the following equation:

$$C_{ss} = \frac{(F)(D/\tau)}{Cl}$$

where C_{ss} is the steady-state concentration, F is bioavailability (1 for immediate-release VPA; 0.9 for sustained-release VPA), D is dose in milligrams, τ is dosing interval in hours, and Cl is clearance (5–10 mL/hr/kg). A steady-state concentration of 50 mcg/mL is a reasonable target, and choosing a clearance of 10 mL/hr/kg would give us a conservative recommendation. So for this patient, the dose of extended-release VPA given every 12 hours that would achieve a C_{ss} of 50 mcg/mL (or 0.05 mg/mL) would be:

$$D = \frac{(C_{ss})(Cl)(\tau)}{F}$$

$$= \frac{(0.05 \text{ mg/mL})(10 \text{ mL/hr/kg} \times 80 \text{ kg})(12 \text{ hr})}{1} = 480 \text{ mg}$$

This dose can be rounded up to 500 mg every 12 hours. The timing of a serum level can be determined by calculating the half-life:

$$t_{\frac{1}{2}} = \frac{(0.693)}{k} \quad \text{and} \quad Cl = (k)(V_d)$$

$$t_{1/2} = \frac{(0.693)(V_d)}{Cl} = \frac{(0.693)(0.15 \text{ L/kg} \times 80 \text{ kg})(1,000 \text{ mL/L})}{10 \text{ mL/hr/kg} \times 80 \text{ kg}} = 10.4 \text{ hr}$$

To obtain a true steady-state concentration, a VPA level should be checked in 3–5 half-lives, so a level can be checked after 52 hours (10.4 × 5 = 52 hr).

CASE 2: VPA DRUG INTERACTION THAT DECREASES LEVELS

A 42-year-old man is seen in the infectious diseases clinic for a two-month follow-up for his treatment of tuberculosis. He has a history

TABLE 19-3	Valproic Acid Drug Interactions	
Drugs That DECREASE VPA Concentration	**Drugs That May INCREASE VPA Concentration**
Bile acid–binding resins – decreased absorption	Aspirin (high dose) – protein binding displacement/decreased intrinsic clearance
Carbamazepine – hepatic metabolism induced	
Carbapenem antibiotics – multiple mechanisms	Cimetidine – hepatic metabolism inhibited
Lamotrigine – hepatic metabolism induced	
Phenytoin – hepatic metabolism induced	Macrolides – unknown mechanism
Phenobarbital – hepatic metabolism induced	Felbamate – hepatic metabolism inhibited
Rifampin – hepatic metabolism induced	
Ritonavir – hepatic metabolism induced	
Sevelamer – decreased absorption	

of seizures for which he takes Depakote 500 mg PO BID and hypertension for which he takes metoprolol XL 100 mg PO daily. He takes Rifater® (rifampin, isoniazid/pyrazinamide) 6 tablets PO daily for his infection. He reports an increase in seizure activity in the last few weeks. A serum level is collected and is reported to be 20 mcg/mL (his serum level 2 months ago was 60 mcg/mL).

Height = 70 inches

Weight = 92 kg

QUESTION

What approach is needed to address the patient's increase in seizure activity?

Answer:

VPA is metabolized by glucuronidases in the liver and rifampin is a potent inducer of these enzymes. A 40 percent increase in clearance can result from concomitant use of rifampin or its derivatives, and its effect can be seen relatively quickly. To adjust for this interaction, a higher daily dose can be given (increase to 2 g/day or 20 mg/kg/day), and the dosing interval can be shortened to 6 hours (500 mg PO q6h). A serum trough level can be obtained in 3–4 days to ensure attainment of therapeutic concentrations if no seizures are noted beforehand. Once the rifampin therapy is complete, the VPA can be decreased to the previous regimen of 500 mg PO every 12 hours. The timing of this change may be difficult to predict. It is reasonable to wait until mild symptoms of toxicity occur (e.g., drowsiness), which signal a down-regulation of enzymes responsible for VPA metabolism with subsequent increase in serum levels. Another option would be obtaining a serum level in weekly intervals to document the increase in serum VPA concentrations before decreasing to the previous dose.

Other agents that can induce hepatic enzyme activity and thus decrease the steady-state serum concentrations of VPA include phenytoin,[18,19,20] lamotrigine,[21] and carbamazepine. As seizure control sometimes requires more than a single agent, anticonvulsants that induce or inhibit each other's metabolism[15,22,23] should be closely monitored for clinical effect as well as therapeutic serum concentrations.

CASE 3: DOSING IN RENAL DYSFUNCTION

JJ is a 54-year-old woman admitted with acute kidney injury from interstitial nephritis. Her baseline serum creatinine is 0.9 mg/dL, and currently it is 2.3 mg/dL. She has a history of seizures for which she takes Depakote 250 mg PO TID.

QUESTION

What is the best recommendation for dose adjustments in a patient with renal insufficiency?

Answer:

Only 3 percent of VPA is excreted unchanged by the kidneys. Dosing adjustment in renal impairment is unnecessary. However, patients with chronic renal dysfunction have altered protein binding, usually as a result of low albumin and retention of serum proteins that may displace VPA from its binding sites. The result may be increased free fraction of VPA with typically normal total VPA levels. Therapeutic drug monitoring using free VPA levels may be

necessary to prevent unnecessary dosage increases and subsequent toxicities.

CASE 4: DOSING IN HEMODIALYSIS

SB is a 58-year-old man with end-stage renal disease on hemodialysis three times weekly. He has a new diagnosis of migraine headaches and was prescribed Depakote ER 500 mg PO daily.

QUESTION

What modifications, if any, are required to manage his VPA therapy?

Answer:

The qualities of a drug that affect its ability to be dialyzed include its molecular weight, protein binding, volume of distribution, and water solubility. Hemodialysis tends to decrease VPA serum concentrations by about 20 percent, but no supplemental doses are recommended. Protein binding may be decreased in renal failure patients, resulting in low to normal total serum levels, but higher than expected free concentrations. If signs of concentration-related toxicity are seen (e.g., increased somnolence, dizziness, tremor, thrombocytopenia), a free level should be checked because total levels may be misleading. No standard therapeutic range is established for valproic acid used for migraine prophylaxis, so in this situation adjusting the dose to maintain serum levels at ~50 mcg/mL seems reasonable because a disproportionately higher free fraction may occur with higher total concentrations leading to toxicity.

CASE 5: DOSING IN HEPATIC FAILURE

A 57-year-old man with a history of cirrhosis is currently being seen for treatment of acute partial seizures. He was on phenobarbital when he developed Stevens-Johnson Syndrome and is being considered for valproic acid therapy. His liver function tests are as follows: alkaline phosphatase (ALP) 250 IU/L, aspartate transaminase (AST) 135 IU/L, alanine transaminase (ALT) 167 IU/L, albumin (Alb) 2.1 g/dL, total bilirubin (TBIL) 1.9 mg/dL, and direct bilirubin (DBIL) 0.9 mg/dL. His INR is 1.8 and he has mild ascites and Grade I encephalopathy. He weighs 80 kg.

QUESTION

What dose of VPA would you recommend?

Answer:

The use of VPA in patients with severe liver disease is not typically recommended due to the incidence of fatal hepatotoxicity, especially in children younger than 2 years of age. The pharmacokinetics of VPA have been studied in patients with acute hepatitis and alcoholic cirrhosis. The volume of distribution is increased (0.2 L/kg) as a result of lower albumin production and the clearance is decreased (0.5 L/hr) due to intrinsic hepatocellular damage.[24] As a result, dosing must be decreased in patients with hepatic impairment. Total serum levels are typically normal with a higher free fraction that may necessitate free level monitoring. Initial dosing of VPA in patients with hepatic impairment is difficult due to the lack of clear laboratory markers of liver function similar to creatinine clearance used to adjust doses in patients with renal dysfunction. The Child-Pugh score has been used to help guide dosing in patients with hepatic failure and takes into consideration several laboratory markers and clinical signs. Based on scoring, patients fall into category A, B, or C, with C denoted as having the most severe liver disease. In general, patients who fall into category B or C tend to require a 20–30 percent decrease in their drug dosing. VPA is contraindicated for patients in category C, but can be dose adjusted for patients in category B if VPA is the only viable option for therapy. This patient has a Child-Pugh score of 9, so a decrease in the initial VPA dosing would be reasonable. Using literature-based dosing of 10 mg/kg/day, we can estimate his daily dose as 800 mg (10 mg/kg/day × 80 kg). After decreasing this by 20 percent for his hepatic function, we calculate his new adjusted daily dose to be 640 mg, which can be rounded up to 250 mg three times daily or the solution can be used for more precise dosing (e.g., 210 mg three times daily).

Using an estimated clearance of 0.5 L/hr from Klotz's study, we can calculate another regimen using an 8-hour dosing interval and a desired steady-state concentration of 50 mcg/mL (or 50 mg/L):

$$D = \frac{(C_{ss})(Cl)(\tau)}{F} = \frac{(50 \text{ mg/L})(0.5 \text{ L/hr})(8 \text{ hr})}{1} = 200 \text{ mg}$$

This dose can be rounded up to 250 mg to utilize the tablets, or the solution can be used for more precise dosing. Therapeutic drug monitoring is recommended in these patients due to the decrease in clearance and need for dosing adjustments to prevent toxicity. The half-life can be calculated as follows:

$$T_{1/2} = \frac{(0.693)(V_d)}{Cl} = \frac{(0.693)(0.2 \text{ L/kg} \times 80 \text{ kg})}{0.5 \text{ L/hr}} = 22 \text{ hr}$$

A steady-state serum level can be obtained in 3–5 half-lives or after 110 hours (~5 days).

CASE 6

A 35-year-old woman comes in with status epilepticus. She weighs 68 kg and is 5 foot 2 inches. Calculate an intravenous loading dose and oral maintenance dose for valproic acid therapy. Use both literature-based dosing and population-based dosing strategies for the maintenance dosing.

Answer:

First, calculate a loading dose to be given intravenously. The range in the literature is 21–28 mg/kg, so choosing 25 mg/kg:

$$LD = 25 \text{ mg/kg} \times 68 \text{ kg} = 1,700 \text{ mg}$$

The total dose can be infused at a rate of 3 mg/kg/min, or over 8 minutes.

Method 1: Based on literature, the initial dosing range is 10–15 mg/kg/day. Treatment for status epilepticus is usually aggressive, so use the upper limit:

MD = 15 mg/kg/day = 15 mg/kg/day × 68 kg = 1,020 mg/day, rounded to 1,000 mg/day or 500 mg every 12 hours

Method 2: Using population-based pharmacokinetic parameters, we can calculate volume of distribution and clearance to determine dose:

V_d = 0.15 L/kg × 68 kg = 10.2 L

Cl = 10 mL/hr/kg × 68 kg = 680 mL/hr, or 0.68 L/hr

$$D = \frac{(C_{ss})(Cl)(\tau)}{F} = \frac{(50 \text{ mg/L})(0.68 \text{ L/hr})(12 \text{ hr})}{1} = 408 \text{ mg}$$

This dose can be rounded up to 500 mg every 12 hours.

	Volume of Distribution (V_d)	Clearance (Cl)	Half-Life ($t_{1/2}$)
TABLE 19-4 Valproic Acid Pharmacokinetic Parameters			
Neonates[25] > 10 days old > 2 weeks old	0.28 L/kg	11 mL/kg/hr	10–67 hr 7–13 hr
Children[26,27] < 2 years 2–4 years > 4 years	0.13 L/kg	24.5 mL/kg/hr 19.9 mL/kg/hr 12.7 mL/kg/hr	11 hr
Adults[28]	0.14–0.23 L/kg	7–12 mL/kg/hr	6–17 hr
Elderly[29]	0.16 L/kg	7.5 mL/kg/hr	15.3 hr

CASE 7

A 6-year-old boy is seen in the clinic for new-onset absence seizures. The neurologist decides to start valproic acid therapy. He weighs 40 pounds. Calculate a maintenance regimen using the Depakote Sprinkles formulation.

Answer:

Step 1: Calculate the patient's estimated volume of distribution and clearance. Using the values from Table 19-4 and converting the weight into kilograms (40 pounds = 18.2 kg):

$$V_d = 0.13 \text{ L/kg} \times 18.2 \text{ kg} = 2.4 \text{ L}$$
$$Cl = 12.7 \text{ mL/hr/kg} \times 18.2 \text{ kg} = 231 \text{ mL/hr}$$

Step 2: Aiming for a steady-state concentration of 50 mg/L, we can calculate a maintenance dose to be given every 12 hours:

$$D = \frac{(C_{ss})(Cl)(\tau)}{F}$$
$$= \frac{(50 \text{ mcg/mL})(1 \text{ mg/1,000 mcg})(231 \text{ mL/hr})(12 \text{ hr})}{1} = 138.6 \text{ mg}$$

This result can be rounded to 125 mg every 12 hours.

CASE 8

An 80-year-old man is seen in the intensive care unit for chronic renal failure and malnutrition. He has a history of partial seizures for which he is taking valproic acid. His last known seizure was several weeks ago and a spot electroencephalograph (EEG) was read as negative for seizure activity. His current total serum VPA level is only 30 mcg/mL. The intensivist would like to increase his dose to raise his serum level to therapeutic concentrations. What do you recommend? What other factors need to be considered?

Answer:

Valproic acid displays saturable protein binding, and this patient has many reasons to have altered protein binding—advanced age, renal failure, and malnutrition (low albumin). As a result, the free fraction of VPA is increased, which could lead to an increase in free concentration of VPA. This increase may explain the clinical control of his seizures despite a low serum total level. A change in dose may not be necessary unless evidence of poor seizure control or toxicity is noted. A free VPA level may be prudent if available, as well as a liver profile and albumin. His list of medications should be checked for possible drug interactions with VPA.

VALPROIC ACID LOADING DOSES FOR ACUTE MANIA

Divalproex sodium is FDA approved for the acute treatment of manic or mixed episodes at initial doses of 750 mg daily (~ 10 mg/kg in a 70 kg patient) in divided doses or 25 mg/kg once daily when given as extended-release tablets (e.g., Depakote® ER) and titrated as rapidly as possible to the desired clinical effect.[30-31] After the initial dose of valproic acid for acute mania, treatment doses of valproic acid are 20 mg/kg and are titrated to a clinical response and or a target valproic acid level. The maximum valproic acid dose is 60 mg/kg/daily, but may be exceeded when valproic acid metabolism is increased due to interactions with hepatic enzyme-inducing medications. Titrating the dose of valproic acid upward may be accomplished by increasing the dose by 5–10 mg/kg every 2–4 days or weekly. Without a loading dose and using a slow titration dosing regimen to minimize valproic acid adverse effects, achieving the valproic acid dose and or level that yields a clinical response may take up to several weeks. The antimanic effects of valproic acid are most pronounced within 1–4 days of achieving a serum concentration of 50 mcg/mL or greater.[32] In patients treated with divalproex sodium for acute mania, trough valproic acid levels from 50 to 125 mcg/mL have achieved the desired clinical effects.[30-31] In patients treated with extended-release divalproex sodium for acute mania, slightly higher trough valproic acid levels from 85 to 125 mcg/mL have achieved the desired clinical effects.[30-31] Maintenance valproic acid therapy for initial responses and the prevention of new manic episodes beyond 3–4 weeks are less evidence based and not well-established in controlled clinical trials. Occasionally, the daily dose for maintenance valproic acid therapy may be effective at less than the doses used for acute treatment of mania.

Valproic acid is generally not administered as an oral loading dose due to intolerable gastrointestinal and CNS adverse effects. However, rapid oral loading with oral divalproex sodium has been studied in the management of psychiatric disorders such as mania and has been used safely with minimal adverse effects and a rapid response. Generally, patients can be loaded rapidly with 20-30 mg/kg of divalproex sodium for acute mania or maintenance treatment, administered as the full loading dose on the first day in a single or divided dose or may be administered gradually over 2 days.[33-34] The 2-day rapid divalproex oral loading dose is administered starting with a lower dose on day 1 and the full dose on day 2. Administering the rapid divalproex oral loading dose gradually over 2 days may be preferred over the full dose on the first day because it may cause less gastrointestinal and CNS adverse effects and is easier to tolerate. After the loading dose is complete, the dose should be titrated to achieve a response or a target valproic acid trough level of 50 mcg/mL. Divalproex loading doses of 20 mg/kg or greater generally consistently achieve valproic acid serum levels above 50 mcg/mL.

As a general rule for most drugs, oral loading doses are best administered via liquid dosage forms in order to bypass dissolution—the rate-limiting step of absorption—and achieve faster absorption than tablets and capsules. However, due to the high incidence of valproic acid-induced gastrointestinal adverse effects, valproic acid syrup should not be used for loading doses. In order to minimize gastrointestinal adverse effects, valproic acid loading doses should be administered with the divalproex sodium dosage form (tablets or capsules).

CASE 9: VALPROIC ACID ORAL LOADING DOSES FOR ACUTE MANIA

A 55-year-old, 70-kg, Caucasian man is experiencing agitation, pressured speech, and racing thoughts, and is to be loaded with valproic acid for the management of mania. The medical team would like the patient to receive a rapid valproic acid oral loading dose of 20 mg/kg. Design a rapid valproic acid oral loading dose regimen for this patient.

Answer:

The patient may be started on valproic acid 15 mg/kg on day 1 and then titrated to 20 mg/kg on day 2.

Step 1. Calculate the patient's valproic acid loading dose to begin with 15 mg/kg actual body weight for day 1.

$$\text{Valproic acid loading dose} = (15 \text{ mg})(70 \text{ kg})$$
$$\text{Valproic acid loading dose} = 1,050 \text{ mg}$$

The loading dose for day 1 is 500 mg divalproex sodium twice daily.

Step 2. Calculate the patient's valproic acid loading dose to the target goal of 20 mg/kg actual body weight for day 2.

$$\text{Valproic acid loading dose} = (20 \text{ mg})(70 \text{ kg})$$
$$\text{Valproic acid loading dose} = 1,400 \text{ mg}$$

The loading dose for day 2 may be rounded up to 1,500 mg daily, and may be administered as 500 mg divalproex sodium three times daily or 750 mg twice daily.

Alternatively, the entire divalproex loading dose may be administered on the first day by calculating the patient's valproic acid loading dose to the target goal of 20 mg/kg actual body weight.

$$\text{Valproic acid loading dose} = (20 \text{ mg})(70 \text{ kg})$$
$$\text{Valproic acid loading dose} = 1,400 \text{ mg}$$

The loading dose may be rounded up to 1,500 mg daily and is 500 mg divalproex sodium three times daily or 750 mg twice daily or 1,500 mg as a one-time single dose.

In order to minimize adverse effects, the medical team preferred the 2-day rapid oral loading dose regimen; hence, this patient should be loaded with divalproex sodium 500 mg twice daily for day 1, and 500 mg three times daily, or 750 mg twice daily for day 2. The treatment dose for acute mania will begin on day 3 with a daily dose of 20 mg/kg or 750 mg twice daily titrated upward to a response or to achieve a valproic acid serum trough level of 50 mcg/mL.

CASE 10: VALPROIC ACID ORAL LOADING DOSES USING A 2-DAY REGIMEN FOR ACUTE MANIA

A 43-year-old, 50-kg, Caucasian woman is distractible, agitated, irritable, and becoming aggressive. She is to be loaded with valproic acid for the management of acute mania. The medical team would like the patient to receive a rapid valproic acid oral loading dose of 30 mg/kg over 2 days. Design a rapid valproic acid oral loading dose regimen for this patient.

Answer:

The patient may be started on valproic acid 20 mg/kg on day 1 and then titrated to 30 mg/kg on day 2.

Step 1. Calculate the patient's valproic acid oral loading dose to begin with 20 mg/kg actual body weight for day 1.

$$\text{Valproic acid loading dose} = (20 \text{ mg})(50 \text{ kg})$$
$$\text{Valproic acid loading dose} = 1,000 \text{ mg}$$

The loading dose for day 1 is 500 mg divalproex sodium twice daily.

Step 2. Calculate the patient's loading dose to the target goal of 30 mg/kg actual body weight for day 2.

$$\text{Valproic acid loading dose} = (30 \text{ mg})(50 \text{ kg})$$
$$\text{Valproic acid loading dose} = 1,500 \text{ mg}$$

The loading dose for day 2 is 750 mg divalproex sodium twice daily.

The patient will receive a rapid oral loading dose of valproic acid using the gradual 2-day regimen and will be placed on divalproex sodium tablets 500 mg twice daily for day 1 and 750 mg twice daily for day 2. The treatment dose for acute mania will begin on day 3 with a daily dose of 20 mg/kg or 750 mg twice daily titrated upward to a response and/or to achieve a valproic acid serum trough level of 50 mcg/mL.

CASE 11: VALPROIC ACID ORAL LOADING DOSES USING A 2-DAY REGIMEN FOR ACUTE MANIA

A 66-year-old, 65-kg, African-American man has a history of bipolar disorder and is experiencing a mixed episode with grandiosity and aggressive behavior. The patient is to be loaded with valproic acid for the management of a bipolar mixed episode. The medical team would like the patient to receive a rapid valproic acid oral loading dose of 25 mg/kg over 2 days. Design a rapid valproic acid oral loading dose regimen for this patient.

Answer:

The patient may be started on oral valproic acid 15 mg/kg on day 1 and then titrated to 25 mg/kg on day 2.

Step 1. Calculate the patient's loading dose to begin with 15 mg/kg actual body weight for day 1.

$$\text{Valproic acid loading dose} = (15 \text{ mg})(65 \text{ kg})$$
$$\text{Valproic acid loading dose} = 975 \text{ mg}$$

The valproic acid oral loading dose for day 1 may be rounded up to 1,000 mg and is 500 mg divalproex sodium twice daily.

Step 2. Calculate the patient's valproic acid oral loading dose to the target goal of 25 mg/kg actual body weight for day 2.

$$\text{Valproic acid loading dose} = (25 \text{ mg})(65 \text{ kg})$$
$$\text{Valproic acid loading dose} = 1,625 \text{ mg}$$

The loading dose for day 2 may be rounded down to 1,500 mg and is 750 mg divalproex sodium twice daily.

The patient will receive a rapid oral loading dose of valproic acid using the gradual 2-day regimen and will be placed on divalproex sodium tablets 500 mg twice daily for day 1 and 750 mg twice daily for day 2. The treatment dose for acute mania will begin on day 3 with a daily dose of 20 mg/kg or 750 mg twice daily titrated upward to a response and/or to achieve a valproic acid serum trough level of 50 mcg/mL.

CASE 12: VALPROIC ACID ORAL LOADING DOSES USING EXTENDED-RELEASE DIVALPROEX SODIUM FOR ACUTE MANIA

A 51-year-old, 60-kg, Hispanic man has a history of bipolar disorder, is experiencing grandiosity, is easily agitated and increasingly aggressive, and is exhibiting abusive behavior. The patient is to be loaded with valproic acid for the management of acute mania. The medical team would like the patient to receive a rapid valproic acid oral loading dose with extended-release tablets at 25 mg/kg. Design a rapid valproic acid oral loading dose regimen with extended-release tablets for this patient.

Answer:

The patient may be started on extended-release divalproex sodium 25 mg/kg as a one-time loading dose on day 1.

Step 1. Calculate the patient's loading dose to begin with 25 mg/kg actual body weight for day 1.

$$\text{Valproic acid loading dose} = (25 \text{ mg})(60 \text{ kg})$$
$$\text{Valproic acid loading dose} = 1,500 \text{ mg}$$

The loading dose for day 1 is 1,500 mg divalproex sodium extended-release once daily. The patient may be started on day 2 with a treatment dose of extended-release divalproex sodium.

VALPROIC ACID INTRAVENOUS LOADING DOSES FOR ACUTE MANIA

Intravenous valproic acid has been used effectively for the treatment of manic symptoms.[35-37] The intravenous valproic acid dosage form retains the rapidity of an oral valproic acid loading dose and minimizes the gastrointestinal disturbances from oral loading. Intravenous valproic acid may be more effective than oral valproic acid due in part to a quick saturation of plasma protein binding sites, resulting in higher peak valproic acid serum levels.[35,37] Indeed, according to some reports, intravenous valproic acid may be effective in patients who previously were nonresponsive to oral valproic acid.[35]

Intravenous valproate is not associated with injection site injuries; it is devoid of cardiotoxicity and associated with minimal sedation or respiratory depression. Valproate cannot be administered intramuscularly because it may cause severe muscle tissue damage. The bioavailability of intravenous valproate and oral valproic acid or divalproex sodium is 100 percent, allowing for an easy intravenous to oral switch. Initial doses of intravenous valproate are 20–30 mg/kg/day and should be administered every 6–8 hours.

CASE 13: INTRAVENOUS VALPROATE LOADING DOSES FOR ACUTE MANIA

A 72-year-old, 67-kg, Caucasian male nursing home resident has a history of bipolar disorder and is on quetiapine. The patient is experiencing a manic episode and is known to respond to intravenous valproate for his bouts of mania. The medical team would like to load the patient with intravenous valproate at a dose of 30 mg/kg/day. Design a loading dose regimen for intravenous valproate.

Answer:

Step 1. Calculate the patient's intravenous valproate loading dose at 30 mg/kg actual body weight for day 1.

$$\text{Valproic acid loading dose} = (30 \text{ mg})(67 \text{ kg})$$
$$\text{Valproic acid loading dose} = 2,010 \text{ mg}$$

The loading dose may be rounded down to 2 g daily and is administered as 500 mg intravenous valproate every 6 hours. Each 500 mg dose of intravenous valproate may be administered over 60 minutes or at a rate of less than 20 mg/minute. The patient may be started on day 2 with a treatment dose of divalproex sodium.

REFERENCES

1. Dutta S, Zhang Y. Bioavailability of divalproex extended-release formulation relative to the divalproex delayed-release formulation. *Biopharm Drug Dispos.* 2004;25:345–352.
2. Morton LD, O'Hara KA, Coots BP, Pellock JM. Safety of rapid intravenous valproate infusion in pediatric patients. *Pediatr Neurol.* 2007;36:81–83.
3. Ramsay RE, Cantrell D, Collins SD, et al. Safety and tolerance of rapidly infused Depacon. A randomized trial in subjects with epilepsy. *Epilepsy Res.* 2003;52:189–201.

4. Wheless JW, Vazquez BR, Kanner AM, Ramsay RE, Morton L, Pellock JM. Rapid infusion with valproate sodium is well tolerated in patients with epilepsy. *Neurology*. 2004;63:1507–1508.

5. Bauer LA, Davis R, Wilensky A, Raisys V, Levy RH. Diurnal variation in valproic acid clearance. *Clin Pharmacol Ther*. 1984;35:505–509.

6. Bauer LA, Davis R, Wilensky A, Raisys V, Levy RH. Valproic acid clearance: Unbound fraction and diurnal variation in young and elderly adults. *Clin Pharmacol Ther*. 1985;37:697–700.

7. Klotz U, Antonin KH. Pharmacokinetics and bioavailability of sodium valproate. *Clin Pharmacol Ther*. 1977;21:736–743.

8. Gugler R, von Unruh GE. Clinical pharmacokinetics of valproic acid. *Clin Pharmacokinet*. 1980;5:67–83.

9. Levy RH, Cenraud B, Loiseau P, et al. Meal-dependent absorption of enteric-coated sodium valproate. *Epilepsia*. 1980;21:273–280.

10. Zaccara G, Messori A, Moroni F. Clinical pharmacokinetics of valproic acid—1988. *Clin Pharmacokinet*. 1988;15:367–389.

11. Benet L, Sheiner L. Design and optimization of dosage regimens: Pharmacokinetic data. In: Goodman-Gilman A, ed. *The Pharmacological Basis of Therapeutics*. New York: Macmillan; 1985:1663–1733.

12. Monaco F, Piredda S, Mutani R, Mastropaolo C, Tondi M. The free fraction of valproic acid in tears, saliva, and cerebrospinal fluid. *Epilepsia*. 1982;23:23–26.

13. Nau H, Rating D, Koch S, Hauser I, Helge H. Valproic acid and its metabolites: placental transfer, neonatal pharmacokinetics, transfer via mother's milk and clinical status in neonates of epileptic mothers. *J Pharmacol Exp Ther*.1981;219:768–777.

14. Gomez Bellver MJ, Garcia Sanchez MJ, Alonso Gonzalez AC, Santos Buelga D, Dominguez-Gil A. Plasma protein binding kinetics of valproic acid over a broad dosage range: therapeutic implications. *J Clin Pharm Ther*. 1993;18:191–197.

15. Lai ML, Huang JD. Dual effect of valproic acid on the pharmacokinetics of phenytoin. *Biopharm Drug Dispos*. 1993;14:365–370.

16. Nau H, Loscher W. Valproic acid and metabolites: pharmacological and toxicological studies. *Epilepsia*. 1984;25(Suppl 1):S14–22.

17. Venkataraman V, Wheless JW. Safety of rapid intravenous infusion of valproate loading doses in epilepsy patients. *Epilepsy Res*. 1999;35:147–153.

18. Perucca E, Hebdige S, Frigo GM, Gatti G, Lecchini S, Crema A. Interaction between phenytoin and valproic acid: plasma protein binding and metabolic effects. *Clin Pharmacol Ther*. 1980;28:779–789.

19. Frigo GM, Lecchini S, Gatti G, Perucca E, Crema A. Modification of phenytoin clearance by valproic acid in normal subjects. *Br J Clin Pharmacol*. 1979;8:553–556.

20. Riva R, Albani F, Contin M, et al. Time-dependent interaction between phenytoin and valproic acid. *Neurology*. 1985;35:510–515.

21. Pisani F, Di Perri R, Perucca E, Richens A. Interaction of lamotrigine with sodium valproate. *Lancet*. 1993;341:1224.

22. Tsanaclis LM, Allen J, Perucca E, Routledge PA, Richens A. Effect of valproate on free plasma phenytoin concentrations. *Br J Clin Pharmacol*. 1984;18:17–20.

23. Bauer LA, Harris C, Wilensky AJ, Raisys VA, Levy RH. Ethosuximide kinetics: Possible interaction with valproic acid. *Clin Pharmacol Ther*. 1982;31:741–745.

24. Klotz U, Rapp T, Muller WA. Disposition of valproic acid in patients with liver disease. *Eur J Clin Pharmacol*. 1978;13:55–60.

25. Irvine-Meek JM, Hall KW, Otten NH, Leroux M, Budnik D, Seshia SS. Pharmacokinetic study of valproic acid in a neonate. *Pediatr Pharmacol (New York)*. 1982;2:317–21.

26. Hall K, Otten N, Irvine-Meek J, et al. First-dose and steady-state pharmacokinetics of valproic acid in children with seizures. *Clin Pharmacokinet*. 1983;8:447–455.

27. Sanchez-Alcaraz A, Quintana MB, Lopez E, Rodriguez I. Valproic acid clearance in children with epilepsy. *J Clin Pharm Ther*. 1998;23:31–34.

28. Bowdle AT, Patel IH, Levy RH, Wilensky AJ. Valproic acid dosage and plasma protein binding and clearance. *Clin Pharmacol Ther*. 1980;28:486–492.

29. Perucca E, Grimaldi R, Gatti G, Pirracchio S, Crema F, Frigo GM. Pharmacokinetics of valproic acid in the elderly. *Br J Clin Pharmacol*. 1984;17:665–669.

30. Lexi-Comp, Inc. Valproic acid drug information. In: Rose BD, ed. *UpToDate Medicine*. Wellesley, MA; 2014.

31. McEvoy GK, Snow ED, eds. *AHFS: Drug Information*. Bethesda, MD: American Society of Health-System Pharmacists; 2012:2317–2325.

32. Keck PE Jr, McElroy SL, Tugrul KC, Bennett JA. Valproate oral loading in the treatment of acute mania. *J Clin Psychiatry*. 1993;54(8):305–308.

33. Ghaleiha A, Haghighi M, Sharifmehr M, Jahangard L, Ahmadpanah M, Bajoghli H, Holsboer-Trachsler E, Brand S. Oral loading of sodium valproate compared to intravenous loading and oral maintenance in acutely manic bipolar patients. *Neuropsychobiology*. 2014;70(1):29–35.

34. McElroy SL, Keck PE Jr, Tugrul KC, Bennett JA. Valproate as a loading treatment in acute mania. *Neuropsychobiology*. 1993;27(3):146–149.

35. Grunze H, Erfurth A, Amann B, Giupponi G, Kammerer C, Walden J. Intravenous valproate loading in acutely manic and depressed bipolar I patients. *J Clin Psychopharmacol*. 1999;19(4):303–309.

36. Duggal HS, Jagadheesan K, Gupta S, Basu S, Akhtar S, Nizamie HS. Intravenous valproate: a new perspective in the treatment of manic symptoms. *Indian J Psychiatry*. 2002;44(2):173–176.

37. Jagadheesan K, Duggal H, Gupta S, Basu S, Ranjan S, Sandil R, Akhtar S, Nizamie SH. Acute antimanic efficacy and safety of intravenous valproate loading therapy: an open-label study. *Neuropsychobiology*. 2003;47(2):90–93.

20

Vancomycin

DENISE E. RICCOBONO, PharmD

MARICELLE O. MONTEAGUDO-CHU, PharmD, BCPS

Vancomycin is a glycopeptide antibiotic, approved by the FDA in 1958, which is slowly bactericidal against most gram-positive organisms. It is active against *Staphylococci* (including penicillin- and oxacillin-resistant strains), *Streptococci, Enterococci,* and other gram-positive organisms. It exerts its bactericidal effect by complexing with the D-alanyl-D-alanine portion of the peptide precursor units on the outer surface of the cell membrane and interferes with cell wall synthesis.

During the first few decades of clinical use, vancomycin demonstrated consistent activity against gram-positive bacteria and became the drug of choice to treat most methicillin-resistant *Staphylococcus aureus* (MRSA) infections. However, due to the emergence and increased prevalence of vancomycin-resistant *Enterococci* (VRE), vancomycin intermediate (VISA) and resistant *S. aureus* (VRSA), and heterogenous VISA (hVISA), our confidence in vancomycin as a reliable bactericidal agent has decreased, motivating a renewed interest in appropriate utilization and optimal dosing of vancomycin.[1-3]

DOSING

Due to limited pharmacokinetic studies done when vancomycin was first approved in the late 1950s, it appears that the original intravenous dosing of 1,000 mg every 12 hours or 500 mg every 6 hours was derived arbitrarily. Also, the serum therapeutic ranges accepted for vancomycin of 5–10 mg/L were originally established as guidelines for dosage adjustments in patients with renal failure and was not validated by clinical outcomes. Because vancomycin was thought to be a time-dependent killer and sensitive vancomycin MICs (minimum inhibitory concentration) were ≤4 mg/L, these values were considered acceptable.[2,3]

It is more recently recommended that weight-based dosing be used to dose vancomycin, especially in more moderate/severe infections, and that dosing intervals be adjusted according to renal function.[1] Depending on severity of infection, doses for patients with normal renal function range from 10–15 mg/kg administered intravenously every 8–12 hours. In clinical practice, doses are derived using weight-based dosing via dosing nomograms or by pharmacokinetic calculations. For the purpose of this chapter, we will be discussing vancomycin pharmacokinetic calculations for the adult patient.

PHARMACOKINETICS/PHARMACODYNAMICS

Vancomycin is poorly absorbed from the gastrointestinal tract so it is only given intravenously when treating systemic infections (exception: treatment of *Clostridium difficile*–associated colitis with oral vancomycin). Vancomycin serum concentration-time profile has been described using one-, two-, and three-compartment pharmacokinetic models. The half-life of the first distributive phase is approximately 0.4 hours where as the half-life of the second distributive phase is about 1.6 hours. Plasma protein binding varies and ranges from 30–55 percent.[1,3,4] The volume of distribution is variable and depends on many things such as fluid status, disease state, and age; range is from 0.4–1.0 L/kg.[5-8] The elimination half-life is approximately 6 hours, and can be prolonged up to 7 days in patients with renal failure. Approximately 70–90 percent of the drug is excreted unchanged in the kidney by glomerular filtration. The remainder is excreted by tubular secretion and nonrenal routes.[1,3]

Pharmacokinetic and pharmacodynamic studies have concluded that maximizing the area under the curve/MIC (AUC/MIC) ratio when dosing vancomycin gives optimal efficacy for treating *S. aureus* infections. An AUC/MIC ratio of ≥400 has been advocated as a target to achieve clinical effectiveness with vancomycin against *S. aureus*.[1,9] A higher target value may be necessary with higher bacterial density at site of infection and may vary depending on site of infection.[1,10]

The susceptibility breakpoint of vancomycin for *S. aureus*, set by the Clinical and Laboratory Standards Institute (CLSI), is 2 mg/L, meaning that all *S. aureus* isolates with MICs of 2 mg/L or less are susceptible to vancomycin, and MICs above 2 are intermediate or resistant. Despite these breakpoints, some reports have suggested that patients infected with *S. aureus* isolates with vancomycin MICs of 1–2 mg/L are less likely to have treatment success with vancomycin compared with those who have lower MICs.[1,11-16] Studies have also suggested that low vancomycin serum trough levels (<10 mg/L) may predict therapeutic failure and even have the potential to contribute to the emergence of hVISA and VISA.[1,13,17] For these reasons, it is recommended by current guidelines that vancomycin trough concentrations should be maintained above 10 mg/L and, for complicated infections, 15–20 mg/L.[1] Trough concentrations in this range should be able to achieve AUC/MIC ratio of ≥400 if the MIC ≤1 mg/L. When vancomycin MIC for *S. aureus* is ≥1.5 mg/L, treatment with an alternative agent (other than vancomycin) may be necessary.

PHARMACOKINETIC CALCULATIONS

Vancomycin pharmacokinetics are complex and although they are best described by a two- or three-compartment model, in the clinical setting it is more practical (due to limited sampling) to dose and monitor vancomycin using one-compartment model kinetics.

Challenges associated with calculating population pharmacokinetics include the following[18]:

1. selecting the best dosing weight

2. estimating the vancomycin clearance from creatinine clearance (CrCl)

3. determining the appropriate weight to estimate CrCl

4. estimating appropriate CrCl in patients with diminished muscle mass and the elderly (e.g., SCr <0.7)

5. determining volume of distribution which can be highly variable

CLEARANCE

Vancomycin is eliminated primarily in the kidney via glomerular filtration, and its clearance is correlated with the patient's CrCl. In multiple studies, the vancomycin clearance has been shown to be approximately 70–90 percent of CrCl.[3,4,6,7] The first step in calculating a vancomycin dose is to calculate the patient's weight parameters and estimate the patient's CrCl. Then, estimate the patient's vancomycin clearance (Cl_{vanco}).

Equation 1[19]:   Males: IBW = 2.3 × (inches >60) + 50
Females: IBW = 2.3 × (inches >60) + 45.5

where IBW = ideal body weight (kg).

For the purposes of this chapter, persons whose total body weight is >120 percent above their ideal body weight, adjusted body weight (ABW) will be used to calculate CrCl. If total body weight is less than ideal body weight, use total body weight instead of ideal body weight for the calculation.

Equation 2:   ABW = (0.4 × (TBW – IBW)) + IBW

where ABW = adjusted body weight (kg) and TBW = total body weight (kg).

Equation 3[20]: CrCl (mL/min) using Cockcroft Gault (CG):

$$\text{Males: } \frac{(140 - \text{Age}) \times \text{IBW}}{72 \times \text{SCr}}$$

$$\text{Females: } \frac{(140 - \text{Age}) \times \text{IBW} \times 0.85}{72 \times \text{SCr}}$$

where SCr = serum creatinine (mg/dL).

Equation 4: CL_{vanco} = (70% to 90%) × CrCL

where

CL_{vanco} = vancomycin clearance (L/hr)

CrCl = creatinine clearance (L/hr)

Certain patients have low creatinine excretion for age and body weight due to low muscle mass or muscle atrophy. Normal SCr is approximately >0.7 mg/dL. In these patients whose SCr is below normal, SCr maybe falsely low and if it is used to calculate CrCl using CG, it can give an artificially high CrCl. Those who are likely to have falsely low SCr include persons who are malnourished (albumin <3.0 g/dL), bedbound (such as ventilator patients or paraplegics), elderly (≥65 years), and those on chronic steroids or those with certain chronic diseases (such as muscular wasting diseases).[2,20] In clinical practice, practitioners frequently round up the SCr to a normal SCr of 0.8 or 1.0 mg/dL. In certain patients, rounding the SCr up to 1.0 mg/dL may result in an underestimation of the patients CrCl and can lead to administration of a suboptimal dose (underdosing). Underdosing can be potentially dangerous in critically ill or septic patients. For patients fitting the previous descriptions, the authors of this chapter recommend increasing the SCr to 0.8 mg/dL, and in the elderly ≥65 years, to increase SCr to 1.0 mg/dL (for purposes of calculating CrCl using CG). In these patients, it is important to monitor renal function closely and to obtain vancomycin serum levels. A patient whose normal SCr is 0.4 may be in renal failure or may be dehydrated if their SCr suddenly increases to 1.0, for example.

VOLUME OF DISTRIBUTION

Vancomycin's volume of distribution (V_d) ranges from 0.4 to 1.0 L/kg; however, V_d is variable and depends on many patient factors. Assessing V_d is often the most difficult step. Independent factors shown to affect V_d are gender, age, and weight. Females, elderly, and obese patients are known to have a higher vancomycin V_d per IBW.[5] Other factors such as fluid status (dehydration vs. fluid overload), disease state (e.g., hematologic malignancy), or illness severity (critically ill, septic shock) also affect the distribution of vancomycin.[21-24] Vancomycin V_d as high as 1.68 L/kg has been described in critically ill ICU patients.[22]

When calculating vancomycin population V_d, a number of methods can be utilized. Some use-specific formulas (see the following examples) and others use an average of 0.7 L/kg. The patient's total body weight is used for the calculation, unless otherwise specified. For the purpose of this chapter, we will use the V_d formula by Matzke (median value) seen in the following chart. If the patient's fluid status is known to be abnormal (dehydration or fluid overload), instead of using any equation, we will use either the low or high end of the V_d range (0.4–1.0 L/kg),because equations do not take volume status into account.

CrCl	>60 mL/min	10–60 mL/min	<10 mL/min
Mean V_d	0.72 L/kg	0.89 L/kg	0.9 L/kg
Median V_d	0.56 L/kg	0.84 L/kg	0.84 L/kg

Data from Matzke GR et al.[6]

Ducharme and colleagues[5] provide the following calculations:

Men: V_d(L) = 0.44(IBW) + 0.26(EBW) + 0.32(age)
Women: V_d(L) = 0.48(IBW) + 0.33(EBW) + 0.25(age)

where EBW = excess body weight (kg); (EBW = TBW – IBW).

The following equation comes from Rushing and Ambrose.[25]

$$V_d(L) = 0.17(\text{age}) + 0.22(\text{TBW}) + 15$$

ELIMINATION RATE CONSTANT AND ELIMINATION HALF-LIFE

After calculating the CrCl, Cl_{vanco}, and V_d, the next step is to calculate the elimination rate constant (K) and elimination half-life ($T_{1/2}$). Vancomycin dosing interval usually approximates the $T_{1/2}$.

Equation 5: $$K = \frac{Cl_{vanco}\ (L/hr)}{V_d}$$

where K = elimination rate constant (h^{-1}) and V_d = volume of distribution (L).

Equation 6: $$T_{1/2} = \frac{0.693}{K}$$

where $T_{1/2}$ = elimination half-life (h).

STEADY STATE

Steady state is the point at which the rate of drug administration is equal to the rate of drug elimination and the concentration of drug is constant. This time is the most optimal for obtaining vancomycin levels. It is based on the drug's half-life and occurs after approximately 4–5 half-lives.

Vancomycin levels should be obtained at steady state. Vancomycin peak levels should be obtained 1 hour or more after the dose has finished infusing in order to allow adequate time for drug distribution, and trough levels should be obtained approximately 0–30 minutes before the next dose.

LOADING DOSE

Administration of a vancomycin loading dose is an important step in trying to achieve a serum concentration that approaches the steady-state maximum concentration. It ensures that we achieve an adequate AUC on day 1 of therapy.[2] Attaining steady state is especially important for those patients who have a large volume of distribution or who have a diminished CrCl and long $T_{1/2}$. The target peak or initial plasma concentration (C°) is 30–40 mg/L.

Equation 7:
$$LD = C° \times V_d$$

where LD = loading dose (mg) and C° = initial plasma concentration (mg/L).

Alternatively, in clinical practice many people use 25–30 mg/kg loading doses in critically ill patients.[1]

MAINTENANCE DOSE

After calculating a loading dose, the next step is to calculate a maintenance dose that will give you an approximate peak and trough that you desire (when at steady state). In general, you will want your vancomycin peak to be between 25–40 mg/L and your trough to be 10–20 mg/L. For complicated, severe, or deep-seated infections, it is recommended to aim for a trough of 15–20 mg/L.

Equation 8[26]:
$$C_{SSmax} = \frac{(Dose/t') \times (1 - e^{-Kt'})}{V_d \times K \times (1 - e^{-K\tau})}$$

where C_{SSmax} = maximum concentration at steady state (mg/L); Dose = dose in mg*; t' = infusion time in hours; and τ = dosing interval in hours. *When calculating doses, it is best to round to the nearest 250 mg, and rounding up is preferred.

Equation 9:
$$C_{SSmin} = C_{SSmax} \times (e^{-K(\tau - t')})$$

where C_{SSmin} = minimum concentration at steady state (mg/L).

Vancomycin is administered intravenously and is compatible in normal saline (0.9% sodium chloride) and dextrose 5% water (D5W). If vancomycin is administered too quickly or if it is too concentrated, it is known to cause a histamine-like reaction known as red-man syndrome and may also cause thrombophlebitis. If long-term therapy is required or if higher concentrations are used, it is necessary for the patient to have a central line. Usual concentrations approximate 5 mg/mL and historically have been 1,000 mg in 100 mL infused over 1 hour, but vary per institution. At the author's institution, 500 mg per 100 mL infused over 1 hour; 750 mg per 150 mL infused over 1.5 hours; 1,000–1,500 mg in 250 mL infused over 2 hours; and >1,500 mg in 500 mL infused over ≥3 hours.

CASE STUDIES

CASE 1

AJ is a 56-year-old female who is brought into the ER by EMS with shortness of breath, chest pain, and cough × 7 days. She went to her PMD a few days ago for this problem and was started on levofloxacin, however it was not helping and she was feeling worse. In the ER her temperature was 104° F and her WBC was 17,000 cells/mm³. CXR shows right lower lobe infiltrates. AJ has hypertension, diabetes, and hepatitis C (with moderate ascites). ER attending wants to start the patient on vancomycin (along with other antibiotics) and asks you for a dose.

Height: 5′3″

Weight: 130 lbs

SCr: 1.2 mg/dL

Step 1: Calculate CrCl and vancomycin clearance.

$$IBW = (2.3 \times 3) + 45.5 \qquad TBW = \textbf{59 kg}$$
$$IBW = \textbf{52.4 kg}$$

Because patient's weight is <120 percent IBW, use IBW for calculating CrCl.

$$CrCl = \frac{(140 - 56) \times 52.4 \times 0.85}{72 \times 1.2}$$

$$= 43.3 \text{ mL/min, or } \textbf{2.6 L/hr}$$

Note: To convert from mL/min to L/hr, multiply by 0.06.

Calculate vancomycin clearance (mean = 80%).

$$\textbf{Cl}_{vanco} = (70\% \text{ to } 90\%) \times CrCl \text{ L/hr}$$
$$= 0.8 \times 2.6 \text{ L/hr}$$
$$= \textbf{2.08 L/hr}$$

Step 2: Calculate V_d.

Multiple formulas can be used to calculate V_d, however, none of them take fluid status into consideration. Because we know that fluid accumulation can affect V_d, and this patient has ascites (increased volume status), it may be more appropriate to choose a larger V_d of 0.9 L/kg in this example.

$$V_d = 0.9 \times TBW$$
$$= 0.9 \times 59$$
$$= \textbf{53.1 L}$$

Step 3: Calculate K and $T_{1/2}$.

$$K = \frac{Cl_{vanco} \text{ (L/hr)}}{V_d \text{ (L)}}$$

$$= \frac{2.08 \text{ L/hr}}{53.1 \text{ L}}$$

$$= \textbf{0.039 h}^{-1}$$

$$T_{1/2} = \frac{0.693}{K \text{ (h}^{-1})}$$

$$= \frac{0.693}{0.039}$$

$$= \textbf{17.8 h}$$

Step 4: Calculate a loading dose.

$$LD \text{ (mg)} = C° \text{ (mg/L)} \times V_d \text{(L)}$$
$$= 30 \times 53.1$$
$$= 1,593 \text{ mg}$$

Round to **1,750 mg** given as a one-time dose.

Step 5: Calculate a maintenance dose.

Based on population parameters, pick a dose that you think the patient will need and then plug it into MD formula, adjusting as necessary. For patient AJ, because we are treating pneumonia, we are aiming to achieve a vancomycin trough of 15–20 mg/L. We will start out trying a dose of 1,250 mg (infused over 2 hours) given every 24 hours.

$$C_{SSmax} = \frac{(Dose/t') \times (1 - e^{-Kt'})}{V_d \times K \times (1 - e^{-K\tau})}$$

$$= \frac{(1,250 / 2) \times (1 - e^{-0.039 \times 2})}{53.1 \times 0.039 \times (1 - e^{-0.039 \times 24})}$$

$$= \frac{(625) \times (1 - 0.92)}{53.1 \times 0.039 \times (1 - 0.39)}$$

$$= \textbf{39.68 mg/L}$$

$$C_{SSmin} = C_{SSmax} \times e^{-K(\tau-t')}$$
$$= 39.68 \times e^{-0.039 \times (24-2)}$$
$$= 16.82 \approx \textbf{17 mg/L}$$

So if we start this patient on 1,250 mg vancomycin given every 24 hours, we can expect approximately a peak of 40 mg/L and a trough of 17 mg/L, which is within our target range.

CASE 2

CK is a 35-year-old male who lives in a nursing home and is admitted to the hospital for altered mental status and fever and was started on piperacillin/tazobactam for empiric treatment of a urinary tract infection. On day 2 the urine culture came back positive for gram-positive cocci. Repeat blood cultures remained negative. Patient has a PMH of paraplegia s/p gun wound three years ago. PMD wants to start the patient on vancomycin until the cultures are finalized and asks you for a dose.

Height: 5′10″

Weight: 145 lbs

SCr: 0.4 mg/dL

Albumin: 2.5 g/dL

Step 1: Calculate CrCl and vancomycin clearance.

$$IBW = (2.3 \times 10) + 50 \qquad TBW = \textbf{65.9 kg}$$
$$IBW = 73 \text{ kg}$$

Because patient's weight is <IBW, use TBW for calculating CrCl. With a SCr <0.7 mg/dL for a bedbound patient with an albumin of 2.5 g/dL, round up the SCr to 0.8 mg/dL to compensate for the low muscle mass.

$$CrCl = \frac{(140 - 35) \times 65.9}{72 \times 0.8}$$
$$= 120.1 \text{ mL/min, or } \textbf{7.2 L/hr}$$

Note: To convert from mL/min to L/hr, multiply by 0.06.

Calculate vancomycin clearance: (mean = 80%).

$$Cl_{vanco} = (70\% \text{ to } 90\%) \times CrCl \text{ L/hr}$$
$$= 0.8 \times 7.2 \text{ L/hr}$$
$$= \textbf{5.8 L/hr}$$

Step 2: Calculate V_d.

Derived from Matzke's calculations:

$$V_d = 0.56 \times TBW$$
$$= 0.56 \times 65.9 \text{ kg}$$
$$= \textbf{36.90 L}$$

Step 3: Calculate K and $T_{1/2}$.

$$K = \frac{Cl_{vanco} \text{ (L/hr)}}{V_d \text{ (L)}}$$

$$= \frac{5.8 \text{ L/hr}}{36.90 \text{ L}}$$

$$= \textbf{0.157 h}^{-1}$$

$$T_{1/2} = \frac{0.693}{K \text{ (h}^{-1})}$$

$$= \frac{0.693}{0.157}$$

$$= \textbf{4.4 h}$$

Step 4: Calculate a loading dose.

$$LD \text{ (mg)} = C° \text{ (mg/L)} \times V_d \text{ (L)}$$
$$= 30 \times 36.90$$
$$= 1,107 \text{ mg}$$

Round to **1,250 mg** given as a one-time dose.

Step 5: Calculate a maintenance dose.

Based on population parameters, pick a dose that you think the patient will need and then plug it into the MD formula, adjusting as necessary. For patient CK, because we are treating a complicated UTI, we are aiming to achieve a vancomycin trough of approximately 10–15 mg/L. We will start out trying a dose of 1,000 mg (infused over 2 hour) given every 8 hour.

$$C_{SSmax} = \frac{(Dose/t') \times (1 - e^{-Kt'})}{V_d \times K \times (1 - e^{-K\tau})}$$

$$= \frac{(1,000/2) \times (1 - e^{-0.157 \times 2})}{36.90 \times 0.157 \times (1 - e^{-0.157 \times 8})}$$

$$= \frac{(500) \times (1 - 0.73)}{36.90 \times 0.157 \times (1 - 0.28)}$$

$$= 32.4 \text{ mg/L}$$

$$C_{SSmin} = C_{SSmax} \times e^{-K(\tau-t')}$$
$$= 32.4 \times e^{-0.157 \times (8-2)}$$
$$= 12.6 \approx \textbf{13 mg/L}$$

So if we start this patient on 1,000 mg vancomycin given every 8 hours, we can expect approximately a peak of 32 mg/L and a trough of 13 mg/L, which is within the target range.

CASE 3

BA is a 48-year-old male who lives in a nursing home and is admitted to the hospital for fever, chills, and worsening left leg cellulitis. Blood cultures drawn in the nursing home the day before were positive for gram-positive cocci in clusters. In the ER his temperature was 101°F and his WBC was 20,000 cells/mm³. Patient has a PMH of diabetes, hypertension, CAD, and CVA. The ID consultant wants to start the patient on vancomycin and asks you for a dose.

Height: 5′8″

Weight: 200 lbs

SCr: 1.4 mg/dL

Step 1: Calculate CrCl and vancomycin clearance.

$$IBW = (2.3 \times 8) + 50 \qquad TBW = \textbf{90.9 kg}$$
$$IBW = 68.4 \text{ kg}$$
$$90.9/68.4 = 133\%$$

Because patient's weight is >120 percent IBW, use ABW for calculating CrCl.

$$ABW \text{ (kg)} = (0.4 \times (TBW - IBW)) + IBW$$
$$= \textbf{77.4 kg}$$

$$CrCl = \frac{(140 - 48) \times 77.4}{72 \times 1.4}$$

$$= 70.6 \text{ mL/min or 4.2 L/hr}$$

Note: To convert from mL/min to L/hr, multiply by 0.06.

Calculate vancomycin clearance (median = 80%).

$$Cl_{vanco} = (70\% \text{ to } 90\%) \times CrCl \text{ L/hr}$$
$$= 0.8 \times 4.2 \text{ L/hr}$$
$$= \textbf{3.4 L/hr}$$

Step 2: Calculate V_d.

Derived from Matzke's calculations:

$$V_d = 0.56 \times TBW$$
$$= 0.56 \times 90.9 \text{ kg}$$
$$= \textbf{50.9 L}$$

Step 3: Calculate K and $T_{1/2}$.

$$K = \frac{Cl_{vanco} \text{ (L/hr)}}{V_d \text{ (L)}}$$

$$= \frac{3.4 \text{ L/hr}}{50.9 \text{ L}}$$

$$= \textbf{0.067 h}^{-1}$$

$$T_{1/2} = \frac{0.693}{K \text{ (h}^{-1})}$$

$$= \frac{0.693}{0.067}$$

$$= \textbf{10.34 h}$$

Step 4: Calculate a loading dose.

$$LD \text{ (mg)} = C° \text{ (mg/L)} \times V_d \text{(L)}$$
$$= 30 \times 50.9$$
$$= 1,527 \text{ mg}$$

Round to **1,500 mg** given as a one-time dose.

Step 5: Calculate a maintenance dose.

Based on population parameters, pick a dose that you think the patient will need and then plug into MD formula. Adjust as necessary. For patient BA, because we are treating severe cellulitis with bacteremia in a diabetic patient (decreased tissue perfusion of vancomycin), we are aiming to achieve a vancomycin trough of approximately 15–20 mg/L. We will start out trying a dose of 1,000 mg (infused over 2 hours) given every 12 hours.

$$C_{SSmax} = \frac{(Dose/t') \times (1 - e^{-K t'})}{V_d \times K \times (1 - e^{-K\tau})}$$

$$= \frac{(1000/2) \times (1 - e^{-0.067 \times 2})}{50.9 \times 0.067 \times (1 - e^{-0.067 \times 12})}$$

$$= \frac{(500) \times (1 - 0.87)}{50.9 \times 0.067 \times (1 - 0.45)}$$

$$= 34.57 \text{ mg/L}$$

$$C_{SSmin} = C_{SSmax} \times e^{-K(\tau - t')}$$
$$= 34.57 \times e^{-0.067 \times (12 - 2)}$$
$$= 17.69 \approx 18 \text{ mg/L}$$

So if we start this patient on 1,000 mg vancomycin given every 12 hours, we can expect a peak of approximately 35 mg/L and a trough of 18 mg/L, which is within our target range.

PATIENT-SPECIFIC PHARMACOKINETICS

Equation 10: $\qquad K = \dfrac{\ln (C1/C2)}{\Delta t} \quad$ or $\quad K = \dfrac{\ln (C1/C2)}{\tau - (t' + t^2 + t^3)}$

where

C1 = observed peak

C2 = observed trough

Δ t = difference in time between C1 and C2 within the same dosing interval

τ = dosing interval

t' = infusion time

t^2 = time between peak drawn and the end of the infusion

t^3 = time between trough drawn and true trough

Equation 11: $\qquad C_{peak} = C1 \times e^{(+K \times t2)}$

where C_{peak} = true peak (end of vanco infusion).

Equation 12: $\qquad C_{trough} = C2 \times e^{(-K \times t3)}$

where C_{trough} = true trough.

Equation 13: $\qquad V_d = \dfrac{(Dose/t') \times (1 - e^{-Kt'})}{K \times [C_{peak} - (C_{trough} \times e^{-Kt'})]}$

CASE 1 (CONT.)

On day 4 of therapy, the team decides to check vancomycin levels for AJ. Because estimated $T_{1/2}$ was 18 hours, 5 ×18 hours = 90 hours = 3.75 days; it should now be at steady state. At this point, respiratory cultures have returned positive for MRSA with a vancomycin MIC of 1 mg/L. AJ is clinically responding, fever is improving with decreased respiratory symptoms, and WBC is trending downward. Labs are stable, and after hydration, SCr has decreased to 0.9 mg/dL.

Height = 5′3″

Weight = 130 lbs

SCr = 0.9 mg/dL

AJ receives vancomycin 1,250 mg once daily at 10:00 AM. A peak level drawn on day 4 of therapy at 2:00 PM was 30.5 mg/L and a trough level drawn on day 5 of therapy at 8:30 AM was 13.0 mg/L.

QUESTION

What is the patient's true peak and trough? Is this dose adequate to achieve a trough of ≥15 mg/L? If not, calculate a dose to achieve this target trough.

Answer:

Step 1: Calculate patient-specific K.

$$K = \frac{\ln (C1/C2)}{\Delta t} \qquad \text{or} \qquad K = \frac{\ln (C1/C2)}{\tau - (t' + t^2 + t^3)}$$

$$K = \frac{\ln (30.5/13.0)}{\text{(diff. between 2 PM and 8:30 AM)}} \qquad \text{or} \quad K = \frac{\ln (30.5/13.0)}{24 - (2 + 2 + 1.5)}$$

$$K = \frac{0.85}{18.5 \text{ h}}$$

$$= \textbf{0.046 h}^{-1}$$

Step 2: Calculate true peak and true trough.

$$C_{peak} = C1 \times e^{(+K \times t2)}$$
$$= 30.5 \times e^{(+0.046 \times 2)}$$
$$= \textbf{33.44 mg/L}$$

$$C_{trough} = C2 \times e^{(-K \times t3)}$$
$$= 13.0 \times e^{(-0.046 \times 1.5)}$$
$$= \textbf{12.13 mg/L}$$

Step 3: Calculate true V_d, Cl, and $T_{1/2}$.

$$V_d = \frac{(Dose/t') \times (1 - e^{-Kt'})}{K \times [C_{peak} - (C_{trough} \times e^{-Kt'})]}$$

$$= \frac{(1,250/2) \times (1 - e^{-0.046 \times 2})}{0.046 \times [33.44 - (12.13 \times e^{-0.046 \times 2})]}$$

$$= \frac{(625) \times (1 - 0.91)}{0.046 \times (33.44 - 11.04)}$$

$$= \textbf{54.6 L}$$

$$Cl_{vanco} = V_d \times K$$
$$= 54.6 \text{ L} \times 0.046 \text{ h}^{-1}$$
$$= \textbf{2.5 L/h}$$

$$T_{1/2} = \frac{0.693}{0.046}$$
$$= \textbf{15.1 h}$$

Step 4: Calculate new vancomycin dose using patient-specific PK. We will start by trying 1,000 mg every 18 hours (infused over 2 hours).

$$C_{SSmax} = \frac{(Dose/t') \times (1 - e^{-Kt'})}{V_d \times K \times (1 - e^{-K\tau})}$$

$$= \frac{(1,000/2) \times (1 - e^{-0.046 \times 2})}{54.6 \times 0.046 \times (1 - e^{-0.046 \times 18})}$$

$$= \frac{(500) \times (1 - 0.91)}{54.6 \times 0.046 \times (1 - 0.44)}$$

$$= \textbf{31.9 mg/L}$$

$$C_{SSmin} = C_{SSmax} \times e^{-K(\tau - t')}$$
$$= 31.9 \times e^{-0.046 \times 16}$$
$$= 31.9 \times 0.48$$
$$= \textbf{15.3 mg/L}$$

CASE 2 (CONT.)

On day 3 of therapy, the team decides to check vancomycin levels for CK. If estimated $T_{1/2}$ was 4.4 hours, 5 × 4.4 hours = 22 hours ≈ 1 day, it should now be at steady state. Urine cultures return and are growing MRSA and E. coli. Blood cultures remain negative and patient is clinically responding. Labs have remained stable.

Height = 5′10″

Weight = 145 lbs

SCr = 0.4 mg/dL

CK receives vancomycin 1,000 mg every 8 hours at 6:00 AM, 2:00 PM, and 10:00 PM. A peak level drawn on day 3 of therapy at 5:00 PM was 40.8 mg/L and a trough level drawn on day 3 of therapy at 1:30 PM was 29.5 mg/L.

What is the patient's true peak and trough? Is this dose adequate to achieve a trough of 10–15 mg/L? If not, calculate a dose to achieve this target trough.

Answer:

Step 1: Calculate patient-specific K.

Because the peak and trough were not in the same line, you will have to move over the trough level from 1:30 PM to 9:30 PM in order to calculate the Δt. Because it is steady state, this can be done.

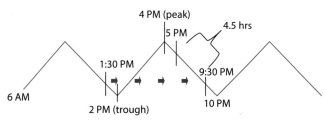

$$K = \frac{\ln (C1/C2)}{\Delta t} \quad \text{or} \quad K = \frac{\ln (C1/C2)}{\tau - (t' + t^2 + t^3)}$$

$$K = \frac{\ln (40.8/29.5)}{(\text{diff. between 5 PM \& 9:30 PM})} \quad \text{or} \quad \frac{\ln (40.8/29.5)}{8 - (2 + 1 + 0.5)}$$

$$K = \frac{0.32}{4.5 \text{ h}}$$

$$= \textbf{0.071 h}^{-1}$$

Step 2: Calculate true peak and true trough.

$$C_{peak} = C1 \times e^{(+K \times t2)}$$
$$= 40.8 \times e^{(+0.071 \times 1)}$$
$$= \textbf{43.8 mg/L}$$

$$C_{trough} = C2 \times e^{(-K \times t3)}$$
$$= 29.5 \times e^{(-0.071 \times 0.5)}$$
$$= \textbf{28.5 mg/L}$$

Step 3: Calculate true V_d, Cl, and $T_{1/2}$.

$$V_d = \frac{(Dose/t') \times (1 - e^{-Kt'})}{K \times [C_{peak} - (C_{trough} \times e^{-Kt'})]}$$

$$= \frac{(1000/2) \times (1 - e^{-0.071 \times 2})}{0.071 \times [43.8 - (28.5 \times e^{-0.071 \times 2})]}$$

$$= \frac{(500) \times (1 - 0.87)}{0.071 \times (43.8 - 24.8)}$$

$$= \textbf{48.1 L}$$

$$Cl_{vanco} = V_d \times K$$
$$= 48.1 \text{ L} \times 0.071 \text{ h}^{-1}$$
$$= \textbf{3.4 L/h}$$

$$T_{1/2} = \frac{0.693}{0.071}$$
$$= \textbf{9.8 h}$$

Step 4: Calculate new vancomycin dose using patient-specific PK.

It appears we overestimated CK's CrCl and underestimated his V_d. In bedbound patients with decreased muscle mass, it is more difficult to estimate renal function by means of CrCl formulas. For this reason, it is important to monitor these patients' serum vancomycin levels and adjust doses as necessary. We will start by trying 1,000 mg every 12 hours (infused over 2 hours).

$$C_{SSmax} = \frac{(Dose/t') \times (1 - e^{-Kt'})}{V_d \times K \times (1 - e^{-K\tau})}$$

$$= \frac{(1000/2) \times (1 - e^{-0.071 \times 2})}{48.1 \times 0.071 \times (1 - e^{-0.071 \times 12})}$$

$$= \frac{(500) \times (1 - 0.87)}{48.1 \times 0.071 \times (1 - 0.43)}$$

$$= \textbf{33.3 mg/L}$$

$$C_{SSmin} = C_{SSmax} \times e^{-K(\tau - t')}$$

$$= 33.3 \times e^{-0.071 \times 10}$$

$$= 33.3 \times 0.49$$

$$= \textbf{16.3 mg/L}$$

Because the patient has a UTI, we do not necessarily need to shoot for a trough of 15–20 mg/L. A trough above 10 mg/L will suffice; therefore, you can recommend a dose of 1,000 mg given every 12 hours or 750 mg given every 12 hours.

OPTIMIZING AUC$_{24}$ / MIC RATIO

As previously discussed, targeting a vancomycin AUC/MIC ratio ≥400 helps to achieve maximal efficacy when treating MRSA infections. To ensure that a selected dosing regimen has met this target, the AUC24 can be approximated by calculating the dose given over a 24 hour period and dividing it by the patient's vancomycin clearance.

CASE 3 (CONT.)

Patient was receiving 1,000 mg every 12 hours infused over 2 hours.

An AUC/MIC ratio can be estimated by using the following equation:

Equation 14[7,9]:

$$AUC_{24} = \frac{Dose}{Cl_{vanco}}$$

$$= \frac{2,000 \text{ mg}}{3.4 \text{ L/h}}$$

$$= 588 \text{ mg} \cdot \text{h/L}$$

If MIC was 0.5 mg/L:

$$AUC_{24}/MIC = 588 \text{ mg} \cdot \text{h/L}/0.5 \text{ mg/L} = 1,176$$

If MIC was 1.0 mg/L:

$$AUC_{24}/MIC = 588 \text{ mg} \cdot \text{h/L}/1.0 \text{ mg/L} = 588$$

If MIC was 2.0 mg/L:

$$AUC_{24}/MIC = 588 \text{ mg} \cdot \text{h/L}/2.0 \text{ mg/L} = 294$$

If the MIC of vancomycin to *S. aureus* was ≤1, the AUC$_{24}$/MIC would be 588 or greater, which meets our target of ≥400.[9]

VANCOMYCIN DOSING IN PATIENTS UNDERGOING RENAL REPLACEMENT THERAPIES

Patients with either acute or chronic kidney disease have significant changes in the pharmacokinetics of vancomycin due to the increased V_d and decreased total drug clearance. The V_d of vancomycin in patients with chronic kidney disease is affected by alterations in plasma protein binding (due to low albumin) and variation in fluid status, as well as other patient-specific factors mentioned earlier.

Both the renal and nonrenal clearance of vancomycin are affected in patients with impaired renal function. Vancomycin is excreted primarily via glomerular filtration, so in patients with end-stage renal disease (ESRD) the elimination half-life of the drug is prolonged to 54–180 hours.[6] As mentioned earlier, the nonrenal

TABLE 20-1	Vancomycin Clearances with Various Types of Dialysis and Dialyzer Membranes	
Types of Dialysis	**Membranes**	**CL$_{HD}$ (mL/min)**
Low-flux hemodialysis	Cuprophane	9.6–15[37–39]
High-flux hemodialysis	Polysulfone	44.7–130.7[35,37,38,41,42]
	Polyacrylonitrile	47–58.4[37,39,40]
	Cellulose triacetate	49.2–111.4[43]
Continuous venovenous hemodiafiltration	Acrylonitrile	10–17[34]
Continuous venovenous hemofiltration	Acrylonitrile	5.8–13.4[45]
	Polymethylmethacrylate	7.5–27[45]
	Polysulfone	5.2–22.1[45]

clearance of vancomycin in patients with normal renal function is about 10–30 percent of the total drug clearance. However, in patients with ESRD undergoing hemodialysis, the nonrenal clearance of vancomycin is reduced to 5–6 mL/min.[6,33]

The vancomycin dosing regimen in patients undergoing renal replacement therapies (RRT)—intermittent hemodialysis (IHD) and continuous renal replacement therapy (CRRT)—can vary depending on their residual renal function, type of dialysis, dialyzer membrane or filter composition, and blood flow rate being used. The type of dialysis membrane used is crucial in determining the impact of vancomycin removal during RRT. The dialysis membrane can be a combination of low or high efficiency with low or high flux. *High efficiency* refers to using membranes with larger surface area, which removes small-size solutes such as urea. Low-flux hemodialysis (LFHD) membranes have smaller pores and lower ultrafiltration coefficients as compared to the high flux hemodialysis (HFHD) membranes. The LFHD membrane, such as cuprophane, is relatively impermeable to drugs with molecular weight greater than 1,000 daltons.[34] Because vancomycin has a molecular size of 1,500 daltons, the removal of the drug using LFHD is almost negligible, allowing for at least once weekly dosing intervals. Unlike LFHD, HFHD uses a membrane (such as polysulfone) with large pore sizes. HFHD is efficient in removing molecules that have a molecular weight of 10,000 daltons or less.[34] Hence, the removal of vancomycin during HFHD is significantly large, about 25–50 percent.[35,36] Table 20-1 provides some examples of low- and high-flux dialyzer membranes used in IHD and CRRT and their respective vancomycin clearances found in the literature. Keep in mind that the variance in vancomycin clearance found between the different types of dialysis membranes may also be due to patients' residual renal function as well as the duration of dialysis session.

INTERMITTENT HEMODIALYSIS

As mentioned earlier, the elimination half-life of vancomycin in ESRD patients is prolonged for at least 54 hours. Assuming the steady state is reached after four to five half-lives, steady state will not be reached until after 216–270 hours or after 9–11 days of therapy. Therefore, to ensure a sufficient area under the curve (AUC) on day 1 of therapy, loading doses should be given to all patients.[6]

Due to the minimal amount of vancomycin cleared by the LFHD membrane, the dosing interval is much longer in LFHD as compared to HFHD. The usual maintenance dose in patients undergoing LFHD is 1,000 mg intravenous every 5–14 days, depending on the target prehemodialysis serum concentration. On the other hand, patients on HFHD can receive vancomycin 500–1,000 mg after each hemodialysis session.[46] Vancomycin doses can be calculated by phamacokinetic calculations utilizing LD and MD equations seen previously or by using dosing algorithms based on pre-HD concentrations. One example of a vancomycin dosing algorithm

TABLE 20-2	Revised Vancomycin-Dosing Algorithm for Patients Receiving Three-Times Weekly High-Flux Hemodialysis
HD Session No.	Intervention
1	Give vancomycin 1,000 mg after hemodialysis.
2	Give vancomycin 500 mg after hemodialysis.
3	If prehemodialysis vancomycin concentration is: • >20 mg/L, withhold one dose of vancomycin • 5–20 mg/L, give 500 mg after hemodialysis • <5 mg/L, give 1,000 mg after each hemodialysis session
4	Give vancomycin 500 mg after hemodialysis (or 1,000 mg based on session 3).
5	If the dose was held or changed in session 3, determine prehemodialysis vancomycin concentration and follow dosing guideline per session 3. If the dose was not held or changed, give 500 mg.
6	Give vancomycin 500 mg after hemodialysis (or 1,000 mg based on session 5).
7	Determine prehemodialysis vancomycin concentration, interpret, and follow dosing guideline per session 3.
8	Give vancomycin 500 mg after hemodialysis (or 1,000 mg based on session 7).
9	Give vancomycin 500 mg after hemodialysis (or 1,000 mg based on session 7).

Used with permission from Pai AB, Pai MP. Vancomycin dosing in high flux hemodialysis: A limited-sampling algorithm. *Am J Health-Syst Pharm.* 2004;61:1812–1816.

in patients undergoing HFHD is provided in Table 20-2.[47] In this algorithm, Pai and Pai formulated dosing recommendations based on their patients' predialysis drug concentration obtained before each session.[47] It is important to note that at least 20 percent of samples in the study were subtherapeutic vancomycin concentration of $\leq$10 mg/L.

CASE 4

BT is a 40-year-old female diagnosed with left heel cellulitis. Patient has a wound drainage that is positive with MRSA sensitive to vancomycin. Patient has ESRD and is currently receiving hemodialysis on Mondays, Wednesdays, and Fridays from 8 AM to 12 PM. The dialysis clinic that she goes to uses a cuprophane, a low-flux hemodialysis membrane, with a reported vancomycin clearance of 0.58 L/h.

Height = 5′5″

Weight = 60 kg

Provide a loading dose with an initial concentration of 30 mg/L and maintenance dose with a peak and trough concentrations of 30–40 mg/L and 10–15 mg/L, respectively, for the patient.

Step 1: Determine the loading dose of vancomycin.

The dose for this patient should be determined using Equation 7. Because the patient is ESRD, we will use 0.84 L/kg (derived from Matzke) to calculate the V_d.

$$V_d = 0.84 \text{ L/kg} \times 60 \text{ kg}$$
$$= 50.4 \text{ L}$$
$$LD = C° \times V_d$$
$$= 30 \times 50.4$$
$$= 1,512 \text{ mg, or } \textbf{1,500 mg}$$

Note: Doses should be rounded to the nearest 250 mg.

Step 2: Calculate K.

Assuming the patient has no residual renal function and the vancomycin clearance is 5 mL/min (or 0.3 L/h), calculate the K:

$$K \text{ (h}^{-1}) = Cl_{vanco} / V_d$$
$$= 0.30 / 50.4$$
$$= \textbf{0.006/h}$$

Step 3: Determine the half-life.

$$T_{1/2} = 0.693/K$$
$$= 0.693/0.006$$
$$= \textbf{115.5 h (or 4.8 days)}$$

In 5 days, patient is scheduled for another HD session. A pre-HD concentration of 15 mg/L was measured.

Step 4: Calculate the replacement dose.

Equation 15a:

$$\text{Replacement dose} = Vd \times TBW \times (C° - C_{preHD})$$
$$= 0.84 \times 60 \times (30 - 15)$$
$$= \textbf{756 mg, or 750 mg}$$

CASE 5

MC is 73-year-old male who was sent to the ER for a possible MRSA bacteremia secondary to an infected central line on Tuesday. Patient is ESRD and has been on hemodialysis three times a week (every Monday, Wednesday, and Friday) for 5 years. While in the ER, he was given a loading dose of vancomycin 1,750 mg intravenously. On the following day after he finished his dialysis session, the team administered a dose of vancomycin 1,000 mg. The team obtained a predialysis vancomycin concentration on Friday of 16 mg/L. If the percent removal of vancomycin after HFHD is 35 percent, determine the postdialysis concentration and replacement dose after each session.

Height = 5′9″

Weight = 70 kg

Step 1: Calculate the initial plasma concentration that will be achieved with the loading dose.

$$C° = LD/ V_d$$
$$= \frac{1,750}{(0.84)(70)}$$
$$= 29.76 \text{ mg/L}$$

Step 2: Estimate the postdialysis concentration of vancomycin using Equation 15b. Of note, this equation does not factor any other methods of drug removal other than dialysis. However, because the estimated nonrenal clearance of vancomycin in ESRD is minimal, the percentage of drug removal is insignificant.

Equation 15b[4]:

$$C_{postdialysis} = C_{predialysis} \times (100 - \text{percent drug removal after HFHD})$$
$$= 16 \times (100\% - 35\%)$$
$$= \textbf{10.4 mg/L}$$

Step 3: Assume that the initial vancomycin concentration after a loading dose of vancomycin 1,750 mg is 29.8 mg/L, and estimate the replacement dose using Equation 15c.

Equation 15c[48]:

$$\text{Replacement dose} = V_d \times TBW \times (C^0 - C_{postdialysis})$$
$$= 0.84 \times 70 \times (29.76 - 10.4)$$
$$= 1,138.37 \text{ mg, or } \textbf{1,250 mg}$$

Vancomycin 1,250 mg after HFHD will be given to this patient. However, to ensure that we are targeting an appropriate trough level, another prehemodialysis concentration can be obtained. Based on the level, we may continue or change the dosage regimen.

CONTINUOUS RENAL REPLACEMENT THERAPY

Continuous renal replacement therapy (CRRT) is frequently used to treat critically ill patients with acute or chronic renal failure. In comparison to intermittent hemodialysis, CRRT is better tolerated in unstable patients and is effective in removing solutes during a 24-hour dialysis session. The variants of CRRT commonly used in critically ill patients are CVVHD, CVVH, and CVVHDF.

Diffusion and convection are the two mechanisms used in CRRT when removing fluids, waste products, or drugs. Diffusion is a process of removal in which solutes move through the concentration gradients between the blood and the dialysate across the semipermeable hemodialysis membrane. Convection, on the other hand, refers to the removal of a large amount of water across a large-pore dialysis membrane into the ultrafiltrate compartment, dragging along with it solutes dissolved in the water, which occurs irrespective of concentration gradient or molecular size. Conventional intermittent hemodialysis (IHD) and continuous venovenous hemodialysis (CVVHD) are primarily diffusion, whereas continuous venovenous hemofiltration (CVVH) uses convection. The continuous venovenous hemodiafiltration (CVVHDF) uses both convection and diffusion in removing drug and solutes, resulting in greater drug removal compared to the other RRT. The variables that affect drug clearances during CRRT are the drug's molecular weight, permeability to pass through the membrane or sieving coefficient (SC), and the renal replacement techniques being used. (i.e., convection and/or diffusion methods; blood, dialysate, and ultrafiltration flow rates; and duration of CRRT).

Because CVVH uses a convective method, its vancomycin clearance is dependent on SC and ultrafiltration rate (UFR) as shown in Equation 16.[34] The SC is the ratio of drug concentration in the ultrafiltrate to the prefilter plasma concentration. Table 20-3 lists some examples of SC of vancomycin for a particular hemodialysis membrane.[49] If the SC is not known, the unbound fraction (f_u) of the drug can also be substituted as seen in the Equation 16a.[34] The vancomycin clearance via CVVHD, on the other hand, is primarily diffusion, so its drug removal can be estimated by multiplying the dialysate flow rate (DFR) and SC as seen in Equation 17.[34] CVVHDF is a combination of diffusion and convection methods; therefore, the clearance of vancomycin can be predicted using Equation 18 provided that the DFR is less than 33 mL/min and the blood flow rate is at least 75 mL/min.[34]

Using the estimated vancomycin CRRT clearance, a once-daily regimen can be determined using Equation 19.[49] Another way to empirically dose vancomycin in patients during CRRT is provided in Table 20-4.[50] To ensure that the calculated vancomycin trough level is at target, the clinician should obtain a level at least 24 hours after the start of therapy and then obtain another after level after steady state is reached after the fourth dose.

TABLE 20-3 Examples of Sieving Coefficient During CRRT for Vancomycin[49]

Filter Membrane	Sieving Coefficient
Acrylonitrile copolymer	0.70
Polysulfone	0.68
Polymethylmethacrylate	0.86

TABLE 20-4 Dosing Recommendations for Vancomycin during CRRT[50]

Loading Dose for CRRT	Maintenance Dose for CRRT		
	CVVH	CVVHD	CVVHDF
15–25 mg/kg	10–15 mg/kg q24–48h	10–15 mg/kg q24h	7.5–10 mg/kg q12h

Equation 16[34]: $$CL_{CVVH} (L/h) = UFR (L/h) \times SC$$

Equation 16a[34]: $$CL_{CVVH} (L/h) = UFR (L/h) \times f_u$$

Equation 17[34]: $$CL_{CVVHD} (L/h) = UFR (L/h) \times SC$$

Equation 18[34]: $$CL_{CVVHDF} (L/h) = (UFR + DFR) \times SC$$

Equation 19[49]:

$$Dose (mg/24\ hr) = C_{pSS} \times Total\ clearance[(CL_{CRRT} + CL_{NR} + CL_{vanco}) \times 24\ hr]$$

where

C_{pSS} = steady-state plasma concentration

CL_{CRRT} = drug clearance during CRRT

CL_{NR} = nonrenal clearance (for anuric patients, the weighted mean is 16 mL/min (range: 9–35 mL/min))

CL_{vanco} = residual renal clearance in L/h × 0.8

CASE 6

A 56-year-old male who developed an acute renal injury (ARI) after an abdominal surgery will be undergoing a CVVH to remove edema and to correct an electrolyte imbalance. Due to his ARI, he is only making a urine output of 200 mL in 24 hours. He currently weighs 200 lbs with an approximate preadmission weight of 170 lbs. His estimated creatinine clearance is 10 mL/min. The ultrafiltration rate of the CVVH is set at 0.5 L/h with Polysulfone (SC 0.68) as the filter membrane being used.

Soon after the patient had started the CVVH therapy, he developed fever and catheter-related infection. The medical team is concerned about a possible MRSA bacteremia, and they would like to initiate vancomycin to the patient empirically.

QUESTION

Provide a loading and maintenance dosing regimen for the patient. For the maintenance dose that you calculated, what are the estimated peak and trough levels?

Answer:

Step 1: Calculate the loading dose. Use the current weight of 200 lbs to obtain the V_d. Because the patient is fluid-overloaded, it may also be appropriate to increase the V_d to 1 L/kg. However, as the fluid is removed and his weight approaches its baseline, the dose should then be adjusted. The initial target concentration should be at least 30 mg/L.

$$Loading\ dose = (C°)(V_d)(TBW)$$
$$= (30)(1)(90.9)$$
$$= 2,720\ mg,\ or\ \mathbf{2,750\ mg}$$

Step 2: Calculate the total clearance. Assume, patient's nonrenal clearance is 16 mL/min because he is anuric. However, if this patient's acute renal failure is prolonged, the assumed CL_{NR} will further decrease over time.

Total clearance = $CL_{CRRT} + CL_{NR} + CL_{vanco}$

$$CL_{CVVH} = UFR \times SC$$
$$= 0.5 \times 0.68$$
$$\mathbf{= 0.34 \ L/h}$$

$$CL_{NR} = 16 \ mL/min \times 0.06$$
$$\mathbf{= 0.96 \ L/h}$$

$$CL_{Vanco} = 10 \ mL/min \times 0.8 \times 0.06$$
$$\mathbf{= 0.48 \ L/h}$$

Total clearance = $CL_{CRRT} + CL_{NR} + CL_{vanco}$

$$= 0.34 + 0.96 + 0.48$$
$$\mathbf{= 1.78 \ L/h}$$

Step 3: Calculate the maintenance dose. Assume that the vancomycin steady-state plasma concentration to be targeted is 20 mg/L.

Maintenance dose (mg/24 hr) = $C_{pSS} \times$ (Total clearance $\times$ 24 hr)

$$= 20 \times 1.78 \times 24$$
$$= 854.4 \ mg, \ or \ \mathbf{1,000 \ mg \ every \ 24 \ hours}$$

Step 4: With the preceding CVVH vancomycin dosing regimen, calculate the estimated peak and trough levels.

$$K = Cl / V_d$$
$$= 1.78/90.9$$
$$\mathbf{= 0.02 \ / \ h}$$

$$C_{SSmax} = \frac{(Dose/t')(1 - e^{-Kt'})}{(V_d)(k)(1 - e^{-K\tau})}$$

$$= \frac{(1,000/2)(1 - e^{-(0.02)(2)})}{(90.9)(0.02)(1 - e^{-(0.02)(24)})}$$

$$\mathbf{= 28.99 \ mg/L}$$

$$C_{SSmin} = C_{SSmax} \ (e^{-K(\tau - t')})$$
$$= 28.99(e^{-(0.02)(24 - 2)})$$
$$\mathbf{= 18.55 \ mg/L}$$

SAMPLING OF VANCOMYCIN IN PATIENTS UNDERGOING HEMODIALYSIS

It is evident that vancomycin concentrations rebound at the end of HFHD. A plasma profile of vancomycin concentration versus time showed that levels are significantly lowered during a HFHD session, which later increased as the session ended after 3–6 hours.[46] This phenomenon is thought to be a result from the movement of vancomycin from plasma protein-binding sites rather than peripheral compartments. Postdialysis rebound does not occur during low-flux hemodialysis or continuous renal replacement therapy. The total body clearance of vancomycin during CRRT almost remains constant, so trough level can be obtained at any time during continuous hemodialysis. However, if dialysis is stopped and vancomycin treatment still needs to be continued, then the plasma concentration must be determined 4–6 hours after stopping the drug and before readministration of any drug.[46] For high-flux hemodialysis, vancomycin levels should not be drawn within 6 hours after high-flux hemodialysis session, and pre-HFHD trough levels are recommended.

PERITONEAL DIALYSIS

The continuous ambulatory peritoneal dialysis (CAPD) and automated peritoneal dialysis (APD) are the two types of peritoneal dialysis. During CAPD, the dialysate fluid is left to dwell in the patient's peritoneal cavity overnight for 4–6 hours, during which it will absorb the waste products from the blood through the peritoneum. The dialysate fluid is drained out manually during the day and the process is repeated four times daily. APD, on the other hand, is the opposite of CAPD where the long dwell of the dialysate solution occurs during the day, and the solution is replaced by a dialysis machine overnight while the patient sleeps. Patients on APD are usually attached to the machine for 8–10 hours a day.

Vancomycin administration in peritoneal dialysis patients can either be intraperitoneally or intravenously. Intraperitoneal dosing decreases the risk of infusion-related syndrome, and if the patient has peritonitis, it will provide a direct delivery of the drug to the site of infection. In patients without peritonitis, it is expected that 50 percent of the drug will be absorbed during a 4- to 6-hour dwell-time.[55] In patients with peritonitis, however, the absorption of vancomycin is closer to 90 percent.[55] Therefore, when dosing vancomycin intravenously in peritoneal dialysis patients without peritonitis, the dose should be approximately 50 percent of the intraperitoneal dose.[54] In a study by Morse and colleagues, administering a single vancomycin dose of 30 mg/kg intraperitoneally during CAPD achieved a serum level of 15 ± 3.6 mg/L and 21 ± 1.7 mg/L after 72 hours and 24 hours of dosing, respectively.[54] These levels were found to be comparable after a single intravenous vancomycin dose of 15 mg/kg, targeting serum levels of 15.4 ± 3.1 mg/L and 19.8 ± 4.9 mg/L after 72 hours and 24 hours of dosing, respectively. The recommended vancomycin dosing regimens by International Society for Peritoneal Dialysis (ISPD) for intermittent and continuous peritoneal dialysis during CAPD and intermittent APD are summarized in Table 20-5.[56] Keep in mind that the dosing interval of vancomycin during peritoneal dialysis may vary from the ISPD guidelines, depending on the patient's residual renal function, peritoneal dialysis type, and target serum levels. To prepare vancomycin-containing dialysate bag for CAPD and APD intermittent dosing, the calculated dose is diluted in a 2-liter dialysate bag and dwells for at least 6 hours for it to be effectively absorbed into the systemic circulation.

CASE 7

A 60-year-old woman (60-kg) on CAPD has been empirically started on vancomycin 1,750 mg intravenously for peritonitis treatment.

TABLE 20-5	Intraperitoneal Dosing of Vancomycin in CAPD and APD[56]				
Continuous Ambulatory Peritoneal Dialysis[a]			**Automated Peritoneal Dialysis***		
Intermittent	**Continuous (per exchange)**				
	Loading Dose	**Maintenance Dose**	**Loading Dose**	**Maintenance Dose**	
15–30 mg/kg every 5–7 days	1,000 mg/L	25 mg/L	30 mg/ kg in long dwell	15 mg/kg IP in long dwell every 3-5 days[b]	

[a]In patients with residual renal function, increasing the dose by 25 percent may be necessary.
[b]These dosing intervals will aim to keep serum levels above 15 mg/L.

QUESTION

What is the replacement dose of vancomycin if the trough level, obtained 4 days after dosing, is 15 mg/L?

Answer:

The measured trough level of 15 mg/L is appropriate for treating this patient's infection, so keeping this level is desirable. Equation 15c can be used to determine a replacement dose. This dosing formula is used to target peak or initial vancomycin concentration from the actual trough (C_{TROUGH}). In this case, the initial vancomycin concentration after giving a loading dose of 1,750 mg is 34.72 mg/L. Because the patient is on peritoneal hemodialysis, we will assume that the V_d is 0.84 L/kg.

$$Dose = V_d(TBW)(C° - C_{TROUGH})$$
$$= 0.84 \times 60 \times (34.7 - 15)$$
$$= 992.88 \text{ mg, or } \mathbf{1,000 \text{ mg}}$$

Although we were able to determine the replacement dose of vancomycin for this patient, it is still advisable to repeat serum levels in 4 days to ensure levels remain above 15 mg/L. If, however, the repeated level goes below the target, we recommend decreasing the dosing interval by 1 day, and then repeat levels in 3 days.

ADVERSE DRUG EVENTS

NEPHROTOXICITY AND OTOTOXICITY

The old vancomycin preparation in the 1950's contained a substantial amount of impurities that made the drug highly ototoxic and nephrotoxic. However, with modern production techniques those impurities were removed thus lessening these toxicities to a certain extent.

The exact mechanism of vancomycin-induced nephrotoxicity (VIN) has not been fully elucidated; but it is speculated that it may be due to complement activation and increased oxidative stress in the renal proximal tubules.[57] Various literature define VIN as either an increase in the SCr level of ≥ 0.5 mg/dL or 50 percent from baseline; or decrease in creatinine clearance to <50 mL/min or a decrease of >10 mL/min from a baseline of CrCl of <50 mL/min. In the 1980s, VIN was reported in 0–5 percent of patients, but when vancomycin is coadministered with other nephrotoxic agents, the VIN rates increase to as high as 35 percent.[58,59] Other factors that have been shown to increase the incidence of VIN include high doses of vancomycin, ≥ 4 grams per day,[60] extended duration of therapy,[61] and high target trough levels.[61,62]

Vancomycin-induced ototoxicity (VIO) has been documented in case reports but is less commonly reported as an adverse drug event compared to VIN. VIO can either be reversible or irreversible, depending on the vancomycin serum concentrations. Reversible ototoxicity is generally associated with vancomycin serum levels greater than 40 mg/L and irreversible damage with greater than 80 mg/L.[63] The ototoxicity associated with vancomycin is characterized by damage in the auditory nerve causing full deafness in all frequencies.[64] The high-frequency sensory hairs in the cochlea are affected first, then the middle- and low-frequency hairs. Once the hair cell degenerates, the deafness produced is irreversible and permanent. Therefore, if a patient starts complaining of loss of acuity to high-frequency sounds and tinnitus, which are regarded as prominent signs of VIO, vancomycin therapy should be discontinued. Factors associated with VIO other than high serum levels are concomitant use of ototoxic agents and age (middle-aged patients have higher risk).[65]

VANCOMYCIN-INDUCED THROMBOCYTOPENIA

Thrombocytopenia is a well-recognized adverse event associated with vancomycin use and has an estimated frequency of 2–3 percent.[66,67] Vancomycin-induced thrombocytopenia (VIT) may be caused by a vancomycin and platelet membrane glycoprotein IIb/IIIa complex, which in turn stimulates the production of vancomycin-dependent immunoglobulin G (IgG) antibodies and leads to platelet destruction via complement activation.[68] Von Drygalski and others found that patients with vancomycin-dependent antibodies had a median percentage decrease in platelet count from baseline of 95 percent (range: 76–99%) while on vancomycin therapy.[68] In this study, the median nadir platelet count was 10,000 count per mm³ (range: 1,000–60,000 count per mm³) after 7 days (range: 3–27 days) of treatment. Although, the VIT was found to be reversible after discontinuation of treatment, the median time required for the platelet level to return to at least 150,000 count per mm³ after stopping vancomycin was 7.5 days (range: 4–17).

HYPERSENSITIVITY REACTIONS

Red man syndrome (RMS) and anaphylaxis are the two types of hypersensitivity reactions associated with vancomycin. RMS is an infusion-related reaction common to vancomycin, especially if the drug is infused at a rapid rate. RMS is an anaphylactoid reaction caused by the release of histamine from mast cells and basophils found in the skin, lung, gastrointestinal tract, myocardium, and vascular system.[69,70] The incidence of RMS varies from 3.7 percent[71] to 47 percent[72] in infected patients, and rates up to 90 percent[69] have been seen in healthy volunteers when a 1,000 mg dose was infused over 1 hour.

RMS can manifest with generalized flushing, pruritus, and erythematous rash involving the face, neck, and upper torso.[73] In severe cases, patients may also present with hypotension, chest pain, and dyspnea.[73] RMS can occur after infusion of the first dose of vancomycin or at any time during vancomycin therapy. It can appear as early as 4–10 minutes after the start of infusion or can occur after the infusion has completed. The IDSA vancomycin guideline suggests that infusion of vancomycin can be given safely at a rate no faster than 500 mg/hr.[1] If RMS occurs, the vancomycin infusion should be stopped immediately and diphenhydramine 50 mg intravenous or oral given to the patient. If hypotension occurs, intravenous fluid bolus and/or vasopressor may also be given. Once the rash and itching resolves, the vancomycin infusion can be resumed at a slower rate to avoid recurrence of RMS.

The other type of hypersensitivity reaction to vancomycin is an IgE-mediated systemic anaphylaxis. In order for a patient to have this reaction, he or she has to have previous exposure to vancomycin to elicit an IgE antibody response against the drug.[73] The vancomycin-specific IgE antibodies then bind to mast cells and basophils and with subsequent exposure to vancomycin a cross-linking of cell-bound IgE occurs causing mast cell and or basophil to degranulate. When mast cells and basophils de granulate, vasoactive mediators such as histamine, leukotrienes, prostaglandins, and platelet-activating factors are released. Manifestations of a anaphylaxis reaction may include urticaria, angioedema, hypotension, and/or bronchospasm. These reactions can be life threatening unless emergent care is obtained. If anaphylaxis occurs, epinephrine 0.3 mg intramuscular or 1:1,000 strength is the first-line agent of therapy. Future use of vancomycin should be avoided in these patients.

REFERENCES

1. Rybak M, Lomaestro B, Rotschafer JC, et al. Therapeutic drug monitoring of vancomycin in adult patients: A consensus review of the American Society of Health Systems Pharmacist, the Infectious Diseases Society of America, and the Society of Infectious Diseases Pharmacists. *Am J Health-Syst Pharm.* 2009;66:82–98.

2. DeRyke CA. Alexander DP. Optimizing vancomycin dosing through pharmacodynamic assessment targeting area under the concentration time curve / minimum inhibitory concentration. *Hosp Pharm.* 2009;44:751–765.

3. Wilhelm MP, Estes L. Vancomycin. *Mayo Clinic Proceedings.* 1999;74:928–935.

4. Moellering RC. Pharmacokinetics of vancomycin. *J Antimicrob Chemother* 1984;14(suppl D):43–52.

5. Ducharme MP, Slaughter RL, Edwards DJ. Vancomycin pharmacokinetics in a patient population: Effect of age, gender, and body weight. *Ther Drug Monit.* 1994;16:513–518.

6. Matzke GR, McGory RW, Halstenson CE, Keane WF. Pharmacokinetics of vancomycin in patients with various degrees of renal function. *Antimicrob Agents Chemother.* 1984;25(4):433–437.

7. Rodvold KA, Blum RA, Fischer JH, et al. Vancomycin pharmacokinetics in patients with various degrees of renal function. *Antimicrob Agents Chemother.* 1988;32(6):848–852.

8. Rotschafer JC, Crossley K, Zaske DE, et al. Pharmacokinetics of vancomycin: Observations in 28 patients and dosing regimens. *Antimicrob Agents Chemother.*1982;22(3):391–394.

9. Moise–Broder PA, Forrest A, Birmingham MC, Schentag JJ. Pharmacodynamics of vancomycin and other antimicrobials in patients with *Staphylococcus aureus* lower respiratory infections. *Clin Pharmacokin.* 2004;43(13):925–942.

10. Craig WA, Andes DR. Invivo pharmacodynamics of vancomycin against VISA, heteroresistant VISA, and VSSA in the neutropenic murine thigh-infection model. Paper presented at 46th ICAAC, 2006. Abstr A-644. American Society for Microbiology, Washington, DC.

11. Sakoulas G, Moise-Broder PA, Schentag J, et al. Relationship of MIC and bactericidal activity to efficacy of vancomycin for treatment of methacillin resistant *Staphylococcus aureus* bacteremia. *J Clin Microbiol.* 2004;42:2398–2402.

12. Hidayat LK, Hsu DI, Quist R, et al. High-dose vancomycin therapy for methicillin-resistant *Staphylococcus aureus* Infection: Efficacy and toxicity. *Arch Intern Med.* 2006;166:2138–2144.

13. Howden BP, Ward PB, Charles PG, et al. Treatment outcomes for serious infections caused by methicillin-resistant *Staphylococcus aureus* with reduced vancomycin susceptibility. *Clin Infect Dis.* 2004;38:521–528.

14. Moise PA, Sakoulas G, Forrest A, et al. Vancomycin in-vitro bactericidal activity and its relationship to efficacy in clearance of methicillin-resistant *Staphylococcus aureus* bacteremia. *Antimicrob Agents Chemother.* 2007;51:2582–2588.

15. Soriano A, Marco F, Martinez JA, et al. Influence of vancomycin minimum inhibitory concentration on the treatment of methicillin-resistant *Staphylococcus aureus* bacteremia. *Clin Infect Dis.* 2008;46: 193–200.

16. Lodise TP, Graves J, Graffunder E, et al. Relationship between vancomycin MIC and failure among patients with methicillin-resistant *Staphylococcus aureus* bacteremia treated with vancomycin. *Antimicrob Agents Chemother.* 2008;52:3315–3320.

17. Sakoullas G, Gold HS, Cohen RA, et al. Effects of prolonged vancomycin administration on methicillin-resistant *Staphylococcus aureus* in a patient with recurrent bacteremia. *J Antimicrob Chemother.* 2006;57:699–704.

18. Murphy JE, Gillespie DE, Bateman CV. Predictability of vancomycin trough concentrations using seven approaches for estimating pharmacokinetic parameters. *Am J Health-Syst Pharm.* 2006;63: 2365–2370.

19. Devine BJ. Gentamicin therapy. *Drug Intell Clin Pharm.* 1974;8: 650–655.

20. Cockcroft DW, Gault MH. Predictions of creatinine clearance from serum creatinine. *Nephron.* 1976;16(1):31–41.

21. Revilla N, Martin-Suarez A, Paz Perez M, et al. Vancomycin dosing assessment in intensive care unit patients based on population pharmacokinetic/pharmacodynamic simulation. *Br J Clin Pharmacol.* 2010;70(2):201–212.

22. del Mar Ferandez de Gatta Garcia M, Revilla N, Calvo MV, et al. Pharmacokinetic/pharmacodynamic analysis of vancomycin in ICU patients. *Intensive Care Med.* 2007;33:279–285.

23. Llopis-Salvia P, Jimenez-Torres NV. Population pharmacokinetic parameters of vancomycin in critically ill patients. *J Clin Pharm Ther.* 2006;31:447–454.

24. Santos Buelga D, del Mar Fernandez de Gatta M, Herrera EV, et al. Population pharmacokinetic analysis of vancomycin in patients with hematologic malignancies. *Antimicrob Agents Chemother.* 2005;49:4934–4941.

25. Rushing TA, Ambrose PJ. Clinical application and evaluation of vancomycin dosing in adults. *J. Pharm Technol.* 2001;17:33–38.

26. Sawchuk RJ, Zaske DE. Pharmacokinetics of dosing regimens which utilize multiple intravenous infusions: Gentamicin in burn patients. *J Pharmacokinet Biopharm.* 1976;4(2):183–195.

27. Blouin RA, Bauer LA, Miller DD, et al. Vancomycin pharmacokinetics in normal and morbidly obese subjects. *Antimicrob Agents Chemother.* 1982;21(4):575–580.

28. Ryback MJ, Albrecht LM, Berman JR, et al. Vancomycin pharmacokinetics in burn patients and intravenous drug abusers. *Antimicrob Agents Chemother.* 1990;34(5):792–795.

29. Dolton M, Xu H, Cheong E, et al. Vancomycin pharmacokinetics in patients with severe burn injuries. *Burns.* 2010;36:469–476.

30. Krogstad DJ, Moellering RC, Greenblatt DJ. Single dose kinetics of intravenous vancomycin. *J Clin Pharmacol.* 1980;197–201.

31. Lee E, Winter ME, Boro MS. Comparing two predictive methods for determining serum vancomycin concentrations at a Veterans Affairs Medical Center. *Am J Health-Syst Pharm.* 2006;63:1972–1975.

32. Mohr JF, Murray BE. Point: Vancomycin is not obsolete for the treatment of infection caused by methicillin-resistant Staphylococcus aureus. *Clin Infect Dis.* 2007;44:1536–1542.

33. Moellering RC, Krogstad DJ, Greenblatt DJ. Vancomycin therapy in patients with impaired renal function: a nomogram for dosage. *Ann Intern.* 1981;94:343–346.

34. Matze GR. 2009. Principles of drug therapy in patients with reduced kidney function. In Greenberg A and Cheung AK (Eds.). *Primer on Kidney Diseases,* 5th ed. Philadelphia, PA: Saunders Elsevier.

35. Foote EF, Dreitlein WB, Steward CA, Kapoian T, Walker JA, Sherman RA. Pharmacokinetics of vancomycin when administered during high flux hemodialysis. *Clin Nephrol.*1998;50:51–55.

36. Mason NA, Neudeck BL, Welage LS, et al. Comparison of 3 vancomycin dosage regimens during hemodialysis with cellulose triacetate dialyzers: Postdialysis versus intradialytic administration. *Clin Nephrol.* 2003;60:96–104.

37. Alwakeel J, Najjar TA, al-Yamani MJ, Huraib S, al-Haider A, Abuaisha H. Comparison of the effects of three haemodialysis membranes on vancomycin disposition. *Int Urol Nephrol.* 1994;26:223–228.

38. Lanese DM, Alfrey PS, Molitoris BA. Markedly increased clearance of vancomycin during hemodialysis using polysulfone dialyzers. *Kidney Int.* 1989;35:1409–1412.

39. Torras J, Cao C, Rivas MC, Cano M, Fernandez E, Montoliu J. Pharmacokinetics of vancomycin in patients undergoing hemodialysis with polyacrylonitrile. *Clin Nephrol.* 1991;36:35–41.

40. Zoer J, Schrander-van der Meer AM, van Dorp WT. Dosage recommendation of vancomycin during hemodialysis with highly permeable membranes. *Pharm World Sci.* 1997;19:191–196.

41. Pollard TA, Lampasona V, Akkerman S, Tom K, Hooks MA, Mullins RE, Maroni BJ. Vancomycin redistribution dosing recommendations following high-flux hemodialysis. *Kidney Int.* 1994;45:232–237.

42. Touchette MA, Patel RV, Anandan JV, Dumler F, Zarowitz BJ. Vancomycin removal by high-flux polysulfone hemodialysis membranes in critically ill patients with end-stage renal disease. *Am J Kidney Dis.* 1995;26:469–474.

43. Welage LS, Mason NA, Hoffman EJ, et al. Influence of cellulose triacetate hemodialysis on vancomycin pharmacokinetics. *J Am Soc Nephrol.* 1995;6:1284–1290.

44. Bellomo R, Ernest D, Parkin G, Boyce N. Clearance of vancomycin during continuous arteriovenous hemodiafiltration. *Crit Care Med.* 1990;18:181–183.

45. Joy MS, Matzke GR, Frye RF, Palevsky PM. Determinants of vancomycin clearance by continuous venovenous hemofiltration and continuous venovenous hemodialysis. *Am J Kidney Dis.* 1998;31:1019–1027.

46. Launay-Vacher V, Izzedine H, Mercardal L, Gilbert D. Clinical review: Use of vancomycin n haemodialysis patients. *Crit Care.* 2002;6(4): 313–316.

47. Pai AB, Pai MP. Vancomycin dosing in high flux hemodialysis: A limited-sampling algorithm. *Am J Health-Syst Pharm.* 2004;61:1812–1816.

48. Ambrose PJ, Winter ME. Vancomycin. In Winter ME (Ed.). *Basic Clinical Pharmacokinetics,* 5th ed. Baltimore, MD: Lippincott Williams and Wilkins, 2010.

49. Joy MS, Matze GR, Armstrong DK, Marx MA, Zarowitz BJ. A primer on continuous renal replacement therapy for critically ill patients. *Ann Pharmacother.* 1998;32:362–375.

50. Heintz BH, Matzke GR, Dager WE. Antimicrobial dosing concepts and recommendations for critically ill adult patients receiving continuous renal replacement therapy or intermittent hemodialysis. *Pharmacother.* 2009;29(5):562–577.

51. Macias WL, Mueller BA, Scarim SK. Vancomycin pharmacokinetics in acute renal failure: Preservation of non-renal clearance. *Clin Pharmacol Ther.* 1991;50:688–694.

52. Reetze-Bonorden P, Bohler J, Kohler C, Schollmeyer P, Keller E. Elimination of vancomycin in patients on continuous arteriovenous hemodialysis. *Contrib Nephrol.* 1991;93:135–139.

53. Davies SP, Azadian BS, Kox WJ, Brown EA. Pharmacokinetics of ciprofloxacin and vancomycin in patients with acute renal failure treated by continuous hemodialysis. *Nephrol Dial Transplant.* 1992;7:848–854.

54. Santre C, Leroy O, Simon M, Georges H, Guery B, Beuscart C, Beaucaire G. Pharmacokinetics of vancomycin during continuous hemodiafiltration. *Intensive Care Med.* 1993;19:347–350.

55. Morse GD, Farolino DF, Apicella MA, Walshe JJ. Comparative study of intraperitoneal vancomycin pharmacokinetics during continuous ambulatory peritoneal dialysis. *Antimicrob Agents Chemother.* 1987;31: 173–177.

56. Kam-Tao Li P, Szeto CC, Piraino B, et al. Peritoneal dialysis-related infections recommendations: 2010 update. *Perit Dial Int.* 2010;30:393–423.

57. Hazlewood KA, Brouse SD, Pitcher WD, Hall RG. Vancomycin-associated nephrotoxicity: Grave concern or death by character assassination? *Am J Med.* 2010;123(2):182.e1–182e7.

58. Downs NJ, Neihart RE, Dolezal JM, Hodges GR. Mild nephrotoxicity associated with vancomycin use. *Arch Intern Med.* 1989;149(8):1777–1781.

59. Sorrell TC, Collignon PJ. A prospective study of adverse reactions associated with vancomycin therapy. *J Antimicrob Chemother.* 1985;16(2):235–241.

60. Lodise TP, Lomaestro B, Graves J, Drusano GL. Larger vancomycin doses (at least four grams per day) associated with an increased incidence of nephrotoxicity; *Antimicrob Agents Chemother.* 2008;52(4):1330–1336.

61. Rybak MJ, Albrecht LM, Boike SC, Chandreasekar PH. Nephrotoxicity of vancomycin, alone and with an aminoglycoside. *J Antimicrob Chemother.* 1990;25(4):679–687.

62. Lodise TP, Patel N, Lomaestro BM, et al. Relationship between initial vancomycin concentration-time profile and nephrotoxicity among hospitalized patients. *Clin Infect Dis.* 2009;49:507–514.

63. Saunders NJ. Why monitor peak vancomycin concentrations? *Lancet.* 1994;344:1748–1750.

64. Bailie GR, Neal D. Vancomycin ototoxicity and nephrotoxicity: A review. *Med Toxicol Adverse Drug Exp.* 1988;3(5):376–386.

65. Forouzesh A, Moise PA, Sakoulas G. Vancomycin ototoxocity: A reevaluation in an era of increasing vancomycin doses. *Antimicrob Agents Chemother.* 2009;53(2):483–486.

66. Borland CD, Farrar WE. Reversible neutropenia from vancomycin. *JAMA.* 1979;242:2392–2393.

67. Keserwala HH, Rahill WJ, Amaram N. Vancomycin-induced neutropenia [letter]. *Lancet.* 1981;1(8235):1423.

68. Von Drygalski A, Curtis BR, Bougie DW, McFarland JG, et al. Vancomycin-induced thrombocytopenia. *NEJM.* 2007;356:904–910.

69. Polk RE, Healy DP, Schwartz LB, Rock DT, Garson ML, Roller K. Vancomycin and the RMS: Pharmacodynamics of histamine release. *J Infect Dis.* 1988;157:502–507.

70. DeShazo RD, Kemp SF. Allergic reactions to drugs and biologic agents. *JAMA.* 1997;278:1895–1906.

71. O'Sullivan TL, Ruffing MJ, Lamp KC, Warbasse LH, Ryback MJ. Prospective evaluation of red man syndrome in patients receiving vancomycin. *J Infect Dis.* 1993;168:773–776.

72. Wallace MR, Mascola JR, Oldfield EC. Red man syndrome: incidence, etiology, and prophylaxis. *J Infect Dis.* 1991;164:1180–1185.

73. Wazny LD, Daghigh B. Desensitization protocols for vancomycin hypersensitivity. Ann *Pharmacother.* 2001;35:1458–1464.

CHAPTER 21

Warfarin

VALERY L. CHU, BS, PharmD, BCACP, CACP, AE-C
HELENE C. MALTZ, BS, PharmD, BCPS

OVERVIEW

Following the isolation of hemorrhagic agents from spoiled sweet clover hay in the 1930s and development of 3-phenyacetyl ethyl, 4-hydroxycoumarin as a rat poison in 1948, warfarin has been the primary oral anticoagulant used in North America since its approval for medical use in 1954.[1] Even following the availability of new oral anticoagulant classes, it is widely used for its various indications including prophylaxis and treatment of venous thrombosis and pulmonary embolism, prophylaxis and treatment of thromboembolic complications of atrial fibrillation and heart valve replacement, and postmyocardial infarction (MI) reduction in the risk of death, recurrent MI, and thromboembolic events such as stroke or systemic embolization.[2]

Warfarin, a vitamin K antagonist (VKA), inhibits the C1 subunit of vitamin K epoxide reductase (VKORC1) complex, preventing the regeneration of vitamin K_1 epoxide. This interferes with the carboxylation and activation of vitamin K-dependent clotting factors, factors II, IV, IX, and X (Figure 21-1).[2-4] At the same time, carboxylation of the natural anticoagulants proteins C and S is inhibited as well.[4] This effect can be reversed with the administration (pharmacologically or nutritionally) of vitamin K_1, which is also called phytonadione.[4] Prolongation of the prothrombin time (PT) is seen with warfarin therapy, and a standardized measurement of this effect, the international normalized ratio (INR), is utilized for warfarin monitoring because it has been shown to correlate with efficacy.[2,5,6]

PHARMACOKINETICS

Warfarin has nearly 100 percent oral bioavailability, achieving peak concentrations within 4 hours of administration.[2] Its volume of distribution is small, 0.14 L/kg, and is limited by 99 percent protein binding, primarily to albumin.[2,4] Commercially available warfarin products are equal, racemic mixtures of the R and S enantiomers.[4] The S-warfarin enantiomer is five times more potent. It is primarily metabolized by cytochrome P-450 (CYP) 2C9, and in part by CYP 2C19. The less potent R-warfarin enantiomer is metabolized by CYP 1A2 and CYP 3A4.[7] The products of metabolism are inactive and 92 percent excreted in the urine.[2] The pharmacokinetic half-life of warfarin is 36–42 hours[2,4]; therefore, ≥4 days is required to achieve steady-state concentrations of any given warfarin dose. However, the chief pharmacodynamic effect of warfarin is caused by its inhibition of factor II (thrombin). The full effect of warfarin is therefore determined by the half-life of factor II (60–72 hours), so complete factor II inhibition can take 10 days or more to achieve.[4] It is for the same reason that when warfarin is initiated, its antithrombotic effect is not realized until at least 5 days of treatment

has elapsed. Therefore, overlap with another form of anticoagulation with a faster onset, historically unfractionated or low molecular weight heparin, is required for the first 5 days *and* until the INR produced by warfarin therapy is in the therapeutic range for 2 consecutive days.[4,7] Since complete factor II inhibition can take 10 days or more to achieve, and close monitoring of the extent and rate of anticoagulation achievement is warranted during initiation.

ADVERSE EFFECTS

The major adverse effect associated with warfarin use is bleeding, including fatal intracranial and gastrointestinal (GI) hemorrhages.[2] High-intensity anticoagulation, older age, variable coagulation control, history of GI bleeds, hypertension, cerebrovascular disease, anemia, malignancy, trauma, renal impairment, liver function impairment, and genetic predisposition to over-anticoagulation are risk factors for bleeding. Because of the possibility of bleeding, it is imperative that any modifiable risk factors are eliminated or reduced prior to initiation of warfarin therapy, appropriate monitoring of anticoagulation is performed, and the benefit of anticoagulation outweighs the risk for each patient.[2,4,6]

Other serious adverse effects include tissue necrosis early in warfarin therapy and systemic atheroemboli or cholesterol microemboli presenting as "purple toe syndrome." Less serious reactions include vasculitis, elevations in liver enzymes, GI complaints, and allergic reactions, which may be related to the dyes used in the tablets.[2,8]

DOSING STRATEGIES

Initiation of warfarin therapy can follow two general approaches: the use of a dose considered to be a prediction of the ultimate maintenance dose or use of a higher dose initially (often given the inaccurate moniker of "loading dose") in an attempt to more rapidly identify the anticipated dose of warfarin to achieve target INR. Estimations of eventual maintenance doses must account for vast inter- and intrapatient variability discussed in the following section. It is also possible, through the use of various nomograms, to quickly titrate a given warfarin dose upward to the necessary maintenance dose based on the early INR response. It is essential that qualified, experienced clinicians are available to interpret the early INR response appropriately to improve patient outcomes.[9-11]

Several nomograms for dosing warfarin in the initiation stages of therapy have been developed. In 1999, a comparison of 5 mg and 10 mg initiation doses used to treat inpatients with heterogeneous indications found that patients in the 5 mg group were more likely to achieve stable anticoagulation within days 3–5 than those receiving the 10 mg dose (relative risk, 2.22, 95% confidence

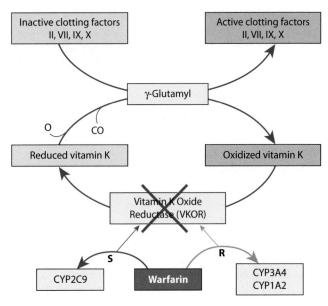

FIGURE 21-1. Mechanism of action of warfarin.

TABLE 21-1	Factors That Increase or Reduce Warfarin Dose Requirements[2,4,5,7,14]	
Factor	Warfarin Dose Requirement	Mechanism
Genetic variation		
CYP 2C9*2 or *3	Reduced	Impaired metabolism of S-warfarin
VKORC1 haplotype A	Reduced	Preexisting impairment of VKORC1 activity
Increased age	Reduced	Multiple: hypoalbuminemia, decreased dietary/absorbed vitamin K, drug interactions due to polypharmacy
Hepatic dysfunction	Reduced	Reduced synthesis of coagulation factors
High fever	Reduced	Increased catabolism of coagulation factors
Hypothyroidism	Increased	Reduced metabolism of coagulation factors
Hyperthyroidism (natural or drug-induced)	Reduced	Increased catabolism of coagulation factors
Increased dietary vitamin K	Increased	Bypassing of VKORC1 through warfarin-insensitive pathway
Reduced dietary vitamin K	Reduced	Potentiation of inhibition of VKORC1
Drug interactions	Variable	*See Table 21-2 and text section on Drug Interactions.*
Alcohol ingestion: acute	None or Reduced	Inhibition of warfarin metabolism (binge drinking)
Alcohol ingestion: chronic	Variable	Induced metabolism or concomitant hepatic dysfunction

TABLE 21-2	Suggested Maintenance Warfarin Daily Doses Based on Genotypes[2]					
	CYP2C9					
VKORC1	*1/*1	*1/*2	*1/*3	*2/*2	*2/*3	*3/*3
GG	5–7 mg	5–7 mg	3–4 mg	3–4 mg	3–4 mg	0.5–2 mg
AG	5–7 mg	3–4 mg	3–4 mg	3–4 mg	0.5–2 mg	0.5–2 mg
AA	3–4 mg	3–4 mg	0.5–2 mg	0.5–2 mg	0.5–2 mg	0.5–2 mg

interval (CI) 1.30–3.70 [P <0.003]). Over-anticoagulation was less likely in the 5 mg group, although this difference did not reach statistical significance.[6] Conversely, a randomized clinical trial in 2003 of outpatients with venous thromboembolism and a mean age of approximately 55 years found that those receiving a 10 mg initial dose reached a therapeutic INR 1.4 days earlier than those receiving a 5 mg dose (P <0.001) and a higher percentage of patients on the 10 mg dose were therapeutic by day 5 (83% vs 46%, P <0.001). No differences in bleeding or INRs greater than 5 were noted between the groups.[12] Therefore, the 9th Antithrombotic Therapy and Prevention of Thrombosis: American College of Chest Physicians (ACCP) Evidence-Based Clinical Practice Guidelines recommend the second approach with an initial dose of 10 mg daily for the initial 2 days for otherwise stable outpatients with no risk factors for excessive warfarin sensitivity, followed by dosing adjustments made based on INR measurements.[10] Were hospitalized, elderly patients with comorbidities to receive the same dosage, it may result in over-anticoagulation, so more conservative doses may be warranted in such cases.

DOSING VARIABILITY

While warfarin therapy is individualized through monitoring of the INR response to specific dosage regimens in each patient, the selection of an initial dose, as a prediction of the resultant maintenance dose, is complicated by wide intra- and interpatient variability. Up to 10-fold interpatient variability has been reported,[5,13] and many factors, both predictable and unpredictable, are responsible for the disparity (Table 21-1).[4,5]

GENETICS

Because of significant genetic variability in CYP 2C9 enzymatic activity, individuals with CYP 2C9*2 and CYP 2C9*3 variant alleles have reduced enzymatic clearance of S-warfarin. Variability in VKORC1, resulting in baseline ineffective coagulation, exists as well.[2] The Food and Drug Administration (FDA) suggests that genetic variations can be considered when a dosing regimen is selected, with expected maintenance doses based on genotype presentation provided by Bristol-Myers Squibb, manufacturer of Coumadin® brand of warfarin (Table 21-2)[2]; however, the current

ACCP guidelines do not recommend genetic testing prior to warfarin initiation.[10] Studies assessing the application of pharmacogenetic data to the selection of a warfarin dose have been conducted. The International Warfarin Pharmacogenetics Consortium[13] conducted a validation cohort of 1,009 subjects and found that an algorithm incorporating variations in CYP 2C9 and VKORC1 was significantly better at correctly predicting the warfarin dose for patients requiring ≤21 mg (low dose) or ≥49 mg (high dose) of warfarin per week (49.3% vs. 33.3% and 24.8% vs. 7.2%, both P <0.001, respectively) as compared to a clinical algorithm without genetic information. However, no significant benefit was seen for patients requiring intermediate weekly doses. The authors propose that patients requiring low or high weekly doses of warfarin would benefit from such an algorithm since they may otherwise be over- or under-anticoagulated. On the other hand, in a prospective, observational study of 214 subjects, Li et al.[5] found that even though accounting for genetic variations can assist with dose requirement prediction, in most cases the same information can be gleaned from close, expert monitoring of early INR response. Furthermore, not all variability is reflected by genetic testing and clinical evaluation of INR response would, therefore, be required in any case.

AGE

It is widely accepted that the elderly have increased sensitivity to warfarin, requiring lower weekly doses than younger individuals.[14] In a prospective and retrospective cohort including 2,359 subjects ≥80 years of age, Garcia et al.[14] found that the average weekly warfarin dose decreased by 0.4 mg per year (95% confidence interval

(CI), 3.8–5.3; P <0.001). The mechanism for this effect is not completely clear but may involve a combination of hypoalbuminemia, reduced vitamin K intake or GI absorption, and drug interactions due to polypharmacy.[14] Furthermore, the time to achieve an anticoagulation effect is delayed by approximately 24–36 hours in the elderly.[15] The elderly are also more susceptible to bleeding complications with warfarin use, and reversal of anticoagulation takes longer in the elderly as well.[14]

The standard nomograms often used for initiating warfarin therapy may overestimate the dose required for the elderly, placing them at risk for bleeding complications. Therefore, age-adjusted nomograms have been developed, including one by Gedge et al.[15] In an age-stratified, randomized prospective study of 120 individuals over the age of 65, the investigators found that while their age-adjusted, low-dose warfarin induction regimen took longer to achieve a therapeutic INR than the comparator nomogram[16] (patients 65–75 years of age: 4.6 ± 1.6 days vs. 3.8 ± 0.8 days, P = 0.03; patients >75 years of age: 4.5 ± 1.4 days vs. 3.5 ± 0.7 days, P = 0.03), use of the age-adjusted regimen resulted in a slightly longer duration of time spent in the therapeutic range (patients 65–75 years of age: 3.0 ± 1.3 days vs. 2.7 ± 1.3 days, P = 0.03; patients >75 years of age: 2.9 ± 1.1 days vs. 2.4 ± 1.3 days, P = 0.04) and significantly fewer INRs >4.5 in the first 8 days.

Roberts et al.[17] hypothesized that the standard 5 mg starting doses, considered nonloading initiation doses at the time the study was conducted, may overshoot the actual maintenance dose requirement of elderly patients. They found that 73 patients (30 of whom were >75 years of age) dosed with an age-adjusted nomogram were able to quickly achieve a stable therapeutic INR without significant over-anticoagulation (INR >4.0). A nonsignificant trend of patients with albumin levels <3 gm/dL requiring lower doses was seen as well.

CLINICAL CONDITIONS

The clinical status of any individual can also change depending on comorbid conditions, concomitant medications, alterations in dietary vitamin K intake, and alcohol use. Hepatic dysfunction can ultimately result in reduced production of coagulation factors, causing an enhanced response to warfarin and increased risk of bleeding.[4] A similar effect is seen with high fevers or hyperthyroidism, both hypermetabolic states that enhance degradation of coagulation factors.[4] The metabolism of coagulation factors can be reduced in the hypothyroid state, requiring increased doses. This effect can disappear once the hypothyroidism is corrected and a euthyroid state is achieved.[18]

Inconsistent vitamin K intake can affect warfarin's therapeutic effect. Excessive intake can counteract the desired effect of warfarin because dietary vitamin K can bypass VKORC1 through a warfarin-insensitive pathway. A diet deficient in vitamin K, which can result from decreased overall intake as seen with sick patients given antibiotics that deplete vitamin K-producing bacteria in the GI tract, fat malabsorption, or intravenous diets lacking adequate vitamin K supplementation, can be associated with increased sensitivity to warfarin's effects.[4] Because the INR represents the therapeutic effect of a given warfarin dosage regimen in a specific patient, and dosage adjustments are made to titrate warfarin to the desired INR, the actual quantity of vitamin K consumed, whether it is low, moderate, or high, is not relevant as long as the intake remains stable. With consistency comes a more predictable warfarin dose-INR response; therefore, large variations in the amount of vitamin K ingested should be avoided.

DRUG INTERACTIONS

Alterations in response to warfarin may result from interactions with numerous medications. Several distinct and overlapping mechanisms are responsible for these interactions as well as the inability to predict the outcome of the interactions precisely in many cases.[7] Medications can affect the metabolic clearance of warfarin by affecting CYP 2C9, 2C19, 1A2, and/or 3A4. Inhibition of CYP 2C9 is most significant as it affects the more potent S-warfarin.

Interactions involving the GI tract can occur as well. Some medications may bind to warfarin in the GI tract, preventing or reducing its absorption and resultant efficacy. Broad-spectrum antibiotics, especially if used for a long duration, can impair endogenous vitamin K synthesis through disruption of the normal flora of the GI tract, potentiating the effect of warfarin.[7]

Pharmacodynamic interactions can result from coadministration of warfarin with agents that also impair hemostasis (antiplatelet or anticoagulant agents) or increase hemorrhagic potential (gastric irritants). The cumulative consequence of these additive effects is an increased bleeding risk.[7]

Finally, because warfarin is highly protein-bound, displacement interactions can enhance warfarin's effects until equilibrium with serum concentrations can be reestablished.[4,7]

Given the known pharmacokinetic and pharmacodynamic mechanisms by which warfarin may interact with other agents, it is possible to anticipate potential drug-drug interactions (Table 21-3). Among the numerous published reports of interactions with warfarin, most are single case reports with confounding factors. Holbrook et al. performed an exhaustive review of the available evidence and summarized the likelihood of interactions occurring with select agents, but noted that lack of published data did not preclude the possibility of an interaction, especially in instances of theoretical mechanisms for interaction.[7]

Even though in theory it is best to avoid possible interactions, especially those considered major and highly probable, a risk versus benefit assessment in some situations may favor the use of potentially interacting medications. For interactions that may alter warfarin level and the INR, the INR test serves as a useful tool to measure the magnitude of the interaction so that in most cases, interactions are manageable with more frequent measurement of the INR, close monitoring for signs and symptoms of bleeding, and the reestablishment of an appropriate warfarin maintenance dose accounting for the interacting medication.[7]

MONITORING

Warfarin prolongs the PT, which reflects the extent of the inhibition of factors II, VII, and X. The test relies on the addition of calcium and thromboplastin to citrated plasma. However, due to variability in the potency of different batches of thromboplastin, the INR, a means of standardizing the PT values, is now used in lieu of PT. The INR calculation converts the ratio of a patient's PT to that of the mean normal PT accounting for the responsiveness of the specific thromboplastin used in the laboratory conducting the assay of the VKA effect on coagulation factors. This responsiveness is the International Sensitivity Index (ISI) and the formula used is as follows[4]:

$$INR = (patient\ PT/mean\ normal\ PT)^{ISI}$$

The ACCP guidelines recommend an INR between 2.0 and 3.0 for venous thromboembolic and atrial fibrillation indications and an INR between 2.5 and 3.5 for mitral valve replacement. Because the target range is the condition at which optimization of desired efficacy converges with acceptable toxicity risk, the time in target range (TTR) should be maximized.[10]

Historically, even though inpatients are generally monitored daily, for outpatient therapy, the INR is monitored once or twice weekly until the warfarin dose is determined and INR stability is

Agent	Theoretical Mechanism(s)	Effect on INR[a]	Effect on Bleed Risk[a]	Likelihood of Interaction[b,c]
Acarbose	Unknown	↑	↑	++
Acetaminophen	Competitive substrate for CYP 1A2	↑	↑	+++
Amiodarone	CYP 1A2 and 2C9 inhibition	↑	↑	+++
Amoxicillin/clavulanate	Unknown	↑	↑	+++
Aspirin	Additive bleed risk	0	↑	++
Azole antifungals	CYP 2C9, 2C19, +/− 3A4 inhibition	↑	↑	0 / ++ / +++
Barbiturates	CYP 2C9 +/− 3A4 induction	↑	0	+++
Carbamazepine	CYP 2C9 and 3A4 induction	↑	0	+++
Celecoxib	Competitive substrate for CYP 2C9	↑	↑	++
Cholestyramine	Reduce bioavailability	↑	0	+++
Cimetidine	CYP 1A2, 2C19, and 3A4 inhibition	↑	↑	+++
Ciprofloxacin	CYP 1A2 and 3A4 inhibition	↑	↑	+++
Citalopram	CYP 1A2 inhibition	↑	↑	+++
Clarithromycin	CYP 3A4 inhibition	↑	↑	++
Cotrimoxazole	CYP 2C9 inhibition, competitive substrate for CYP 2C9 and 3A4	↑	↑	+++
Diltiazem	CYP 3A4 inhibition	↑	↑	+++
Fenofibrate	CYP 2C9 and 3A4 inhibition	↑	↑	+++
Fish oil	Enhanced antiplatelet effect	↑	↑	+++
Fluorouracil	CYP 2C9 inhibition	↑	↑	++
Fluvastatin	CYP 2C9 inhibition	↑	↑	++
Fluvoxamine	CYP 1A2, 2C19, and 2C9 inhibition	↑	↑	++
Gemfibrozil	CYP 2C9 and 3A4 inhibition	↑	↑	+
Grapefruit juice	CYP 3A4 inhibition	↑	↑	++
Isoniazid	CYP 1A2 and 3A4 inhibition	↑	↑	+++
Ketoconazole	CYP 3A4 inhibition	↑	↑	0
Mercaptopurine	Unknown	↓	0	+++
Mesalamine	Additive bleed risk, unknown	0	↑ / ↓	+++
Metronidazole	CYP 2C9 inhibition	↑	↑	+++
NSAIDs	Additive bleed risk	0	↑	++ / +++
Orlistat	Reduced vitamin K absorption	↑	↑	+
Phenytoin	CYP 1A2 and 3A4 induction	↓	0	++
Protease inhibitors	CYP 3A4 inhibition	↑	↑	+ / ++
Ribavirin	Unknown	↓	0	+++
Rifampin	CYP 1A2, 2C19, 2C9, and 3A4 induction	↓	0	+++
Sertraline	CYP 2C9 inhibition	↑	↑	+++
Simvastatin	CYP 3A4 inhibition	↑	↑	++
Tamoxifen	Competitive substrate for CYP 2C9 and 3A4	↑	↑	++
Tramadol	Competitive substrate for CYP 3A4	↑	↑	++
Trazodone	Competitive substrate for CYP 3A4	↓	0	+++
Zileuton	CYP 1A2 and 3A4 inhibition	↑	↑	+++

TABLE 21-3   Select Drug Interactions with Warfarin[7,19-21]

[a]↑, Increased; ↓, Decreased; 0, No effect

[b]Estimation based on systematic evaluation of published reports by Holbrook and colleagues[7]

[c]+++, Highly probable; ++, Probable; +, Possible[7]

achieved. This monitoring regimen is followed by testing every 4 weeks. The current ACCP guidelines recommend monitoring the INR at intervals of up to 12 weeks for patients with consistently stable INRs.[10,11] This recommendation is partially based on a randomized, noninferiority trial of 250 patients at a stable warfarin dose for 6 months.[22] The authors found no significant difference in TTR between the 4-week group and the 12-week group (74.1% ± 18.8% vs. 71.6% ± 20.0%; noninferiority P = 0.020). Significantly fewer dosage adjustments were necessary in the 12-week group and no significant differences in bleeding or thromboembolic complications. One caveat to this recommendation is that contact with anticoagulation staff was maintained at 4-week intervals, even for those with INR monitoring every 12 weeks.

A study conducted by Witt et al.[23] describes clinical factors that can predict which patients may be more likely to have highly stable INRs and may be monitored on a less frequent basis. These factors included age over 70 and the absence of diabetes mellitus, heart failure, or concomitant estrogen therapy.

Should single outlying INRs occur during routine monitoring, a repeat INR should be conducted within 1 to 2 weeks to confirm whether dosage adjustments are clinically necessary.[10]

BRAND VERSUS GENERIC FORMULATIONS

Warfarin is a medication with a narrow therapeutic range, with the possibility of slight increases or decreases in therapeutic effect resulting in over-anticoagulation and bleeding or under-anticoagulation

TABLE 21-4	Warfarin Dosage Strengths and Colors[2]
Dose strength	Color
1 mg	Pink
2 mg	Lavender
2.5 mg	Green
3 mg	Tan
4 mg	Blue
5 mg	Peach
6 mg	Teal
7.5 mg	Yellow
10 mg	White

and thrombotic complications. Warfarin also requires individualized, careful titration of the dose to patient-specific therapeutic INR. Because of the serious consequences of slight variations in bioavailability for such medications, concern over the bioequivalence of different formulations of warfarin, including the differences between brand name and generic products, has arisen. A recent systematic review of relevant literature was conducted by Dentali and colleagues[24] to assess whether significant consequences occur following switches between brand-name and generic warfarin. They found that overall, generic products that met FDA requirements for bioequivalence had no clinically significant differences in safety or efficacy when compared with brand-name products; INR results as well as thromboembolic and bleeding outcomes were evaluated. The authors recommended close monitoring should switches between products occur and switches should be infrequent so additional monitoring should not be necessary if patients remain at a stable warfarin dose. Available dose strengths are consistent between brand-name and generic manufacturers, as are the colors of the tablets (Table 21-4).

REVERSAL OF ANTICOAGULATION

EMERGENT REVERSAL FOR BLEEDING OR INCREASED BLEEDING RISK

As previously mentioned, the major complication of warfarin therapy is bleeding and administration of vitamin K can counteract the effects of warfarin and can, therefore, be used as an antidote. A major bleeding event in a patient receiving warfarin is a medical emergency and supratherapeutic INRs are associated with an increased risk for bleeding.

The urgency of warfarin reversal depends on various clinical factors, particularly the occurrence of active bleeding. Therefore, the ACCP recommendations for elevated INRs are stratified based on the degree of INR elevation and presence or absence of major bleeding. A study conducted by Crowther et al.[25] illustrated that no clinical benefit, measured by a difference in the frequency of bleeding, thromboembolism, or death, was seen when the outcomes of those with elevated INRs but no active bleeding who received low-dose vitamin K were compared to those who received placebo. Because of this and other similar studies, the ACCP guidelines currently suggest that no vitamin K be administered for INRs between 4.5 and 10.0 with no evidence of bleeding.[10] For those on warfarin with INRs >10.0 and no evidence of bleeding, a low dose of 2.5 mg of oral vitamin K is suggested because of the significant hemorrhagic risk.[10]

For those experiencing VKA-associated major bleeding, previous ACCP recommendations included the administration of fresh frozen plasma (FFP), which is effective if dosed appropriately but incurs several significant complications and barriers to use. The current recommendations favor the administration of 4-factor prothrombin complex concentrate (PCC) along with 5–10 mg of vitamin K administered as a slow intravenous injection over FFP.[10] Routine supportive care should be administered as well.

The time necessary for supratherapeutic INRs to decline to a value within the therapeutic range is dependent on several clinical factors. The risk factors for persistent INR elevation were evaluated in a retrospective cohort study by Hylek et al.[26] that reviewed follow-up INRs drawn 2 days after an INR >6.0 was recorded. The study demonstrated that the risk of the subsequent INR remaining >4.0 was increased in patients of greater age (odds ratio [OR] per decade of life, 1.18 [95% CI, 1.01–1.38]), with higher index INR value (odds ratio per unit, 1.25 [95% CI, 1.14–1.37]), in patients with decompensated heart failure (OR, 2.79 [95% CI, 1.30–5.98]), and with a concomitant active cancer diagnosis (OR, 2.48 [95% CI, 1.11–5.57]). The same risk was decreased in patients who required larger weekly warfarin doses (adjusted OR per 10 mg warfarin, 0.87 [95% CI, 0.79–0.97]), indicating they are less sensitive to warfarin's effects.

BRIDGING THERAPY IN THE PERIOPERATIVE PERIOD

When patients receiving warfarin therapy are scheduled for surgical procedures that entail a significant risk of bleeding, it is recommended that the warfarin be discontinued 5 days prior to surgery and restarted 12–24 hours after surgery, once hemostasis is achieved.[27] This process allows for the effects of warfarin to be minimized while the surgical bleeding risk is greatest. In cases where patients are at a high thrombotic risk, including some patients with mitral valve replacement, atrial fibrillation, and venous thromboembolism, and the lack of anticoagulation during the pre- and postprocedure period entails a substantial risk of clot development, bridging with another anticoagulant that is shorter acting and more rapidly effective upon reinstitution of antithrombotic therapy is recommended. The shorter-acting agent is then stopped closer to the actual procedure time and can be restarted after hemostasis is achieved and until warfarin's full antithrombotic effects are reestablished.[27]

For minor dental procedures, 2–3 days cessation of warfarin therapy is sufficient, and for minor dermatological and cataract surgeries, warfarin therapy can continue unchanged.[27]

CASE STUDIES

CASE 1: INITIATION IN INPATIENT SETTING

TE is a 60-year-old male who presents to the emergency department complaining of swelling and pain in his left leg for one week, with onset of shortness of breath and sharp chest pain last night. Computed tomography (CT) studies confirm acute pulmonary embolism (PE) and proximal deep vein thrombosis (DVT). His past medical history is significant only for hypertension and dyslipidemia (for which he takes lisinopril, chlorthalidone, and simvastatin). Chemistry, metabolic panel, and blood counts are within normal limits. He is hypotensive so the decision is made to admit TE to a medical floor. For the acute venous thromboembolism (VTE), he is started on warfarin and enoxaparin to overlap at least 5 days.

Height = 6′0″

Weight = 120 kg

Answer:

In the setting of CVA prevention secondary to chronic atrial fibrillation, the time frame to establish effective anticoagulation is generally less urgent. Although it depends on the individual level of risk for CVA, overlap with heparin is usually not needed. Selecting a starting dose of warfarin based on the patient's estimated maintenance dose is appropriate. If INRs cannot be closely monitored (e.g., every 3 days), initiating at a more conservative dose may be prudent.

AF is relatively elderly, has mild-to-moderate heart failure, and takes atorvastatin, all characteristics that suggest a lower maintenance dose. If the expectation is to evaluate an INR one week after therapy initiation, AF may be started on 2–2.5 mg daily of warfarin, with further dose adjustments made based on INR results in one week's time. This approach reduces the burden of more frequent INR monitoring, with the trade-off of potentially extending the time required to establish the maintenance warfarin dose.

CASE 4: MAINTENANCE DOSE ADJUSTMENT

A Single Out-of-Range INR in an Otherwise Stable Patient

AF has been stabilized on warfarin 5 mg daily for chronic atrial fibrillation for the past 5 months, with INR monitoring every 4 weeks. Her last 3 INRs have been in her target 2.0–3.0 range (2.31, 2.84, 2.67). Today, she reports for routine INR monitoring and the result is 1.72. On questioning, she claims no recent change in medications, vitamin K-rich food intake, or medical conditions. She does not recall any recent missed doses of warfarin.

QUESTION

How should AF's warfarin dose be adjusted?

Answer:

One of the pitfalls of warfarin dosing inexperience is the tendency to react to any out-of-range INR by changing the dose. The result is needless dose changes that reduce time in therapeutic range and potentially compromising anticoagulation efficacy and/or safety. An out-of-range INR should always trigger the clinician to (1) carefully rule out any recent changes and factors that could impact warfarin, including and especially medication adherence, and (2) review the patient's recent INR and warfarin dosing history for trends.

A single out-of-range INR, particularly if close to the target range (<0.5 above or below), does not always warrant a warfarin dose change. AF has an established recent record of INR stability on the same warfarin dose and no readily identifiable changes that may interact with warfarin. In this case, she should continue to take warfarin 5 mg daily but her follow-up time should be shortened to 1–2 weeks to verify whether she is experiencing a true trend requiring a dose change.

Two or Three Consecutive Out-of-Range INRs, Consistently High or Low

At her next follow-up, AF's INR is 1.86, and her warfarin dose was maintained at 5 mg daily. At today's follow-up, her INR is 1.64, and she again reports no relevant changes to warfarin dosing, medications, diet, and medical conditions.

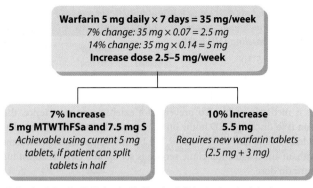

M=Monday, T=Tuesday, W=Wednesday, Th=Thursday, F=Friday, Sa=Saturday, S=Sunday

FIGURE 21-2. Adjusting warfarin maintenance dose for a low INR.

QUESTION

How should AF's warfarin dose be adjusted?

Answer:

When two or three consecutive INRs consistently fall out-of-range at the upper or lower end of the target INR range, a dose change is usually appropriate. The target INR is typically the center of the range, so that even with mild fluctuations in INRs, the patient will remain in the target range most of the time. For AF, an INR of 2.5 should be targeted, especially given her high CVA risk based on CHADS2 risk score.[29] Her recent INRs (1.72, 1.96, and 1.84) support an increase in her warfarin dose.

For INRs that are within 0.5–1.0 from the target result of 2.5, the warfarin dose may be increased between 7–14 percent of the total weekly dose (Figure 21-2).

To evaluate the effect of a dose change, AF's INR should be rechecked sooner. With multiple INRs supporting the need for a dose increase, and a relatively small dose increase being made, the INR could be evaluated in two weeks to increase the likelihood of assessing the new dose's full effect. An INR checked after one week may be premature, but is reasonable based on suspicion of patient unreliability in following instructions and/or a desire to be sure the dose change is trending appropriately.

Single Out-of-Range INR by >0.5 in an Otherwise Stable Patient

At her new maintenance warfarin 5.5 mg daily dose, AF experiences a period of stable INRs in her target 2.0–3.0 range. At today's visit, her INR is 3.9 and she reports no relevant changes to warfarin dosing, medications, diet, and medical conditions.

QUESTION

How should AF's warfarin dose be adjusted?

Answer:

Whether an INR is slightly or further out of target range, the clinician must still (1) carefully rule out any recent changes and factors that could impact warfarin, including and especially medication adherence, and (2) review the patient's recent INR and warfarin dosing history for trends.

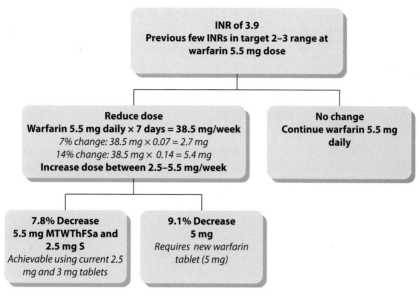

FIGURE 21-3. Adjusting warfarin maintenance for an elevated INR.

In this case, AF's INR of 3.9 is a larger excursion from target range. Given the previously stable INRs and warfarin dose and if an interacting factor cannot be identified from patient history, these are two possible interventions (Figure 21-3).

If the warfarin dose is reduced, follow-up should preferentially be within one week to evaluate the initial effect. Follow-up time is largely guided by urgency of maintaining time in therapeutic range and degree of predictability of next INR. In this case, AF's unexpectedly high INR that is also >0.5 out of target range warrants closer follow-up even after a dose reduction, so a one-week evaluation is prudent.

Lowering the dose is not the only option. Considering the high INR of 3.9 was unexpected and no etiology was identified, it is also reasonable to maintain the same dose and reevaluate to see whether it is a true trend that requires a dose change. AF's high CVA risk is a consideration, and a reason to hold off on a dose reduction. AF could be instructed to hold today's warfarin dose to allow the INR to trend back down to target range, then resume her usual 5.5 mg daily dose. In this case, however, the INR should be evaluated within one week in case a dose reduction is warranted.

CASE 5: DRUG INTERACTIONS— AMIODARONE, A CYP INHIBITOR

IR is a 65-year-old male on warfarin for chronic atrial fibrillation, stabilized for the past few months at warfarin 6 mg daily to target an INR range of 2.0–3.0. Secondary to frequent episodes of symptomatic palpitations, his cardiologist is initiating amiodarone 400 mg twice daily today, to be reduced to 400 mg once daily in 2 weeks, then 200 mg daily in 4 weeks.

QUESTION

How should IR's warfarin dose be adjusted?

Answer:

Amiodarone interacts with warfarin, frequently and substantially, leading to greatly reduced warfarin doses to maintain the target INR range. It is an inhibitor of CYP 1A2, 2C9, and 3A4 enzymes, reducing metabolism of both enantiomers of warfarin, thus increasing warfarin concentrations and its anticoagulant effect.

The pharmacokinetics of amiodarone further complicates the interaction. It has a prolonged and highly variable time of onset, maximal effect, and elimination if therapy is withdrawn. These factors are often critical in deciding how to monitor and manage warfarin dosing with interacting agents. Because amiodarone requires a long period to achieve steady-state effect, the full effect of the interaction may not be realized for several weeks, hence weekly INR follow-up and dose adjustments should be planned for the next 4 weeks, possibly as long as 8 weeks.

The interaction appears to be dose-dependent. Sanoski et al.[30] observed a strong inverse correlation (r2 = 0.94, p <0.005) between amiodarone dose and warfarin dose, and suggested reducing warfarin dose by approximately 40 percent, 35 percent, 30 percent, and 25 percent for amiodarone maintenance doses of 400, 300, 200, and 100 mg daily, respectively. Although IR's target maintenance amiodarone dose is 200 mg daily, it is reasonable to expect a stronger initial interaction related to the loading dose.

IR's warfarin dose should be preemptively lowered today, given the high likelihood and degree of interaction. An initial dose reduction of 10–20 percent is reasonable. Possible regimens for the first week include warfarin 5 mg daily, a 16.7 percent reduction, or warfarin 3 mg MWF (Monday, Wednesday, Friday) and 6 mg STThSa (Sunday, Tuesday, Thursday, Saturday), a 21.4 percent reduction.

IR's INR should be assessed in one week to determine magnitude of the initial interaction. If the INR is <2.0, the dose could be increased up to 10 percent or left unchanged if very close to 2.0. If the INR is between 2.0–3.0, the dose could be left unchanged or reduced by <10 percent. If the INR is >3.0, the dose could be reduced by 10–15 percent. In all cases, the INR should be assessed again in one week.

As IR's amiodarone dose is tapered to his target 200 mg once daily after one month, it can be expected that warfarin requirements may increase at that time, although not to his 6 mg maintenance dose prior to amiodarone therapy. Therefore, I.R. will likely require close INR monitoring for up to 8 weeks to establish his new maintenance warfarin dose on amiodarone 200 mg daily.

CASE 6: DRUG INTERACTIONS— CARBAMAZEPINE, A CYP INDUCER

BA is a 65-year-old female on warfarin for bilateral acute DVTs 5 months ago, and stabilized at warfarin 8.5 mg daily to target an INR 2.0–3.0. She has been on long-standing carbamazepine therapy for a single grand mal seizure that she could recall, at a dose of 200 mg every 8 hours. Her neurologist instructs BA with a taper protocol (week 1–2: 200 mg every 12 hours; week 3–4: 100 mg every 12 hours), with the intention of discontinuing carbamazepine in 4 weeks.

QUESTION

How should BA's warfarin dose be adjusted?

Answer:

The antiepileptic agent carbamazepine is a potent inducer of CYP 3A4 and moderate inducer of CYP 2C9, therefore, increasing the metabolic clearance of both enantiomers of warfarin. Patients taking warfarin and carbamazepine concurrently will require higher warfarin doses to maintain an INR in the target range. Less appreciated than interactions that occur when an interacting agent is added to warfarin therapy are those when such agents are discontinued.

BA's current maintenance warfarin dose reflects the induction effect of carbamazepine. When the latter is discontinued, B.A. will likely need a dose reduction. The month-long tapering schedule further complicates the reversal of the interaction.

If the magnitude of carbamazepine's induction effect on BA's warfarin dose is unknown (i.e., carbamazepine was initiated and stabilized prior to warfarin therapy), it will be prudent to begin monitoring INRs weekly, and making dose adjustments as needed. Induction interactions are unlikely to reverse as quickly as inhibition, so it is unnecessary to preemptively reduce her dose.

CASE 7: WARFARIN REVERSAL—BLEEDING

LB is a 55-year-old male on warfarin for prevention of recurrent VTE, stabilized on warfarin 11.5 mg daily for over a year to target an INR range of 2.0–3.0. He has been medically stable, with no changes in medications, for the past year. His concomitant medications include docusate, senna, lactulose, and pantoprazole. Today, he calls the clinic to report experiencing malaise and coughing for the past 2 days, and today coughed up brownish, coffee-ground material twice. He denies observing other signs and symptoms of bleeding.

QUESTION

What do you advise LB to do?

Answer:

Coffee-ground emesis suggests upper GI bleeding, and constitutes an emergency that must be promptly evaluated. LB should be instructed to take no further warfarin doses and immediately present for emergency care. If the medical assessment confirms GI bleeding, phytonadione 5–10 mg by slow intravenous infusion is indicated regardless of the INR to reverse warfarin. The use of a 4-factor PCC may be considered to rapidly reestablish normal hemostasis, especially in life-threatening bleeds, while FFP is an alternate adjunct if PCCs are unavailable.

CASE 8: WARFARIN REVERSAL—ELECTIVE

BH is a 67-year-old male on warfarin for atrial fibrillation, stabilized on warfarin 7 mg daily for >6 months but recently had his dose adjusted to 6 mg, to target an INR range of 2.0–3.0. His other medical conditions include hypertension and dyslipidemia. He is undergoing workup for prostate cancer and is scheduled for a prostate biopsy in 2 weeks. His primary care provider (PCP) clears him for the procedure but requests your assistance with the perioperative management of anticoagulation.

QUESTION

What do you recommend?

Answer:

Prostate biopsy is a procedure that entails a high bleeding risk, and therefore requires full reversal of warfarin. Assuming BH's current INR is within target range, he will need to hold warfarin 5 days prior to the biopsy to allow his INR to decline to baseline. An INR should be assessed on the day of the biopsy to ensure it is safe to proceed. Warfarin may be restarted after the biopsy, on the same day if hemostasis is achieved, as its onset of action requires several days.

BH has a low to moderate risk of CVA, with a CHADS2 risk score of 2. The use of bridge therapy with a short-acting parenteral anticoagulant will not confer significant benefit, so BH can simply hold warfarin therapy. It may be considered, however, if both BH and his PCP strongly preferred the added protection against thrombosis.

HOMEWORK CASES

CASE 1

TS is a 56-year-old female on warfarin for prevention of recurrent VTE, stabilized for the past few months at warfarin 7.5 mg daily to target an INR range of 2.0–3.0. At her PCP appointment today, she reports a 3-day history of burning pain on urination and urgency, but no fever or flank pain. Her PCP prescribes cotrimoxazole DS 160 mg/800 mg every 12 hours for 3 days for urinary tract infection (UTI).

QUESTION 1

By what mechanisms does cotrimoxazole interact with warfarin?

Answer:

Sulfamethoxazole is a CYP 2C9 inhibitor, a competitive substrate of both CYP 2C9 and CYP 3A4, and may displace warfarin from protein-binding sites.

QUESTION 2

What effect is anticipated with the addition of cotrimoxazole to stable warfarin therapy?

Answer:

Cotrimoxazole may potentiate warfarin's hypoprothrombinemic effect, increasing the INR and bleeding risk.

QUESTION 3

How should TS's warfarin dose be adjusted?

Answer:

Duration of concomitant therapy is relevant. With only three days of therapy, the duration of the interaction is limited. It is preferable to use an alternate agent with no interaction potential to treat the UTI. If an alternate is not possible, consider holding warfarin on day 1 preemptively, then continue the same maintenance dose.

QUESTION 4

When should TS's INR be reevaluated?

Answer:

The INR should be reevaluated on day 3–4 to determine the extent of the interaction, and to allow for another warfarin dose adjustment, if needed. It is anticipated that TS may resume her usual warfarin 7.5 mg dose thereafter.

CASE 2

DW is an 83-year-old female who was hospitalized with an acute CVA with new finding of atrial fibrillation. Her past medical history is significant for anemia, hypertension, type 2 diabetes, chronic kidney disease, and peripheral vascular disease. Her medications on admission were aspirin 81 mg daily, fosinopril 20 mg daily, insulin glargine 30 units subcutaneously daily, and sitagliptin 25 mg daily. She is started on unfractionated heparin for anticoagulation and diltiazem for rate control. Lab work show chronically elevated serum creatinine of 1.8–2.0, low albumin level, and anemia. Her baseline INR is 0.8.

Height = 5'2"
Weight = 55 kg

QUESTION 1

What is an appropriate warfarin dose to initiate for DW?

Answer:

Consider warfarin 5–7.5 mg daily. DW is at high risk for CVA (CHADS2 risk score of 5) but also high bleed risk, which demands a balanced approach. If INRs may be monitored daily in this inpatient setting, it increases the safety of a higher dose initiation.

QUESTION 2

Estimate DW's maintenance warfarin dose. Indicate the patient characteristics that influenced this estimate.

Answer:

Relevant patient characteristics that suggest DW will need a lower dose include advanced age, multiple comorbidities, possible malnutrition, low height and weight, and diltiazem therapy. A reasonable guess without pharmacogenomics information may be that DW's warfarin maintenance dose is 2.5 mg daily.

QUESTION 3

What drug interactions, if any, are of concern?

Answer:

Diltiazem is a moderate inhibitor of CYP 3A4, which affects the less potent warfarin R-enantiomer. In theory, it may potentiate warfarin. Aspirin is an antiplatelet that independently increases bleeding risk. In combination with warfarin, a higher bleeding risk may be anticipated.

CASE 3

IU is a 45-year-old male on warfarin for prevention of CVA and systemic embolism for a prosthetic mitral valve replacement. He has been stabilized on warfarin 4 mg daily for the past 3 months to target INR 2.5–3.5. He presents to clinic ahead of schedule to see his PCP, reporting 3 days of fever, productive cough, and no appetite. He has taken only over-the-counter acetaminophen (4–6 tablets a day) to self-treat. IU is diagnosed with viral bronchitis and advised to drink fluids, take bed rest, and prescribed an antitussive. His INR is today is 5.8. IU reports no unusual signs or symptoms of bleeding and denies any change in prescription medications.

QUESTION 1

What may have contributed to IU's elevated INR?

Answer:

Fever and illness, poor oral intake, and large doses of acetaminophen may all potentiate warfarin effect and INR result.

QUESTION 2

Should IU be given phytonadione (vitamin K) to manage his elevated INR? If so, at what dose, route, and frequency?

Answer:

The use of phytonadione in the absence of bleeding is discouraged, as the absolute risk of bleeding in the time required for the INR to decline back within target range with phytonadione is not reduced compared to without it. In particular, IU is anticoagulated for a high thrombosis risk condition with a higher INR target, and the use of phytonadione may cause his INR to fall below target range.

QUESTION 3

How should IU's warfarin dose be adjusted?

Answer:

Warfarin should be held for 1–2 days to allow the INR to decline back into the target range. Because of great intervariability between patients in the time needed to decay the INR, reevaluate the INR after the dose hold to determine further intervention. As long as the suspected factors for elevating IU's INR remain, frequent INR monitoring and probable temporary reduction in warfarin dose will be needed.

REFERENCES

1. Mueller RL, Scheidt S. History of drugs for thrombotic disease. Discovery, development, and directions for the future. *Circulation*. 1994;89:432–449.

2. Coumadin [package insert]. Bristol-Myers Squibb Pharma Company, Princeton, NJ, October 2011. Available at: http://packageinserts.bms.com/pi/pi_coumadin.pdf (accessed February 25, 2013).

3. Nutescu EA, Shapiro NL, Chevalier A, Amin AN. A pharmacologic overview of current and emerging anticoagulants. *Clev Clin J Med*. 2005;72:S2–S6.

4. Hirsh J, Fuster V, Ansell J, Halperin JL. American Heart Association/American College of Cardiology Foundation guide to warfarin therapy. *Circulation*. 2003;107:1692–1711.

5. Li C, Schwarz UT, Ritchie MD, Roden DM, Stein CM, Kurnik D. Relative contribution of CYP2C9 and VKORC1 genotypes and early INR response to the prediction of warfarin sensitivity during initiation of therapy. *Blood*. 2009;113:3925–3930.

6. Crowther MA, Ginsberg JB, Kearon C, et al. A randomized trial comparing 5-mg and 10-mg warfarin loading doses. *Arch Intern Med*. 1999;159:46–48.

7. Holbrook AM, Pereira JA, Labiris R, et al. Systematic overview of warfarin and its drug and food interactions. *Arch Intern Med*. 2005;165:1095–1106.

8. Spyropoulos AC, Hayth KA, Jenkins P. Anticoagulation with anisindione in a patient with a warfarin-induced skin eruption. *Pharmacotherapy*. 2003;23:533–536.

9. Dager WE. Initiating warfarin therapy. *Ann Pharmacother*. 2003;37:905–908.

10. Holbrook A, Schulman S, Witt DM, et al. Evidence-based management of anticoagulation therapy: Antithrombotic therapy and prevention of thrombosis, 9th ed: American College of Chest Physicians evidence-based clinical practice guidelines. *Chest*. 2012;141:e152S–e184S.

11. Ageno W, Gallus AS, Wittkowsky A, Crowther MA, Hylek EM, Palareti G. Oral anticoagulant therapy: Antithrombotic therapy and prevention of thrombosis, 9th ed: American College of Chest Physicians evidence-based clinical practice guidelines. *Chest*. 2012;141:e44S–e88S.

12. Kovacs MJ, Rodger M, Anderson DR, et al. Comparison of 10-mg and 5-mg warfarin initiation nomograms together with low-molecular-weight heparin for outpatient treatment of acute venous thromboembolism. *Ann Intern Med*. 2003;138:714–719.

13. International Warfarin Pharmacogenetics Consortium, Klein TE, Altman RB, Eriksson N, et al. Estimation of the warfarin dose with clinical and pharmacogenetic data. *N Engl J Med*. 2009;360:753–764.

14. Garcia D, Regan S, Crowther M, Hughes RA, Hylek EM. Warfarin maintenance dosing patterns in clinical practice: Implications for safer anticoagulation in the elderly population. *Chest*. 2005;127:2049–2056.

15. Gedge J, Orme S, Hampton KK, Channer KS, Hendra TJ. A comparison of a low-dose warfarin induction regimen with the modified Fennerty regimen in elderly inpatients. *Age Ageing*. 2000;29:31–34.

16. Fennerty A, Dolben J, Thomas P, et al. Flexible induction dose regimen for warfarin and prediction of maintenance dose. *Br Med J (Clin Res Ed)*. 1984;288:1268–1270.

17. Roberts GW, Helboe T, Nielsen CBM, et al. Assessment of an age-adjusted warfarin initiation protocol. *Ann Pharmacother*. 2003;37:799–803.

18. Bucerius J, Joe AY, Palmedo H, Reinhardt MJ, Biersack, H-J. Impact of short-term hypothyroidism on systemic anticoagulation in patients with thyroid cancer and Coumadin therapy. *Thyroid*. 2006;16(4):369–374.

19. Food and Drug Administration. Drug development and drug interactions: Table of substrates, inhibitors and inducers. Available at: http://www.fda.gov/Drugs/DevelopmentApprovalProcess/DevelopmentResources/DrugInteractionsLabeling/ucm093664.htm (accessed June 24, 2013).

20. Flockhart DA. Drug interactions: Cytochrome P450 drug interaction table. Indiana University School of Medicine (2007). Available at: http://medicine.iupui.edu/clinpharm/ddis/table.aspx (accessed March 4, 2013).

21. Buckley MS, Goff AD, Knapp WE. Fish oil interaction with warfarin. *Ann Pharmacother*. 2004;38(1):50–52.

22. Schulman S, Parpia S, Stewart C, Rudd-Scott L, Julian JA, Levine M. Warfarin dose assessment every 4 weeks versus every 12 weeks in patients with stable international normalized ratios. *Ann Intern Med*. 2011;155:653–659.

23. Witt DM, Delate T, Clark NP, et al. Outcomes and predictors of very stable INR control during chronic anticoagulation therapy. *Blood*. 2009;114:952–956.

24. Dentali F, Donadini MP, Clark N, et al. Brand name versus generic warfarin: A systematic review of the literature. *Pharmacotherapy*. 2011;31:386–393.

25. Crowther MA, Ageno W, Garcia D, et al. Oral vitamin K versus placebo to correct excessive anticoagulation in patients receiving warfarin. *Ann Intern Med*. 2009;150:293–300.

26. Hylek EM, Regan S, Go AS, Hughes RA, Singer SE, Skates SJ. Clinical predictors of prolonged delay in return of the international normalized ratio to within the therapeutic range after excessive anticoagulation with warfarin. *Ann Intern Med*. 2001;135:393–400.

27. Douketis JD, Spyropoulos AC, Spencer FA, et al. Perioperative management of antithrombotic therapy: Antithrombotic therapy and prevention of thrombosis, 9th ed: American College of Chest Physicians evidence-based clinical practice guidelines. *Chest*. 2012;141:e326S–e350S.

28. Kearon C, Akl EA, Comerota AJ, et al. Antithrombotic therapy for VTE disease, 9th ed: American College of Chest Physicians evidence-based clinical practice guidelines. *Chest*. 2012;141:e419S–494S.

29. Gage BF, Waterman AD, Shannon W, Boechler M, Rich MW, Radford MJ. Validation of clinical validation schemes for predicting stroke: Results from the National Registry of Atrial Fibrillation. *JAMA*. 2001;285:2864–2870.

30. Sanoski CA, Bauman JL. Clinical observations with the amiodarone/warfarin interaction: Dosing relationships with long-term therapy. *Chest*. 2002;121:19–23.

CHAPTER

22

Erythropoietin-Stimulating Agents

TIMOTHY NGUYEN, PharmD, FASCP, BCPS, CCP
VIJAY LAPSIA, MD
SARA S. KIM, PharmD, BCOP

OVERVIEW

Erythropoietic stimulating agents (ESA) are recombinant and synthetic erythropoietin (EPO). They are structurally and biologically similar to endogenous EPO and are used in the management of various types of anemia. Drugs in this class are epoetin alfa, darbepoetin alfa, and peginesatide. ESAs work by stimulating the bone marrow to produce red blood cells. Epoetin alfa, sometimes referred to as recombinant human erythropoietin (rHuEPO), is an exogenous EPO manufactured by recombinant DNA technology, and it was approved by the Food and Drug Administration (FDA) in 1989. It contains a 165-amino acid sequence with three N-linked and one O-linked carbohydrate changes and has the same biological effects as endogenous EPO.[1,2] It has a molecular weight of 30,400 daltons and is produced by mammalian cells.

Darbepoetin alfa (DA), a hyperglycosylated epoetin alfa analogue, contains five N-linked carbohydrate chains, two more than epoetin alfa, and has the same mechanism of action as rHuEPO.[3,4] Compared with epoetin alfa, darbepoetin alfa has a threefold increased serum half-life and allows extended dosing intervals.[4-6] The additional N-linked carbohydrate chains increased the molecular weight of darbepoetin from 30.4 to 37.1 daltons, and the carbohydrate contribution to the molecule corresponding increased from 40 percent to approximately 52 percent.[7]

Peginesatide is a synthetic pegylated peptide. It stimulates the EPO receptor similar to the endogenous hormone EPO and rHuEPO. Peginesatide is produced using chemistry rather than recombinant DNA technology. Its amino acid sequence is completely different from EPO and yet still able to activate the EPO receptor and stimulates erythropoiesis.[8] In the summer of 2014, the manufacturer suspended peginesatide production due to post marketing reports of serious hypersensitivity reactions that may be life-threatening or fatal.

The FDA approved ESAs for the treatment of anemia resulting from chronic kidney disease, anemia in certain types of cancer patients receiving myelosuppressive chemotherapy, certain treatments for human immunodeficiency virus (HIV), and also to reduce the number of blood transfusions during and after certain major surgeries.[8,19,20] ESAs are also reportedly being used off-label for various conditions, including myelodysplastic syndrome,[9] critically ill patients,[10,11] chronic heart failure,[12] anemia of chronic disease,[13] chronic hepatitis C virus infection,[14] and anemia in low birth weight infants.[15]

PHARMACOKINETICS

rHuEPO has a relatively short terminal half-life of 4–8 hours in humans, and it needs to be administered two to three times a week.[16] Compared with rHuEPO, the EPO analogue darbepoetin-alfa carries two additional glycosylation sites that permit a higher degree of

glycosylation. Consequently, darbepoetin alfa has a longer half-life of 25.3–48.8 hours in humans,[5] and greater in vivo biological activity, which allows for less frequent administration.[17] Unlike rHuEPO or darbepoetin alfa, peginesatide comprises a peptide sequence that is dimerized and linked to a two-branched 20-kDa PEG moiety, thus prolonging systemic circulation and reducing enzymatic degradation.[18] This characteristic permits a once-monthly dosing schedule. (See Tables 22-1 through 22-4.)

DOSING CONSIDERATIONS

Adequate iron supply is necessary for maintaining an optimal response to ESA therapy. Prior to and during ESA therapy, a patient's iron stores, including transferrin saturation (TSAT) and serum ferritin, should be evaluated. Virtually all patients will eventually require supplemental iron to increase or maintain TSAT to levels that will adequately support erythropoiesis stimulated by ESA. The FDA recommends using the lowest dose possible to avoid RBC transfusions.

rHuEPO administered subcutaneously (SC) is more efficacious than intravenous (IV) administration. The required dose of rHuEPO administered via IV is usually 25 percent to 30 percent higher than SC administration to achieve a similar erythropoietic response. The reason is thought to be due to a rapid decline in rHuEPO concentration (i.e., below the threshold necessary for erythropoiesis) after IV administration.[21] In contrast, dosage requirements of darbepoetin-alfa do not appear to differ between the IV and SC routes of administration. The dose of DA is apparently equivalent between the IV and SC administration.

Dose reduction or increase by approximately 25 percent is suggested to maintain goal Hb levels. Significant variability in responsiveness in various patient populations makes it wise to individualize patient treatment (Table 22-5).

In normal subjects, plasma EPO levels range from 0.01 to 0.03 units/mL and increase 100- to 1,000-fold during hypoxia or anemia.[22] Responsiveness to rHuEPO therapy in HIV-infected patients is dependent on the endogenous serum EPO level prior to treatment. Patients with endogenous serum EPO levels ≤500 mUnits/mL and receiving a dose of zidovudine ≤4,200 mg/week may respond to rHuEPO therapy. Patients with endogenous EPO levels >500 mUnits/mL do not appear to respond to rHuEPO therapy.[19] In patients with CKD, serum EPO level is expected to be low, therefore it has no diagnostic value. Neither does it influence the starting dose or any adjustment in dosing of ESAs

TABLE 22-1	ESAs Pharmacokinetics Data[8,19,20]			
Drug		**rHuEPO**	**Darbepoetin**	**Peginesatide**
Half-Life	IV	4–13 hours	21–22	25 ± 7.6 hours
	SC	19–25 hours	42–70	53 ± 17.7 hours

TABLE 22-2 ESAs Dosing Information[8,19,20]

Generic Name (Brand name)	Epoetin alfa (Epogen, Procrit)	Darbepoetin alfa (Aranesp)	Peginesatide (Omontys)
Indication	CKD	CKD and Dialysis	Adult CKD on dialysis
Dosing	Adults: 50–100 units/kg IV or SC three times weekly Peds: 50 units/kg IV or SC three times weekly	Dialysis: 0.45 mcg/kg IV or SC weekly Nondialysis: 0.75 mcg/kg SC every 2 weeks	Initially, 0.04 mg/kg once monthly
Indication	Zidovudine-treated HIV	n/a	n/a
Dosing	Adults: 100 units/kg IV or SC weekly for 8 weeks	n/a	n/a
Indication	Chemotherapy-associated anemia in cancer		n/a
Dosing	Adults: 150 units/kg SC three times weekly or 40,000 units SC weekly Peds: 600 units/kg IV weekly (max 40,000 units weekly)	2.25 mcg/kg SC weekly or 500 mcg SC every 3 weeks	n/a
Indication	Surgery	n/a	n/a
Dosing	Adults: 300 units/kg SC daily for 10 days prior to surgery, day of surgery, and 4 days after surgery, or 600 units/kg weekly starting 3 weeks prior to, and on day of surgery	n/a	n/a

IV, intravenous; kg, kilogram; SC, subcutaneous

in such patients; these agents may have some use, however, in patients with anemia secondary to chronic illness. In addition, regression of left ventricular hypertrophy (LVH) is a known benefit of initiation of treatment with ESAs.

The FDA also stated that health care professionals who prescribe ESAs for anemia in cancer patient for chemotherapy-induced anemia must (1) complete a online training module that covers the use of ESAs; (2) be enrolled in the ESA APPRISE (Assisting Providers and Cancer Patients with Risk Information for the Safe Use of ESAs) Oncology program following completion of the training module and obtain provider enrollment number; (3) sign the patient/health care professional acknowledgment form prior to initiation of ESA therapy; and provide a copy of the signed consent form to the patient.[23]

Other monitoring parameters include hemoglobin (Hb), iron indices, folic acid, cyanocobalamin levels, and red blood cells profiles.

SIDE EFFECTS

All ESAs prescribed must be part of a Risk Evaluation and Mitigation Strategy (REMS) to ensure the safe use of these drugs.

The FDA mandated that the patients be provided with material and guidance to understand the risks associated with ESAs. For patients with cancer, these risks include the following:

1. ESA may cause tumors to grow faster.
2. ESA use may be associated with earlier death.
3. ESAs may cause some patients to develop blood clots and serious heart problems such as a heart attack, heart failure, or stroke.

TABLE 22-4 Adult Dosing Conversion from EPO, DA, to Peginesatide[8,19,20]

EPO to Peginesatide (CKD on Dialysis: Initial peginesatide once monthly based on estimated weekly EPO dose; administer first dose 1 week after the last dose of EPO)		DA to Peginesatide (CKD on Dialysis: Initiate peginesatide once monthly at the next scheduled DA dose)	
units/week	mg/month	mcg/week	mg/month
<2,500	2	<12	2
2,500–4,300	3	12–18	3
4,300–6,500	4	18–25	4
6,500–8,900	5	25–35	5
8,900–13,000	6	35–45	6
13,000–19,000	8	45–60	8
19,000–33,000	10	60–95	10
33,000–68,000	15	95–175	15
68,000 or greater	20	175 or greater	20

CKD, chronic kidney disease; EPO, rHuEPO; DA, darbepoetin alfa

TABLE 22-3 Adult Dosing Conversion Between EPO and DA[8,19]

Previous Weekly EPO Dose (units/week)	Predicted Weekly DA Dose (mcg/week)
<1500	6.25
1,500–2,499	6.25
2,500–4,999	12.5
5,000–10,999	25
11,000–17,999	40
18,000–33,999	60
34,000–89,999	100
≥90,000	200

EPO, rHuEPO; DA, darbepoetin alfa

For this reason, ESA therapy is not indicated for treatment of chemotherapy-induced anemia (CIA) if the patient is receiving chemotherapy for curative intent.

Patients with or without cancer should be informed that the use of ESAs can increase the risk of stroke, heart attack, heart failure, blood clots, and death. All patients receiving ESAs are instructed to read the medication guide to understand the benefits and risks of using an ESA, and to discuss with their health care professional any questions they may have. Also, patients with cancer will need to sign an acknowledgment form that states that they have talked with their health care professional about the risks associated with ESAs. This form must be signed before patients begin a course of ESA treatment. Patients without cancer will be asked to get blood tests while using ESAs to help guide the course of therapy and lower the risk of serious adverse events.

Side effects include vascular-access thrombosis, seizures, hypertension, and others. ESAs are rated pregnancy category C. In addition, some patients have developed anti-EPO antibodies due to immunogenicity, which can reduce the benefit of taking epoetin alfa.[17] ESA-related pure red cell aplasia (PRCA) is a rare but potentially life-threatening condition. The presence of neutralizing antibodies has been observed and most cases have been associated with darbepoetin and rHuEPO given SC in patients with CKD, and treated for hepatitis C infection with interferon and ribavirin.[17,19]

TABLE 22-5 Monitoring

	Hemoglobin Levels	
	Food and Drug Administration (FDA)	Kidney Disease: Improving Global Outcomes (KDIGO)
CKD not on dialysis	• Consider initiating ESA only when Hb <10 g/dL and the need to assess for RBC-related transfusion • If Hb >10 g/dL, decrease or stop ESA; use the lowest ESA dose to avoid RBC transfusion	• Individualized consideration before initiation ESA therapy if Hb <10 g/dL
CKD on dialysis	• Initiate ESA when Hb <10 g/dL • If Hb approaches or exceeds 11 g/dL, decrease or stop ESA therapy	• Initiate ESA therapy if Hb 9–10 g/dL; avoid Hb falling below 9 g/dL • Maintenance: in general, ESA therapy is not suggested if Hb >11.5 g/dL
Oncology related	• Initiate ESA if Hb <10 g/dL and at least 2 additional months of planned chemotherapy • Use the lowest dose to avoid RBC transfusion	n/a
Zidovudine treated-HIV	• Withhold EPO if Hb >12 g/dL	n/a

CONTRAINDICATIONS/WARNINGS

CONTRAINDICATIONS

ESAs are contraindicated in patients with uncontrolled hypertension and hypersensitivity to any of the components including albumin (human) and mammalian cell-derived products.

WARNINGS

All ESAs carry serious Black box warnings. Insufficient Hb response to ESA therapy may indicate a greater risk for cardiovascular events and mortality than in other patients, based increased risks for death and serious cardiovascular events in controlled clinical trials of patients with cancer.[24] These events included myocardial infarction, stroke, congestive heart failure, and hemodialysis vascular access thrombosis. A rate of Hb rise >1 g/dL over two weeks may contribute to these risks. A higher incidence of DVT was documented in patients receiving rHuEPO who were not receiving prophylactic anticoagulations.[19]

Hyporesponsiveness to ESA can also occur if Hb does not increase despite being adequately dosed. Contributing factors to hyporesponsiveness may include iron deficiency, chronic blood loss, hemolysis, malignancy, infectious and inflammatory conditions, severe malnutrition, vitamin deficiency, severe hyperparathyroidism, and other conditions.[25]

ESA therapies have changed the treatment of anemia in CKD and various patient settings. Clinicians should be informed of ESA prescribing profiles and side effects in order to effectively manage ESA therapies and at the same time avoid serious consequences associated with its use.

CASE STUDIES

CASE 1: ESA AND CKD PREDIALYSIS

A 77-year-old Caucasian man with long-standing hypertension, diabetes, and a 20-year history of tobacco smoking presents for evaluation of CKD. Recently he had an episode of acute angina for which he underwent cardiac catheterization. At that time he was found to have CKD (serum creatinine 2.4 mg/dL) and was advised follow up with outpatient nephrology. He is otherwise well, denies fatigue or reduced exercise capacity, and has quit smoking several months ago. On laboratory evaluation serum hemoglobin was 10.5 mg/dL.

QUESTION

How would you manage the patient's anemia?

Answer:

At this time, the patient is asymptomatic and although the Hb is low (anemia in CKD is diagnosed when the Hb concentration is <10 g/dL),[19] available evidence suggests little to no benefit to be gained by raising the Hb over 10 mg/dL in diabetic patients with ESA naive CKD not yet on dialysis. If this patient was awaiting a kidney transplant reducing the need for blood transfusions (to prevent the development of antibodies) would be a concern, however, that is not the case at this time.

Additional evaluation for other correctable causes of anemia—including gastrointestinal losses, inflammatory states, and nutritional deficiencies including folate, Vitamin B12 and iron—should be completed. Once the cause of the anemia is identified to be due to his chronic disease a more in-depth risk-benefit discussion specifically in terms of the minimal benefit in quality of life (QOL) and the heightened risk of stroke would be appropriate.

Follow -Up in 3 Months

On further evaluation, patient was found to have TSAT of 20 percent, ferritin 125 ng/mL, reticulocyte count of 1.2 percent, and no evidence of blood loss (fecal occult blood test negative times three).

QUESTION

What is the next step in the management?

Answer:

Iron therapy is underutilized in patients with CKD. TSAT of less than 20 percent and/or serum ferritin levels <200 ng/nL generally indicate iron deficiency. Iron supplementation is recommended for adult patients with CKD if TSAT is ≤30 percent and ferritin is ≤500 ng/ml, because in the CKD population higher saturation and ferritin levels are desirable to ensure that patients are iron replete.

Follow -Up in 6 Months

Hemoglobin level is now 9.3 mg/dL. Patient now notes some fatigue. Laboratory evaluation suggests adequate iron stores.

QUESTION

What role does ESA have?

Answer:

In practice the use of ESAs in patients with CKD not yet on dialysis is subject to wide variability. The possibility of organ transplantation, patient preferences, and reimbursement limitations must be taken into consideration. It is important to balance the potential benefits of reducing blood transfusions and anemia-related symptoms against the risks of harm in individual patients (e.g., stroke, vascular access loss, hypertension). As per KDIGO,[25] the decision whether to initiate ESA therapy for adult CKD patients not yet on dialysis (CKD ND) with Hb concentration 10 g/dL must be individualized based on the rate of fall of Hb concentration, prior response to iron therapy, the risk of needing a transfusion, the risks related to ESA therapy, and the presence of symptoms attributable to anemia. Once the decision to start the patient on ESA is made, additional decisions include choosing an ESA, initial ESA dose, route and frequency of ESA administration, and an Hb level monitoring schedule.

Additional notes:

Target Hb levels: Should be individualized. ESA therapy in patients with diabetes and CKD have an increased risk of ischemic stroke, thromboembolism, and cancer-related death in patients with a preexisting diagnosis of cancer. Increasingly, clinicians are now targeting Hb levels of 10 to 11 g/dL, aiming for the lower end of the target if they are unlikely to benefit from a QOL perspective.

Frequency of Hb monitoring: At least monthly for patients on ESAs.

Dose of ESA: The initial ESA dose should be determined using the patient's Hb concentration, body weight, and clinical circumstances.

Route and frequency of administration should be determined by the CKD treatment setting and the class of ESA. For CKD ND and patients on peritoneal dialysis (CKD PD), the KDIGO suggests subcutaneous administration of ESA.[25]

CASE 2: ESA AND CKD-HEMODIALYSIS

A 68-year-old African American male with end-stage kidney disease (ESKD) due to diabetes and hypertension is currently receiving hemodialysis (HD) treatment thrice weekly. Lately the patient reports a history of fatigue and lightheadedness for a few weeks. On physical exam, no blood loss is evident, and stool guaiac is negative, BP 130/85 mmHg, HR 75 bpm, and weight is 75 kg. His hemoglobin level is 9.5 g/dL, ferritin is 350 ng/dL, and transferrin saturation (TSAT) is 35 percent.

QUESTION

How would you approach management and evaluation of this patient's anemia?

Answer:

Initial evaluation of anemia and CKD:

- Complete blood count, which should include Hb concentration, red cell indices, white blood cell count, and differential and platelet count
- Absolute reticulocyte count
- Iron indices: Serum ferritin and TSAT levels
- Serum vitamin B12 and folate levels

Initiate ESA therapy with great caution if used at all. An increase in Hb concentration without starting ESA treatment is desired. Do not initiate ESA in CKD patients with active malignancy—in particular

when cure is the anticipated outcome—a history of stroke, or a history of malignancy.

Iron levels are within normal limit, the patient has ESKD and receives HD, therefore, ESKD and HD are the primary causes of anemia. The patient's Hb level is at 9.5 g/dL, and he is experiencing symptoms. According to the latest KDIGO guidelines,[25] the patient would be benefit from ESA therapy. Initiate EPO at 50 units/kg IV three times weekly with HD.

If EPO is utilized:

- Epoetin alfa 3,500 units, IV, three times weekly with dialysis.
- For HD, either IV or SC route may be considered; IV administration will decrease the number of injections to the patient since the patient is receiving HD with access.
- If SC route is initiated, the dose can be decreased by approximately 30 percent (i.e., 2,500 units SC three times weekly).

If DA is utilized:

- Starting dose is 0.45 mcg/kg weekly, and the patient's weight is 75 kg.
- The calculated dose is 33.75 mcg, rounded to the nearest available prefilled dose. In this case, start the patient on 40 mcg SC weekly.

If peginesatide is utilized:

- Initiate at 0.04 mg/kg monthly (i.e., 3 mcg SC monthly).

Monitor:

- Monitor Hb level weekly during initiation and then monthly thereafter.
- Hb level should not increase more than 1 g/dL in any two-week period.
- Monitor iron indices prior to and during ESA therapy.
- Monitor BP regularly.

ESA therapy should be individualized based on the rate of decrease of Hb concentration, prior response to iron therapy, the risk of needing a transfusion, the risks related to ESA therapy, and the presence of symptoms attributable to anemia.

4 Weeks Later

The patient's laboratory results four weeks later were: Hb 10.2 g/dL, ferritin 250 ng/dL, and TSAT 25 percent.

QUESTION

What is the best course of action at this time?

Answer:

Since the patient was started on ESA, ESA took up iron storage for hemoglobin synthesis and the ferritin and TSAT levels decreased. According to the current KDIGO guidelines, maintenance IV iron should be initiated. Iron dextran, iron sucrose, sodium ferric gluconate, ferric carboxymaltose or ferumoxytol are options. IV iron carries risk of anaphylactic reaction and adverse events along with unknown long-term safety profiles.

3 Months Later

Over the next three months, the patient's Hb has been ranging around 10.1 g/dL to 10.8 g/dL. The patient is now asymptomatic and clinically stable.

QUESTION

What is the optimal ESA dose and target Hb level for this patient?

Answer:

Many controversial issues surround the best Hb levels. The KDOQI has slightly different targets compared to the FDA's product labeling. Several revisions were made to the NKF and KDOQI guidelines due to data from the TREAT trials and others trials.[26-30] Patients receiving ESA therapy should be kept on the lowest maintenance ESA dose to avoid the need for receiving blood transfusions. The latest KDIGO guidelines suggest Hb levels not exceeding 11 g/dL with some room for titration up to 11.5 g/dL.[25] This patient is currently on a stable ESA and IV iron regimen, therefore, no change is necessary at the present time.

CASE 3: ESA AND ONCOLOGY

The patient is a 70-year-old female (60 kg) who was diagnosed with Stage IV colorectal cancer two months ago. She presented to oncology clinic to receive second cycle of FOLFOX chemotherapy regimen. She complains of significant fatigue. Today's blood result shows Hb of 7.8 g/dL. Her baseline Hb at the time of diagnosis was 12 g/dL.

QUESTION

Base on the NCCN Guidelines, is ESA therapy indicated for this patient?

Answer:

Yes, ESA therapy is recommended for patients with chemotherapy-induced anemia (CIA) in a noncurative setting. In this setting, the initiation of ESA therapy is recommended if Hb <10 g/dL. The lowest possible dose of ESA should be used to avoid blood transfusion.[31]

QUESTION

What is the manufacturer-recommended initial dose of epoetin alfa or darbepoetin alfa for this patient?

Answer:

For CIA, the initial dose of darbepoetin alfa recommended by the manufacturer is 2.25 mcg/kg per week as SC injection (most often given as 100 mcg SC weekly) or 500 mcg SC every 3 weeks.[20] The recommended initial dose of epoetin alfa is 150 units/kg SC three times weekly or 40,000 units SC weekly.[29]

Six weeks later, the patient returns to the clinic and complains of feeling extremely fatigued. Today's lab results show Hb 8 g/dL, ferritin 500 ng/mL, and TSAT 20 percent.

QUESTION

Based on the NCCN guidelines, how should the management be changed for this patient's CIA?

Answer:

The rise in Hb <1 g/dL over 6 weeks since the patient started ESA therapy indicates that the dose of darbepoetin should be titrated up

to 150 mcg once weekly.[31] Also, addition of IV iron supplementation to ESA therapy is recommended for low iron.[31]

CASE 4: ESA AND ONCOLOGY

The patient, JP, is a 35-year-old male who was diagnosed with Stage III NSCLC six months ago. He presented to the clinic to receive his fifth cycle of adjuvant chemotherapy regimen. The patient complains of shortness of breath and hypotension upon standing up. Today's blood test shows Hb of 9 g/dL.

QUESTION

Based on the NCCN guidelines, is ESA therapy indicated for JP?

Answer

For CIA, ESA therapy is not indicated in curative setting. A number of randomized trials have been shown that the use of ESA in cancer patients increase the risk of thromboembolism and tumor progression or recurrence, and also shortened overall survival.[19,20,31]

Five years later, the patient's tumor has metastasized to the liver and bones. The patient presents to the clinic for a second cycle of chemotherapy regimen. Hb is 11 g/dL.

QUESTION

Based on the NCCN guidelines, should ESA be offered to JP?

Answer:

The NCCN guideline does not recommend initiating ESA therapy for CIA if the Hb is 10 or higher.[19,20,31] For CIA, ESA therapy should only be offered to patients whose Hb <10 g/dL and lowest possible dose of ESA should be used to avoid blood transfusion. ESA therapy should not be offered to a patient who is receiving concomitant chemotherapy with curative intent.

REFERENCES

1. Egrie J, Strickland T, Lane J, et al. Characterization and biological effects of recombinant human erythropoietin. *Immunobiol.* 1986;72: 213–224.
2. Halstenson CE, Macres M, Katz SA, et al. Comparative pharmacokinetics and pharmacodynamics of epoetin alfa and epoetin beta. *Clin Pharmacol Ther.* 1991;50:702–712.
3. Nissenson A. Novel erythropoiesis stimulating protein for managing the anemia of CKD. *Am J Kidney Dis.* 2001;38:1390–1397.
4. Rency MA, Scoble HA, Kim Y. Structural characterization of natural human urinary and recombinant DNA-derived erythropoietin: Identification of des-arginine 166 erythropoietin. *J Biol Chem.* 1987;262:17156–17163.
5. Macdougall IC, Gray SJ, Elston O, et al. Pharmacokinetics of novel erythropoiesis stimulating protein compared with epoetin alfa in dialysis patients. *J Am Soc Nephrol.* 1999;10:2392–2395.
6. Macdougall IC. CERA (continuous erythropoietin receptor activator): A new erythropoiesis stimulating agent for the treatment of anemia. *Curr Hematol Rep.* 2005;4:436–440.
7. Egrie JC, Browne JK. Development and characterization of novel erythropoiesis stimulating protein (NESP). *Br J Cancer.* 2001;84:3–10.
8. Omontys*(pegisenatide) prescribing information. Affymax, Inc., Palo Alto, CA. Available at: www.omontys.com (accessed February 12, 2013).
9. Santini V. Treatment of low-risk myelodysplatic syndrome: Hematopoietic growth factors erythropoietins and thrombopoietins. *Semin Hematol.* 2012;49(4):295–303

10. Corwin HL, Gettinger A, Rodriguez RM, et al. Efficacy of rHuEPO in the critically ill patient: A randomized controlled trial. *JAMA*. 2002;288:2827–2835.

11. Corwin HL, Gettinger A, Fabian TC, et al. Efficacy and safety of EPO in critically ill patients. *N Engl J Med*. 2007;357:965–976.

12. Silverberg DS, Wexler D, Sheps D, et al. The effect of correction of mild anemia in severe, resistant congenital heart failure using subcutaneous erythropoietin and intravenous iron: A randomized controlled study. *J Am Coll Cardiol*. 2001;37:1775–1780.

13. Weiss G, Goodnough LT. Anemia of chronic disease. *N Engl J Med*. 2005;352:1011–1023.

14. Dieterich DT, Wasserman R, Brau N, et al. Once-weekly epoetin alfa improves anemia and facilitates maintenance of ribavirin dosing in hepatitis C virus-infected patients receiving ribavirin plus interferon alfa. *Am J Gastroenterology*. 2003;98:2491–2499.

15. Arif B, Ferhan K. rHuEPO therapy in low-birth weight preterm infants: A prospective controlled study. *Pediatr Int*. 2005;47:67–71.

16. Faulds D, Sorkin EM. Epoetin (recombinant human erythropoietin): A review of its pharmacodynamic and pharmacokinetic properties and therapeutic potential in anaemia and the stimulation of erythropoiesis. *Drugs*. 1989;38(6):863–899.

17. Bunn HF. New agents that stimulate erythropoiesis. *Blood*. 2007;109(3):868–737.

18. Woodburn KW, Holmes CP, Wilson SD, et al. Absorption, distribution, metabolism, and excretion of peginesatide, a novel ESA, in rats. *Xenobiotica*. 2011;42(7):660–670.

19. Epogen®(Epoetin alfa) Prescribing information. Available at: www.epogen.com/pdf/epogen_pi.pdf (accessed February 5, 2013).

20. Aranesp®(darbepoetin alfa) prescribing information. Available at: www.aranesp.com/pdf/aranesp_PI.pdf (accessed February 5, 2013).

21. Macdougall IC. Optimizing the use of erythropoietic agents—pharmacokinetic and pharmacodynamic considerations. *Nephrol Dial Transplant*. 2002;17(suppl 5):66–70.

22. Graber S, Krantz S. Erythropoietin alfa and the control of red cell production. *Ann Rev Med*. 1978;29:51–66.

23. U.S. Food and Drug Administration. Postmarketing drug safety information for patients and providers. Approved Risk Evaluation and Mitigation Strategies (REMS). Available at: http://www.fda.gov/Drugs/DrugSafety/PostmarketDrugSafety InformationforPatientsandProviders/ucm109375.htm (accessed January 9, 2013).

24. Nordstrom B, et al. Use of ESAs among chemotherapy patients with Hb exceeding 12 g/dL. *J Manag Care Pharm*. 2008;14(9):858–869.

25. Kidney Disease: Improving Global Outcomes (KDIGO) Anemia Work Group. KDIGO Clinical Practice Guideline for Anemia in Chronic Kidney Disease. *Kidney Int Suppl*. 2012;2:279–335.

26. Pfeffer MA, Burdmann EA, Chen CY, et al. A trial of darbepoetin alfa in type 2 diabetes and chronic kidney disease. *N Engl J Med*. 2009;361:2019–2032.

27. Singh AK, Szczech L, Tang KL, et al. Correction of anemia with epoetin alfa in chronic kidney disease. *N Engl J Med*. 2006;355:2085–2098.

28. Lau JH, Gangji AS, Rabbat CG, Brimble KS. Impact of hemoglobin and erythropoietin dose changes on mortality: A secondary analysis of results from a randomized anemia management trial. *Nephrol Dial Transplant*. 2010;25:4002–4009.

29. Besarab A, Bolton WK, Browne JK, et al. The effects of normal as compared with low hematocrit values in patients with cardiac disease who are receiving hemodialysis and epoetin. *N Engl J Med*. 1998;339:584–590.

30. Drueke TB, Locatelli F, Clyne N, et al. Normalization of hemoglobin level in patients with chronic kidney disease and anemia. *N Engl J Med*. 2006;355:2071–2084.

31. National Comprehensive Cancer Network. Cancer and treatment-related anemia. Version 1.2013. Available at: http://www.nccn.org/professionals/physician_gls/pdf/anemia.pdf (accessed February 5, 2013).

23

Direct Thrombin Inhibitors

ERIN E. MANCL, PharmD, BCPS
STACY A. VOILS, PharmD, MS, BCPS

OVERVIEW OF INTRAVENOUS DIRECT THROMBIN INHIBITORS

Intravenous (IV) direct thrombin inhibitors (DTIs), including argatroban, bivalirudin, and lepirudin have been developed and evaluated for the treatment of heparin-induced thrombocytopenia (HIT), acute coronary syndrome (ACS), percutaneous coronary intervention (PCI), and venous thromboembolism (VTE). DTIs exert their anticoagulant effect by binding directly to thrombin, thereby inhibiting both soluble and fibrin-bound thrombin.[1] The direct binding to thrombin produces an anticoagulant effect independent of antithrombin (AT) activity. The ability to bind to fibrin-bound thrombin may be particularly advantageous in the setting of an active clot, such as a coronary thrombosis, because fibrin-bound thrombin can stimulate further clotting activity. In addition, compared to heparin-based regimens, DTIs may offer a more predictable anticoagulant effect due to their lack of binding to other plasma proteins. Furthermore, DTIs are a mainstay therapy in patients with HIT because they are not associated with immune-mediated thrombocytopenia.

DTIs were developed after the discovery of hirudin, a peptide first isolated from the salivary glands of medicinal leeches.[2,3] Currently, three IV DTIs are approved for use in North America: argatroban, bivalirudin, and lepirudin. However, as of May 31, 2012, the manufacturer of lepirudin discontinued production and distribution of lepirudin.[4] At the time of writing this chapter, no other manufacturers were producing lepirudin; therefore, its current use in practice is limited and will likely cease once supply is exhausted.

PHARMACOKINETICS

ARGATROBAN

Argatroban is a small (molecular weight 500 kDa) synthetic DTI administered as a continuous IV infusion due to its limited bioavailability if administered orally.[5] Upon initiation of an infusion, anticoagulant effect is seen immediately. The volume of distribution is approximately 174–180 mL/kg, with protein binding observed at 20 percent and 35 percent to albumin and alpha-1-acid glycoprotein, respectively. Argatroban is hepatically cleared primarily via hydroxylation and aromatization of the 3-methyltetrahydroquinoline ring. Minor metabolism to four known metabolites through cytochrome (CYP)-450 3A4/5 has been observed. Plasma concentration of metabolite M1 is 0–20 percent parent drug concentration, and this metabolite has a pharmacodynamics effect three–five times weaker than argatroban. Metabolites M2 to M4 are found in low quantities and are pharmacodynamically inactive. Total clearance ranges from 4.7 to 5.1 mL/kg/min at doses up to 40 mcg/kg/min, but

such clearance is reduced to 1.9 mL/kg/min in hepatic impairment. The elimination half-life of argatroban is approximately 39–51 minutes but extends to 181 minutes in patients with hepatic dysfunction (defined as Child-Pugh score >6). Therefore, dose adjustment and close monitoring in patients with hepatic impairment are essential. Approximately 20 percent of argatroban is removed through hemodialysis.

BIVALIRUDIN

Bivalirudin is a 20-amino-acid semisynthetic polypeptide analog of hirudin administered as a continuous IV infusion.[6] Although not usually administered subcutaneously, the bioavailability of bivalirudin is approximately 40 percent when given in this manner. When administered as an IV infusion, bivalirudin is also relatively rapid acting with anticoagulant effects seen immediately upon therapy initiation. The volume of distribution is approximately 200 mL/kg. Other than thrombin, bivalirudin does not bind to any other proteins in the plasma. Bivalirudin is cleared renally and through plasma esterase. Approximately 20 percent of bivalirudin is eliminated unchanged in the urine. Most of this elimination (70%) is observed within 2 hours after IV administration. The remaining clearance occurs through proteolytic cleavage in the plasma. Overall drug clearance decreases as glomerular filtration rate (GFR) decreases. Observed clearance rates are 3.4 mL/min/kg, 2.7 mL/min/kg, 2.8 mL/min/kg, and 1 mL/min/kg for patients with GFR of >60 mL/min, 30–59 mL/min, 10–29 mL/min, and dialysis-dependent off dialysis, respectively. These clearance rates correlate with an elimination half-life of approximately 25 minutes, 22 minutes, 34 minutes, and 57 minutes. In dialysis-dependent patients, the observed half-life is approximately 3.5 hours as approximately 25 percent of bivalirudin is cleared through hemodialysis.

LEPIRUDIN

Lepirudin is typically administered as a continuous IV infusion, but when given subcutaneously, the bioavailability is near 100 percent.[7] The exact volume of distribution is not well-quantified, but it is known to distribute into extracellular fluids. Approximately 35 percent of lepirudin is excreted in the urine as unchanged drug. Clearance in healthy patients is approximately 174 mL/min compared to 2.7 mL/min in patients undergoing hemodialysis. Notably, total body clearance is also dependent on gender and age, with clearance reduced by 25 percent in women and 20–25 percent in elderly. The elimination half-life ranges 0.8–2 hours in patients with normal renal function, but can be as prolonged as 107 hours in severe renal insufficiency. Lepirudin is cleared through high-flux dialyzers, and dialysis has been successfully used to reduce concentrations to therapeutic levels in cases of excessive dosing.

DOSING[6]

ARGATROBAN

Argatroban is mainly used in the treatment and prevention of thrombosis in patients with HIT, but it is also less commonly used in PCI and coronary thrombosis.[5] In the prophylaxis and treatment of HIT with or without thrombosis, the American College of Chest Physicians (ACCP) guidelines recommend an initial infusion rate of 1–2 mcg/kg/min adjusted to maintain a steady-state activated partial prothrombin time (aPTT) of 1.5–3 times the initial baseline value.[5,8] Institution-specific protocols often vary in their titration recommendations but, in general, the aPTT is checked 2 hours after initiation or any rate change. If the aPTT is below goal range, a 20 percent increase in rate is recommended whereas if the aPTT is above range, the infusion is held for 2 hours before resuming at 50 percent lower rate. If the aPTT is significantly elevated (e.g., >150 seconds), it is appropriate to repeat the aPTT to ensure adequate decrease before resuming therapy at a reduced rate. Due to reduced clearance in patients with hepatic disease, the recommended initial dosage is 0.5 mcg/kg/min with titration to an aPTT 1.5–3 times the initial baseline. It has also been observed that critically ill patients, with and without hepatic dysfunction, have an impaired clearance of argatroban. In a study of critically ill patients, an argatroban dosing nomogram was developed and evaluated for ability to achieve and maintain goal therapeutic aPTT ranges.[9] In this study, the time to stabilization of aPTTs was 27 hours using an initial dose of 0.5 mcg/kg/min and titrating to a goal aPTT range of 45–90 seconds. In the critically ill population, the aPTT was checked at 4 hours after initiation and each dose adjustment, an increase from the usual 2 hours in healthy patients. Therefore, it is reasonable and highly recommended to start at a reduced dose (~25% usual dose for healthy patients) in patients with critical illness and/or hepatic impairment. Empiric dose adjustments are not necessary in noncritically ill patients with isolated renal impairment. Observational data suggest that no dose adjustment is required for obese patients (body mass index up to 51 kg/m^2); therefore, argatroban should be dosed using actual body weight.[10]

Although less commonly used compared to bivalirudin, argatroban is sometimes used in the treatment of coronary artery thrombosis or in patients undergoing PCI, especially in patients identified to have or be at risk for HIT. In PCI, argatroban is administered with an initial bolus of 350 mcg/kg given over 3–5 minutes, followed by a continuous infusion ranging 15–30 mcg/kg/min, usually titrated to a goal-activated clotting time (ACT).[5] Infusion rates higher than 40 mcg/kg/min are usually reserved for patients with thrombus formation during procedure, dissection, or impending abrupt closure.

If administered for the medical treatment of an acute myocardial infarction, the recommended dose of argatroban is 100 mcg/kg bolus over 1 minute followed by a continuous infusion of 1–3 mcg/kg/min titrated to a goal aPTT of 50–85 seconds.[11]

BIVALIRUDIN

Bivalirudin is used in patients undergoing PCI for unstable angina or acute MI and in patients with HIT who require PCI.[6] When used in PCI, bivalirudin is typically initiated with a 0.75 mg bolus dose followed by a continuous infusion of 1.75 mg/kg/hr.[12] The infusion can be maintained for the duration of the procedure and titrated as needed to a goal ACT. If used as adjunct therapy in patients receiving thrombolytics, an infusion of 0.5 mg/kg/hr with subsequent decrease to 0.1 mg/kg/hr after 12 hours has been used with success.[13] Dose reduction is recommended for patients with renal insufficiency.[6] In patients with a creatinine clearance of 30–59 mL/

minute, the bolus dose should be omitted and an infusion at 1.75 mg/kg/hr should be given. If the creatinine clearance is less than 30 mL/min, then the bolus dose is omitted and the initial infusion rate is reduced to 1 mg/kg/hr. Finally, in hemodialysis patients, the recommended infusion rate is 0.25 mg/kg/hr.

Although bivalirudin is not FDA-approved for the treatment of HIT, it has been utilized in the setting of HIT with or without thrombosis. ACCP guidelines recommend use of bivalirudin in patients with HIT if they require cardiac surgery intervention.[8] In addition, due to limitations with argatroban as well as evidence suggesting equal effectiveness,[14] bivalirudin is frequently used in the management of HIT in noncardiac surgery patients as well. In this setting, bivalirudin is initiated as a continuous infusion rate of 0.15–0.2 mg/kg/hr and titrated to a goal aPTT 1.5–2.5 times the baseline.[8] The aPTT can be checked 2 hours after initiation and any subsequent dose adjustment. Like other IV DTIs, titration of bivalirudin varies by institution-specific protocols and clinical practice, but in general, when the aPTT is less than goal range, the infusion is increased by 20 percent. If the aPTT is elevated, the infusion is held for 2 hours before resuming at 50 percent infusion rate. In addition, several studies have demonstrated a reduced dose requirement in patients with renal insufficiency.[15-17] The average dose required for creatinine clearance of >60 mL/min, 30–60 mL/min, and <30 mL/min was 0.13, 0.08, and 0.05 mg/kg/hr, respectively.[16] In addition, intermittent hemodialysis, sustained low-efficiency daily diafiltration, and continuous renal replacement therapy patients required 0.07, 0.09, and 0.07 mg/kg/hr, respectively. Therefore, empiric dose reduction should be strongly considered in this population. Furthermore, in critically ill patients with and without renal impairment, similar dose reductions are recommended. Observational data suggest bivalirudin can be safely initiated at 0.14 mg/kg/hr in critically ill patients with isolated hepatic impairment, 0.03–0.05 mg/kg/hr in those with renal or combined hepatic and renal impairment, and 0.03–0.04 mg/kg/hr in patients receiving continuous renal replacement therapy.[18] Finally, bivalirudin should be dosed on actual body weight, even in obese individuals. In a retrospective review of 135 patients treated with bivalirudin for HIT, dosing with actual body weight was not associated with reduced effectiveness or increased adverse event rates in an obese population (body mass index >30 kg/m^2).[19]

Bivalirudin has been administered subcutaneously for the prevention of DVT in orthopedic surgery patients who have undergone major hip or knee surgery.[20] In this setting, bivalirudin 1 mg/kg subcutaneously every 8 hours was more effective than lower doses (0.3–1 mg/kg every 12 hours).

LEPIRUDIN

When lepirudin was available, it was primarily used for the treatment of HIT with or without thrombosis. According to the ACCP guidelines, the initial recommended infusion rate is 0.15 mg/kg/hr with an optional initial bolus dose of 0.4 mg/kg in the case of perceived life-threatening thrombosis.[21] A lepirudin infusion is normally adjusted to achieve a target range of aPTT 1.5–2.5 times higher than baseline.[8] In patients with renal failure, ACCP guidelines recommend initiating the infusion at a rate based on the serum creatinine value. For a serum creatinine of <1.02 mg/dL, 1.02–1.58 mg/dL, 1.58–4.42 mg/dL, and >4.52 mg/dL, the recommended initial rate is 0.1, 0.05, 0.01, and 0.005 mg/kg/hr, respectively. Furthermore, in a small study of 10 patients receiving lepirudin during hemodialysis, doses ranged from 0.008 to 0.125 mg/kg/hr.[22]

In rare clinical scenarios, lepirudin has been administered subcutaneously for the treatment of VTE. When administered in this fashion, a dose of 1.25 mg/kg given subcutaneously twice daily into the abdominal wall was found to be safe and effective.[23]

MONITORING

Although IV DTIs affect prothrombin time (PT), the aPTT is used to monitor response to DTI therapy. The aPTT is prolonged during DTI therapy since thrombin inhibition leads to a decrease in platelet activation and other clotting factors activated by thrombin. Infusions of IV DTIs are normally titrated to a goal aPTT range above baseline (usually 1.5–2.5 times). It is important to note that the dose-response relationship is not linear, as a plateau of the aPTT is sometimes observed at higher doses of the DTIs. In addition, the commercially available aPTT reagents will vary in their sensitivities to each DTI. The ecarin clotting time (ECT) yields a more linear dose-response relationship, but this test is not widely available, nor has it been consistently studied in clinical trials. Furthermore, all IV DTIs affect the international normalized ratio (INR) to a variable extent specific to the DTI. At therapeutic doses, argatroban has the greatest effect on the INR. For patients transitioning to vitamin K antagonist therapy, it is recommended to continue overlap until the INR is 4 before discontinuing the argatroban infusion.[5] Once the infusion is stopped, a repeat INR in 4–6 hours should be checked to assess the INR when therapeutic concentrations of argatroban are no longer present. Alternatively, some centers utilize testing of the factor X levels during anticoagulation bridging. If the factor X level is <45 percent, the INR value is more likely to remain above 2 when argatroban has been fully eliminated.

ADVERSE EFFECTS

The most common adverse effects reported with all IV DTIs are hemorrhagic complications. The risk of any major bleeding complication associated with intravenous DTIs was observed in clinical trials to vary from 1–11 percent.[5-7] These complications include events such as major and minor gastrointestinal bleeding, retroperitoneal bleeding, and intracranial hemorrhage. In a retrospective analysis, bleeding risk factors associated with argatroban therapy included major surgery prior to or during therapy, dosing weight >90 kg, total bilirubin >3 mg/dL, and baseline platelets ≤70,000 per mL.[24]

In addition to bleeding, lepirudin is also associated with antibody development during therapy.[7] Formation of antihirudin antibodies occurs in approximately 40–70 percent of patients who receive lepirudin for HIT. The antibody-lepirudin complexes can alter the pharmacokinetics of the drug, usually resulting in prolonged clearance of lepirudin. This impaired elimination may enhance the anticoagulant effect. In a prospective evaluation of patients with HIT treated with lepirudin, the development of antibodies was dependent on duration of treatment and was associated with enhanced anticoagulant effect, although no difference was noted in rates of major bleeds.[25]

REVERSAL OF ANTICOAGULANT EFFECT OF INTRAVENOUS DTI

No specific antidote exists for the reversal of IV DTIs. Fortunately, due to the relatively short half-lives of the available agents, ceasing the infusion results in fairly rapid termination of the anticoagulant effects. Therefore, if an adverse effect such as bleeding occurs, it is recommended to stop the infusion and maintain supportive care with blood products as needed. In addition, it has been demonstrated in several case reports that administration of recombinant factor VIIa (rVIIa) as salvage therapy can reverse the anticoagulant activity of IV DTIs.[26,27] The risks of thrombosis with administration of rVIIa must be considered in the individual patient.

OVERVIEW OF ORAL DIRECT THROMBIN INHIBITORS

Although vitamin K antagonists and heparins have been the mainstay therapy for anticoagulation in atrial fibrillation and prevention or treatment of VTE, they have several limitations. Administration of heparins is limited to IV or subcutaneous routes, which can be difficult for compliance and patient mobility. Furthermore, warfarin requires frequent monitoring because it has a narrow therapeutic index and is associated with many drug and food interactions. As a result, research efforts have focused on developing orally bioavailable anticoagulants that require less frequent monitoring. Ximelagatran was one of the first oral DTIs to be approved for use in Europe, but was eventually voluntarily withdrawn from the market due to associated risk of severe liver toxicity.[28] In the United States, dabigatran etexilate is the first and only currently available oral DTI. It is currently FDA-approved for stroke prevention in nonvalvular atrial fibrillation and for the treatment and prevention of recurrent VTE.[29]

PHARMACOKINETICS

After oral administration, dabigatran has a bioavailability of approximately 3–7 percent.[29] Dabigatran is supplied in a capsule form that contains dabigatran etexilate mesylate pellets. After absorption, these pellets are hydrolyzed to form dabigatran, the active moiety. Notably, the bioavailability increases by 75 percent if the capsule is opened or tampered with. Therefore, dabigatran capsules should not be opened, chewed, crushed, or broken prior to administration. Dabigatran absorption is delayed if taken with food, but the overall extent of absorption or bioavailability remains unchanged.[30] Dabigatran is approximately 35 percent bound to plasma protein and has an associated volume of distribution of 50–70 L.[29] Dabigatran is not metabolized by cytochrome P-450 enzymes and also does not induce or inhibit their activity. A small percentage of dabigatran is subject to glucuronidation. Four different active acyl glucuronide metabolites are formed, each accounting for less than 10 percent of total plasma concentrations of dabigatran. Renal elimination accounts for approximately 80 percent of overall dabigatran clearance. In healthy individuals with normal renal function, the elimination half-life of dabigatran is 12–17 hours.[31] In an open-label pharmacokinetic study, following a single dose of 150 mg, the dabigatran half-life increased in mild renal impairment (creatinine clearance 50–80 mL/min) to 16.6 hours, in moderate renal impairment (creatinine clearance 30–50 mL/min) to 18.7 hours, in severe renal impairment (creatinine clearance <30 mL/min) to 27.5 hours, and in hemodialysis to 34.1 hours.[32] After a single dose, it was observed that dabigatran is cleared up to 68 percent by hemodialysis. In a case report of a patient who was taking dabigatran chronically prior to a cardiac surgery, a session of preoperative hemodialysis for 2.5 hours successfully reduced the thrombin time (TT) from 90.6 seconds to 60.2 seconds.[33] Surgery was completed without complication.

DOSING

Dabigatran is FDA-approved for the prevention of stroke in patients with nonvalvular atrial fibrillation based on the results of the Randomized Evaluation of Long-Term Anticoagulant Therapy (RE-LY) trial.[34] For this indication, the recommended dose is 150 mg twice daily, a dose associated with relative risk reduction in developing a stroke or systemic embolism compared to warfarin. For patients with a creatinine clearance of 15–30 mL/min or patients receiving concomitant P-glycoprotein inhibitors such as dronedarone or systemic ketoconazole, the dose should be reduced to 75 mg twice daily.[29] Dabigatran use should be avoided in patients with a creatinine clearance less than 15 mL/min or in patients with a creatinine clearance of 15–30 mL/min who are also receiving concomitant P-glycoprotein inhibitors.

The most recent ACCP guidelines do not recommend oral DTI or factor Xa inhibitor therapy over warfarin or low-molecular-weight heparin for the treatment of VTE.[35] Dabigatran is FDA approved for the treatment and prevention of recurrent VTE. In the RE-COVER trial, dabigatran at a dose of 150 mg twice daily was noninferior to warfarin in the rate of VTE and VTE-related death in patients who had an acute, symptomatic deep vein thrombosis or pulmonary embolism.[36]

Finally, dabigatran has also been evaluated for the prevention of VTE in orthopedic patients who have undergone a major hip or knee surgery. In the RE-MOBILIZE and RE-MODEL trials, dabigatran was compared to enoxaparin in patients who had undergone total knee replacements while in the RENOVATE and RENOVATE-II trials, patients had undergone total hip replacements.[37-40] Dabigatran demonstrated noninferiority to enoxaparin in RE-MODEL, RENOVATE, and RENOVATE-II, but failed to demonstrate noninferiority in the RE-MOBILIZE trial. Notably, the dose of dabigatran utilized in these trials was 220 mg once daily, a dosage form not currently available for use in the United States.

DOSING WHILE TRANSITIONING TO OR FROM OTHER ANTICOAGULANTS

When converting to dabigatran from warfarin, it is recommended to discontinue warfarin and initiate dabigatran therapy when the INR is less than 2.[29] If converting from dabigatran to warfarin, recommendations differ based on renal function. For a patient with a creatinine clearance of greater than 50 mL/min, 30–50 mL/min, and 15–30 mL/min, warfarin should be initiated 3, 2, and 1 day(s) prior to stopping dabigatran, respectively. It is important to note that because dabigatran can sometimes contribute to an elevated INR, the INR in the first 2 days after discontinuation of dabigatran may not be due to the effects of warfarin alone.

When converting to dabigatran from a parenteral anticoagulant, initiation of dabigatran therapy should occur at the time of the next scheduled dose of the parenteral anticoagulant or as soon as the continuous infusion is stopped.[29] If converting from dabigatran to a parenteral anticoagulant, it is recommended to initiate the parenteral anticoagulant 12 hours after the last dabigatran dose in patients with a creatinine clearance greater than 30 mL/min and 24 hours after the last dose if the creatinine clearance is less than 30 mL/min.

In the perioperative period, dabigatran discontinuation is based on renal function and bleeding risk of the procedure.[29] If the creatinine clearance is greater than 50 mL/min, dabigatran should be discontinued 2–4 days prior to a high bleed risk procedure and 1 day prior to a standard bleed risk procedure. If the creatinine clearance is 30–50 mL/min, the recommended timing of discontinuation extends to 4 and 2 days, respectively. Finally, if the creatinine clearance is less than 30 mL/min, dabigatran should be stopped 6 days before a high bleed risk procedure and 2–5 days before a standard bleed risk procedure.[41]

MONITORING

Prior to initiation and periodically during treatment with dabigatran, renal function must be assessed in order to guide dosing. Although no specific frequency recommendation exists, it is essential to check renal function prior to initiation and elective surgery as well as

during situations where renal function may have declined, such as acute illness. In contrast to warfarin therapy, routine monitoring for extent of anticoagulant effect is not required with dabigatran use. However, if needed, the ACCP guidelines recommend aPTT and thrombin time (TT) tests to assess level of anticoagulation associated with dabigatran in patients experiencing bleeding or requiring invasive procedures.[42] The aPTT can be prolonged with dabigatran use, but the relationship between the aPTT and dabigatran plasma concentrations is curvilinear.[31,43] As such, at higher concentrations of dabigatran, the aPTT flattens rather than increasing proportionately. The TT is a direct measure of DTI activity and correlates with dabigatran plasma concentrations in a linear fashion. However, the TT assay may not be useful in emergency scenarios if excessive dabigatran concentrations are suspected because the maximum measurement of the test can be exceeded by dabigatran concentrations of greater than 600 ng/mL. Therefore, TT assay is useful to detect presence of any concentration of dabigatran. Finally, similar to IV DTIs, the ECT assay is prolonged in a linear correlation with serum plasma levels of dabigatran. Limitations of this assay include availability of test and its use is currently limited to research trials.

ADVERSE EFFECTS

The most common adverse effects associated with dabigatran use are dyspepsia and bleeding complications.[29] In clinical trial, rates of dyspepsia were found to be approximately 11.8 percent in patients taking 150 mg twice daily.[34] This dosage was associated with a relatively higher discontinuation rate compared to warfarin. Hemorrhagic complications occurred at similar rates to that of warfarin in the RE-LY trial. Any type of bleeding occurred in 16.6 percent of patients, while major bleeding and life-threatening bleeding occurred in 3.3 percent and 1.7 percent, respectively. Patients identified to be at highest risk of bleeding complications include those with renal impairment. A post-hoc analysis demonstrated a significant increase in major bleeding with dabigatran compared to warfarin (5.4% vs 3.3%) in patients with a creatinine clearance less than 50 mL/min.[44]

REVERSAL

Current ACCP guidelines do not provide a recommendation for reversal of dabigatran, but do state that rVIIa and prothrombin complex concentration (PCC) may be useful based on animal and in vitro models.[42] In addition, hemodialysis and early administration of activated charcoal may have a role in reducing systemic concentrations of dabigatran. Following dabigatran administration in animals, PCC corrected the aPTT, ECT, and TT and prevented expansion of intracerebral hemorrhage.[45] However, in a study in healthy human volunteers, 4-factor PCC did not reverse the effects of dabigatran.[46] In an *ex vivo* study involving healthy volunteers, *activated* PCC (aPCC) corrected thrombin generation parameters following a single dose of dabigatran.[47] Given limited data, it is reasonable to consider PCC, aPCC, or rVIIa use in the setting of a life-threatening bleed associated with dabigatran.

CASE STUDIES

CASE 1: SUSPECTED HIT

KT is a 65-year-old male admitted for shortness of breath and right-sided lower extremity edema. Lower extremity Doppler ultrasonography imaging demonstrates evidence of acute deep vein thrombosis, and pulmonary angiography demonstrates acute pulmonary embolism. KT is admitted to a general medicine service initiated on a heparin infusion. Initial relevant labs: SCr 2.1, AST 20, ALT 19, INR 1, PT 12.2 s, aPTT 23 s, platelet count is 305,000/m³. Four days into the admission, KT's platelet count has decreased to 94,000/m³ and HIT is suspected.

Height = 5′9″

Weight = 82 kg

QUESTION 1

What anticoagulation therapy should KT be switched to?

Answer:

KT's heparin therapy should be discontinued due to the possibility of HIT. As alternate anticoagulant therapy, an intravenous direct thrombin inhibitor should be initiated. In KT's case, argatroban is most appropriate since his liver function is normal. Bivalirudin could be utilized; however, careful adjustments would be necessary because KT's kidney function is impaired.

QUESTION 2

At what dose should the new anticoagulant be started? How should it be monitored and adjusted?

Answer:

Argatroban therapy should be initiated at 2 mcg/kg/min (164 mcg/min) and titrated to a goal aPTT of 1.5–3 times the baseline. If KT were more critically ill or had impaired liver dysfunction, the initial dose should be reduced to 0.5 mcg/kg/min (41 mcg/min). The aPTT can checked 2 hours after initiation or any rate change. Hospitals often have institution-specific protocols, such as the following:

aPTT below goal range (<1.5 times baseline)	Increase infusion rate by 20%	Recheck aPTT 2 hours after rate change
aPTT within goal range (1.5–3 times baseline)	No change to infusion rate	Recheck aPTT in 6 hours
aPTT above goal (<2 times goal range)	Hold infusion for 1 hour, then resume at 50% lower rate	Recheck aPTT 2 hours after resumed therapy
aPTT above goal (>2 times goal range)	Hold infusion for 2 hours and resume at 50% lower rate once aPTT is within goal range	Recheck aPTT every 2 hours until within goal range, then recheck aPTT 2 hours after resumed infusion

QUESTION 3

KT's aPTT is checked 2 hours after starting new therapy, and it is 24 s. How should the infusion be adjusted?

Answer:

For KT, the goal aPTT range is 1.5–3 times the baseline, or 34.5–72 s. Because the initial aPTT is below goal (and following the sample protocol given), the infusion rate should be increased by 20 percent to 2.4 mcg/kg/min (196.8 mcg/min). A repeat aPTT should be checked 2 hours after the rate change.

CASE 2: ARGATROBAN BRIDGING TO WARFARIN

In the previous case, KT is diagnosed with HIT based on positive HIT antibody and serotonin release assay tests. KT is maintained on

the argatroban infusion for anticoagulant therapy. When preparing for discharge, warfarin therapy is initiated at 5 mg daily. Pertinent labs the day warfarin therapy is initiated include INR 2.1, PT 16.2 s, aPTT 48 s.

QUESTION 4

How long should warfarin and argatroban therapy be overlapped? When can argatroban be safely discontinued?

Answer:

ACCP guidelines recommend vitamin K antagonist therapy be overlapped with parenteral anticoagulation therapy for at least 5 days and until the INR is >2.[35] In the case of overlapping warfarin with argatroban therapy, it is important to recognize that argatroban causes an elevation in the INR. Note KT's INR prior to starting warfarin therapy is 2.1, which is entirely due to the anticoagulant effect of argatroban. Warfarin should be initiated and overlapped for at least 5 days and argatroban can be discontinued when the INR is >4. Upon discontinuation of argatroban, it is recommended to repeat the INR 4–6 hours later to ensure the INR is within goal range (2–3). If the repeat INR is >2, no further argatroban therapy is needed, but if it is <2, argatroban may need to be resumed.

CASE 3: ARGATROBAN DOSE ADJUSTMENT/ DOSE ADJUSTMENT FOR ORGAN DYSFUNCTION/CRITICALLY ILL

AG is a 57-year-old male with a history of stroke-related to atrial fibrillation, coronary artery disease, and recent HIT with associated VTE. He is admitted to the intensive care unit (ICU) with severe pneumonia. Warfarin was stopped upon hospital admission and not resumed due to planed tracheostomy placement surgery. Two days after surgery, AG was still in the ICU and placed on an argatroban infusion to bridge to warfarin therapy. The infusion was ordered to be adjusted to an aPTT of 1.5–3 times the baseline.

Height = 6′0″

Weight = 77 kg

QUESTION 5

What dose of argatroban is recommended for this patient? How should argatroban be monitored?

Answer:

This patient is critically ill and argatroban dosing requirements have been shown to be decreased in this population compared to noncritically ill patients.[9] The initial dose of argatroban should be no greater than 0.5 mcg/kg/min with monitoring of the aPTT 4 hours after initiation and with any dosing change. In critically ill patients with multiple organ dysfunction, heart failure, anasarca, or postcardiac surgery, argatroban should be initiated at no greater than 0.25 mcg/kg/min due to reports of extremely reduced dosage requirements in these patients.

CASE 4: BIVALIRUDIN AND RENAL IMPAIRMENT

JS is a 68-year-old female with a history of coronary artery disease, hypertension, end-stage renal disease (hemodialysis 3 times weekly), and HIT without thrombosis secondary to heparin therapy who is admitted for mitral valve replacement and coronary artery bypass graft (CABG) surgery. JS is initiated on bivalirudin for anticoagulation therapy during the procedure. Postoperatively, JS is admitted to the cardiac surgery intensive care unit and requires resumption of bivalirudin for the anticoagulation of her mechanical mitral valve. Pertinent labs: SCr 3.7, INR 1, PT 11.8 s, aPTT 26 s.

Height = 5′3″

Weight = 65 kg

QUESTION 6

What dose of bivalirudin should be initiated? How should bivalirudin therapy be monitored and adjusted?

Answer:

Because JS is dialysis-dependent, bivalirudin should be initiated at 0.05 mg/kg/hr (3.25 mg/hr) based on available evidence in patients with severe renal impairment.[16] The infusion should be titrated to a goal aPTT of 1.5–2.5 times the baseline, or 39–65 s. The aPTT should be checked 2 hours after initiation and any infusion rate adjustment.

QUESTION 7

Two days later, JS becomes acutely ill with a hospital-acquired pneumonia and requires vasopressor therapy. The nephrology service recommends continuous renal replacement therapy (CRRT) for management of JS's end-stage renal disease while she is hemodynamically unstable. The bivalirudin infusion is held in order to obtain access for CRRT therapy. Upon resumption, on what dose of bivalirudin should JS be started?

Answer:

Based on available data, patients receiving CRRT required 0.03–0.07 mg/kg/hr of bivalirudin to achieve therapeutic aPTT ranges.[15-17] Due to acute illness and change in dialysis therapy, it is reasonable to resume the bivalirudin at 0.03 mg/kg/hr and titrate to goal aPTT range. The aPTT can be checked 2 hours after initiation and any rate adjustment; however, due to the prolonged half-life observed in critically ill patients with concomitant renal impairment, it may be reasonable to extend this time to 4 hours.

CASE 5: DABIGATRAN DOSE ADJUSTMENT

RH is a 65-year-old male with a past medical history of atrial fibrillation and chronic obstructive pulmonary disease (COPD) admitted to the general medicine service for an acute COPD exacerbation. Medications include amiodarone 200 mg daily, fluticasone/salmeterol inhaler twice daily, albuterol inhaler as needed, and dabigatran 150 mg twice daily, all of which are resumed upon hospital admission. Pertinent labs: SCr 2.2 (estimated creatinine clearance 30 mL/min).

QUESTION 8

What adjustments should be made to the dabigatran dose? What if dronedarone was added to the patient's regimen and amiodarone discontinued?

Answer:

Because renal elimination accounts for most of the clearance of dabigatran, caution should be undertaken when administering this medication to patients with renal insufficiency due to prolonged duration of action and increased risk of bleeding.[29] In this patient, the half-life of dabigatran would be expected to be approximately double as compared to healthy individuals. Therefore, the dose should be empirically decreased to 75 mg bid, with close monitoring for signs and symptoms of bleeding. Dabigatran is not recommended in patients with an estimated creatinine clearance less than 30 mL/min who are receiving P-glycoprotein inhibitors such as dronedarone.

CASE 6: ORAL DTI BRIDGING

AD is a 77-year-old male with a past medical history of hypertension, dyslipidemia, and nonvalvular atrial fibrillation (anticoagulated with dabigatran) who has a scheduled colonoscopy in two weeks. The gastroenterologist would like AD to hold his anticoagulation before the procedure in case any biopsy samples need to be taken (standard bleeding risk). Pertinent labs: SCr 0.71, INR 1.1, PT 11.3 s, aPTT 38 s.

Height = 6′0″

Weight = 80 kg

QUESTION 9

What instructions should AD be given regarding holding and resuming his dabigatran around the colonoscopy?

Answer:

The holding of dabigatran prior to a scheduled procedure is determined by the patient's renal function and the bleeding risk of the procedure.[29] In this situation, the possibility of needing a biopsy during colonoscopy is associated with a standard bleed risk (vs. a high bleed risk). In addition, AD's creatinine clearance is estimated to be 98 mL/min based on his age and SCr. Taken together, AD should hold his dabigatran doses the day before the procedure and resume the day after the procedure.

QUESTION 10

How would your answer differ if AD's SCr was 1.5?

Answer:

If AD's serum creatinine was 1.5, his estimated creatinine clearance would be 46 mL/min and therefore, his dabigatran doses should be held for **two** days prior and then resumed the day after procedure.

REFERENCES

1. Majerus PW, Tollefsen DM. Anticoagulant, thrombolytic, and antiplatelet drugs. In: Goodman & Gilman's The Pharmacological Basis of Therapeutics, 10th ed. New York: McGraw-Hill, 2001.
2. Toschi V, Lettino M, Gallo R, Badimon JJ, Chesebro JH. Biochemistry and biology of hirudin. Coron Artery Dis. 1996;7(6):420–428.
3. Wallis RB. Hirudins: From leeches to man. Semin Thromb Hemost. 1996;22(2)185–196.
4. American Journal of Health-System Pharmacists. Discontinued Drug Bulletin. Available at: http://www.ashp.org/drugshortages/notavailable/bulletin.aspx?id=924 (accessed January 15, 2013).
5. Argatroban [package insert]. Research Triangle Park, NC: GlaxoSmithKline, 2012.

6. Bivalirudin [package insert]. Parsippany, NJ: The Medicines Company, 2012.

7. Lepirudin [packager insert]. Montville, NJ: Bayer HealthCare Pharmaceuticals, 2010.

8. Linkins LA, Dans AL, Moores LK, et al. Treatment and prevention of heparin-induced thrombocytopenia: Antithrombotic therapy and prevention of thrombosis, 9th ed: American College of Chest Physicians evidence-based clinical practice guidelines. Chest. 2012;141(2)(suppl):e495S–e530S.

9. Keegan SP, Gallagher EM, Ernst NE, et al. Effects of critical illness and organ failure on therapeutic argatroban dosage requirements in patients with suspected or confirmed heparin-induced thrombocytopenia. Ann Pharmacother. 2009;43(1):19–27.

10. Rice L, Hursting MJ, Baillie GM, et al. Argatroban anticoagulation in obese versus nonobese patients: Implications for treating heparin-induced thrombocytopenia. J Clin Pharmacol. 2007;47(8):1028–1034.

11. Vermeer F, Vahanian A, Fels PW, et al. Argatroban and alteplase in patients with acute myocardial infarction: The ARGAMI Study. J Thromb Thrombolysis. 2000;10:233–240.

12. Stone GW, Witzenbichler B, Guagliumi G, et al. Bivalirudin during primary PCI in acute myocardial infarction. N Engl J Med. 2008;358(21):2218–2230.

13. Lidon RM, Theroux P, Lesperance J, et al. A pilot, early angiographic patency study using a direct thrombin inhibitor as adjunctive therapy to streptokinase in acute myocardial infarction. Circulation. 1994;89:1567–1572.

14. Skrupky LP, Smith JR, Deal EN, et al. Comparison of bivalirudin and argatroban for the management of heparin-induced thrombocytopenia. Pharmacotherapy. 2010;30(12):1229–1238.

15. Wisler JW, Washam JB, Becker RC. Evaluation of dose requirements for prolonged bivalirudin administration in patients with renal insufficiency and suspected heparin-induced thrombocytopenia. J Thromb Thrombolysis. 2012;33(3):287–295.

16. Tsu LV, Dager WE. Bivalirudin dosing adjustments for reduced renal function with or without hemodialysis in the management of heparin-induced thrombocytopenia. Ann Pharmacother. 2011;45(10):1185–1192.

17. Runyan CL, Cabral KP, Riker RR, et al. Correlation of bivalirudin dose with creatinine clearance during treatment of heparin-induced thrombocytopenia. Pharmacotherapy. 2011;31(9):850–856.

18. Kiser TH, Fish DN. Evaluation of bivalirudin treatment for heparin-induced thrombocytopenia in critically ill patients with hepatic and/or renal dysfunction. Pharmacotherapy. 2006;26(4):452–460.

19. Tsu LV, Dager WE. Comparison of bivalirudin dosing strategies using total, adjusted, and ideal body weights in obese patients with heparin-induced thrombocytopenia. Pharmacotherapy. 2012;32(1):20–26.

20. Ginsberg JS, Nurmohamed MT, Gent M, et al. Use of hirulog in the prevention of venous thrombosis after major hip or knee surgery. Circulation. 1994;90:2385–2389.

21. Garcia DA, Baglin TP, Weitz JI, et al. Parenteral anticoagulants: Antithrombotic therapy and prevention of thrombosis, 9th ed: American College of Chest Physicians evidence-based clinical practice guidelines. Chest. 2012;141(2)(suppl):e24S–e43S.

22. Bucha E, Nowak G, Czerwinski R, et al. R-hirudin as anticoagulant in regular hemodialysis therapy: Finding of therapeutic R-hirudin blood/plasma concentrations and respective dosages. Clin Appl Thromb Hemost. 1999;5(3):164–170.

23. Schiele F, Lindgaerde F, Eriksson H, et al. Subcutaneous recombinant hirudin (HBW 023) versus intravenous sodium heparin in treatment of established acute deep vein thrombosis of the legs: a multicentre prospective dose-ranging randomized trial. Thromb Haemost. 1997;77(5):834–838.

24. Doepker B, Mount KL, Ryder LJ, et al. Bleeding risk factors associated with argatroban therapy in the critically ill. J Thromb Thrombolysis. 2012;l34(4):491–498.

25. Eichler P, Friesen HJ, Lubenow N, Jaeger B, Greinacher A. Antihirudin antibodies in patients with heparin-induced thrombocytopenia treated with lepirudin: Incidence, effects on aPTT, and clinical relevance. Blood. 2000;96(7):2373–2378.

26. Oh JJ, Akers WS, Lewis D, et al. Recombinant factor VIIa for refractory bleeding after cardiac surgery secondary to anticoagulation with the direct thrombin inhibitor lepirudin. Pharmacotherapy. 2006;26(4):569–577.

27. Nagle EL, Tsu LV, Dager WE. Bivalirudin for anticoagulation during hypothermic cardiopulmonary bypass and recombinant factor VIIa for iatrogenic coagulopathy. Ann Pharmacother. 2011;45(9):e47.

28. Lee WM, Larrey D, Olsson R, et al. Hepatic findings in long-term clinical trials of ximelagatran. Drug Saf. 2005;28(4):351–370.

29. Dabigatran [package insert]. Ridgefield, CT: Boehringer Ingelheim Pharmaceuticals, Inc., 2012.

30. Stangier J, Eriksson BI, Dahl OE, et al. Pharmacokinetic profile of the oral direct thrombin inhibitor dabigatran etexilate in healthy volunteers and patients undergoing total hip replacement. J Clin Pharmacol. 2005;45(5):555–563.

31. Stangier J, Rathgen K, Stahle H, et al. The pharmacokinetics, pharmacodynamics and tolerability of dabigatran etexilate, a new oral direct thrombin inhibitor, in healthy male subjects. Br J Clin Pharmacol. 2007;64(3):292–303.

32. Stangier J, Rathgen K, Stahle H, et al. Influence of renal impairment on the pharmacokinetics and pharmacodynamics of oral dabigatran etexilate: An open-label, parallel-group, single-centre study. Clin Pharmacokinet. 2010;49(4):259–268.

33. Wanek MR, Horn ET, Elapavaluru S, et al. Safe use of hemodialysis for dabigatran removal before cardiac surgery. Ann Pharmacother. 2012;46:epub.

34. Connolly SJ, Ezekowitz MD, Yusuk S, et al. Dabigatran versus warfarin in patients with atrial fibrillation. N Engl J Med. 2009;361:1139–1151.

35. Kearon C, Akl EA, Comerota AJ, et al. Antithrombotic therapy for VTE disease: Antithrombotic therapy and prevention of thrombosis, 9th ed: American College of Chest Physicians evidence-based clinical practice guidelines. Chest. 2012;141:e419s–e494s.

36. Schulman S, Kearon C, Kakkar AK, et al. Dabigatran versus warfarin in the treatment of acute venous thromboembolism. N Engl J Med. 2009;361(24):2342–2352.

37. Ginsberg JS, Davidson BL, Comp PC, et al. Oral thrombin inhibitor dabigatran etexilate vs. North American enoxaparin regimen for prevention of venous thromboembolism after knee arthroplasty surgery. J Arthroplasty. 2009;24(1):1–9.

38. Eriksson BI, Dahl OE, Rosencher N, et al. Oral dabigatran etexilate vs. subcutaneous enoxaparin for the prevention of venous thromboembolism after total knee replacement: The RE-MODEL randomized trial. J Thromb Haemost. 2007;5(11):2178–2185.

39. Eriksson BI, Dahl OE, Huo MH, et al. Oral dabigatran versus enoxaparin for thromboprophylaxis after primary total hip arthroplasty (RE-NOVATE II*). A randomised, double-blind, non-inferiority trial. Thromb Haemost. 2011;105(4):721–729.

40. Eriksson BI, Dahl OE, Rosencher N, et al. Dabigatran etexilate versus enoxaparin for prevention of venous thromboembolism after total hip replacement: A randomised, double-blind, non-inferiority trial. Lancet. 2007;370(9591):949–956.

41. Fawole A, Daw HA, Crowther MA. Practical management of bleeding due to the anticoagulants dabigatran, rivaroxaban, and apixaban. Cleve Clin J Med 2013;80:443–451.

42. Ageno W, Gallus AS, Wittkowsky A, et al. Oral anticoagulant therapy: Antithrombotic therapy and prevention of thrombosis, 9th ed: American College of Chest Physicians evidence-based clinical practice guidelines. Chest. 2012;141(2 suppl):e44s–e88s.

43. van Ryn J, Stangier J, Haertter S, et al. Dabigatran etexilate—a novel, reversible, oral direct thrombin inhibitor: Interpretation of coagulation assays and reversal of anticoagulant activity. Thromb Haemost. 2010;103(6):1116–1127.

44. Eikelboom JW, Wallentin L, Connolly SJ, et al. Risk of bleeding with 2 doses of dabigatran compared with warfarin in older and younger patients with atrial fibrillation: An analysis of the randomized evaluation of long-term anticoagulant therapy (RE-LY) trial. Circulation. 2011;123(21):2363–2372.

45. Zhou W, Schwarting S, Illanes S, et al. Hemostatic therapy in experimental intracerebral hemorrhage associated with the direct thrombin inhibitor dabigatran. Stroke. 2011;42(12):3594–3599.

46. Eerenberg ES, Kamphuisen PW, Sijpkens MK, et al. Reversal of rivaroxaban and dabigatran by prothrombin complex concentrate: A randomized, placebo-controlled, crossover study in healthy subjects. Circulation. 2011;124(14):1573–1579.

47. Marlu R, Hodaj E, Paris A, Albaladejo P, Cracowski JL, Pernod G. Effect of non-specific reversal agents on anticoagulant activity of dabigatran and rivaroxaban: A randomised crossover ex vivo study in healthy volunteers. Thromb Haemost. 2012;108(2):217–224.

CHAPTER

24

Pharmacokinetic Considerations in Oncology

ALICE C. CEACAREANU, PharmD, PhD
ZACHARY A.P. WINTROB, MSc

DOXORUBICIN

The anthracycline age began over half century ago, when a soil sample harvested near the Castel del Monte in Italy revealed *Streptomyces peucetius*, a new bacterial strain producing a bright red pigment that was found to have good activity against murine tumors. A mutated strain of *S. peucetius* was found to produce a different red compound that was named Adriamycin, after the Adriatic Sea. Today, also known as doxorubicin (DOXO), this prototype compound remains one of the most prescribed antineoplastic agents. Currently, more than 2,000 known DOXO analogues provide invaluable clinical and research applicability.

DOXO has an exceptional chemical reactivity and is able to react with several molecules within the cell, leading to a variety of toxic effects, all of which contribute to its unique antineoplastic efficacy. Beginning with polymerase inhibition and DNA intercalation and ending with perturbation of calcium homeostasis, DOXO finds itself a place in most antineoplastic combo regimens.[1-5]

In order to relate DOXO dosing to its therapeutic effect or occurrence of toxicity, a number of physiologically based pharmacokinetic (PBPK) models have been tested to allow for simulation and prediction of therapeutic drug or metabolite levels.[6] Roughly a decade ago, Gustafson and colleagues developed a DOXO PBPK model capable to predict PK alterations in special human populations; however, despite its invaluable utility, this model is largely underutilized for clinical benefit.[6] The model described here is available as a complete model code from Gustafson and others. We provide this information with the hope of promoting its utilization in direct patient care.

1. Tissue compartment mass balance:

$$dA_T/dt = Q_T(C_A - C_{V-T})$$
$$C_{V-T} = A_T/[\ V_T + (T_{DNA} \times V_T)/(K_{DNA} + C_{V-T})$$
$$+ (T_{CAL} \times V_T)/(K_{CAL} + C_{V-T})\ ]$$

2. Blood compartment mass balance:

$$dA_B/dt = \Sigma Q_T \times C_{V-T} - (Q_C - Q_L) \times C_A - Q_L \times C_{BL}$$
$$C_A = A_B/V_B \times (1 - F_B)$$
$$C_{BL} = A_B/V_B$$

3. DOXO metabolism by aldo-keto reductases:

$$dAM_{AKR}/dt = (V_{MAX-AKT} \times C_{V-T})/(K_{M-AKT} \times C_{V-T})$$

4. DOXO metabolism by aglycone:

$$dAM_{AG}/dt = K_{MET-AG} \times C_{V-T} \times V_T$$

5. Amount of DOXO eliminated in urine (U):

$$dAE_U/dt = F_{FILT} \times Q_K \times C_A + (V_{MAX-PGP-K} \times C_{BL})/(K_{M-PGP-K} + C_{BL})$$

6. Amount of DOXO eliminated in feces (F):

$$dAE_F/dt = [(V_{MAX-PGP-L} \times C_{V-L})/(K_{M-PGP-L} + C_{V-L})]$$
$$+ [(V_{MAX-PGP-G} \times C_{V-G})/(K_{M-PGP-G} + C_{V-G})]$$

NOMENCLATURE[8]

Q: Blood flow (L/h)

A: Amount of drug (mols)

V: Tissue volume (L)

C_A: Arterial blood concentration of free DOXO (M)

C_V: Venous blood concentration of total DOXO leaving tissues (M)

C_{BL}: Arterial blood concentration of total DOXO (M)

F_B: Fraction of DOXO bound to plasma proteins

T_{DNA}: Tissue-specific DNA binding capacity for DOXO (M)

T_{CAL}: Tissue-specific cardiolipin binding capacity for DOXO (M)

K_{DNA}: Binding affinity of DOXO for DNA (M)

K_{CAL}: Binding affinity of DOXO for cardiolipin (M)

AM: Amount metabolized (mols)

AE: Amount excreted (mols)

V_{MAX}: Maximum rate of activity (mols/hr/L tissue)

K_M: Michaelis's constant (M)

K_{MET}: First-order metabolic rate constant (h^{-1} kg tissue^{-1})

F_{FILT}: Fraction renal blood flow filtered at the glomerulus

Subscripts:

T: Generic tissue compartment

C: Total cardiac output

L: Liver

K: Kidney

G: Gut

B: Blood

AKR: Aldo-keto reductase

AG: Aglycone

PGP: P-glycoprotein

Given DOXO's liver metabolism and bile elimination, dose reduction was considered a logical approach in cases with hepatic disease or liver metastases. However, dose reduction requirement has never been validated in patients with liver dysfunction and little is known about its actual clinical benefit. We provide here evidence indicating the main rationale for or against dose adjustment in various clinical circumstances.

To date a whole body of clinical practice has widely adopted DOXO dose reduction by 50 percent and 75 percent, respectively, in patients with moderately and severely impaired liver function, based on evidence provided from clinical trials research involving not more than 17 patients with liver dysfunction.[7-9] Roughly two decades ago, a study including 64 patients with nonlymphocytic leukemia that evaluated the relationship between pretreatment liver function and DOXO PK indicated similar plasma levels, incidence of toxicity and complete response rate in patients with mild pretreatment liver impairment receiving full dose of DOXO and in those with normal hepatic function. Individuals with impaired liver function in which a dose reduction has been applied displayed lower plasma concentrations and less toxicity, but no significant difference in response rate when compared to those receiving full dose.[10] Although beyond the study's main goal, whether the lower-dose group encountered a shorter duration of response and survival remains unknown. Interestingly a number of subsequent studies, evaluating altogether roughly 40 patients with liver impairment, reported either normal plasma profiles or moderately increased AUC for DOXO and doxorubicinol, not justifying dose adjustment in patients with liver dysfunction receiving full DOXO dose.[11-14] A significantly increased AUC and prolonged half-life time was associated with bilirubin levels sixfold higher than normal.[14]

Considering these data together with the evidence of anthracycline-induced cardiomyopathy unveils interesting clues. The recommended maximum cumulative lifetime dose of 450–550 mg/m² DOXO and 400–550 mg/m² daunorubicin was the result of a documented frequency of 5 percent of patients developing congestive cardiac failure when treated with this dose. Although cardiac failure incidence up to 50 percent was observed in cases receiving 1,000 mg/m², a significant improvement was found to be associated with administration of a weekly dose or >24-hour continuous infusion as opposed to bolus.[15,16] Potentially the cause for lower cardiotoxicity incidence observed in a modified administration schedule is the additional time that allows the slow formation and elimination of doxorubicinol. Its formation was shown to be slower in patients with elevated bilirubin and at least one study (4 out of 31 cases with impaired liver function) reported prolonged half-life time.[14] Mildly abnormal liver function tests did not affect DOXO clearance and toxicity, and it is likely that any dose reduction for bilirubin levels lower than 3 are likely going to result in decreased effectiveness. High bilirubin levels have been associated with higher AUC.[13,14] However, DOXO toxicities appear to be related to the peak plasma concentration rather than the AUC.[17] Thus, weekly dosing administered by slow continuous infusion may provide a survival advantage over dose reduction, especially in populations with preexisting cardiac disease or concomitant or prior mediastinal or chest wall irradiation in which the maximum cumulative dose will already be reduced. In such patients who also present with impaired liver function or liver metastasis, further dose reduction should be cautiously considered.

CASE STUDIES

CASE 1

A 48-year-old Caucasian woman with a history of successfully treated breast cancer, roughly a decade ago, is diagnosed with acute myelogenous leukemia (AML). She is initiated on Ara-C standard dose (100 mg/m²) for 7 days and is to begin daunorubicin 45 mg/m² for 3 days upon clarification of the total cumulative anthracycline dose received during her breast cancer treatment. A discussion with the oncologist who treated her for breast cancer reveals that her initial treatment included a total DOXO dose of 825 mg. He also indicates

that his dosing was guarded due to patient's history of hepatitis B and associated risk for liver failure due to virus activation. Her current liver function tests are as follows: AST = 112, ALT = 98, Alk Phos = 232, TBili = 1.7, DBili = 0.7, Albumin = 3.4.

Height = 173 cm

Weight = 212 kg

QUESTION 1

Is daunorubicin a viable option in this patient?

Answer:

Daunorubicin is a significant component of the AML antineoplastic treatment; however, its use is limited by the cumulative lifetime dose of any anthracycline ever administered in that patient, regardless of the time frame since last utilization (including childhood, if applicable).

Because she received DOXO for breast cancer treatment, the utilized equivalent of daunorubicin should be calculated. Her dose per body surface area should be calculated according to her current actual body weight.[18]

QUESTION 2

Has she reached her lifetime cumulative dose?

Answer:

$$\text{DOXO Mwt} = 543.5 \text{ g/mol}$$
$$\text{Daunorubicin Mwt} = 564 \text{ g/mol}$$
$$825 \text{ mg DOXO} = 825 \text{ mg}/543.5 \text{ mg} \times \text{mmol}^{-1} = \sim1.5 \text{ mmols DOXO}$$

Following the chemistry law of Avogadro, 1 mol of DOXO contains the same number of molecules as 1 mol of daunorubicin. Thus, 1.5 mmols DOXO = 1.5 mmols daunorubicin.

We can now convert mmols daunorubicin into mg:

$$1.5 \text{ mmols daunorubicin} = 1.5 \; \cancel{\text{mmol}} \times 564 \text{ mg} \times \cancel{\text{mmol}^{-1}}$$
$$= 846 \text{ mg daunorubicin equivalent used for breast cancer treatment}$$

The correct answer is that patient has NOT yet reached the daunorubicin lifetime cumulative dose.

QUESTION 3

How many anthracycline cycles could she take advantage of without increasing the risk of hepatitis B reactivation?

Answer:

The patient's current BSA can be calculated with the formula:

$$\text{BSA (m}^2\text{)} = 0.007184 \times \text{Height (cm)}^{0.725} \times \text{Weight (kg)}^{0.425}$$
$$= 0.007184 \times (173)^{0.725} \times (212)^{0.425}$$
$$= \sim 2.94 \text{ m}^2$$

Thus, since her lifetime cumulative dose for daunorubicin is 550 mg/m², she could in theory receive a total of 550 mg × m⁻² × 2.94 m² = 1,617 mg. Considering she already received a daunorubicin equivalent of 846 mg, she could theoretically receive up to 1,617 – 846 = 771 mg daunorubicin.

Her planned daunorubicin dose is 45 mg/m² daily for 3 days (cycle 1). The expected dose utilization per cycle will be:

$$45 \text{ mg/m}^2 \times 2.94 \text{ m}^2 \times 3 \text{ days (cycle)} = \sim397 \text{ mg/cycle}$$

Based on her liver function tests (emphasis on low albumin and slightly elevated bilirubin), it is possible that she may benefit from administration of a lower dose instead of a full 45 mg/m² dose. A 25 percent dose reduction will allow administration of a guarded amount of anthracycline, less likely to reactivate the dormant hepatitis B virus, and also potentially allow two cycles of Ara-C + daunorubicin combination regimen, known for its increased effectiveness as compared to Ara-C alone.

CARBOPLATIN

Carboplatin holds the advantage in therapy with significantly lower numbers of nonhematological toxicities as compared to cisplatin (Figure 24-1).[19] The benefit of much less nephrotoxicity and peripheral neuropathy and the similar cytotoxic activity as cisplatin facilitated the gradually increased carboplatin utilization over the last decades. With thrombocytopenia as the main dose-limiting toxicity, pretreatment renal function rather than kidney toxicity affects the extent of thrombocytopenia. Therefore, close therapeutic drug monitoring should be conducted routinely for carboplatin treatment.[20,21] Renal clearance is directly associated to the glomerular filtration rate (GFR), potentially due to the lack of active renal secretion and near exclusive filtration through the glomerulus. The antineoplastic activity and toxicity will then be determined mainly by the administered dose and the pretreatment GFR. Calvert and colleagues were able to demonstrate in a retrospective study that AUC was linearly related to dose only when GRF changes have been accounted for.[22] The initial *Calvert formula*, Dose (mg) = AUC × (1.2 × GFR + 20), was tested on 18 patients as part of the phase I evaluation. A PK prospectively designed study of 31 patients was then conducted to evaluate the dosage formula. Observed and predicted AUC values have been plotted together, demonstrating a good correlation (correlation coefficient r = 0.886, P<0.00001).

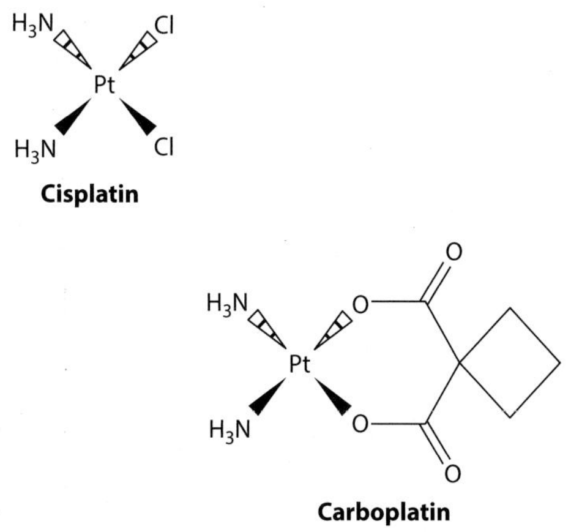

FIGURE 24-1. Structurally, carboplatin is both larger than cisplatin and less potent. The structural differences cause carboplatin to have a lower membrane permeability which results in carboplatin doses being much higher; with respect to metabolism it is also less reactive. Pharmacokinetically, this manifests in the form of a longer half-life than cisplatin and a much larger fraction being recovered in urine. Despite undergoing minimal metabolism, carboplatin is able to yield cisplatin upon incubation in solution with sodium chloride. This makes it hard to identify whether or not the portion that is not recovered unchanged in urine is the result of metabolism or simply a chemical reaction with circulating chloride ions.

TABLE 24-1	Guidelines recommended maximum carboplatin doses per target AUCs	
Target AUC	**Max Carboplatin Dose**
6	900 mg
5	750 mg
4	600 mg

In order to increase precision of the dose calculation, the nonrenal clearance for the tested cases has been measured as the difference between the renal and the total plasma clearance, with the assumption that the nonrenal clearance is constant. The formula generated was:

$$\text{Dose (mg)} = \text{AUC} \times (A \times \text{GFR} + B)$$

where A is the ratio of GFR to the renal clearance of the drug and B is the nonrenal clearance. The formula basically suggests that the nonrenal clearance is independent of patient characteristics.

Today A is assumed to equal 1 and, although the estimation of creatinine clearance is higher than GFR, the two values are used interchangeably for calculation of the dose by using the *Calvert formula*.

$$\text{Total carboplatin dose (mg)} = \text{Target AUC} \times (\text{GFR} + 25)$$

The National Cancer Institute's Cancer Therapy Evaluation Program recently published an action letter on AUC-based dosing of carboplatin guidelines. Through this letter it advises that GFR used in the *Calvert formula* should not exceed 125 mL/min, thus capping the maximum carboplatin dose based on target AUC (Table 24-1).

This update has prompted the Gynecologic Oncology Group (GOG) to use Cockcroft-Gault instead of Jelliffe formula for GFR estimation. Because Cockcroft-Gault formula can still overestimate renal function in obese and elderly patients and further lead to carboplatin overdosing, GOG has recommended that in patients with abnormally low creatinine, a minimum serum creatinine value of 0.7 mg/dL should be used when estimating GFR. This value also accounts for the newer creatinine assay calibration system based on isotope dilution mass spectrometry.

CASE 2

A 74-year-old Caucasian male with a history of stage IIB nonsmall cell lung cancer, status postlobectomy one week ago, is to be started on carboplatin and paclitaxel for five cycles. He is a thin, frail man who tolerated surgery well and has unremarkable labs. The most recent serum creatinine level of 0.4 mg/dL. The oncologist wants patient to be dosed for an AUC of 5 and receive 150 mg/m² paclitaxel.

Height = 181 cm

Weight = 65 kg

QUESTION 1

What are the doses in mg to be administered in this patient?

Answer:

This dosage requires knowing the patient's GFR, which can be sufficiently estimated by calculating the patient's creatinine clearance based on the Cockcroft-Gault method. Because the serum creatinine level is <0.7 mg/dL, as per guidelines, 0.7 mg/dL should be used in its place in this calculation:

$$\text{CrCl} = [(140 - \text{Age in years}) \times (\text{Ideal body weight in kg}) \times (0.85, \text{ if female})]/(72 \times \text{Serum creatinine in mg/dL})$$

where

Ideal body weight for men in kg = 50 + [2.3 × (Height in inches – 60)]

Ideal body weight for women in kg = 45.5 + [2.3 × (Height in inches – 60)]

Therefore:

$$CrCl = \{(140 - 74) \times [50 + 2.3(181/2.54 - 60)]\}/(72 \times 0.7)$$

$$= 99.4 \text{ mL/min}$$

Using the Clavert formula:

$$\text{Target dose in mg} = 5 \times (99.4 + 25)$$

$$= 622 \text{ mg}$$

Thus the target dose for each cycle to target an AUC of 5 is 622 mg, assuming that the patient's serum creatinine does not exceed 0.7 mg/dL.

METHOTREXATE

Methotrexate (MTX) history dates back to 1947 when Sidney Farber succeeded in extending the life of children with leukemia. Today, MTX is one of the most widely used drugs with large applicability in the treatment of various diseases, including cancer. Its utilization in oncology applies to treatment of both solid and hematologic malignancies, including osteosarcoma, breast, lung, stomach, bladder, head and neck cancers, as well as leukemia and lymphoma.

MTX is an antimetabolite drug that enters the cell primarily via the reduced folate carrier, an endocytic uptake mechanism, activated by MTX binding to the folate receptor. However, at extracellular concentrations above 20 μM MTX is able to enter the cell by passive diffusion in addition to active transport.[23] Upon its penetration into the cell, MTX inhibits the conversion of dihydrofolate to tetrahydrofolate by competitive inhibition of dihydrofolate reductase.[24] Methylated tetrahydrofolate is essential for the conversion of deoxyuridine monophosphate to deoxythymidine monophosphate by thymidylate synthase through reductive methylation. Subsequent phosphorylation of deoxythymidine monophosphate yields thymidine triphosphate, one of the four nucleotides used in DNA synthesis.[25] By inhibiting the upstream production of substrates essential for DNA synthesis and repair, MTX inhibits cell growth, thereby inducing apoptosis in rapidly proliferating cancer cells.

In addition to inhibiting DNA synthesis, MTX can be polyglutamated by folypolyglutamate synthetase. Long-chain polyglutamated MTX then also interferes with *de novo* purine synthesis and inhibits RNA production by inhibiting glycinamide ribunucleotide transformylase, the enzyme that catalyzes the transfer of a formyl group from formyl tetrahydrofolate to glycinamide ribonucleotide. Importantly, the inhibition of this reaction prevents the production of formyl-glycinamide ribonucleotide, a purine precursor, and tetrahydrofolate, preventing the downstream biosynthesis of inosine monophosphate.[26] Polyglutamated MTX also provides the advantage of an increased intracellular mean residence time, thereby allowing a greater intracellular exposure. However, polyglutamates can be cleaved by γ-glutamyl hydrolase yielding a lower number of glutamates bound to MTX.[23] Both MTX and its polyglutamates have dramatically greater affinity, between 1,000- and 10,000-fold, for dihydrofolate reductase than does dihydrofolate, its natural substrate.[24,27] However, in order to have the desired effect MTX must first make it to the tumor cell. This process, for oral formulations, requires absorption from the gut into the blood stream and then surviving the "first-pass effect" of the liver before it reaches the tumor.

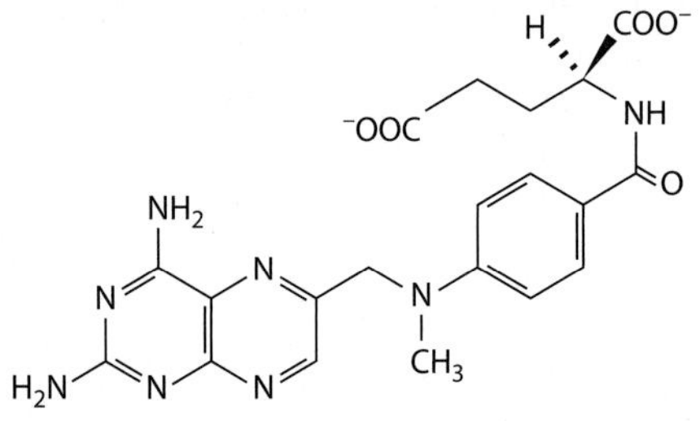

FIGURE 24-2. The structure of MTX at physiologic pH. The α-carboxyl group has a pKa of 4.70 ± 0.10 and the γ-carboxyl group has a pKa of 3.36 ± 0.20.[28] At pH values of 5.5–8, MTX is anionic, thus predominantly absorbed by saturable active transport in the gut.

The structure of MTX is charged at physiologic pH (Figure 24-1). Both carboxyl groups, as well as nitrogen 1 and 10, are deprotonated at physiologic pH and thus MTX is anionic with a negative 2 charge.[27,28] As a result MTX is prevented from easily diffusing across intestinal membranes and thus the primary method of absorption is active transport. This transport is saturable and, therefore, creates an inverse relationship between bioavailability and dose whereby the bioavailability of MTX decreases with high doses. Gastrointestinal bacteria are also responsible for metabolizing approximately 5 percent of the dose before it is ever absorbed. Bioavailability of oral MTX ranges from as low as 12 percent at doses exceeding 40 mg/m² to almost 90 percent at doses less than one quarter of that, but high MTX doses used in cancer treatment typically range from 1 to 12 g/m², which necessitate intravenous infusion (Figure 24-2).

MTX has also been demonstrated to be a substrate for a number of efflux and chemo-resistant transporters from the ATP-binding cassette (ABC) superfamily of membrane transporters, including multidrug-resistant protein 2 (MRP2)[29] and breast cancer resistance protein (BCRP).[30,31] These transporters play a major role in the distribution of MTX throughout the body. While biliary clearance is only a minor route of elimination, responsible for less that 10 percent of MTX clearance, MRP2 is expressed in a number of tissues and tumors.[32-35] Overexpression and overactive alleles of efflux transporters, such as the BCRP encoded by a single nucleotide polymorphism C >T (rs717620) in the 5' untranslated region, result in approximately a 30 percent increase in clearance and 40 percent increase in volume of distribution.[31] Even though these alleles are associated with preventing delayed elimination, the main risk factor for toxicity, they are also associated with decreased exposure, the main risk factor for relapse and death.

Regardless of transporter variation, the predominant route of elimination for MTX is glomerular filtration with approximately 90 percent of the dose being eliminated unchanged in the urine.[36] The predominance of renal excretion raises real concerns regarding nephrotoxicity. Due to the relatively high pKa of MTX and its metabolite 7-hydroxy MTX, it may become protonated in low-pH urine, which can result in precipitation and kidney injury. For this reason, urine alkalization is mandatory prior to MTX infusion. Genetic polymorphisms in transporters are also associated with delayed elimination by the kidney. The most profound is a common functional C667T substitution in methylenetetrahydrofolate reductase. This polymorphism does not directly affect secretion by the kidney; it is rather an upstream target of MTX therapy. It is nonetheless associated with a 50 percent increase in half-life, a threefold increase in AUC, and a fourfold decrease in glomerular filtration rate.[37]

The most employed tool to prevent toxicity and prevent underdosing is now utilization of therapeutic drug monitoring algorithms that have been developed using pharmacokinetic-based Bayesian estimation. For years, associations between pharmacokinetics and both disease response and toxicity have been studied with some conflicting results. Reports dating back to 2004 suggest that pharmacokinetic parameters such as AUC and C_{max} are useful for predicting outcomes, as well as toxic side effects such as mucositis.[38-41] Other reports indicate that pharmacokinetic monitoring was of little benefit for predicting outcomes or toxicity.[42] What is important to recognize is that the study by Martelli and colleagues, who found little benefit, used a maximum dose of 4.5 g/m² over 24 hours, while the studies by others had maximum doses of 8–12 g/m² over the same time frame. The effect is that the AUCs achieved in the study by Martelli did not reach the threshold set by previous studies to detect the improved outcomes. The threshold suggested by Aquerreta and colleagues is an AUC of 4,000 mmol·hr/L, while Martelli had a mean AUC of 1,810 mmol·hr/L with a range of 622–4,964 mmol·hr/L. At the opposite end, other studies that also have difficulty discriminating benefit in survival use a default dosing of 12 g/m² that only observes AUCs between 10,000 and 16,000 mmol·hr/L.[43]

Regardless, when taken together, all the studies share similar survival AUC relationships. Despite the studies not finding significant differences in survival based on the quartiles or median splits they observed, the Kaplan-Meier survival curves for the AUCs observed are comparable to those of the relevant quartile observed by those that found a difference. That is to say, regardless of the study, an AUC of 4,000 mmol·hr/L has comparable survival to another AUC of 4,000 mmol·hr/L. This finding builds a strong rationale for pharmacokinetic dosing of MTX.

MTX concentrations are well described by a two-compartment mammillary model with an alpha and beta phase of elimination. The alpha phase is typically short and thus most sampling schemes miss it entirely because dosing algorithms are based on pharmacokinetic parameters at 24 and 48 hours postinfusion. As a result, little is reported about the alpha phase except that the half-life during this elimination phase is approximately 3.5 hours in patients with normal elimination as compared to the terminal half-life seen during the beta phase of approximately 12.5 hours. The main driver

of the half-life is clearance, commonly measured during the beta phase to be between 8 and 11 L/hr,[41,44-46] and predicted by Equation 1 where Cl_{MTX} is the clearance of MTX, Cl_{Cr} is the creatinine clearance in mL/min as calculated by the Cockroft-Gault method with a maximum value of 140 mL/min, and BSA is body surface area in m² as calculated by the DuBois and DuBois method.[47]

$$\text{Equation 1: } Cl_{MTX} = 10.8 \frac{l}{hr} \times \left[\frac{Cl_{cr}}{95 \frac{mL}{min}} \right]^{0.28} \times \left[\frac{BSA}{1.75 m^2} \right]^{0.15}$$

When dosing MTX, however, it is impractical to routinely monitor blood levels as one would in a pharmacokinetic study and, therefore, the implementation of sparse sampling at either 24 hours or 48 hours is used to assess whether a patient is having delayed elimination. In such cases, the dose can be adjusted for future administrations but leucovorin rescue must be initiated to offset the MTX toxicity that is likely to be experienced in cases of delayed elimination. Table 24-2 summarizes the published studies regarding delayed elimination of MTX and dose or leucovorin rescue adjustment.

Only Pauley and colleagues present a method used for dose optimization based on a target steady-state concentration (C_{pSS}) during infusion. This method increased the number of patients within the desired range by approximately 17 percent. Such a method requires gathering pharmacokinetic data at multiple time points, at least three or four, during a previous round of MTX therapy to fit using a two-compartment mammillary infusion model that can then be used to target a dose for a particular C_{pSS} range. The proposed sampling strategy included a level drawn just prior to infusion, at 6 hours, at 23 hours, and at 42 hours. The draw at 23 hours was just prior to the end of the 24-hour infusion, and likely to be considered a confirmation of the calculated C_{pSS}. Using the pharmacokinetic information gathered during the previous MTX administration and model fitting, specifically BSA normalized clearance, one can target the next dose using Equation 2.

TABLE 24-2 Summary of MTX PK-based dosing recommendations

Author	Dose (g/m²)	Infusion Duration (hr)	AUC Range (μmol·hr/L)	C₂₄ (μmol/L)	C₄₈ (μmol/L)	Recommendation
Joerger, M. et al.	0.5 then 3	0.25 then 3	486–1,710	5	N/A	C₂₄ 5–7, −5% of dose; C₂₄ 7–9, −15% of dose; C₂₄ 9–12, −25% of dose; C₂₄ >12, −35% of dose
Comandone, A. et al.	12	4	3,477.1–12,681.2	N/A	N/A	Default leucovorin rescue 8 mg/m² q6h for 3 days beginning 24 hr after MTX initiated, do not consider dose reduction, rather prolong posthydration to 48 hr or more.
Monjanel-Mouterde, S. et al.	1.5	4	290.5–1,177.3	0.2	0.2	Default leucovorin rescue 25 mg q6h for 24 hr starting 18 hr after MTX initiated. If MTX concentration is >0.2 at 36 hr, increase rescue duration to 36 hr, and if still >0.2 at 48 hr, extend leucovorin rescue duration to 48 hr or until methorexate is <0.2, whichever is longer.
Pauley, J. et al.	2.5 or 5	24 or 24	Not reported		1ᵃ	Default leucovorin rescue 10 mg/m² or 15 mg/m² q6h × 5 for 2.5 or 5 g/m² MTX, respectively, starting 42 hr after MTX initiated. If MTX >1 at 42 hr, continue leucovorin until MTX <0.1. If side effects develop (↑ serum creatinine, mucositis, pleural effusion/ascites), continue until methotrexate undetectable (<0.03).
Piard, C. et al.	5	24	Not reported	0.2	0.2	Default leucovorin rescue 12 mg/m² q6h until MTX <0.2 or at least 3 doses, whichever is greater, started 36 hr after MTX initiated.

C₂₄ is the MTX concentration at 24 hr and C₄₈ is the MTX concentration at 48 hr.
ᵃRecorded at 42 hr not 48 hr.

Equation 2: Targeted dose $\frac{mg}{m^2}$

$$= \frac{\text{Infusion length (hr)} \cdot \text{Predicted clearance} \left(\frac{L}{hr \cdot m^2}\right) \cdot C_{pSS}\left(\frac{\mu mol}{L}\right)}{\left[2.2 \cdot \left(1 - \text{Fraction loading dose}\right)\right]}$$

Where the infusion length is the total infusion time in hours minus the infusion time of the loading dose in hours, the fraction loading dose is given by Equation 3, and predicted clearance is given by either the previously measured value or Equation 4 if targeting a C_{pSS} >33 μM with a previously measured clearance <7.5 L/hr·m².

Equation 3: $\frac{\text{Amount of loading dose}}{\text{Amount of total dose}}$

Equation 4: $10^{4.349 + 0.1152 \cdot \text{Log(Previous Clearance)} - 0.3422 \cdot SrCr - 0.239 \cdot \text{Bilirubin} - 0.000582 \cdot SGPT}$

where the previous clearance and the predicted clearance are both BSA normalized, SrCr is the serum creatinine in units of mg/dL, bilirubin is in units of mmol/L, and SGPT is the serum glutamic pyruvic transaminase in units of units/L.

It is important to note the units of the target dose are mg/m² not g/m² and so represent one place where a dosing error could be made because MTX is typically dosed as g/m² not mg/m². Furthermore, the drug concentration in the central compartment of a two-compartment infusion model, while the infusion is running, is described by Equation 5, where Q is the infusion rate, α and β are the initial phase and the terminal phase residual slopes, respectively, and k_{21} is the first-order exchange rate constant between the peripheral compartment and the central compartment.

Equation 5: $\frac{Q}{V_1(\alpha - \beta)}\left[\frac{\left(k_{21} - \beta\right)\left(1 - e^{-\beta t}\right)}{\beta} - \frac{\left(k_{21} - \alpha\right)\left(1 - e^{-\alpha t}\right)}{\alpha}\right]$

If we set the time equal to infinity, Equation 5 reduces to Equation 6.

Equation 6: $\frac{Q \cdot k_{21}}{V_1 \cdot \alpha \cdot \beta}$

Because the elimination rate constant, k_e, is equal to $(\alpha \times \beta)/k_{21}$ and with the assumption that the concentration at time infinity is steady state, if the assumption that the MTX concentration at 23 hours is also steady state holds, then by substitution we obtain Equation 7.

Equation 7: $\text{Clearance} = \frac{\text{Infusion rate}}{C_{23 hr}}$

The equation allows an estimation of the previous clearance knowing only one steady-state MTX concentration and the infusion rate for use in the dose adjustment calculated by Equation 2. Pauley and colleagues point out that if the calculated target dose is more than a 50 percent increase or decrease, then the dose change should be limited to no more than 50 percent. Important to note is that Equation 7 assumes linear elimination kinetics, which may not necessarily be true. Tubular reabsorption is saturable at doses as low as 7.5 mg. Also the metabolism to 7-hydroxy-MTX and subsequent biliary excretion are also saturable, but the doses employed in the oncology setting exceed 7.5 mg by about 100- to 3,000-fold and biliary excretion is responsible for less than 10 percent of the total clearance, so it seems likely that any error introduced by Equation 7 would be negligible.[48,49] Nonlinearity can also be introduced by

saturable protein binding, and MTX is known to be albumin bound. However, Lee and colleagues demonstrated that in analbuminemic rats, MTX had the same fraction bound to plasma proteins because the lack of albumin binding was able to be compensated by β-plus and γ-globulins. Furthermore, plasma protein binding has been demonstrated to be linear for MTX at concentrations ranging from 100 pM to 1 mM, ranges that could be expected to be observed in MTX treatment, with 1 mM being about five- to tenfold higher than a C_{pSS} targeted by a 24-hour infusion.[50]

CASE 3

A 17-year-old male, junior basketball player, presents with worsening right leg pain after a physically challenging game. The leg is now swelling, and he reports no falls. Consistent with the young man's report, X-ray shows no fracture, but a destructive lesion raises the suspicion of a potential malignancy. Magnetic resonance imaging and needle biopsy further confirmed the diagnosis of nonmetastatic osteosarcoma in his proximal right tibia. He is started on four cycles of high-dose methotrexate (HDMTX) with leucovorin rescue and two cycles of cisplatin and daunorubicin, which he tolerates well. Each HDMTX involved 20 g MTX over 4 hours. Patient experienced delayed clearance initially, but clearance improved after the following three cycles. The tumor has been subsequently resected and he underwent an allograft placement. His postsurgery serum creatinine has been 0.8 mg/dL, thus chemotherapy was resumed postsurgery with two additional cycles of HDMTX. After the sixth cycle, patient developed acute nephrotoxicity; serum creatinine at the end of the cycle reaching 5.9 mg/dL. Plasma MTX concentration were 1,500 umol/L at 24 hours postinfusion, 510 umol/L at 48 hours, and 270 umol/L at 72 hours. Patient was treated with aggressive hydration, diuresis, and 1,500 mg leucovorin intravenously every 6 hours since the last MTX dose.

QUESTION 1

Assuming the renal function remains unchanged, when are the MTX levels expected to drop below 0.1 umol/L?

Answer:

Because MTX follows two-compartment kinetics and these concentrations are log linear, we can calculate the terminal half-life as ln(2)/β where β is the terminal residual slope. The actual concentrations are plotted in Figure 24-3.

$$\beta = [\ln (C1) - \ln (C2)] /(t_2 - t_1)$$
$$= [\ln (510) - \ln (270)]/(72 \text{ hr} - 48 \text{ hr})$$
$$= 0.636/24 \text{ hr}$$

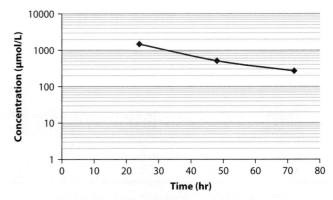

FIGURE 24-3. Terminal (β Phase) Plasma MTX Concentrations vs. Time

So:

$$\beta = 0.027 \text{ h}^{-1}, \text{ therefore the half-life is:}$$
$$T_{1/2} = \text{Ln}(2)/0.027\text{h}^{-1}$$
$$= 0.693/0.027$$

The terminal half-life of MTX in this patient is 25 hours and 40 minutes.

We will next target to learn how many half-lives are necessary to reach 0.1 μmol/L.

Because the fraction remaining at N half-lives is given by the equation

$$1/2^n$$

which should be equal with the fraction 0.1 μmol/L/270 μmol/L, where 270 is the last observed MTX level.

$$0.1/270 = 1/2^n$$
$$2^n = 2,700$$
$$n = \log_2 (2,700)$$
$$n = 11.4$$

Therefore, it will take 11.4 half-lives to reach 0.1 μmol/L or

$$11.4 \times 25.666 \text{ hr}$$
$$= 292 \text{ hr}, 36 \text{ min}$$

or approximately 12 days, 4 hours, and 36 minutes.

PEMETREXED

Pemetrexed (PMTX) is a novel antifolate used in the treatment of mesothelioma and non-small lung cancer. Like MTX, PMTX is an antimetabolite drug that inhibits dihydrofolate reductase, thymidylate synthase, and glycinamide ribonucleotide formyltransferase. It is predominantly cleared via renal filtration with 70 percent to 90 percent of the dose being excreted unchanged in the urine within 24 hours,[51] and as a result, drug-drug interactions that can affect PMTX elimination need to be avoided in patients with impaired renal function. PMTX, however, has a higher affinity than methotrexate for folypoly-γ-glutamate synthase, which results in prolonged intracellular exposure to PMTX polyglutamates. PMTX also follows a two-compartment model, though many use a three-compartment model, and has a terminal half-life of 1–4 hours with a BSA normalized clearance of 2.3 L/hr·m². [52-54] However, because of the toxicities observed during the phase I clinical trials, PMTX is dosed at 500 mg/m² and modified based on toxicities observed in the patient as defined in Table 24-3.

With regard to renal impairment, no adjustment is necessary if the patient's creatinine clearance, as calculated by the Cockcroft and Gault method, is >45 mL/min. However, PMTX is not recommended in patients with a creatinine clearance less than 45 mL/min, and caution should be used in concomitant medication with drugs that may decrease PMTX clearance when the patient's creatinine clearance is below 80 mL/min.

5-FLUOROURACIL

Despite the successful addition of targeted therapy, alone or in combination 5-fluorouracil (5-FU) remains the cornerstone drug of colorectal cancer treatment for the past five decades and is prescribed as a first-line therapy in nearly all patients.[56,57] The

TABLE 24-3 PMTX dose modification based on empiric treatment[55]

Worst Toxicity Observed in Previous Cycle	Modified PMTX Dose (% of Previous Dose) or Recommended Action
Grade 4 neutropenia (ANC <500/mm³)	75%
≥Grade 3 thrombocytopenia	75%
≥Grade 3 diarrhea or any diarrhea requiring hospitalization	75%
Other Grade 3 organ/nonhematologic toxicity	75%
Any thrombocytopenic bleeding (platelets <50,000/mm³)	50%
Grade 3 or 4 mucositis	50%
≥Grade 3 neurotoxicity	Discontinue
≥Grade 3 toxicity after two prior dose reductions	Discontinue
Any occurrence of Stevens-Johnson syndrome or toxic epidermal necrolysis	Discontinue
Other Grade 4 organ/nonhematologic toxicity	Discontinue
Symptoms suggesting pneumonitis	Hold and investigate, discontinue if confirmed

years following the introduction of the biological therapies in colorectal cancer show new patterns of chemotherapy utilization. 5-FU-oxaliplatin regimens' utilization as first-line therapy in metastatic colorectal cancer (mCRC) patients rose from 55 percent in 2004 to more than 70 percent in 2007 and remained steady until 2011, the time of the most recent review.[58]

Similarly to other chemotherapies, 5-FU has a narrow therapeutic window, its effectiveness is influenced by a significant interindividual variability in exposure and clearance. The most closely associated PK parameter with tumor kill effect is total drug exposure or AUC.[59,60] For this reason, continuous infusion is preferred to the bolus administration because only one sample needs to be collected, usually at steady state (>2 hr into the infusion). The calculation of the AUC, under the assumptions of the well-stirred model, requires the steady-state concentration (C_{SS}) and the time of continuous infusion (T_{CI}), in hours:

$$\text{AUC} = C_{SS} \times T_{CI}$$

Target AUC may vary based on the type of tumor treated and required 5-FU distribution. However, neutropenia, diarrhea, mucositis, and hand-foot syndrome are adverse events associated with an AUC >30 mg*h/L in most solid tumors treated with 5-FU. AUC is well correlated with response rate and stable disease in patients administered continuous infusion,[61] but also with disease-free survival in individuals receiving bolus 5-FU+Leucovorin as adjuvant in early-stage colon cancer.[62]

Although age does not affect 5-FU PK,[63] its interindividual variation is the result of several pharmacogenetic variants leading to differences in absorption, distribution, metabolism, and clearance. Up to 100-fold interindividual PK variability has been reported in patients treated with 5-FU and identified as mainly due to the BSA-based dosing, which remains the main cause of poor outcomes.[64] Two separate studies found a complete lack of association between BSA and 5-FU clearance.[65,66] Thus, with less than one third of the treated patients achieving optimal drug levels and nearly half being in fact underdosed,[67] routine monitoring has been repeatedly recommended since the beginning of the previous decade. More recently, Capitain and colleagues provided one of the most reliable evidences to date, showing that PK-guided 5-FU therapy offers significant clinical advantage in mCRC.[65,68] Safety and efficacy of PK-guided 5-FU dosing was compared to the standard BSA-based dose adjustment in 118 patients with mCRC receiving FOLFOX (folinic acid, fluorouracil, and oxaliplatin) regimen. Distribution of grade 3 and 4 adverse events among the two study groups favored considerably the PK-guided dosing method. PK-adjusted 5-FU allowed dose intensification and demonstrated improved efficacy and toxicity as well as 9-to-20-fold fewer adverse events, such as diarrhea and mucositis.[66,69] The Capitain study also indicated that PK-adjusted 5-FU therapy can result in lower cost when compared to the cost of targeted therapies. A PK-optimized 5-FU exposure remains constant regardless of the administration mode, schedule, or combination with other therapeutic agents.

Despite already having a clinically proven 5-FU target level and dose adjustment algorithms to bring plasma concentrations into the desired range, the analytical methods remain time-consuming and costly, requiring extensive sample preparation and full-time technicians—all of which have delayed significantly the widespread adoption of a PK-based dosing approach in 5-FU treatment. Semiquantitative cell-based assays used initially for the assessment of 5-FU PK were replaced by gas and then high-pressure liquid chromatography, which remained the most common used method of drug level determination until recently. At present, a new 5-FU immunoassay by Saladax Biomedical, Inc., was proven to provide rapid and equally reliable results, as well as being easy to integrate into daily clinical practice.[69-71] While requiring only 10 uL of plasma, this immunoassay involves extremely selective monoclonal antibodies shown to have <1 percent cross-reactivity for 5-FU's main metabolite, dihydro-5-FU and <0.05 percent for capecitabine.

The current 5-FU dose adjustment approach established by Gamelin and colleagues from the French cancer facility, Centre Paul Papin, indicate that a BSA-based dose be administered during the first treatment cycle, followed by PK-guided dose adjustments to maintain an AUC 20–25 mg*h/L, regardless of the mode of administration, for all the subsequent treatment cycles. This dosing method has been applied thus far to roughly 5,000 patients every year following the treatment algorithm presented in Table 24-4[72]:

Using this dose adjustment algorithm, target AUC has been achieved after four cycles and the mean dose leading to target AUC was 1,790 mg/m^2/wk, and ranged from 765 mg/m^2 to 3,300 mg/m^2.[72] Without PK monitoring and dose optimization, only 4 of 49 individuals receiving BSA-based therapy had an AUC within the target range, reinforcing the need for optimized dosing in patients treated with 5-FU.

5-FU DOSE ADJUSTMENT IN PATIENTS WITH DIHYDROPYRIMIDINE DEHYDROGENASE DEFICIENCY

Dihydropyrimidine dehydrogenase (DPD) is the rate-limiting enzyme responsible for 5-FU conversion to dihydrofluorouracil, its inactive metabolite. Approximately 80 percent of the total administered 5-FU dose is DPD-inactivated. This enzyme is ubiquitous in various tissue across the human body, and its activity presents a great variability due to genetic polymorphism.[73] Although observed in less than 3 percent of the population, marked deficiencies may lead to polyvisceral toxicity and are frequently lethal.[74] Complete DPD deficiency is an autosomal-transmitted disease, also known as "syndrome of familial pyrimidinuria or uraciluria." The disease is usually asymptomatic, although neurologic abnormalities have been reported. The clinical value of DPD activity has not been appreciated until the findings reported by Lu and others when 21 and 4 out 360 patients with breast cancer were identified to have low and profoundly decreased DPD activity, respectively, which is suggestive of DPD deficiency.[75] With regard to 5-FU toxicity potentially due to DPD deficiency, today we know that half of patients experiencing 5-FU toxicity have no documented alterations in the DPD gene. Thus, other factors also contribute to 5-FU metabolism and toxicity. Currently, no approved DPD activity measurement test is available in the United States. The question of whether a test dose of 5-FU should be administered before or instead of the BSA-based dose during the first cycle of treatment has not been evaluated to date. By using the Gamelin dosing algorithm, it is likely that abnormally high steady-state concentrations acquired in DPD-deficient cases would be immediately detected upon measurement of the first plasma level, and subsequent reductions, including holding a dose, would be reasonable approaches for clinical management.

5-FU DOSE ADJUSTMENT IN PATIENTS WITH IMPAIRED RENAL AND LIVER FUNCTION

Three cohorts of patients with various degrees of organ dysfunction (SCr 1.5–3 mg/dL, SBili 1.5–5 mg/dL, SBili >5 mg/dL) were studied for 5-FU PK associated with the administration of a 24-hour continuous infusion.[76] All patients could be safely treated without any dose adjustment.

TABLE 24-4	Major adverse effects of NMBA			
	In the Absence of Toxicity		**In the Presence of Toxicity (WHO grade scale)**	
5-FU Plasma Concentration (µg/L)	AUC (mg·h·L^{-1})	5-FU Dose Adjustment (± % of previous dose)		
<500	<4	+70	Grade 2 toxicity:	
500–1,000	4 to <8	+50	Dose decreased by 200 mg	
1,000–1,200	8 to <10	+40		
1,200–1,500	10 to <12	+30	Grade 3 toxicity:	
1,500–1,800	12 to <15	+20	Hold dose for 1 week, then dose decreased by 300 mg	
1,800–2,200	15 to <18	+10		
2,200–2,500	18 to <20	+5		
2,500–3,000	20 to <24	Unchanged		
3,000–3,500	24 to <28	−5		
3,500–3,700	28 to <31	−10		
>3,700	>31	−15		

CASE 4

A 61-year-old woman was recently diagnosed with a stage 2 locally advanced adenocarcinoma of the rectum (T3N0M0). Total resection of the rectum has been followed by adjuvant 5-FU treatment (500 mg/m²) on days 1 through 5 of weeks 1, 2, 5, 20, and 25. The first two days of chemotherapy were well tolerated, but soon after her third dose she developed a cold tingling sensation between the toes and her gait became unsteady. Neuro exam reported impaired toe and heel walk and absent jerk reflexes, all consistent with a grade 3 toxicity to 5-FU. Her labs show normal DPD activity, thus a 5-FU level has been ordered for evaluation of her drug exposure. It is now day 4 of treatment postsurgery, and the laboratory informs the team that 5-FU level will be available in 3 days. On day 7, the reported 5-FU level is 4,900 ug/L. A new 5-FU blood level obtained on day 14 is reported by the lab as 2,850 ug/L.

Height = 172 cm

Weight = 109 kg

QUESTION 1

What is the appropriate clinical action for 5-FU management on days 4 and 12?

Answer:

Given the grade 3 toxicity confirmed by neurologist and associated with initiation of 5-FU treatment, further drug administration will be on hold for 1 week. Before reinitiation, a new 5-FU level should be drawn.

$$BSA(Dubois) = 0.007184 \times (172)^{0.725} \times (109)^{0.425}$$
$$= 2.20 \text{ m}^2$$

Because BSA >2 m², the 5-FU dose calculation should have been capped at 2×500 mg/m² = 1,000 mg for a BSA of 2 m². Exact dosing for 2.2 m² (2.2×500 mg = 1,100 mg) could have likely led to toxic 5-FU levels.

5-FU therapy will be reinitiated at a lower dose calculated as follows:

$$2 \text{ m}^2 \times 500 \text{ mg} = 1,000 \text{ mg}$$
$$\underline{- \ 300 \text{ mg}}$$
$$700 \text{ mg}$$

A total dose of 700 mg will be reinitiated a week later, after collection of a new drug level.

QUESTION 2

What 5-FU dose should be administered on day 1 of week 5? Why?

Answer:

The level reported for day 14 denotes that therapeutic range has been achieved on the new 5-FU dose (700 mg) and treatment should continue unchanged. Patient should continue to be monitored closely for any adverse events.

CYTARABINE

Cytosine arabinoside (Ara-C) is a structural analogue of deoxycytidine, one of the several nucleosides isolated from the marine sponge *Cryptothethya crypta*,[77] its name being given by the arabinose sugar

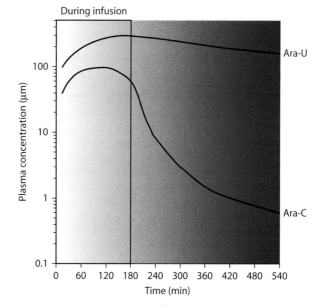

FIGURE 24-4. Simulation of plasma Ara-C and Ara-U concentrations during and after a theoretical 3-hour infusion of 3g/m2 Ara-C administered every 12 hours for 4 doses.

substituted for ribose. The drug was first synthesized in 1959 with the addition of a trans-hydroxyl group in the 2' position,[78] a change made with the intent of targeting subsequent metabolism to a deoxyribose-like sugar.[79] Ara-C cancer cell penetration is a carrier-mediated process[80] upon which the drug undergoes intracellular phosphorylation to cytarabine 5'-triphosphate (CTP), a molecule responsible for inhibition of DNA synthesis and, ultimately, the cell-kill effect. Ara-C plasma levels of 8–10 μmol/L were reported to lead to CTP-saturated cancer cells, an aspect essential for treatment effectiveness.[81] As an S-phase-specific drug, Ara-C's therapeutic effect is dependent on prolonged exposure at a toxic level, a level whose achievement is particularly challenging due to the drug's rapid detoxification to uracil arabinoside, the so called metabolite Ara-U (Figure 24-4).

Ara-C has little to no retention in tissue or blood and is quickly metabolized to a deaminated inactive compound, Ara-U. The antitumor effect of Ara-C is well documented as correlated with increased half-life and, thereby, greater exposure. For this reason standard, 100–200 mg/m², or high, 1–3 g/m², Ara-C doses have to be administered over 2- to 4-hour infusions and repeated every 12 hours to ensure the necessary exposure for a therapeutic effect.[83-85] Capizzi and colleagues have suggested that Ara-U buildup becomes a mechanism of self-potentiation, Ara-U accumulation leading to inhibition of its parent compound's catabolism.[82,85] Apparently, Ara-U is also responsible for the "arrest" of cancer cells in S-phase, thus increasing the activity of the Ara-C kinase to the extent of CTP-level saturation within the cancer cell, and further enhanced tumor kill.[86] Some have suggested that accumulation of circulating Ara-U may also circumvent the occurrence of Ara-C resistance.[82]

One of the unique features of Ara-C toxicity is neurotoxicity, an adverse event reported in up to 40 percent of patients receiving high-dose Ara-C (HiDAC), >2 g/m². Most commonly, neurotoxicity presents as peripheral neuropathy, but cerebellar toxicity, such as dysarthria with truncal and gait ataxia, or more aggravated cerebellar syndrome, such as encephalopathy, psychosis, seizures, and coma, have been reported as well.[87] Median time of neurotoxicity onset was reported to be 5 days (range, 1–10 days) and, although reversible in

TABLE 24-5 Ara-C Dosing Based on Serum Creatinine

Serum Creatinine	ΔCr	Ara-C Dose
<1.49 mg/dL		2 or 3 g/m^2 (per protocol)
1.5–1.99 mg/dL	0.5–1.2 mg/dL	1 g/m^2 per dose
≥2.0 mg/dL	≥1.2 mg/dL	0.1 g/m^2 per dose

most of the cases, fatal instances have been reported in a number of clinical trials.[88-90] Risk factors associated with neurotoxicity post-HiDAC treatment were male gender, age over 50 years, prior or concurrent CNS leukemia, other unrelated CNS disorder or therapy, and renal insufficiency.[87,90] Renal insufficiency, defined as pretreatment creatinine clearance <60 mL/min. All significantly increased the risk for development of neurotoxicity.[87,91] Damon and others indicated that two of the patients who developed neurotoxicity during renal insufficiency subsequently went on receiving HiDAC during periods of normal renal function without recurrence of neurotoxicity. In his study, Damon found that 100 percent of patients with CrCl <20 mL/min who were given HiDAC courses developed neurotoxic symptoms. That number decreased to 86 percent in patients with CrCl between 20 to 40 mL/min, and 60 percent in cases with CrCl of 40 to 60 mL/min.[87] Neurotoxicity only occurred in 8 percent of the cases with pretreatment CrCl >60 mL/min.

Roughly two decades ago, Smith and colleagues developed the first therapeutic dose monitoring algorithm for patients with renal insufficiency receiving HiDAC.[91] Renal impairment was defined as serum creatinine level of 1.5 mg/dL or greater during the HiDAC administration, or a change in creatinine level of at least 0.5 mg/dL from pretreatment baseline.[91] The HiDAC dose adjustment algorithm proposed in the Smith study is described in Table 24-5.

Lindner and colleagues were among the first suggesting that Ara-U accumulation in patients with impaired renal function may be associated with neurotoxicity occurrence due to elevated Ara-U in CSF.[92] Interestingly, when CSF cytidine deaminase levels are low, Ara-C deamination within the CSF is unlikely to lead to toxic levels. Thus, the plasma Ara-U concentrations above a certain level are able to cross blood-brain-barrier, increasing the risk for neurotoxicity. Based on the drug PK as just described, sustained high Ara-C levels are required to achieve desired cancer therapy outcomes, making high-dose Ara-C practice one of the most common approaches for treatment.

Furthermore, in patients with impaired renal function, Ara-U levels decline slowly, changing from a linear to a nonlinear elimination kinetic, while Ara-C level would appear to remain unchanged.[85] Given its intense utilization in treatment of hematologic malignancies, Ara-C continues to be the target of several efforts to improve its timing and scheduling. Because the cytotoxic effect is correlated with longer Ara-C half-life and delayed deamination, research has been focused on the development of Ara-C formulations protected from deamination and also on trials evaluating co-administration with a potent cytidine deaminase inhibitor, tetrahydruridine (THU).[93] When coadministered with Ara-C doses as low as 100 mg/m^2, THU determined an Ara-C plasma exposure of more than 10 umol/L, a concentration only achieved with high-dose Ara-C. However, a significantly decreased volume of distribution and total clearance were also observed. Protection by liposome encapsulation has been initially unsuccessful, primarily due to liposome instability.[94] However, stability improvement was provided by the encapsulation in polyethylene glycol (PEG) derivatives,[95] which marked the beginning of the Ara-C encapsulation *"lamellar"* liposomes, formulations with cytotoxic effect superior to both free drug and other liposome encapsulations. $T_{1/2\beta}$ of the *lamellar* liposome encapsulated Ara-C (DepoCyt') is more than 100-fold longer than the naked drug. Therefore, administration

of intrathecal doses as low as 50 mg can be scheduled every other week in the treatment of lymphomatous meningitis, a malignant infiltration of the leptomeninges (DepoCyt package insert).

CASE 5: (MODIFIED AFTER A CASE REPORT BY RADESKI ET AL.[96])

The patient is a 48-year-old woman with relapsed stage IV-A mantle cell lymphoma and a background of dialysis-dependent end-stage renal disease (ESRD). She was diagnosed 2.5 years ago with lymphoma and treated with six cycles of a modified R-CHOP (rituximab, cyclophosphamide, doxorubicin, vincristine, and prednisone). Complete remission was achieved with clearance of lymphoma cells from blood and bone marrow and resolution of lymphadenopathy. Now she presents with progressive splenomegaly and presence of lymphoma cells in blood and bone marrow, consistent with relapsed mantle cell lymphoma. She is started on Ara-C 1 g/m^2, with patient's body surface area capped at 2 m^2 due to obesity.

Height = 1.66 m

Weight = 111 kg

Following three cycles of single-agent Ara-C, a partial response was achieved with a reduction in splenic size and fewer peripheral circulating lymphoma cells. No neurotoxicity or unexpected adverse events occurred with Ara-C treatment. Given the partial response, treatment with Ara-C and carboplatin has been initiated with a view to a future autologous stem cell transplant.

Ara-C was administered as a 2-hour intravenous infusion and repeated 24 hours later. Five 4-hour dialysis sessions were carried out beginning 3.5 and 2 hours after the end of infusion to ensure removal of Ara-U only. Ara-C disposition was best represented by a two-compartment model and the following information was recorded: Ara-C distribution $t_{1/2}$ = 0.05 h, elimination $t_{1/2}$ = 0.7 h, $AUC_{0-\infty}$ = 6.52 mg*h/L, V_{SS} = 181 L, and Cl = 307 L/hr. For Ara-U, distribution $t_{1/2}$ = 4.1 h, elimination $t_{1/2}$ = 34 h, $AUC_{0-\infty}$ = 757 mg*h/L, V_{SS} = 118 L, and Cl = 2.6 L/hr.

QUESTION 1

Given her ESRD, was this patient a candidate for 0.1 g/m^2 standard Ara-C dose?

Answer:

Due to her ongoing relapse, the standard Ara-C dose will not be a viable option. Additionally, because the patient is dialysis-dependent and the main metabolite of concern, Ara-U, is removable by dialysis, HiDAC is warranted. Moreover, her partial response to HiDAC indicates that a HiDAC-combined regimen (e.g., carboplatin combination) will be the treatment of choice for continuation of her chemo regimen.

QUESTION 2

Knowing that Ara-C molecular weight is 243, find out if the Ara-C dose administered provided sufficient toxic exposure to ensure appropriate tumor kill in this patient.

Answer:

Because Ara-C fits a two-compartment model, we can assume that the relationship CSS = Dose rate/Cl, derived from setting time to infinity in a two-compartment infusion model. We know that her Cl is reported as 307L/h and her dose is 1 g/m2 infused over 2 hours. Using the DuBois and DuBois formula, the patient's BSA is calculated as follows:

$$0.007184 \times (166)^{0.725} \times (111)^{0.425} = 2.16 \text{ m}^2$$

She has a BSA greater than 2 m² and, therefore, her dose would be capped at 2 g

The 2 g dose is infused over 2 hours so the dose rate would be:

$$2 \text{ g/2 hr} = 1 \text{ g/hr or } 1,000 \text{ mg/hr}$$

So her steady-state concentration would be:

$$C_{SS} = (1 \text{ g/hr})/(307 \text{ L/hr})$$
$$= 0.00325 \text{ g/L}$$

This result needs to the be converted to molar concentration:

$$(0.00325 \text{ g/L}) \times (1 \text{ mol/243 g}) = 0.0000134 \text{ mol/L}$$

Finally convert to µmol/L:

$$(0.0000134 \text{ mol/L}) \times (1,000,000 \text{ µmol/1mol}) = 13.4 \text{ µmol/L}$$

But what about time to steady state? The elimination half-life of Ara-C is 0.7 h. So, in 2 hours, almost $2/0.7 = 2.9$ half-lives have elapsed and, therefore, $[100 - (100/2^{2.9})] = -86.6$ percent of C_{SS} has theoretically been achieved. If we round down to 80 percent (0.8) to be conservative we get:

$$0.8 \times (13.4 \text{ µmol/L}) = 10.7 \text{ µmol/L}$$

Because 10.7 µmol/L of Ara-C is greater than the 8–10 µmol/L suggested to provide sufficient toxic exposure, this dose provides enough exposure to cause tumor kill.

CYCLOSPORINE

Officially used as an immunosuppressant to prevent transplant rejection, specifically indicated for allogeneic kidney, liver, and heart transplant,[97] cyclosporine (Cs) does not have a direct indication in oncology. However, despite the lack of a direct indication, Cs is commonly used in hematologic cancer patients undergoing bone marrow or hematopoietic stem cell transplant to prevent graft-versus-host disease.

Cs (known as cyclosporin or ciclosporin) has two forms, cyclosporine and cyclosporine modified. The unmodified form is often called cyclosporine A (or cyclosporin A or ciclosporin A), whereas the modified form simply has "modified" replacing the "A." Confusion regarding the appropriate name began well before it made it to market. CsA, the most commonly used agent and the one that will be discussed in this chapter, simply called Cs henceforth, was originally isolated from the fungus *Tolypocladium inflatum*.[98] However, when it was first isolated from Norwegian soil samples in 1969 by Dr. Hans Peter Frey, *Tolypocladium inflatum* was incorrectly identified as *Trichoderma polysporum*. In 1971, Gams showed that the fungus actually belonged to a new genus and thus renamed it *Tolypocladium inflatum*, the name officially used today, despite it being shown in 1983 that it was actually the same fungus known as *Pachybasium niveum*.[99,100] Under the International Code of Botanical Nomenclature, then, Bissett correctly proposed the new name *Tolypocladium niveum*. This name was never adopted because the immunosuppressive properties of Cs had been discovered in 1972 and by 1983, the year Cs was approved, the consensus was that the Cs-producing fungus was of such commercial value that any naming confusion could be disastrous. Nonetheless, the names used for this fungus today include *Tolypocladium*

inflatum, *Tolypocladium inflatum* Gams, *Hypocladium inflatum gams,* and *Beauveria nivea. Beauveria nivea* arose when von Arx combined the genera *Tolypocladium* and *Beauveria* in 1986. *Beauveria* had seniority in naming due to its greater duration of use, as did *niveum* compared to *inflatum,* yielding *Beauveria nivea.*[101] Nonetheless, sufficient recent evidence suggests that *Tolypocladium* and *Beauveria* are in fact separate genera, and American Type Culture Collection has again begun indexing the Cs-producing fungus as *Tolypocladium inflatum* Gams instead of *Beauveria nivea.*

Cs is a large undecapeptide that is neutral and lipophilic at physiologic pH. As a result it is usually given either via intravenous infusion or as an oral suspension in olive oil formulated as either a gelatin capsule or as a bottled liquid. It exerts its immunosuppressive effect primarily by inhibition the calcineurin pathway through Cs binding to cyclophilins, specifically cyclophilin A. It is only this complex that then binds calcineurin, the effect being that when T cell receptors are stimulated and the intracellular calcium levels rise, activating calmodulin, calmodulin cannot release the autoinhibitory domain of calcineurin. Under normal conditions, calcineurin would then exhibit phosphatase activity responsible for dephosphorylation of nuclear factor of activated T cell (NFAT) family members, specifically NFAT1, NFAT2, and NFAT4. By preventing the dephosphorylation of NFAT family members, they are unable to translocate to the nucleus and activate transcription of genes encoding the cytokines interleukin-2, interleukin-4, and CD40L. Evidence also suggests it may have some upstream inhibition of the Jun N-terminal kinase and the p38 mitogen-activated protein kinase families that can be overwhelmed in instances of acute inflammatory response via a non-calcineurin-mediated pathway.[102]

The T cell inhibition has the desired effect of preventing the adaptive immune system from effectively developing an immune reaction against either the transplant or the host. The side effects of Cs, however, are typically mediated by other actions. Cs, despite clearance being predominantly hepatic, is nephrotoxic in approximately 30 percent of patients.[97] The mechanism behind nephrotoxicity is likely through its stimulation of transforming growth factor beta that causes fibrogenesis in the kidney medulla and subsequent inability of the renal cells to preferentially accumulate compatible organic solutes, such as sorbitol and inositol, for protection from the hypertonic environment. It ultimately results in tubular atrophy and permanent renal damage.[102,103] The nephrotoxicity is exacerbated by Cs-inducing hypertension, likely via sympathetic stimulation of the subdiaphragmatic vagi and low thoracic spinal roots as well as enhancing calcium ion influx to smooth muscle cells causing vasoconstriction.[104,105] Fibrogenesis can be ameliorated by concomitant magnesium supplementation that, though the mechanism is still unclear, is thought to inhibit chemoattractants involved in macrophage infiltration of the medulla, which is necessary for fibrosis.[106,107]

Due to the complexity of its mechanism of action and the barriers it must cross to reach the appropriate sites, Cs pharmacodynamics are particularly challenging. This complexity makes it difficult to define pharmacokinetic parameters that are of great utility in predicting outcomes, a problem compounded by the fact that Cs is large, lipophilic, binds nonlinearly to plasma proteins, and is nonlinearly absorbed by blood cells and predominantly cleared by hepatic metabolism. Despite these challenges some efforts have been made to model Cs pharmacokinetics. Lindholm and Kahan were among the first to report on a large data set with years of follow-up including pharmacokinetic data. The lack of a specific assay to detect Cs and the discovery that whole blood was required to accurately detect Cs, due to sedimentation, significantly impaired researchers. Their study population included renal transplant patients and found that, despite receiving similar doses, a correlation was found between not only C_{max}, trough concentration, and clearance, but also bioavailability, as they pertained to rejection.[108]

The study by Lindholm and Kahan added to the accumulating evidence that increased exposure decreased the rate of rejection; however, their study did not include information about adverse events. Two years earlier Bacigalupo and colleagues had similar results and reported findings regarding the most significant oncologic adverse event, relapse of hematologic malignancy, but they did not performed any pharmacokinetic analysis. Their findings showed that while high-dose cyclosporine significantly decreased the incidence of GVHD, it also significantly increased the rate of hematologic malignancy relapse. This finding began a search for a method of therapeutic drug monitoring that would help to maintain cyclosporine levels in a therapeutic range. Thus, trough-concentration monitoring came into practice whereby the 24-hour postdose concentration in whole blood is monitored. A variety of research shows that the lower limit for the trough concentration to prevent rejection or GVHD is approximately 200 ng/mL, but little study has been conducted regarding a safe upper limit and, as a result, this lower-limit is considered the target of dose titration.[108-110] However, a study by Machishima et al. targeted a trough concentration of 500 ng/mL. Like the standard protocol, all patients were started on a dose of 3 mg/kg/day and the dose titrated to achieve a trough level between 450 and 550 ng/mL, with the final average dose being 3.6 mg/kg/day as a continuous 24-hour infusion, thus making the trough level a steady-state level. Upon switching to oral therapy, the dose was given every 12 hours and then again titrated to maintain a 24-hour trough level between 450 and 550 ng/mL.

The outcome of maintaining a steady-state level between 450 and 500 ng/mL were that 4-year overall survival and disease-free survival were 70.7 percent and 60.9 percent, respectively.[111] These guidelines are markedly different from giving the standard dose of 3 mg/kg/day and only tailoring therapy by dose reduction, 25 percent reduction when serum creatinine doubles as compared to baseline or a 50 percent reduction when it triples. In the latter protocol investigated by Ratanatharathorn et al., 2-year overall survival and disease-free survival were 57.2 percent and 50.4 percent, respectively.[112] Some differences, however, are worth noting between the two studies. The Machishima study only included standard-risk patients, defined as AML in first or second complete remission, CML in first or second chronic phase, nonleukemic myeloproliferative disorders, and myelodysplastic syndromes. In contrast, the Ratanatharathorn study contained both standard-risk and high-risk patients (those not fitting the description of standard risk). The primary adverse event that was associated with targeting a higher trough level was non-dose-limiting increased liver function tests.

It is likely that in the future cyclosporine dosing will target greater exposure, but the debate regarding how to achieve this goal remains. Most therapeutic drug monitoring schemes utilize the trough concentration to guide treatment. Although it seems like a reasonable approach to estimate overall exposure, the fact that absorption kinetics are highly variable make it a tenuous assumption when it comes to oral delivery. The time to T_{max} has been reported as ranging from <1.8 hours to >6 hours.[108] With such variability in T_{max}, using a trough concentration tells little about the actual exposure because it is dependent on both disposition and elimination kinetics. For this reason, some have proposed that monitoring C_{max} may actually be a better measure of exposure.[113] But until a better method of targeting C_{max} is developed, its use seems unfeasible. Another challenge is in converting the intravenous dose to an oral dose; it is done by simply doubling or tripling the daily intravenous dose, per hospital protocol, and then splitting it into two doses taken 12 hours apart. Some evidence indicates that tripling the dose may better target pediatric patients with shorter

bowels and, therefore, reduced bioavailability.[114] It is recommended that a trough level be drawn 24 hours prior to switching to oral medication and 24 hours after the switch for comparison of trough levels in order to titrate the oral dose as quickly as possible.

CASE 6

A 9-year-old girl diagnosed with refractory AML has recently undergone an allogeneic hematopoietic stem cell transplant with her older sister as a donor after failing induction therapy with daunorubicin and TKIs. The family was consulted and informed of the risks associated with transplant and GVHD. She has been receiving 3.3 mg/kg/day cyclosporine via continuous intravenous infusion for about 5 weeks. Her past three trough concentrations were 233 ng/mL, 198 ng/mL, and 248 ng/mL, and she is ready to switch to oral suspension.

QUESTION 1

What starting dose and monitoring would you recommend?

Answer:

Because she is a pediatric patient with a short bowel and decreased bioavailability the IV dose is multiplied by 3 to get the oral dose:

$$3 \times 3.3 \text{ mg/kg/day} = 9.9 \text{ mg/kg/day}$$

This daily total dose, to achieve a greater exposure and decrease the risk of toxicity from a high C_{max}, should be split and given every 12 hours. Therefore:

$$(0.5 \text{ day}/12 \text{ hr}) \times (9.9 \text{ mg/kg/day}) = 4.95 \text{ mg/kg/12 hr}$$

After starting this dose, the 24-hour trough should be compared to the stable trough concentration achieved during prior infusion and the oral dose titrated accordingly.

REFERENCES

1. Taatjes DJ, Gaudiano G, Resing K, Koch TH. Alkylation of DNA by the anthracycline, antitumor drugs adriamycin and daunomycin. *J Med Chem.* 1996;39(21):4135–4138. Epub 1996/10/11.doi:10.1021/jm960519z. PubMed PMID: 8863788.
2. Taatjes DJ, Gaudiano G, Resing K, Koch TH. Redox pathway leading to the alkylation of DNA by the anthracycline, antitumor drugs adriamycin and daunomycin. *J Med Chem.* 1997;40(8):1276–1286. Epub 1997/04/11.doi:10.1021/jm960835d. PubMed PMID: 9111302.
3. Doroshow JH. Role of hydrogen peroxide and hydroxyl radical formation in the killing of Ehrlich tumor cells by anticancer quinones. *Proc Natl Acad Sci USA.* 1986;83(12):4514–4518. Epub 1986/06/01. PubMed PMID: 3086887; PubMed Central PMCID: PMC323764.
4. Oakes SG, Schlager JJ, Santone KS, Abraham RT, Powis G. Doxorubicin blocks the increase in intracellular Ca++, part of a second messenger system in N1E–115 murine neuroblastoma cells. *J Pharmacol Exp Ther.* 1990;252(3):979–983. Epub 1990/03/01. PubMed PMID: 2319480.
5. Bielack SS, Erttmann R, Kempf-Bielack B, Winkler K. Impact of scheduling on toxicity and clinical efficacy of doxorubicin: What do we know in the mid-nineties? *Eur J Cancer.* 1996;32A(10):1652–1660. Epub 1996/09/01. PubMed PMID: 8983270.
6. Gustafson DL, Rastatter JC, Colombo T, Long ME. Doxorubicin pharmacokinetics: Macromolecule binding, metabolism, and excretion in the context of a physiologic model. *J Pharm Sci.* 2002;91(6):1488–1501. Epub 2002/07/13.doi:10.1002/jps.10161. PubMed PMID: 12115848.
7. Benjamin RS. Pharmacokinetics of adriamycin (NSC-123127) in patients with sarcomas. *Cancer Chemother Rep.* 1974;58(2):271–273. Epub 1974/03/01. PubMed PMID: 4830501.

8. Benjamin RS, Wiernik PH, Bachur NR. Adriamycin chemotherapy—Efficacy, safety, and pharmacologic basis of an intermittent single high-dosage schedule. *Cancer*. 1974;33(1):19–27. Epub 1974/01/01. PubMed PMID: 4810094.

9. Superfin D, Iannucci AA, Davies AM. Commentary: Oncologic drugs in patients with organ dysfunction: A summary. *Oncologist*. 2007;12(9):1070–1083. Epub 2007/10/05.doi:10.1634/theoncologist.12–9–1070. PubMed PMID: 17914077.

10. Brenner DE, Wiernik PH, Wesley M, Bachur NR. Acute doxorubicin toxicity. Relationship to pretreatment liver function, response, and pharmacokinetics in patients with acute nonlymphocytic leukemia. *Cancer*. 1984;53(5):1042–1048. Epub 1984/03/01. PubMed PMID: 6692298.

11. Chan KK, Chlebowski RT, Tong M, Chen HS, Gross JF, Bateman JR. Clinical pharmacokinetics of adriamycin in hepatoma patients with cirrhosis. *Cancer Res*. 1980;40(4):1263–1268. Epub 1980/04/01. PubMed PMID: 6244090.

12. Morris RG, Reece PA, Dale BM, Green RM, Kotasek D, Saccoia NC, et al. Alteration in doxorubicin and doxorubicinol plasma concentrations with repeated courses to patients. *Ther Drug Monit*. 1989;11(4):380–383. Epub 1989/01/01. PubMed PMID: 2741185.

13. Johnson PJ, Dobbs N, Kalayci C, Aldous MC, Harper P, Metivier EM, et al. Clinical efficacy and toxicity of standard dose adriamycin in hyperbilirubinaemic patients with hepatocellular carcinoma: relation to liver tests and pharmacokinetic parameters. *Brit J Cancer*. 1992;65(5):751–755. Epub 1992/05/01. PubMed PMID: 1316777; PubMed Central PMCID: PMC1977380.

14. Piscitelli SC, Rodvold KA, Rushing DA, Tewksbury DA. Pharmacokinetics and pharmacodynamics of doxorubicin in patients with small-cell lung cancer. *Clin Pharmacol Ther*. 1993;53(5):555–561. Epub 1993/05/01. PubMed PMID: 8387903.

15. Launchbury AP, Habboubi N. Epirubicin and doxorubicin: A comparison of their characteristics, therapeutic activity and toxicity. *Cancer Treat Rev*. 1993;19(3):197–228. Epub 1993/07/01. PubMed PMID: 8334677.

16. Shan K, Lincoff AM, Young JB. Anthracycline-induced cardiotoxicity. *Ann Intern Med*. 1996;125(1):47–58. Epub 1996/07/01. PubMed PMID: 8644988.

17. Zalupski M, Metch B, Balcerzak S, Fletcher WS, Chapman R, Bonnet JD, et al. Phase III comparison of doxorubicin and dacarbazine given by bolus versus infusion in patients with soft-tissue sarcomas: A Southwest Oncology Group study. *J Natl Cancer Inst*. 1991;83(13):926–932. Epub 1991/07/03. PubMed PMID: 2067035.

18. Griggs JJ, Mangu PB, Anderson H, Balaban EP, Dignam JJ, Hryniuk WM, et al. Appropriate chemotherapy dosing for obese adult patients with cancer: American Society of Clinical Oncology clinical practice guideline. *J Clin Oncol*. 2012;30(13):1553–1561. Epub 2012/04/05. doi:10.1200/JCO.2011.39.9436. PubMed PMID: 22473167.

19. Harrap KR. Preclinical studies identifying carboplatin as a viable cisplatin alternative. *Cancer Treat Rev*. 1985;12(Suppl A):21–33. Epub 1985/09/01. PubMed PMID: 3910219.

20. Calvert AH, Newell DR, Gumbrell LA, O'Reilly S, Burnell M, Boxall FE, et al. Carboplatin dosage: Prospective evaluation of a simple formula based on renal function. *J Clin Oncology*. 1989;7(11):1748–1756. Epub 1989/11/01. PubMed PMID: 2681557.

21. Taguchi J, Saijo N, Miura K, Shinkai T, Eguchi K, Sasaki Y, et al. Prediction of hematologic toxicity of carboplatin by creatinine clearance rate. *Jpn J Cancer Res*. 1987;78(9):977–982. Epub 1987/09/01. PubMed PMID: 3117753.

22. Calvert AH, Harland SJ, Newell DR, Siddik ZH, Harrap KR. Phase I studies with carboplatin at the Royal Marsden Hospital. *Cancer Treat Rev*. 1985;12(Suppl A):51–57. Epub 1985/09/01. PubMed PMID: 3910222.

23. Panetta JC, Yanishevski Y, Pui CH, Sandlund JT, Rubnitz J, Rivera GK, et al. A mathematical model of in vivo methotrexate accumulation in acute lymphoblastic leukemia. *Cancer Chemother Pharmacol*. 2002;50(5):419–428. Epub 2002/11/20.doi:10.1007/s00280-002-0511-x. PubMed PMID: 12439601.

24. Chabner BA, Roberts TG, Jr. Timeline: Chemotherapy and the war on cancer. *Nat Rev Cancer*. 2005;5(1):65–72. Epub 2005/01/05.doi:nrc1529 [pii] 10.1038/nrc1529. PubMed PMID: 15630416.

25. Longley DB, Harkin DP, Johnston PG. 5-fluorouracil: Mechanisms of action and clinical strategies. *Nat Rev Cancer*. 2003;3(5):330–338. Epub 2003/05/02.doi:10.1038/nrc1074nrc1074 [pii]. PubMed PMID: 12724731.

26. Manieri W, Moore ME, Soellner MB, Tsang P, Caperelli CA. Human glycinamide ribonucleotide transformylase: Active site mutants as mechanistic probes. *Biochemistry*. 2007;46(1):156–163. Epub 2007/01/03. doi:10.1021/bi0619270. PubMed PMID: 17198385; PubMed Central PMCID: PMC2518408.

27. Ozaki Y, King RW, Carey PR. Methotrexate and folate binding to dihydrofolate reductase. Separate characterization of the pteridine and p-aminobenzoyl binding sites by resonance Raman spectroscopy. *Biochemistry*. 1981;20(11):3219–3225. Epub 1981/05/26. PubMed PMID: 7018571.

28. Poe M. Acidic dissociation constants of folic acid, dihydrofolic acid, and methotrexate. *J Biol Chem*. 1977;252(11):3724–3728. Epub 1977/06/10. PubMed PMID: 16913.

29. Masuda M, I'Izuka Y, Yamazaki M, Nishigaki R, Kato Y, Ni'inuma K, et al. Methotrexate is excreted into the bile by canalicular multispecific organic anion transporter in rats. *Cancer Res*. 1997;57(16):3506–3510. Epub 1997/08/15. PubMed PMID: 9270020.

30. Volk EL, Rohde K, Rhee M, McGuire JJ, Doyle LA, Ross DD, et al. Methotrexate cross-resistance in a mitoxantrone-selected multidrug-resistant MCF7 breast cancer cell line is attributable to enhanced energy-dependent drug efflux. *Cancer Res*. 2000;60(13):3514–3521. Epub 2000/07/26. PubMed PMID: 10910063.

31. Simon N, Marsot A, Villard E, Choquet S, Khe HX, Zahr N, et al. Impact of ABCC2 polymorphisms on high-dose methotrexate pharmacokinetics in patients with lymphoid malignancy. *Pharmacogenomics J*. 2013;13(6):507–513. Epub 2012/10/17.doi:10.1038/tpj.2012.37. PubMed PMID: 23069858.

32. Faneyte IF, Kristel PM, van de Vijver MJ. Multidrug resistance associated genes MRP1, MRP2 and MRP3 in primary and anthracycline exposed breast cancer. *Anticancer Res*. 2004;24(5A):2931–2939. Epub 2004/11/03. PubMed PMID: 15517899.

33. Hinoshita E, Uchiumi T, Taguchi K, Kinukawa N, Tsuneyoshi M, Maehara Y, et al. Increased expression of an ATP-binding cassette superfamily transporter, multidrug resistance protein 2, in human colorectal carcinomas. *Clin Cancer Res*. 2000;6(6):2401–2407. Epub 2000/06/29. PubMed PMID: 10873092.

34. Ifergan I, Meller I, Issakov J, Assaraf YG. Reduced folate carrier protein expression in osteosarcoma: implications for the prediction of tumor chemosensitivity. *Cancer*. 2003;98(9):1958–1966. Epub 2003/10/30. doi:10.1002/cncr.11741. PubMed PMID: 14584080.

35. Ohishi Y, Oda Y, Uchiumi T, Kobayashi H, Hirakawa T, Miyamoto S, et al. ATP-binding cassette superfamily transporter gene expression in human primary ovarian carcinoma. *Clin Cancer Res*. 2002;8(12):3767–3775. Epub 2002/12/11. PubMed PMID: 12473588.

36. Murashima M, Adamski J, Milone MC, Shaw L, Tsai DE, Bloom RD. Methotrexate clearance by high-flux hemodialysis and peritoneal dialysis: A case report. *Am J Kidney Dis*. 2009;53(5):871–874. Epub 2009/04/03.doi:10.1053/j.ajkd.2009.01.016. PubMed PMID: 19339090.

37. El-Khodary NM, El-Haggar SM, Eid MA, Ebeid EN. Study of the pharmacokinetic and pharmacogenetic contribution to the toxicity of high-dose methotrexate in children with acute lymphoblastic leukemia. *Med Oncol*. 2012;29(3):2053–2062. Epub 2011/06/07.doi:10.1007/s12032-011-9997-6. PubMed PMID: 21644011.

38. Aquerreta I, Aldaz A, Giraldez J, Sierrasesumaga L. Methotrexate pharmacokinetics and survival in osteosarcoma. *Pediatr Blood Cancer*. 2004;42(1):52–58. Epub 2004/01/31.doi:10.1002/pbc.10443. PubMed PMID: 14752795.

39. Hegyi M, Gulacsi A, Csagoly E, Csordas K, Eipel OT, Erdelyi DJ, et al. Clinical relations of methotrexate pharmacokinetics in the treatment for pediatric osteosarcoma. *J Cancer Res Clin Oncol*. 2012;138(10):1697–1702. Epub 2012/06/02.doi:10.1007/s00432-012-1214-2. PubMed PMID: 22652833.

40. Joerger M, Huitema AD, Krahenbuhl S, Schellens JH, Cerny T, Reni M, et al. Methotrexate area under the curve is an important outcome predictor in patients with primary CNS lymphoma: A pharmacokinetic-pharmacodynamic analysis from the IELSG no. 20 trial. *Br J Cancer*. 2010;102(4):673–677. Epub 2010/02/04.doi:10.1038/sj.bjc.6605559 [pii]. PubMed PMID: 20125159; PubMed Central PMCID: PMC2837574.

41. Johansson AM, Hill N, Perisoglou M, Whelan J, Karlsson MO, Standing JF. A population pharmacokinetic/pharmacodynamic model of methotrexate and mucositis scores in osteosarcoma. *Ther Drug Monit*. 2011;33(6):711–718. Epub 2011/11/23.doi:10.1097/FTD.0b013e31823615e1 00007691-201112000-00008 [pii]. PubMed PMID: 22105588.

42. Martelli N, Mathieu O, Margueritte G, Bozonnat MC, Daures JP, Bressolle F, et al. Methotrexate pharmacokinetics in childhood acute lymphoblastic leukaemia: a prognostic value? *J Clin Pharm Ther*. 2011;36(2):237–245. Epub 2011/03/04.doi:10.1111/j.1365-2710.2010.01179.x. PubMed PMID: 21366654.

43. Comandone A, Passera R, Boglione A, Tagini V, Ferrari S, Cattel L. High-dose methotrexate in adult patients with osteosarcoma: Clinical and pharmacokinetic results. *Acta Oncol*. 2005;44(4):406–411. Epub 2005/08/27.doi:M35H585202742110 [pii] 10.1080/02841860510029770. PubMed PMID: 16120550.

44. Monjanel-Mouterde S, Lejeune C, Ciccolini J, Merite N, Hadjaj D, Bonnier P, et al. Bayesian population model of methotrexate to guide dosage adjustments for folate rescue in patients with breast cancer. *J Clin Pharm Ther*. 2002;27(3):189–195. Epub 2002/06/26.doi:402 [pii]. PubMed PMID: 12081632.

45. Holmboe L, Andersen AM, Morkrid L, Slordal L, Hall KS. High-dose methotrexate chemotherapy: Pharmacokinetics, folate and toxicity in osteosarcoma patients. *Br J Clin Pharmacol*. 2012;73(1):106–114. Epub 2011/06/29.doi:10.1111/j.1365-2125.2011.04054.x. PubMed PMID: 21707700; PubMed Central PMCID: PMC3248260.

46. Plard C, Bressolle F, Fakhoury M, Zhang D, Yacouben K, Rieutord A, et al. A limited sampling strategy to estimate individual pharmacokinetic parameters of methotrexate in children with acute lymphoblastic leukemia. *Cancer Chemother Pharmacol*. 2007;60(4):609–620. Epub 2006/12/30.doi:10.1007/s00280-006-0394-3. PubMed PMID: 17195068.

47. Joerger M, Ferreri AJ, Krahenbuhl S, Schellens JH, Cerny T, Zucca E, et al. Dosing algorithm to target a predefined AUC in patients with primary central nervous system lymphoma receiving high dose methotrexate. *Br J Clin Pharmacol*. 2012;73(2):240–247. Epub 2011/08/16. doi:10.1111/j.1365-2125.2011.04084.x. PubMed PMID: 21838788; PubMed Central PMCID: PMC3269583.

48. Lawrence JR, Steele WH, Stuart JF, McNeill CA, McVie JG, Whiting B. Dose-dependent methotrexate elimination following bolus intravenous injection. *Eur J Clin Pharmacol*. 1980;17(5):371–374. Epub 1980/05/01. PubMed PMID: 7418714.

49. Methotrexate (methotrexate sodium) injection, solution [package insert]. Lake Forest, IL: Hospira, Inc., 2008.

50. Lee JH, Lee YJ, Oh E. Pharmacokinetics of drugs in mutant Nagase analbuminemic rats and responses to select diuretics. *J Pharm Pharmacol*. 2014;66(1):2–13. Epub 2013/10/25.doi:10.1111/jphp.12158. PubMed PMID: 24151919.

51. Mita AC, Sweeney CJ, Baker SD, Goetz A, Hammond LA, Patnaik A, et al. Phase I and pharmacokinetic study of pemetrexed administered every 3 weeks to advanced cancer patients with normal and impaired renal function. *J Clin Oncol*. 2006;24(4):552–562. Epub 2006/01/05. doi:JCO.2004.00.9720 [pii] 10.1200/JCO.2004.00.9720. PubMed PMID: 16391300.

52. Zirkelbach JF, Liu Q. Clinical Pharmacology Review: NDA 21-462 Review—Alimta (Pemetrexed). In Pharmacology DoC. 2010.

53. Dickgreber NJ, Sorensen JB, Paz-Ares LG, Schytte TK, Latz JE, Schneck KB, et al. Pemetrexed safety and pharmacokinetics in patients with third-space fluid. *Clin Cancer Res*. 2010;16(10):2872–2880. Epub 2010/05/13.doi:10.1158/1078-0432.CCR-09-3324 1078-0432.CCR-09-3324 [pii]. PubMed PMID: 20460481.

54. Takimoto CH, Hammond-Thelin LA, Latz JE, Forero L, Beeram M, Forouzesh B, et al. Phase I and pharmacokinetic study of pemetrexed with high-dose folic acid supplementation or multivitamin supplementation in patients with locally advanced or metastatic cancer. *Clin Cancer Res*. 2007;13(9):2675–2683. Epub 2007/05/03. doi:13/9/2675 [pii] 10.1158/1078-0432.CCR-06-2393. PubMed PMID: 17473199.

55. ALIMTA (premetrexed disodium) injection [package insert]. Indianapolis, IN, Eli Lilly and Company, 2004.

56. Tournigand C, Andre T, Achille E, Lledo G, Flesh M, Mery-Mignard D, et al. FOLFIRI followed by FOLFOX6 or the reverse sequence in advanced colorectal cancer: A randomized GERCOR study. J *J Clin Oncol*. 2004;22(2):229–237. Epub 2003/12/06.doi:10.1200/JCO.2004.05.113. PubMed PMID: 14657227.

57. Grothey A, Sargent D, Goldberg RM, Schmoll HJ. Survival of patients with advanced colorectal cancer improves with the availability of fluorouracil-leucovorin, irinotecan, and oxaliplatin in the course of treatment. *J Clin Oncol*. 2004;22(7):1209–1214. Epub 2004/03/31. doi:10.1200/JCO.2004.11.037. PubMed PMID: 15051767.

58. Abrams TA, Meyer G, Schrag D, Meyerhardt JA, Moloney J, Fuchs CS. Chemotherapy usage patterns in a U.S.-wide cohort of patients with metastatic colorectal cancer.*J Natl Cancer Inst*.2014;106(2):djt371. Epub 2014/02/11.doi:10.1093/jnci/djt371. PubMed PMID: 24511107.

59. Trump DL, Egorin MJ, Forrest A, Willson JK, Remick S, Tutsch KD. Pharmacokinetic and pharmacodynamic analysis of fluorouracil during 72-hour continuous infusion with and without dipyridamole. *J Clin Oncol*. 1991;9(11):2027–2035. Epub 1991/11/01. PubMed PMID: 1941062.

60. Gamelin EC, Danquechin-Dorval EM, Dumesnil YF, Maillart PJ, Goudier MJ, Burtin PC, et al. Relationship between 5-fluorouracil (5-FU) dose intensity and therapeutic response in patients with advanced colorectal cancer receiving infusional therapy containing 5-FU. *Cancer*. 1996;77(3):441–451. Epub 1996/02/01.doi:10.1002/(SICI)1097-0142(19960201)77:3<441::AID-CNCR4>3.0.CO;2-N. PubMed PMID: 8630950.

61. Hillcoat BL, McCulloch PB, Figueredo AT, Ehsan MH, Rosenfeld JM. Clinical response and plasma levels of 5-fluorouracil in patients with colonic cancer treated by drug infusion. *Brit J Cancer*. 1978;38(6):719–724. Epub 1978/12/01. PubMed PMID: 743489; PubMed Central PMCID: PMC2009832.

62. Di Paolo A, Lencioni M, Amatori F, Di Donato S, Bocci G, Orlandini C, et al. 5-fluorouracil pharmacokinetics predicts disease-free survival in patients administered adjuvant chemotherapy for colorectal cancer. Clin Cancer Res. 2008;14(9):2749–2755. Epub 2008/05/03. doi:10.1158/1078-0432.CCR-07-1529. PubMed PMID: 18451241.

63. Duffour J, Roca L, Bressolle F, Abderrahim AG, Poujol S, Pinguet F, et al. Clinical impact of intesified 5-Fluorouracil-based chemotherapy using a prospective pharmacokinetically-guided dosing approach: Comparative study in elderly and non-elderly patients with metastatic colorectal cancer. *J Chemother*. 2010;22(3):179–185. Epub 2010/06/23. doi:10.1179/joc.2010.22.3.179. PubMed PMID: 20566423.

64. Undevia SD, Gomez-Abuin G, Ratain MJ. Pharmacokinetic variability of anticancer agents. *Natl Rev Cancer*. 2005;5(6):447–458. Epub 2005/06/02.doi:10.1038/nrc1629. PubMed PMID: 15928675.

65. Gamelin E, Boisdron-Celle M, Guerin-Meyer V, Delva R, Lortholary A, Genevieve F, et al. Correlation between uracil and dihydrouracil plasma ratio, fluorouracil (5-FU) pharmacokinetic parameters, and tolerance in patients with advanced colorectal cancer: A potential interest for predicting 5-FU toxicity and determining optimal 5-FU dosage. *J Clin Oncology*. 1999;17(4):1105. Epub 1999/11/24. PubMed PMID: 10561167.

66. Milano G, Etienne MC, Cassuto-Viguier E, Thyss A, Santini J, Frenay M, et al. Influence of sex and age on fluorouracil clearance. J *J Clin Oncology*. 1992;10(7):1171–1175. Epub 1992/07/01. PubMed PMID: 1607921.

67. Saif MW, Choma A, Salamone SJ, Chu E. Pharmacokinetically guided dose adjustment of 5-fluorouracil: a rational approach to improving therapeutic outcomes. *J Natl Cancer Inst*. 2009;101(22):1543–1552. Epub 2009/10/21.doi:10.1093/jnci/djp328. PubMed PMID: 19841331.

68. Capitain O, Asevoaia A, Boisdron-Celle M, Poirier AL, Morel A, Gamelin E. Individual fluorouracil dose adjustment in FOLFOX based on pharmacokinetic follow-up compared with conventional body-area-surface dosing: A phase II, proof-of-concept study. *Clin Colorectal Cancer*. 2012;11(4):263–267. Epub 2012/06/12.doi:10.1016/j.clcc.2012.05.004. PubMed PMID: 22683364.

69. Smith CG, Grady JE, Kupiecki FP. Blood and urine levels of antitumor agents determined with cell culture methods. *Cancer Res*. 1965;25:241–245. Epub 1965/02/01. PubMed PMID: 14264057.

70. Christophidis N, Mihaly G, Vajda F, Louis W. Comparison of liquid- and gas-liquid chromatographic assays of 5-fluorouracil in plasma. *Clin Chem*. 1979;25(1):83–86. Epub 1979/01/01. PubMed PMID: 761385.

71. Beumer JH, Boisdron-Celle M, Clarke W, Courtney JB, Egorin MJ, Gamelin E, et al. Multicenter evaluation of a novel nanoparticle

immunoassay for 5-fluorouracil on the Olympus AU400 analyzer. *Ther Drug Monit.* 2009;31(6):688–694. Epub 2009/11/26.doi:10.1519/JSC.0b013e3181b866d0. PubMed PMID: 19935361.

72. Gamelin E, Delva R, Jacob J, Merrouche Y, Raoul JL, Pezet D, et al. Individual fluorouracil dose adjustment based on pharmacokinetic follow-up compared with conventional dosage: Results of a multicenter randomized trial of patients with metastatic colorectal cancer. J *J Clin Oncol.* 2008;26(13):2099–2105. Epub 2008/05/01.doi:10.1200/JCO.2007.13.3934. PubMed PMID: 18445839.

73. Etienne MC, Lagrange JL, Dassonville O, Fleming R, Thyss A, Renee N, et al. Population study of dihydropyrimidine dehydrogenase in cancer patients. *J Clin Oncol.* 1994;12(11):2248–2253. Epub 1994/11/01. PubMed PMID: 7964939.

74. Harris BE, Carpenter JT, Diasio RB. Severe 5-fluorouracil toxicity secondary to dihydropyrimidine dehydrogenase deficiency. A potentially more common pharmacogenetic syndrome. *Cancer.* 1991;68(3):499–501. Epub 1991/08/01. PubMed PMID: 1648430.

75. Lu Z, Zhang R, Carpenter JT, Diasio RB. Decreased dihydropyrimidine dehydrogenase activity in a population of patients with breast cancer: Implication for 5-fluorouracil-based chemotherapy. *Clin Cancer Res.* 1998;4(2):325–329. Epub 1998/05/14. PubMed PMID: 9516918.

76. Fleming GF, Schilsky RL, Schumm LP, Meyerson A, Hong AM, Vogelzang NJ, et al. Phase I and pharmacokinetic study of 24-hour infusion 5-fluorouracil and leucovorin in patients with organ dysfunction. *Ann Oncol.* 2003;14(7):1142–1147. Epub 2003/07/11. PubMed PMID: 12853359.

77. Bergmann W FR. Contributions to the study of marine products: XXXII. The nuclesides of sponges. *J Org Chem.* 1951;16:981–987.

78. Walwick ER, Dekker CA, Roberts WK. Cyclization during the phosphorylation of uridine and cytidine: A new route to the 02, 2-cyclonucleosides. *Proc Chem Soc.* 1959;53:84.

79. Blasberg R, Molnar P, Groothius D, Patlak C, Owens E, Fenstermacher J. Concurrent measurements of blood flow and transcapillary transport in avian sarcoma virus-induced experimental brain tumors: implications for chemotherapy. *J Pharmacol Exp Ther.* 1984;231(3):724–735. Epub 1984/12/01. PubMed PMID: 6094798.

80. Wiley JS, Jones SP, Sawyer WH, Paterson AR. Cytosine arabinoside influx and nucleoside transport sites in acute leukemia. *J Clin Invest.* 1982;69(2):479–489. Epub 1982/02/01. PubMed PMID: 6948829; PubMed Central PMCID: PMC370998.

81. Plunkett W, Liliemark JO, Estey E, Keating MJ. Saturation of ara-CTP accumulation during high-dose ara-C therapy: Pharmacologic rationale for intermediate-dose ara-C. *Seminars in Oncology.* 1987;14(2 Suppl 1):159–166. Epub 1987/06/01. PubMed PMID: 3589690.

82. Capizzi RL, Yang JL, Cheng E, Bjornsson T, Sahasrabudhe D, Tan RS, et al. Alteration of the pharmacokinetics of high-dose ara-C by its metabolite, high ara-U in patients with acute leukemia. *J Clin Oncology.* 1983;1(12):763–771. Epub 1983/12/01. PubMed PMID: 6668493.

83. Bolwell BJ, Cassileth PA, Gale RP. High dose cytarabine: A review. *Leukemia.* 1988;2(5):253–260. Epub 1988/05/01. PubMed PMID: 3287015.

84. Appelbaum FR, Baer MR, Carabasi MH, Coutre SE, Erba HP, Estey E, et al. NCCN practice guidelines for acute myelogenous leukemia. *Oncology.* 2000;14(11A):53–61. Epub 2001/02/24. PubMed PMID: 11195419.

85. Kern W, Schleyer E, Unterhalt M, Wormann B, Buchner T, Hiddemann W. High antileukemic activity of sequential high-dose cytosine arabinoside and mitoxantrone in patients with refractory acute leukemias. Results of a clinical phase II study. *Cancer.* 1997;79(1):59–68. Epub 1997/01/01. PubMed PMID: 8988727.

86. Chandrasekaran B, Kute TE, Capizzi RL. Deoxypyrimidine-induced inhibition of the cytokinetic effects of 1-beta-D-arabinofuranosyluracil. *Cancer Chem Pharmacol.* 1992;29(6):455–460. Epub 1992/01/01. PubMed PMID: 1568288.

87. Damon LE, Mass R, Linker CA. The association between high-dose cytarabine neurotoxicity and renal insufficiency. *J Clin Oncol.* 1989;7(10):1563–1568. Epub 1989/10/01. PubMed PMID: 2778484.

88. Lazarus HM, Herzig RH, Herzig GP, Phillips GL, Roessmann U, Fishman DJ. Central nervous system toxicity of high-dose systemic cytosine arabinoside. *Cancer.* 1981;48(12):2577–2582. Epub 1981/12/15. PubMed PMID: 7306918.

89. Nand S, Messmore HL, Jr., Patel R, Fisher SG, Fisher RI. Neurotoxicity associated with systemic high-dose cytosine arabinoside. *J Clin Oncol.* 1986;4(4):571–575. Epub 1986/04/01. PubMed PMID: 3457102.

90. Herzig RH, Herzig GP, Wolff SN, Hines JD, Fay JW, Phillips GL. Central nervous system effects of high-dose cytosine arabinoside. *Seminars in Oncology.* 1987;14(2 Suppl 1):21–4. Epub 1987/06/01. PubMed PMID: 3589694.

91. Smith GA, Damon LE, Rugo HS, Ries CA, Linker CA. High-dose cytarabine dose modification reduces the incidence of neurotoxicity in patients with renal insufficiency. *J Clin Oncol.* 1997;15(2):833–839. Epub 1997/02/01. PubMed PMID: 9053511.

92. Lindner LH, Ostermann H, Hiddemann W, Kiani A, Wurfel M, Illmer T, et al. AraU accumulation in patients with renal insufficiency as a potential mechanism for cytarabine neurotoxicity. *Intl J Hematol.* 2008;88(4):381–386. Epub 2008/10/07.doi:10.1007/s12185-008-0171-7. PubMed PMID: 18836794.

93. Kreis W, Chan K, Budman DR, Schulman P, Allen S, Weiselberg L, et al. Effect of tetrahydrouridine on the clinical pharmacology of 1-beta-D-arabinofuranosylcytosine when both drugs are coinfused over three hours. *Cancer Res.* 1988;48(5):1337–1342. Epub 1988/03/01. PubMed PMID: 3342412.

94. Funato K, Yoda R, Kiwada H. Contribution of complement system on destabilization of liposomes composed of hydrogenated egg phosphatidylcholine in rat fresh plasma. *Biochim Biophys Acta.* 1992;1103(2):198–204. Epub 1992/01/31. PubMed PMID: 1543704.

95. Allen TM, Hansen C, Martin F, Redemann C, Yau-Young A. Liposomes containing synthetic lipid derivatives of poly(ethylene glycol) show prolonged circulation half-lives in vivo. *Biochim Biophys Acta.* 1991;1066(1):29–36. Epub 1991/07/01. PubMed PMID: 2065067.

96. Radeski D, Cull GM, Cain M, Hackett LP, Ilett KF. Effective clearance of Ara-U the major metabolite of cytosine arabinoside (Ara-C) by hemodialysis in a patient with lymphoma and end-stage renal failure. *Cancer Chem Pharmacol.* 2011;67(4):765–768. Epub 2010/06/10.doi:10.1007/s00280-010-1373-2. PubMed PMID: 20532508.

97. Sandimmune® soft gelatin capsules (cyclosporine capsules, USP), Sandimmune® oral solution (cyclosporine oral solution, USP), Sandimmune® injection (cyclosporine injection, USP) [package insert]. East Hanover, NJ, Novartis Pharmaceuticals Corporation, 2013.

98. Borel JF, Feurer C, Gubler HU, Stahelin H. Biological effects of cyclosporin A: A new antilymphocytic agent. *Agents Actions.* 1976;6(4):468–475. Epub 1976/07/01. PubMed PMID: 8969.

99. Bissett J. Notes on Tolypocladium and related genera. *Can J Bot.* 1983;61(5):1311–1329.doi:10.1139/b83-139.

100. Gams W. Tolypocladium, eine Hyphomycetengattung mit geschwollenen Phialiden. *Persoonia.* 1971;6(2):185–191.

101. von Arx JA. Tolypocldium, a synonym for Beauveria. *Mycotaxon.* 1986;25(1):153–158.

102. Matsuda S, Koyasu S. Mechanisms of action of cyclosporine. *Immunopharmacology.* 2000;47(2–3):119–125. Epub 2000/07/06. doi:S0162310900001922 [pii]. PubMed PMID: 10878286.

103. Sheikh-Hamad D, Nadkarni V, Choi YJ, Truong LD, Wideman C, Hodjati R, et al. Cyclosporine A inhibits the adaptive responses to hypertonicity: A potential mechanism of nephrotoxicity. *J Am Soc Nephrol.* 2001;12(12):2732–2741. Epub 2001/12/01. PubMed PMID: 11729242.

104. Meyer-Lehnert H, Schrier RW. Potential mechanism of cyclosporine A-induced vascular smooth muscle contraction. *Hypertension.* 1989;13(4):352–360. Epub 1989/04/01. PubMed PMID: 2538392.

105. Lyson T, McMullan DM, Ermel LD, Morgan BJ, Victor RG. Mechanism of cyclosporine-induced sympathetic activation and acute hypertension in rats. *Hypertension.* 1994;23(5):667–675. Epub 1994/05/01. PubMed PMID: 8175178.

106. Okada T, Matsumoto H, Nagaoka Y, Tomaru R, Iwasawa H, Wada T, et al. Clinical evaluation of chronic nephrotoxicity of long-term cyclosporine A treatment in adult patients with steroid-dependent nephrotic syndrome. *Nephrology (Carlton).* 2011;16(3):319–325. Epub 2010/11/17. doi:10.1111/j.1440-1797.2010.01425.x. PubMed PMID: 21077987.

107. Asai T, Nakatani T, Yamanaka S, Tamada S, Kishimoto T, Tashiro K, et al. Magnesium supplementation prevents experimental chronic cyclosporine a nephrotoxicity via renin-angiotensin system independent mechanism. *Transplantation.* 2002;74(6):784–791. Epub 2002/10/05. PubMed PMID: 12364856.

108. Lindholm A, Kahan BD. Influence of cyclosporine pharmacokinetics, trough concentrations, and AUC monitoring on outcome after kidney transplantation. *Clin Pharmacol Ther.* 1993;54(2):205–218. Epub 1993/08/01. PubMed PMID: 8354028.

109. Ghalie R, Fitzsimmons WE, Weinstein A, Manson S, Kaizer H. Cyclosporine monitoring improves graft-versus-host disease prophylaxis after bone marrow transplantation. *Ann Pharmacother.* 1994;28(3):379–383. Epub 1994/03/01. PubMed PMID: 8193430.

110. Kishi Y, Murashige N, Kami M, Miyakoshi S, Shibagaki Y, Hamaki T, et al. Optimal initial dose of oral cyclosporine in relation to its toxicities for graft-versus-host disease prophylaxis following reduced-intensity stem cell transplantation in Japanese patients. *Bone Marrow Transplant.* 2005;35(11):1079–1082. Epub 2005/04/05.doi:1704960 [pii] 10.1038/sj.bmt.1704960. PubMed PMID: 15806118.

111. Machishima T, Kako S, Wada H, Yamasaki R, Ishihara Y, Kawamura K, et al. The safety and efficacy of acute graft-versus-host disease prophylaxis with a higher target blood concentration of cyclosporine around 500 ng/mL. *Clin Transplant.* 2013;27(5):749–756. Epub 2013/09/17. doi:10.1111/ctr.12213. PubMed PMID: 24033855.

112. Ratanatharathorn V, Nash RA, Przepiorka D, Devine SM, Klein JL, Weisdorf D, et al. Phase III study comparing methotrexate and tacrolimus (prograf, FK506) with methotrexate and cyclosporine for graft-versus-host disease prophylaxis after HLA-identical sibling bone marrow transplantation. *Blood.* 1998;92(7):2303–2314. Epub 1998/09/25. PubMed PMID: 9746768.

113. Duncan N, Craddock C. Optimizing the use of cyclosporin in allogeneic stem cell transplantation. *Bone Marrow Transplant.* 2006;38(3):169–174. Epub 2006/06/06.doi:1705404 [pii] 10.1038/sj.bmt.1705404. PubMed PMID: 16751787.

114. Choi JS, Lee SH, Chung SJ, Yoo KH, Sung KW, Koo HH. Assessment of converting from intravenous to oral administration of cyclosporin A in pediatric allogeneic hematopoietic stem cell transplant recipients. *Bone Marrow Transplant.* 2006;38(1):29–35. Epub 2006/05/23.doi:1705402 [pii] 10.1038/sj.bmt.1705402. PubMed PMID: 16715103.

Note: Page numbers followed by *f* indicate figures; those followed by *t* indicate tables